Promoting Self-Management
of Chronic Health Conditions

Promoting Self-Management of Chronic Health Conditions

Theories and Practice

EDITED BY
ERIN MARTZ

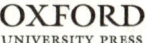

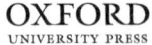

Oxford University Press is a department of the University of Oxford. It furthers
the University's objective of excellence in research, scholarship, and education
by publishing worldwide. Oxford is a registered trade mark of Oxford University
Press in the UK and certain other countries.

Published in the United States of America by Oxford University Press
198 Madison Avenue, New York, NY 10016, United States of America.

© Oxford University Press 2018

All rights reserved. No part of this publication may be reproduced, stored in
a retrieval system, or transmitted, in any form or by any means, without the
prior permission in writing of Oxford University Press, or as expressly permitted
by law, by license, or under terms agreed with the appropriate reproduction
rights organization. Inquiries concerning reproduction outside the scope of the
above should be sent to the Rights Department, Oxford University Press, at the
address above.

You must not circulate this work in any other form
and you must impose this same condition on any acquirer.

Library of Congress Cataloging-in-Publication Data
Names: Martz, Erin, editor.
Title: Promoting self-management of chronic health conditions : theories and practice /
edited by Erin Martz.
Description: Oxford ; New York : Oxford University Press, [2018] |
Includes bibliographical references and index.
Identifiers: LCCN 2017022826 (print) |
LCCN 2017023055 (ebook) | ISBN 9780190606152 (updf) | ISBN 9780190669867 (epub) |
ISBN 9780190606145 (hardback)
Subjects: LCSH: Chronic diseases—Treatment. | Self-care, Health. |
BISAC: PSYCHOLOGY / Clinical Psychology. | MEDICAL / Public Health.
Classification: LCC RC108 (ebook) | LCC RC108 .P76 2018 (print) | DDC 616/.044—dc23
LC record available at https://lccn.loc.gov/2017022826

9 8 7 6 5 4 3 2 1
Printed by Sheridan Books, Inc., United States of America

CONTENTS

About the Editor vii
About the Contributors ix

1. Introduction: Why Study Self-Management? 1
   Erin Martz

2. Defining Self-Management on the Individual Level 10
   Erin Martz

PART I Individual-Level Theories and Interventions to Promote Self-Management

3. Cognitive-Behavioral Therapy to Promote Self-Management 31
   Sharon Eldar, Nora M. Esser, and Stefan G. Hofmann

4. Spreading HOPE: The Development of a Hope-Based Self-Management Intervention 58
   Andy Turner and Faith Martin

5. Illness Intrusiveness and Self-Management of Medical Conditions 80
   Gerald M. Devins and Amy Deckert

6. Motivational Interviewing to Promote Self-Management 126
   Rebecca Phillips, Anne Hogden, and David Greenfield

PART II Research about Specific Chronic Health Conditions

7. Self-Management of Addictive Behaviors 147
   Vanja Radoncic, Betty Marcoux, and Denise Hien

8. Self-Management of Arthritis 171
   Jessica M. Brooks, Kanako Iwanaga, and Fong Chan

9. Self-Management of Burn Injury 197
   James A. Fauerbach and Carisa Perry-Parrish

10. Self-Management of Cancer 225
    Amy Deckert and Gerald M. Devins

11. Self-Management of Cardiac-Related Health Issues 262
    Noa Vilchinsky

12. Self-Management of Diabetes 284
    Jonathan F. Deiches, Emre Umucu, and Fong Chan

13. Self-Management of Epilepsy 319
    Janice M. Buelow and W. Henry Smithson

14. Self-Management of Hearing Impairment 340
    Lucy Handscomb, Gabrielle H. Saunders, and Derek J. Hoare

15. Self-Management of HIV 360
    Faith Martin

16. Self-Management of Multiple Sclerosis 382
    Malachy Bishop and Michael Frain

17. Self-Management of Pain 406
    Thomas Hadjistavropoulos

18. Self-Management of Tinnitus 420
    Erin Martz

19. Self-Management of Vision Impairments 440
    Vicki Blair Drury, Ai Tee Aw, and Priscilla Shiow Huey Lim

PART III Innovative Technology and Techniques to Promote Self-Management

20. Telemedicine 467
    Kristian Kidholm

21. Internet Interventions 482
    Gerhard Andersson

PART IV Promoting Self-Management across the Globe

22. Systemic Models of Self-Management 499
    Erin Martz

Index 521

ABOUT THE EDITOR

Erin Martz has a PhD in Rehabilitation Education and Research and is a Certified Rehabilitation Counselor. She has focused on research coping with and adapting to chronic health conditions and disabilities for the past 20 years. She is a 2017 Fulbright Research Fellow for the U.S. Department of State, works as a research investigator for the U.S. Department of Veterans Affairs, is an assistant professor in the Department of Otolaryngology, Oregon Health and Science University, and runs her own business called Rehability.

ABOUT THE CONTRIBUTORS

Gerhard Andersson, PhD
Medical science professor in Clinical Psychology, clinical psychologist, and psychotherapist
> *Research interests*: The application of information technology in the assessment and treatment of psychiatric and somatic conditions; tinnitus and audiology, including hearing loss, dizziness, and noise sensitivity.

Malachy Bishop, PhD
Professor, Rehabilitation Counseling Program, Department of Early Childhood, Special Education, and Rehabilitation Counseling, University of Kentucky
> *Research interests*: Employment and psychosocial aspects of chronic neurological conditions, including multiple sclerosis, epilepsy, and other chronic neurological conditions; self-management of multiple sclerosis; and the application of quality-of-life research to adaptation to chronic health conditions and disability.

Jessica M. Brooks, PhD, CRC
Postdoctoral Fellow at Dartmouth College and assistant professor at the University of North Texas
> *Research interests*: Psychiatric disorders, chronic pain and other physical disabilities, co-occurring conditions, geriatric mental health services, peer services, health promotion, psychosocial adaptation, and vocational rehabilitation.

Janice M. Buelow, PhD, RN, FAAN
Professor, Science of Nursing Care, Indiana University School of Nursing
> *Research interests*: Promoting and improving self-management in individuals with epilepsy, families of individuals with epilepsy, improving self-management techniques.

Fong Chan, PhD, CRC
Norman L. and Barbara M. Berven Professor of Rehabilitation Psychology and chair of the Department of Rehabilitation Psychology and Special Education at the University of Wisconsin-Madison; director of the Rehabilitation Research and Training Center on Evidence-Based Practice in Vocational Rehabilitation
> *Research interests*: Psychosocial theory and research, demand-side employment, health promotion, and poverty and disability.

Amy Deckert, PhD
Research Fellow, University Health Network, Canada
Research interests: Health behavior change across the cancer trajectory; functional exercise interventions for preemptive symptom control among people living with advanced cancer.

Jonathan F. Deiches, MS, CRC
Doctoral psychology intern, West Virginia University Medicine—University Healthcare
Research interests: Health psychology and behavioral medicine; the role of purpose in life in promoting health behaviors.

Gerald M. Devins, PhD, Clinical Psychology
Senior Scientist, Princess Margaret Cancer Centre; Professor of Psychiatry, University of Toronto; Head, Supportive Care Research, University Health Network
Research interests: Quality of life and the psychosocial impact of medical conditions in (a) illness intrusiveness, the psychosocial impact of chronic and life-threatening medical conditions, and the development of interventions to facilitate adaptation and (b) the sense of self, how this is shaped by medical conditions, and the adaptive implications of these effects.

Vicki Blair Drury, PhD, MCl.Nsg, PGCert Psych,Nsg, Cert. Mens Hlth, BHlthSc(Nsg), BA(Ed), RN, RMHN, OND
Independent scholar, Educare Consulting, Bunbury, Australia
Research interests: Self-management of long-term eye conditions with a focus on individuals with low vision.

Sharon Eldar, PhD
Postdoctoral associate, Department of Psychological and Brain Sciences, Boston University
Research interests: Cognitive-behavioral therapy for individuals with anxiety or depression and the additional effect that positive affect training has on this population.

Nora M. Esser, BS, in progress
Visiting scholar and scientific assistant, Department of Psychological and Brain Sciences, Boston University
Research interests: Disseminating evidence-based treatments to a broader population; stress management, treatment interventions, mental wellness.

James A. Fauerbach, PhD
Associate professor, Department of Psychiatry and Behavioral Science and the Division of Behavioral Medicine at the Johns Hopkins School of Medicine, with joint appointments in the Departments of Physical Medicine and Rehabilitation and Plastic and Reconstructive Surgery
Research interests: Reciprocal and evolving relations between trauma exposure, alterations in appearance (body-image acceptance) and social

adjustment (social stigmatization), and individual differences (e.g., personality, emotion regulation, self efficacy).

Michael Frain, PhD, CRC
Professor, Florida Atlantic University
Research interests: Self-management interventions for people with disabilities, especially multiple sclerosis and veterans.

David Greenfield, PhD
Professor and director of the Australian Institute of Health Service Management, University of Tasmania, Australia
Research interests: Healthcare complex adaptive systems, strategies to improve health services, and the organization of clinical practice.

Thomas Hadjistavropoulos, PhD, ABPP, FCAHS
Professor of psychology and Research Chair in Aging and Health
Research interests: Social and psychological influences on pain; pain communication.

Lucy Handscomb, MSc
Hearing therapist and lecturer in audiology
Research interests: Rehabilitation for adults with acquired hearing loss and tinnitus therapy.

Denise Hien, PhD, ABPP
Professor, Derner Institute for Advanced Psychological Studies, Adelphi University and Adjunct Senior Research Scientist, Columbia University College of Physicians and Surgeons
Research interests: Integrating developmental, affective, and cognitive neuroscience perspectives on traumatic stress; psychotherapy research for trauma-related disorders and addiction; ethnic and cultural factors in the treatment process; maternal aggression and its impact upon adverse child outcomes.

Derek J. Hoare, PhD
Senior Research Fellow (Tinnitus), National Institute for Health Research Nottingham Hearing Biomedical Research Unit; chair of the British Society of Audiology Tinnitus and Hyperacusis Special Interest Group; steering group member of TINNET Working Group 1 (Clinical) to develop pan-European clinical practice guidelines for tinnitus
Research interests: Development of clinical assessment tools and low-intensity psychological and self-help interventions for tinnitus.

Stefan G. Hofmann, PhD
Professor of Psychology, Department of Psychological and Brain Sciences, Boston University
Research interests: The mechanism of treatment change, translating discoveries from neuroscience into clinical applications, and emotion regulation strategies.

Anne Hogden, PhD
Research Fellow, Australian Institute of Health Innovation, Macquarie University
> *Research interests*: Healthcare service delivery; in particular, decision-making and multidisciplinary team processes for people with long-term conditions.

Kanako Iwanaga, MS, in progress
University of Wisconsin-Madison Rehabilitation psychology and vocational rehabilitation.

Kristian Kidholm, PhD
Associate professor and Head of Research at Center for Innovative Medical Research, Denmark
> *Research interests*: Health technology assessment, telemedicine, hospital-based health technology assessment.

Betty Marcoux, MA, in progress
Adelphi University
> *Research interests*: Posttraumatic stress disorder, addictions, anxiety, and depression.

Faith Martin PhD, DClinPsy
Clinical psychologist, South London and the Maudsley NHS Foundation Trust and Honorary Lecturer, University of Bath
> *Research interests*: Self-management of chronic conditions, intervention development methods, conceptualization and measurement of quality of life, and mental health in relation to long-term physical conditions.

Erin Martz, PhD (Book Editor)
Owner of Rehability, Portland, OR, research investigator at Veterans Affairs Portland Health Care System, and assistant professor, Department of Otolaryngology, Oregon Health and Science University
> *Research interests*: Coping with and adapting to chronic health conditions, self-management of chronic health conditions, trauma rehabilitation.

Carisa Perry-Parrish, PhD
Assistant professor, Johns Hopkins School of Medicine, Department of Psychiatry and Behavioral Sciences; Director of Behavior Medicine, Pediatric Burn Program
> *Research interests*: Development of emotion regulation in children and adolescents; role of parents in supporting emotional development and how youth and parents cope with stress, including adjustment to burn injuries in youth; use of mindfulness-based strategies to promote emotion regulation.

Rebecca Phillips, BAppSci (Occupational Therapy) with Honors, PhD
Clinical lecturer, Centre for Health Stewardship, College of Medicine, Biology and Environment, Australian National University
Research interests: Well-being of children and adults with chronic health conditions, with a particular focus on self-management and partnership between clients and clinicians.

Vanja Radoncic, MA
Doctoral candidate in Clinical Psychology, Derner Institute of Advanced Psychological Studies, Adelphi University; research coordinator at Substance Use Research Center, New York State Psychiatric Institute, and Columbia University Medical Center
Research interests: Treatment, research, and training in the areas of addiction and trauma-related disorders.

Gabrielle H. Saunders, PhD
National Center for Rehabilitative Auditory Research Associate Director and Investigator, Veterans Affairs Portland Health Care System; associate professor, Department of Otolaryngology, Oregon Health and Science University
Research interests: Hearing health behavior change and hearing health education though the application of health behavior theory.

Priscilla Shiow Huey Lim, BA (Social Work)
Head, Master Medical Social Worker (Practice Manager), Singapore National Eye Center
Research interests: Vision rehabilitation, low vision, and independent living of visually impaired individuals.

W. Henry Smithson, MB, ChB, MD
Professor of General Practice, University College Cork Ireland and Visiting Professor of Primary Medical Care, University of Sheffield, UK
Research interests: Community care of long-term conditions, how people live with and manage epilepsy, factors relating to death in epilepsy, patterns of medication usage.

Ai Tee Aw, MN, BN, RN, OND
Assistant Director of Nursing, Singapore National Eye Center
Research interests: Low vision, quality of life of both individuals with visual impairments and their caregivers.

Andy Turner, BA Hons, PhD
Professor of Health Psychology
Research interests: Developing, delivering, and evaluating self-management programs for people living with and affected by a long-term health condition; the Help to Overcome Problems Effectively (HOPE) program.

Emre Umucu, MS, CRC
Doctoral candidate, University of Wisconsin-Madison
Research interests: Research methods in rehabilitation, positive psychology, and psychosocial outcome research.

Noa Vilchinsky, PhD
Director of the Psycho-cardiology Research Lab, Department of Psychology, Bar Ilan University
Research interests: Psychocardiology, attachment-related dynamics in chronic health conditions, dyadic coping with chronic health conditions, posttraumatic stress disorder and chronic illness, cultural differences in health behaviors, attitudes toward people with disabilities, and the importance of being treated with respect and dignity in the medical setting.

Promoting Self-Management of Chronic Health Conditions

1

Introduction

Why Study Self-Management?

ERIN MARTZ ■

We propose the formulation of health as the ability to adapt and to self-manage.
—HUBER ET AL. *(2011, p. 3)*

For decades, the World Health Organization (WHO; 1948) has defined health as "a state of complete physical, mental and social well-being and not merely the absence of disease or infirmity" (p. 1). This definition advanced the concept of health in a more positive direction, away from the focus on eliminating diseases. However, Huber and colleagues (2011) pointed out that the WHO's definition needs updating because of its high standard of a "state of complete physical, mental and social well-being," which may not be possible for many people who have chronic health conditions. Huber and colleagues proposed a fundamental shift in the definition of health, moving from the WHO's idealistic definition to a more flexible, practical, and responsive definition of health as being able to adapt and *self-manage* in the context of chronic health conditions. This shift represents an ideal of achieving "complete well-being" to a more reality-based acknowledgement that many people have to deal with one or more chronic health conditions in their lifetimes—and that chronic conditions do not necessarily signify poor health or well-being.

The fundamental goal of the present book is to elaborate on both the theories and the practices that can help individuals with chronic health conditions to become as independent as possible by self-managing their chronic health conditions. Self-management has been defined in many ways (see chapter 2), but, fundamentally, it involves individuals with health conditions taking responsibility for managing their symptoms to the extent that is possible, *while collaborating with healthcare professionals.* The purpose of this book is to investigate the ways that healthcare providers can promote self-management among individuals with chronic health conditions.

The topics discussed in this book include reviews of theoretical models and research on condition-specific, empirically based interventions that promote the self-management of specific chronic health conditions among the adult population. This introductory chapter briefly covers the purpose of this book, what terms are (and are not) used in this book, and the structure of the book. But first, this chapter begins with a discussion of why self-management is an important topic in today's healthcare environment.

WHY PROMOTE SELF-MANAGEMENT?

There are three primary reasons why self-management should be a topic of scientific research and consideration by healthcare providers and healthcare systems.

The Global Increase of Chronic Health Conditions

One of the primary reasons why self-management needs to be promoted is that as the treatment of acute health conditions improves and life expectancy increases, the prevalence of chronic health conditions has risen. Globally, noncommunicable diseases (i.e., chronic health conditions) were "responsible for 68% of the world's 56 million deaths in 2012" (WHO, 2014, p. xi). Chronic health conditions are already the leading cause of death and disability in Europe (Busse, Blümel, Scheller-Kreinsen, & Zentner, 2010). In the United States, *more than 50% of adults have one or more of seven chronic health conditions* (cancer, diabetes, hypertension, stroke, heart disease, pulmonary conditions, and mental health conditions; DeVol et al., 2007). Because this frequency was calculated for only seven chronic health conditions, then the actual prevalence rate for all chronic health conditions would be much higher than 50%. These studies suggest that the challenge of having a chronic health condition is a common issue among the general population.

In addition to the fact that a majority of the US population has at least one chronic health condition, about a quarter of the US population has *more than one* chronic condition (Ward & Schiller, 2012). Ward and Schiller examined the prevalence of multiple chronic conditions (MCC) among US civilian, non-institutionalized adults, using the 2010 National Health Interview Survey (NHIS) dataset. They focused on 10 specific chronic conditions (hypertension, coronary heart disease, stroke, diabetes, cancer, arthritis, hepatitis, weak or failing kidneys, current asthma, or chronic obstructive pulmonary disease). Ward and Schiller found that *26% of US adults had MCC*, which was an increase from

21.8% in 2001. They found higher prevalence rates of MCC among older adults. Ward, Schiller, and Goodman (2014) analyzed the 2012 NHIS dataset and found similar results: approximately half of the US non-institutionalized population reported one of 10 chronic conditions, and 25.5% of them had MCC (i.e., two or more chronic conditions). Because these analyses of the NHIS dataset included only 10 conditions and did not include mental health conditions, Ward et al. acknowledged that their calculations likely *underestimated* the true prevalence of MCC.

The data cited in the previous two paragraphs highlight one reason why it is important to focus on self-management: *the occurrence of chronic health conditions is increasing* among the general population. Yet the increase of chronic health conditions is not the only important indicator of the need to focus on promoting self-management among chronic health conditions. The urgent need to promote self-management arises from the *danger of untreated or unmanaged chronic health conditions*. Seven of the 10 leading causes of death in the United States are chronic health conditions (heart disease, cancer, chronic lower respiratory diseases, cerebrovascular diseases, Alzheimer's disease, diabetes mellitus, and nephritis/nephrotic syndrome/nephrosis; National Center for Health Statistics, 2015).

Costs Associated with Chronic Health Conditions

Another reason why self-management needs to be promoted is that the rising expenditures on healthcare are concomitant with the global increase of chronic health conditions. Of the total US healthcare expenditures, 84% are on individuals with one or more chronic conditions, while 66% of healthcare expenditures are on individuals with two or more chronic conditions (Anderson, 2010). Further, the expenditures in the United States on healthcare are increasing. US spending for healthcare in 2014 amounted to $3.0 trillion, which was 17.5% of the nation's gross domestic product (Martin, Hartman, Benson, Catlin, & National Health Expenditure Accounts Team, 2016).

Not only are there increasing expenditures related to the increase of chronic health conditions, but there are also notable social costs. According to the WHO (2002, p. 11, emphasis added), "Chronic conditions engender *increasingly serious economic and social consequences in all regions and threaten healthcare resources in every country*." Some of the ripple effects of chronic health conditions are experienced as personal and social costs:

> In economic terms, one manifestation of this is that chronic illness degrades society's productive capacity by reducing people's labor output, with people withdrawing from the labor market entirely due to poor health, shifting from full-time to part-time work and/or missing work periodically, accumulating less "human capital" (i.e., knowledge and skills), and being less effective at work ("presenteeism"). (Institute of Medicine, 2012, p. 100)

The annual cost of chronic health conditions to the US economy has been calculated not only due to healthcare expenses but due to reduced productivity. DeVol and Bedroussian (2007) analyzed the impact of seven chronic health conditions (cancer, diabetes, hypertension, stroke, heart disease, pulmonary conditions, and mental health conditions) and found that it was over $1.3 trillion annually in the U.S., based on yearly estimates of $1.1 trillion of lost productivity and $277 billion for treatment.

Time Limitations of Professionals

A third reason why self-management needs to be promoted is the time restrictions of most healthcare professionals (e.g., medical, mental health, and rehabilitation professionals). Most healthcare professionals have limitations on the amount of contact (i.e., frequency and duration) that they are able to have with the individuals that they see in offices, clinics, or hospitals. These professionals provide individuals with chronic health conditions with advice about the current best practices used in treatment. Because of the time-limited nature of healthcare visits, their professional services often are focused primarily on treating problematic symptoms and giving advice about symptom management. Ideally, that level of healthcare would be enough.

However, most chronic health conditions require daily, even hourly, management. Because of the time limitations of healthcare professionals, this necessitates that individuals with chronic health conditions be able to manage their own symptoms, in view that help for managing symptoms is not available constantly to individuals living in community settings. This means that individuals must be taught about their chronic health conditions and given the skills to self-manage as much as possible, while being educated about the parameters of self-treatment. This means they need to know when to seek professional healthcare treatment. Self-management by individuals with chronic health conditions is *not optional but inevitable*, in view that clinicians are "present for only a fraction of the patient's life, and nearly all outcomes are mediated through patient behavior" (Glasgow, Davis, Funnell, & Beck, 2003, p. 563).

PURPOSE OF THIS BOOK

Although healthcare professionals play a vital role in helping individuals with chronic health conditions by providing knowledge about the condition and advise on best practices or evidence-based practices for their fluctuating conditions, most healthcare professionals understand that it is ultimately up to the individuals to take control of managing their chronic health conditions. Yet there is a lot that healthcare professionals can do to promote better self-management. This book discusses multiple aspects of this challenging interpersonal dynamic. It also examines numerous aspects of self-management with the hope that a broad range of this book's content can help healthcare professionals to better understand and facilitate self-management among the individuals with chronic health conditions whom they assist.

This book has a threefold aim: the first aim is to help healthcare professionals to better promote self-management of chronic health conditions by reviewing theoretical models and research on condition-specific, empirically based interventions. The second aim is to help healthcare professionals understand what condition-specific knowledge should be taught to individuals (e.g., in educational interventions), in order to empower them to solve problems related to their specific chronic health condition. The third aim is to help healthcare professionals better understand the range of emotional reactions that can occur at the onset of specific chronic health conditions, in order for professionals to be aware of possible needed areas of intervention and what scientific studies indicate about practices that promote better coping with chronic health conditions.

In summary, this book focuses on mapping out sets of skills, knowledge, and programs that can be used to help facilitate the self-management of a range of chronic health conditions. The models of self-management that are discussed in this book suggest best practices that facilitate the collaboration of healthcare professionals and individuals with chronic health conditions, while empowering the latter to adopt skills for solving problems and handling emotional reactions related to having a chronic health condition.

DEFINITIONS USED IN THIS BOOK

Self-management. A range of self-management definitions are discussed in detail in chapter 2 of this book ("Defining Self-Management on the Individual Level"). Briefly, self-management can be defined as "the active participation by people living with chronic conditions in managing their own health and care. Effective self-management involves the person engaging in activities that protect and promote their health and wellbeing" (Department of Health and Human Services, 2012, p. 5).

One of the earlier definitions of self-management by Corbin and Strauss (1988) involves three components: (a) *medical management,* such as taking medication as prescribed and attending medical appointments; (b) *behavioral management,* such as maintaining or adapting significant chosen life roles after the onset of a chronic health condition; and (c) *emotional management,* such as dealing with the emotional reactions to the onset of a chronic health condition and adapting to its continued or permanent existence.

Chronic health condition: Chronic health condition has been defined as "health problems that require ongoing management over a period of years or decades" (WHO, 2002, p. 11). According to the WHO, the term "chronic condition" expands beyond the traditional perspective that referred only to noncommunicable conditions or "diseases" (e.g., diabetes, cardiovascular disease, and cancer) to include communicable infections (e.g., HIV/AIDS), a variety of mental health conditions (e.g., depression, schizophrenia), and "ongoing impairments in structure" (e.g., amputations, blindness, and joint conditions) as chronic health conditions.

Another definition of chronic health condition includes the following list of qualities:

> Gradual onset; unfolds over time; multivariate causation, changing over time; undulating course, diagnosis often uncertain; prognosis obscure ... no cure; management over time necessary; uncertainty pervasive ... continuous medication use; behavior change (e.g., diet, exercise, leisure); changed social and work circumstances; emotional distress. (Holman & Lorig, 2004, p. 240)

Yet another definition of chronic health condition states: "A chronic condition ... is a condition that is slow in progression, long in duration, and void of spontaneous resolution, and it often limits the function, productivity, and quality of life of those who live with them" (Institute of Medicine, 2012, p. 100).

The term "individual with a chronic health condition" is used in this book, instead of terms like individual with a "chronic disease" or "chronic illness," because the term "chronic health condition" is more representative of a holistic, biopsychosocial approach to disability. Embedded in the terms "chronic illness" and "chronic disease" are references to the "medical model of disability," which focuses on pathology (disease) and its treatment, instead of a holistic view of human functioning and disability. The term "chronic illness" also suggests that the individual is chronically sick, instead of making a distinction that even though one aspect of the individual may not be functioning as expected in the general population, such an individual can still live a dynamic and fulfilling life. These are the primary reasons why the term "chronic health condition," not "chronic illness" or "chronic disease" (except when citing published research, when referring to the "Illness Intrusiveness" theory, or when referring to the disease process underlying a chronic health condition), is used in the present book.

Disuse of the terms "adherence," "compliance," and "patient": The terms "adherence" and "compliance" are not used in this book (other than when citing published research). These two terms reflect a paternalistic or medical model approach to impairment and disability, in which the professionals set up treatment regimens for individuals and those individuals must follow them or are deemed "noncompliant." These terms denote a perspective in which individuals are evaluated based on how much they adhere to or comply with "doctor's orders," even when those orders were not created collaboratively with the individual or when those orders cause individuals discomfort or interfere with their life choices.

Further, the term "patient" is not used in the present book (other than when citing published research), because that term is more reflective of a medical model approach to disability. "Patient" suggests that the person is "sick," instead of a term that emphasizes that an aspect of the person is not functioning as expected for the general population. By using a "person-first" language (e.g., individual with a chronic health condition) in place of the term "patient," a more balanced biopsychosocial perspective of individuals' lives is emphasized, such that the chronic health condition is not highlighted as the focal point of individuals' lives. "Person-first" language implicitly acknowledges that chronic health condition or disability does not have to be "the center of mental gravity" (Livneh & Parker, 2005, p. 19) for individuals who experience one or more chronic health conditions. After all, these individuals are people first, with many roles, interests, and aspects that are not connected to the fact that they have a chronic health condition.

STRUCTURE OF THIS BOOK

This book provides both theoretical and empirically-based approaches. The second chapter of this book ("Defining Self-Management on the Individual Level") discusses a variety of ways of defining self-management. One model is based on a tripartite approach, which includes three areas: (a) the collaboration of healthcare providers in helping individuals manage symptoms of their chronic health conditions, (b) condition-specific education about the typical symptoms and advice about the micro-decisions and actions that the individual with the chronic health condition can take when those symptoms occur, and (c) the coping skills that can be facilitated to address the emotional reactions and stress related to having a chronic health condition. Each chapter in Part II of this book covers these three areas of self-management.

Part I of this book contains chapters that provide theoretical frameworks for promoting behavioral change and health outcomes that are tailored toward helping individuals with chronic health conditions. Several chapters in Part I focus on ideas to facilitate the psychological strength of individuals to take on the responsibility for self-managing their conditions.

Part II of this book contains chapters on the self-management of specific chronic health conditions. These chapters examine published empirical studies, including both basic research and clinical interventions related to managing chronic health conditions. Part II chapters also discuss those programs and interventions that help individuals learn how to make micro-decisions related to their conditions, based on education about the condition and its treatment.

Chapters in Part III cover issues related to the intersection of technology and self-management practices, which healthcare professionals can utilize to help individuals with chronic health conditions. The book concludes with a chapter on systemic models of self-management and its implementation in healthcare systems.

This book has been written to provide a professional resource on self-management of chronic health conditions for healthcare providers, but healthcare recipients may also find this book useful. Ultimately, it is up to healthcare professionals to utilize and implement this knowledge to provide compassionate and effective services to healthcare recipients. Those who have the challenge of living with chronic health conditions can benefit from having healthcare providers who can suggest ideas about self-managing their conditions or provide referrals to evidence-based, condition-specific interventions. As the rates of chronic health conditions continue to increase worldwide, self-management concepts and research can help to provide a roadmap to healthcare professionals in their efforts to help individuals who are dealing with challenge of micro-managing their chronic health conditions.

ACKNOWLEDGMENTS

Thanks go to Dr. Hanoch Livneh for providing feedback on this chapter.

REFERENCES

Anderson, G. F. (2010). *Chronic care: Making the case for ongoing care.* Princeton, NJ: Robert Wood Johnson Foundation.

Busse, R., Blümel, M., Scheller-Kreinsen, D., & Zentner, A. (2010). *Tackling chronic disease in Europe: Strategies, interventions and challenges.* Observatory Studies Series 20. Copenhagen: WHO Regional Office Europe.

Corbin, J. M., & Strauss, A. (1988). *Unending work and care: Managing chronic illness at home.* San Francisco, CA: Jossey-Bass.

Department of Health and Human Services. (2012). *A framework to support self-management.* Retrieved from https://www.dhhs.tas.gov.au/__data/assets/pdf_file/0019/133480/19122012_FINAL_Self_Management_Framework.pdf

DeVol, R., Bedroussian, A., Charuworn, A., Chatterjee, A., Kim, I. K., Kim, S., & Klowden, K. (2007). *An unhealthy America: The economic burden of chronic disease.* Retrieved from https://www.sophe.org/Sophe/PDF/chronic_disease_report.pdf

Glasgow, R. E., Davis, C. L., Funnell, M. M., & Beck, A. (2003). Implementing practical interventions to support chronic illness self-management. *Joint Commission Journal on Quality and Patient Safety, 29*(11), 563–574.

Holman, H., & Lorig, K. (2004). Patient self-management: A key to effectiveness and efficiency in care of chronic disease. *Public Health Reports, 119*(3), 239–243.

Huber, M., Knottnerus, J. A., Green, L., van der Horst, H., Jadad, A. R., Kromhout, D., . . . Schnabel, P. (2011). How should we define health? *BMJ, 343,* 235–237.

Institute of Medicine. (2012). *Living well with chronic illness: A call for public health action.* Retrieved from http://www.nationalacademies.org/hmd/Reports/2012/Living-Well-with-Chronic-Illness.aspx

Livneh, H., & Parker, R. M. (2005). Psychological adaptation to disability perspectives from chaos and complexity theory. *Rehabilitation Counseling Bulletin, 49*(1), 17–28.

Martin, A. B., Hartman, M., Benson, J., Catlin, A., & National Health Expenditure Accounts Team. (2016). National health spending in 2014: Faster growth driven by coverage expansion and prescription drug spending. *Health Affairs, 35*(1), 150–160.

National Center for Health Statistics, Centers for Disease Control and Prevention. (Eds.). (2015). *Health, United States, 2013.* Washington, DC: Government Printing Office.

Ward, B. W., & Schiller, J. S. (2012). Prevalence of multiple chronic conditions among US adults: Estimates from the National Health Interview Survey, 2010. *Preventing Chronic Disease, 10,* E65–E65.

Ward, B. W., Schiller, J. S., & Goodman, R. A. (2014). Multiple chronic conditions among US adults: A 2012 update. *Preventing Chronic Disease, 11,* E62.

World Health Organization. (1948). World Health Organization constitution. Basic Documents 1. Geneva: Author.
World Health Organization. (2002). *Innovative care for chronic conditions: Building blocks for actions: Global report.* Geneva: Author.
World Health Organization. (2014). *Global status report on noncommunicable diseases 2014.* Retrieved from http://www.who.int/nmh/publications/ncd-status-report-2014/en/

2

Defining Self-Management on the Individual Level

ERIN MARTZ ■

The term "self-management" embodies the responsibility that individuals with chronic health conditions have for their own hourly/daily care, which requires them to make continuous decisions related to their conditions while away from the healthcare setting. They are their own "principal caregivers," while healthcare professionals act as their "consultants" (Bodenheimer, Lorig, Holman, & Grumbach, 2002). Because chronic health conditions, by definition (see chapter 1), cannot be cured and will continue for a lengthy (if not lifetime) period of time, self-management will be a "life-time task" (Lorig & Holman, 2003) for most individuals with chronic health conditions.

This chapter examines the range of scientific definitions and models of self-management on an *individual level*, whereas the last chapter of this book covers concepts related to "self-management support," or self-management from a *systems perspective*. This chapter begins with a short discussion of the balancing act of self-management, followed by a brief section on the tripartite model of self-management and then by sections on other ways of defining self-management, how self-management can be distinguished from other terms (e.g., self-care, coping, and adaptation), and how self-management approaches reflect a shift in philosophy. Finally, this chapter ends by suggesting a new model that is an expansion of the tripartite model of self-management.

THE BALANCING ACT OF MANAGING A CHRONIC HEALTH CONDITION

The process of self-managing a chronic health condition involves a continual balancing act among multiple factors (often-fluctuating symptoms, understanding one's health condition and the best ways to manage symptoms, one's views about having a health condition, and one's motivation for implementing healthcare advice given by healthcare professionals). This self-management process is an imperfect one and does not always result in a healthy "equation."

On one side of the self-management equation, individuals have chronic health conditions that they have to manage on a daily basis. This responsibility is no easy task. Most of the burden of self-managing a chronic health condition is on the individuals with chronic conditions because they have to make decisions every day about how to implement healthcare advice for fluctuating symptoms and in new circumstances. These are the *micro-decisions* (Bodenheimer et al., 2002) that they must make throughout the day. They have to learn the necessary condition-specific knowledge (e.g., how to use insulin to manage diabetes or how to reduce seizure frequency with epilepsy) and understand the range of symptoms related to their specific chronic health condition, what those symptoms may indicate, and what actions they should take to address those symptoms. These individuals alone get to *micro-manage* their health. Individuals are "ultimately the primary caregivers" for themselves (Wagner et al., 2005, p. S-10). This unending responsibility can be daunting for some with chronic health conditions.

On the other side of the self-management equation, chronic health conditions require that healthcare providers make *macro-decisions* about how to treat the chronic condition by creating the framework of how to care for the health condition (e.g., a treatment plan). Healthcare providers make the diagnoses and give healthcare advice (e.g., what actions the individual needs to take to treat the chronic health condition), communicating to individuals to help them understand the framework of the treatment plan. These collaborative partnerships may involve shared decision-making between healthcare recipient and provider (Edwards & Elwyn, 2009). Yet, ultimately, it is the individual who must manage the daily, hourly, and even minute-by-minute implementation of that plan.

Forming a collaborative partnership is no easy task for healthcare professionals, in view that the self-management approach is a "complex intervention" (Trappenburg et al., 2013), reflecting that it is a strategy that has numerous components with varying degrees of complexity. Any process that has many "moving pieces" can be complicated to implement, and even more so when the human component of independent-thinking individuals is added. Even though healthcare professionals make the macro-decisions about how to treat a chronic health condition, they have no real control over the behavior of individuals to whom they provide self-management advice. Considering all these factors, it can be challenging for healthcare professionals to motivate individuals to implement the treatment plans, especially if the healthcare providers do not understand self-management approaches.

PERSPECTIVES ON SELF-MANAGEMENT

This section covers a range of definitions of self-management on an individual level, beginning with the tripartite definition of self-management.

A Tripartite Model of Self-Management

The importance placed on various self-management components differ by research teams, and thus definitions of self-management vary widely. Corbin and Strauss (1988) provided one of the first tripartite models of self-management, which many researchers still cite when discussing the definition of self-management. These two researchers proposed that self-management consisted of three components: (a) *medical management*, which involves taking medication as prescribed and attending medical appointments; (b) *behavioral management*, which includes maintaining or changing significant life roles after the onset of a chronic health condition; and (c) *emotional management*, which involves dealing with the emotional reactions to the onset of a chronic health condition and adapting to its continued or permanent existence.

A few years later, Clark et al. (1991) suggested the following three "categories of activities" or "behaviors" in self-management: (a) obtaining sufficient knowledge about one's own condition and treatment choices to make reasonable decisions about one's own care, (b) taking action to manage one's own condition, and (c) coping with emotional reactions to having the condition. Note that Clark et al.'s tripartite concept closely parallels Corbin and Strauss's (1988) perspectives on defining self-management.

Self-Managers

Clark and colleagues (1991) cautioned that self-management involves more than just condition-related education; it involves behavioral integration of that knowledge: "Becoming a better self-manager is linked less to learning facts about a particular condition and more to learning how to set goals, organize resources (including psychic resources), and implement problem-solving strategies" (p. 20). Their views reflected a growing recognition that in the context of chronic condition healthcare, active individuals were needed to help manage the condition outside of the doctor's office. Thus the view of the healthcare recipient as a passive individual who is told what to do by the physician was becoming a dated concept when treating individuals with chronic health conditions. According to Jerant, von Friederichs-Fitzwater, and Moore (2005), passive self-managers had the following characteristics: (a) deferring to healthcare providers, (b) feeling forced to abandon valued roles in life, and (c) using ineffective forms of emotional management (i.e., coping). In contrast, active self-managers displayed the following characteristics (a) collaborating with healthcare providers, (b) striving to maintain valued roles in life, and (c) using consciously chosen coping strategies (Jerant et al., 2005).

The Health Council of Canada (2012) proposed that "good self-managers" are individuals who know the parameters of their responsibilities and who are "actively engaged in their care and are able to make decisions that support their health, including knowing when they can manage on their own and when to seek professional help" (p. 13). Good self-managers also are able to understand their fluctuating symptoms and know what steps to take when they occur. That is, they "monitor and manage symptoms of their condition(s) between healthcare visits; know how to problem-solve or seek help to manage the impact of the condition(s) on their physical, emotional, family, and social life" (Health Council of Canada, 2012, p. 13).

OTHER DEFINITIONS OF SELF-MANAGEMENT

Self-management has been defined in numerous ways that emphasize different aspects, such as the processes or the components. Self-management has been depicted as "a complex dynamic phenomenon consisting of three dimensions: context, process, and outcomes" (Ryan & Sawin, 2009, p. 9). Others noted an array of approaches for defining self-management: a term referring to the processes of self-management, self-management as an intervention program, or the outcomes that result from using self-management practices (Grady & Gough, 2014). The following sections briefly discuss self-management as a process and the components of self-management.

Self-Management as a Process

Because chronic health conditions require ongoing treatment and monitoring, self-management can be viewed as a process. These processes can include both intrapersonal and interpersonal processes that can range from identifying possible health-related problems by recognizing symptoms and managing the emotions triggered by one's chronic health condition to obtaining optimum healthcare by having effective interactions with healthcare providers (Clark et al., 1991).

Other researchers view it from a multidimensional perspective, defining self-management as "the ability of the individual, in conjunction with family, community, and healthcare professionals, to manage symptoms, treatments, lifestyle changes, and psychosocial, cultural, and spiritual consequences of chronic [health conditions]" (Wilkinson & Whitehead, 2009, p. 1145).

Three self-management processes were identified by Schulman and colleagues' (2012) analysis of 101 research studies: (a) focusing on condition-related needs (i.e., health-related needs); (b) activating resources (i.e., assistance from healthcare professionals, family, and community); and (c) living with a chronic health condition (i.e., coping skills, adapting to and integrating the condition and finding meaning). These researchers noted that the trajectory of a health condition and the development of complications or co-occurring health conditions can significantly modify individuals' self-management processes and established routines and, thus, self-management should *not* be viewed as a linear process.

Components of Self-Management

Other models of self-management highlight its components. Several decades ago, Holroyd and Creer (1986) identified the following six *skills* as self-management components: self-monitoring, self-instruction, self-induced stimulus change (e.g., changing the environmental factors that impact the chronic health condition), self-induced response change (e.g., self-reinforcement strategies), relaxation, and decision-making.

Barlow, Wright, Sheasby, Turner, and Hainsworth (2002) reviewed 145 articles on self-management and found eight main components to self-management programs: information, drug-management, symptom-management, management of psychological consequences (e.g., anger, depression, acceptance), lifestyle (including exercise), social support, communication, and a category containing other components (i.e., coping, decision-making, goal-setting, and problem-solving). Other researchers (Lorig & Holman, 2003) proposed that the major self-management components for individuals with chronic health conditions were problem-solving, decision-making, utilizing resources, collaborating with healthcare providers, taking action, and self-tailoring (i.e., adapting self-management skills and knowledge to one's own situation).

Most healthcare researchers and clinicians would agree that individuals need to *take action* to manage their own conditions. The ability to decide what action to take in fluctuating, health-related circumstances involves the skill of *problem-solving*. Researchers began to emphasize that problem-solving was a core skill in self-management education (Bodenheimer et al., 2002; Lorig & Holman, 2003), which they distinguished from traditional chronic health condition education offering information and technical skills (e.g., diabetes education). These researchers pointed out that traditional chronic health condition education helps individuals *define* the problems, while self-management education allows individuals to *identify* their problems and then suggests techniques to help individuals make decisions, take appropriate actions, and change their approaches as they encounter new circumstances.

In Taylor et al.'s (2014) extensive report entitled the *Practical Systematic Review of Self-Management Support for Long-Term Conditions* (PRISMS), they proposed that the following are core components that are likely to be included in self-management interventions for individuals with chronic health conditions:

1. Education: This includes providing information and knowledge about the specific health condition. Regarding the format, there were a variety of formats for the education programs, such as groups, individual meetings, peer or lay-led, computerized or Internet-based, and interventions that included more than one mode.
2. Psychological support: This included a variety of strategies (e.g., problem-solving, action planning, goal-setting, relaxation, cognitive restructuring) to help individuals who are adapting to life after the onset

of a chronic health condition. This adaptation may vary for individuals, depending on the nature of the condition, individuals' beliefs and attitudes, and their social support and financial resources.
3. Support for implementing medication or treatment advice: This may include a healthcare provider giving condition-related advice or feedback about the results of self-monitoring.
4. Practical social support: One purpose of this support is to help individuals better cope, as well as make social adjustments related to their lifestyles. This support may include utilizing peer support or peer mentoring.

Deckert and Devins (see chapter 10 in this book) proposed four levels of self-management targets, which can be used to structure self-management interventions:

1. Primary targets focus on the health condition's trajectory that can be modified by the individual's efforts (e.g., exercise, restricted diets, taking medication).
2. Secondary targets focus on treating symptoms and treatment side effects.
3. Tertiary targets focus on the psychosocial consequences (e.g., depression, quality of life, interpersonal relations).
4. Quaternary targets focus on preventing condition-related complications that can be avoided by means of individuals taking specific actions (e.g., individuals with diabetes attempting to normalize blood-sugar levels in order to avoid complications such as neuropathy or amputation).

Emotional Management

Some self-management research studies do not reference the component of emotional management, favoring instead to emphasize educational and behavioral components (i.e., *knowledge and actions*). While there is a place for the knowledge and action components, most people experience the onset of a chronic health condition as a psychologically-weighted event (i.e., stressful or upsetting). This suggests that if individuals are to be better empowered to self-manage, they must have information on ways of dealing with the psychological stress concomitant with the onset of a chronic health condition. Stress-management strategies can be categorized more broadly as emotional management. Psychological support given to bolster an individual's emotional management can also help to address the numerous barriers that individuals with chronic health conditions may experience, ranging from depression to lack of family or social support (Jerant et al., 2005).

One aspect of emotional management is processing psychological reactions to upsetting events, which includes being aware of and expressing a range of emotions triggered by the onset of a health condition and grieving over impairment-related loss of health and/or functioning (Schulman et al., 2012). Livneh and Antonak (1997) depicted the process of adaptation to chronic health condition and disability as consisting of, in part, being able to deal with the emotional effects of those conditions. Decades of research suggest that adjusting and adapting to a health condition requires accepting changes in one's life and integrating the chronic health condition (Livneh, 2001; Livneh & Antonak, 1997; Schulman et al., 2012; Shontz, 1977; Wright, 1983).

Audulv, Packer, Hutchinson, Roger, and Kephart (2016) examined the overlapping concepts of coping, adaptation, and self-management in the context of a neurological condition and proposed that those three concepts can be viewed as coexisting processes. The following sections briefly suggest distinctions that can be made between the three constructs according to Audulv et al., with additional notes on coping and adaptation added by the present author.

Coping

Lazarus and Folkman (1984) defined coping as the "constantly changing cognitive and behavioral efforts to manage specific external and/or internal demands that are appraised as taxing or exceeding the resources of the person" (p. 141). In the context of chronic health conditions, coping can be viewed as the cognitive, affective, and behavioral attempts to reduce stress related to a disability or a health condition, for which an individual does not necessarily have automatic, adaptive responses (Livneh, 2001). Coping can also be viewed as a psychologically normal response in circumstances that require special psychosocial efforts or are unusually taxing (Costa, Somerfield, & McCrae, 1996). Folkman and Moskowitz (2004) pointed out that individuals' use of adaptive coping strategies should not be regarded as indicative of mastery or resolution of a stressor, given that some situations, like health conditions, involve chronic stress. Thus they proposed that coping should not be viewed as resolving stress—but as *managing* stress.

Adaptation

Livneh (2001) and Livneh and Antonak (1990, 1991, 1997) suggested, based on empirical and clinical research, that there is a multidimensional, nonlinear process of reactions to health condition or disability, which may include negative affectivity like reactions of shock, denial, depression, and anger, as well as more positively weighted emotional, cognitive, and behavioral reactions of acknowledgement and adjustment. Their multidimensional model defines psychosocial adaptation as a dynamic, continuously evolving process that involves an integration of intrapersonal, interpersonal, and environmental elements.

Livneh (2001) and Livneh and Antonak (1997) depicted adaptation as a process in which individuals move toward psychological equilibrium, reintegration, and a reassertion of a positive self-concept after the onset of a health condition. In contrast, coping can be viewed as the short-term strategies that individuals use throughout the day to manage stress, which can facilitate the longer term process of adapting to a chronic health condition (Martz & Livneh, 2007).

SELF-MANAGEMENT

Self-management involves condition-specific actions that are aimed at controlling the symptoms of one's conditions, as well as possible complications and progression of the condition (Audulv et al., 2016). Self-management behaviors are "performed regardless of diagnosis and aim to increase overall health and emphasize living well with a disease" (Audulv et al., p. 6). Further, self-management can be defined as "the tasks that individuals must undertake to live with one or more chronic conditions. These tasks include having the confidence to deal with medical management, role management, and emotional management of their conditions" (Taylor et al., 2014, p. 419).

SELF-MANAGEMENT VERSUS SELF-CARE

According to the Department of Health (2001), the term "self-management" was used during the 1960s and 1970s as part of the self-care movement; at that time, it represented enabling individuals with chronic health conditions to "take more control of their lives by relinquishing involvement with organized healthcare systems" (p. 22). Yet, the latter part of the definition (i.e., relinquishing involvement) was not adopted in scientific research.

Clark et al. (1991) distinguished "self-management" from "self-care" by emphasizing that self-management involves actions that an individual must do in order to reduce the impact of chronic health condition on his or her overall physical health, while self-care involves the actions that healthy people take to avoid chronic health conditions. These authors also emphasized that self-management *requires an ability to cope* with the psychosocial issues that arise from having a chronic health condition. Other researchers distinguished self-management from self-care by stating:

> ["Self-management" can be defined as] those actions individuals and others take to mitigate the effects of a long-term condition and to maintain the best possible quality of life. "Self-care" refers to a wider set of behaviors which both the healthy and the not so healthy take to prevent the onset of illness or disability, and, again to maintain quality of life. (Parsons et al., 2010, pp. 10–11)

Richard and Shea (2011) noted that the distinctions between self-management and self-care are not always clear. They suggested that self-management is a subset of self-care. Yet, for many researchers and clinicians, self-management involves self-monitoring and symptom management, as well as managing the emotional, psychosocial, functional, and physical ramifications of a chronic health condition.

Self-management programs should be distinguished from education or skills training (e.g., diabetes education) provided by healthcare professionals, in that the self-management programs are "designed to allow people with chronic conditions to take an active part in the management of their own condition" (Foster, Taylor, Eldridge, Ramsay, & Griffiths, 2009, p. 3). While healthcare professionals receive extensive clinical and scientific training that allows them to provide healthcare instruction and treatment, individuals with chronic health conditions often receive little instruction about the skills they need for making micro-decisions about their chronic condition as they experience symptom fluctuations in their chronic health condition. Individuals with chronic health conditions need a "toolbox" of knowledge and skills, so that they can problem-solve issues related to their chronic health conditions when healthcare professionals are not accessible to them and by this can be better "self-managers."

It is important to understand that self-management does not exclude health professionals; it includes them as full partners or co-collaborators. Given that individuals with chronic health conditions constantly deal with fluctuating issues, problems, and symptoms related to their health conditions, they need information and clarification about where their healthcare providers's responsibility ends and their responsibility begins.

SELF-MANAGEMENT APPROACHES REFLECTING A SHIFT IN PHILOSOPHY

Historically, healthcare professionals were trained to diagnose and treat acute conditions. This approach to health conditions was called "the medical model" or the "biomedical" philosophy, which focused on correcting pathology, primarily in acute-care settings. The common perception was that healthcare professionals had the final word on medical matters. Wagner and colleagues (2005) depicted that in the acute-care or medical model, professionals were obsessed with identifying and treating physical disease and the doctor had dominance. These researchers advocated for a shift to focus on the person, not the disease, in order to more fully understand health conditions.

In the acute-care healthcare system, when individuals sought healthcare treatment for acute health issues, they were "generally inexperienced and passive recipients of medical care," but with the prevalence of chronic health conditions, the individual seeking healthcare "must become a partner in the process, contributing at almost every decision or action level" (Holman & Lorig, 2000, p. 526). Wagner et al. (2001) also noted that in the acute-care model, the individual had a passive role, because the clinical course and treatment was a few days or weeks; thus there was no urgency to help the individual learn self-management skills. Wagner and colleagues (2005) asserted that the passive individual is less likely to be successful a self-manager.

The acute-care healthcare system has been deemed "paternalistic" in the sense that "the professionals/doctors know best" and thus healthcare recipients were expected to fully implement their advice (Wagner et al., 2005). However, as the prevalence of chronic health conditions continued to rise, there was a need for an approach other than the acute-care model, given that chronic health conditions could not be cured. For many decades, individuals with chronic health conditions and disabilities were socialized into the medical model perspective of impairment and disability, which fostered dependence on professionals, instead of promoting collaboration between healthcare providers and individuals with chronic health conditions (Bodenheimer et al., 2002).

Decades ago, Engel (1977) called for a new kind of medical model: a more holistic one that included the social, psychological, and behavioral components related to health conditions and disability. In 2001, the World Health Organization presented a biopsychosocial model of disability called the International Classification of Functioning, Disability, and Health (ICF). The WHO's ICF model altered the previous WHO model that contained the terms "impairment," "disability," and "handicap" and redefined disability in terms of "impairment," "activity limitation," and "participation restriction." The framework of the ICF was structured as an interactional model, which posited more clearly that disability occurred as an interaction between the person and his or her environment: thus disability was not just a condition inherent in the individual.

The medical model perspective of health conditions is unidimensional by its focus primarily on healing or fixing the particular aspect (i.e., "pathology") of a person that needs a cure or a treatment, and not on the multidimensional person. A biopsychosocial approach to disability and chronic health conditions reflects that individuals can and do live vibrant, productive lives even while having serious, chronic health conditions. This philosophical perspective posits that a chronic health condition or disability does not have to act as the primary identity of an individual's life or does not have to be "the center of mental gravity" of a person (Livneh & Parker, 2005, p. 19). The biopsychosocial perspective of health conditions and disabilities fits well with the movement in rehabilitation and healthcare settings toward addressing the whole person and not just treating an individual's pathology or symptoms.

One research study is worth noting because it compared lay and healthcare providers' understandings of self-management and suggests that many healthcare providers still maintain a medical model perspective (Sadler, Wolfe, & McKevitt, 2014). These researchers found that healthcare providers viewed self-management as including "both a biomedical model of compliance and individual responsibility" (p. 1) but as centrally based on individuals "complying with" advice of their healthcare providers' (i.e., a paternalistic or traditional model of care). In contrast, Sadler and colleagues found that lay people viewed self-management in broader terms that included biomedical, psychological, and social domains, as well as recognition of increased responsibility for individuals with chronic conditions and the need for a collaborative partnership with their healthcare providers.

COLLABORATIVE CARE

Along with a movement toward viewing health condition and disability in more holistic and multidimensional terms, there has been a movement in the past few decades toward collaborative care (Butler et al., 2008). Butler and colleagues noted that the term "collaborative care" has been interchangeably used over the decades with terms such as "integrated care," "complex system interventions," and "multifaceted interventions." Butler et al. clarified that the term "collaborative care" has been used in two different ways: (a) to reflect the need for cooperation among healthcare providers across multiple disciplines and (b) to indicate the alliance between the healthcare provider and the individual with a health issue. The following paragraphs focus on the second use of the term "collaborative care."

An earlier definition of "collaborative care" in the context of health conditions and disabilities was provided by Von Korff, Gruman, Schaefer, Curry, and Wagner (1997), who defined it as containing four components: (a) creating a collaborative definition of problems between healthcare professionals and individuals with chronic health conditions; (b) developing an action plan by healthcare professionals and individuals with chronic health conditions that focus on specific issues; (c) providing self-management training and support services, in order to build skill levels of individuals of chronic health conditions; and (d) following up on contact with healthcare providers, by in-person, telephone, or other means (e.g., virtual contact), in order to enhance self-management.

The role of the healthcare provider has been changing from authoritarian or paternalistic to one of acting as a teacher, partner, and healthcare supervisor (Lorig & Holman, 2003). Bodenheimer et al. (2002, p. 2470) wrote about a new paradigm that was emerging that denoted individuals with chronic health conditions as their own "principal caregivers" and that healthcare professionals were "consultants" to these individuals. These perspectives represented a movement toward collaborative care in which the individual is no longer the passive recipient of care; the healthcare professionals and individuals with chronic health conditions make healthcare decisions together, *with the individuals as experts on their own lives and healthcare professionals as experts on the specific health conditions* (Bodenheimer et al., 2002; Department of Health, 2001). According to the self-management perspective, individuals "accept responsibility to manage their own conditions and are encouraged to solve their own problems *with information, but not orders*, from professionals" (Bodenheimer et al., 2002, p. 2470, emphasis added). The paradigm shift noted by Bodenheimer and colleagues continues to the present day. For example, Foster et al. (2009) observed that healthcare systems are changing from a paternalistic model of care to a partnership model (i.e., a collaborative model of care).

One program reflecting the evolution toward collaborative care was the implementation of the Expert Patients Program by the English government (Department of Health, 2001). This term was utilized as a way to recognize that individuals with chronic health conditions actually knew their own conditions better than healthcare professionals. In this program, self-management programs were "not simply about educating or instructing patients about their condition. ... They are based on developing the confidence and motivation of patients to use their own skills and knowledge to take effective control over life" (Department of Health, 2001, p. 6). The creators of the Expert Patients Program emphasized that it was "not an anti-professional initiative. It is based on partnership" (Department of Health, 2001, p. 7), such that the expertise of healthcare professionals as "essential" in self-management of chronic health conditions. This emphasized that even though self-management programs were shifting more of the decision-making capabilities to individuals with chronic health conditions, the healthcare professional still is and would be a crucial component of the self-management approach.

While the philosophy of collaborative care is empowering, the reality is that not all individuals have the ability to maintain a collaborative partnership with their healthcare provider. In view of that reality, the following three-level categorization of self-management was proposed, which reflected that varying degrees of collaboration will be required by different individuals (Department of Health and Human Services, 2012):

1. Self-directed model of self-management: A person with the chronic condition is able to make informed decisions to effectively self-manage with little input from healthcare professionals.
2. Collaborative model of self-management: Self-management decisions are made in a partnership between the individual and the healthcare provider.
3. Supported model of self-management: The individual's capacity to self-manage is low, and thus a range of strategies and supports are created to support the person's self-management.

EXPANDED TRIPARTITE MODEL OF SELF-MANAGEMENT

As previously mentioned, Corbin and Strauss (1988) proposed a tripartite model of self-management, which included three components: (a) *medical management*, (b) *behavioral management*, and (c) *emotional management*. These researchers defined behavioral management rather broadly by their reference to maintaining "significant life roles." Yet, other definitions of self-management included behavioral management in more concrete terms related to the chronic health condition without the more holistic behavioral concept as Corbin and Strauss proposed. Both Corbin and Strauss's tripartite model and Clark et al.'s (1991) subsequent model contained three cornerstones or targets: *knowledge, actions,* and *coping.* Yet it should be noted that these tripartite definitions of self-management did not emphasize the collaboration between healthcare providers and recipients or highlight other influences of individuals' social or environmental circumstances.

Few multidimensional models exist that represent self-management from the individual's perspective (see chapter 22 of this book for systemic models that have been created to help integrate self-management and chronic health conditions into healthcare systems). However, researchers have proposed definitions that include multidimensional views of self-management on an individual level. This is evident in Barlow's definition cited by Barlow and colleagues (2002), which reflects a biopsychosocial approach:

Self-management refers to the individual's ability to manage the symptoms, treatment, physical and psychosocial consequences and lifestyle changes inherent in living with a chronic condition. Efficacious self-management encompasses ability to monitor one's condition and to affect the cognitive, behavioral, and emotional responses necessary to maintain a satisfactory quality of life (p. 178).

Miller, Lasiter, Ellis, and Buelow (2015) conducted a hybrid concept analysis of 111 articles on self-management and proposed that a multidimensional perspective is needed on self-management. They wrote that self-management was

[A] fluid, iterative process during which patients incorporate *multidimensional strategies* that meet their self-identified needs to cope with chronic disease within the context of their daily living. Strategies are multidimensional because they require the individual to incorporate intrapersonal, interpersonal, and environmental systems . . . to maximize wellness. (pp. 158–159, emphasis added)

Miller and colleagues also asserted that self-management involves complex systems with many layers, such that a two-dimensional or linear perspective (e.g., focusing on the health-related actions and outcomes of an individual) is not the best way to understand the complexity of self-management.

The following model (by this chapter's author) proposes an expansion of the tripartite model of self-management, building on the three components of *knowledge, actions,* and *emotions*. The expanded tripartite model of self-management includes both internal (i.e., the individual with a chronic condition) and external (i.e., resources outside the individual) components.

A. Acquisition of Condition-Specific Knowledge
Internal: An individual with a chronic condition will need knowledge about his or her specific condition and its treatment plan in order to make a range of decisions to micro-manage it. The individual obtains condition-specific knowledge from a variety of possible sources, including self-education (e.g., "bibliotherapy" or reading books about one's condition and its treatment, self-education may also include seeking information on the Internet). An array of knowledge is needed, including how to handle some of the daily or frequently occurring symptoms of condition-related issues, what self-management skills are typically utilized related to their chronic conditions, and what the individual's responsibilities entail related to his or her health condition. The individual learns the parameters of his or her micro-management responsibilities and thus has the knowledge about when to seek advice and/or support from healthcare professionals.

External: The individual learns condition-specific knowledge by means of communication with healthcare providers, as well as individual instruction or group training from a healthcare provider about the specific condition. The provider–individual collaboration typically involves an exchange of information and advice, in order for the individual to understand the treatment plan, based on the provider's knowledge of the best treatment practices. As individuals learn how to self-monitor the symptoms of their health conditions, they can provide feedback to their healthcare provider, who can then discuss with them how the treatment plan could be altered to adjust for the symptoms. Thus, fundamentally, this collaboration is about the exchange of knowledge, information, and ideas between the healthcare provider and recipient.

B. Application of Knowledge

This refers to the action-related or behavioral components of self-managing.

Internal: The individual integrates condition-specific knowledge (gained by self-study or from advice and information given by a healthcare provider) into the micro-managing of his or her health condition. This may require learning problem-solving skills to address a range of health-related issues that may arise during the micro-managing of one's condition. The component also involves decision-making for managing the specific issues created by the chronic health condition. Problem-solving strategies can help individuals tailor the condition-specific knowledge to their unique circumstances; that provides greater flexibility in implementing the treatment plan, because not all best practices for a specific health condition are appropriate for every individual.

External: The measurable behavioral aspects (e.g., blood-glucose averages, blood pressure, number of seizures per month) related to one's chronic health condition may be monitored by one's healthcare provider as an indication of how well the individual is able to self-manage: The provider can suggest strategies to improve targeted health-outcomes.

As part of the behavioral dynamics, the individual learns the parameters of his or her micro-management responsibilities and will know when to reach out for advice and/or support from healthcare professionals. The "application of knowledge" aspect is also represented when the individual utilizes healthcare resources from the environment and community to bolster self-management.

C. Psychosocial Integration

Internal: The individual uses coping strategies to manage the range of emotions that may be triggered after the onset of a chronic health disorder. Either the individual already has appropriate coping strategies to deal with condition-related stress or else learns stress-management skills from self-study or other sources. This aspect of self-management also reflects the individual's integrating the fact of having a chronic

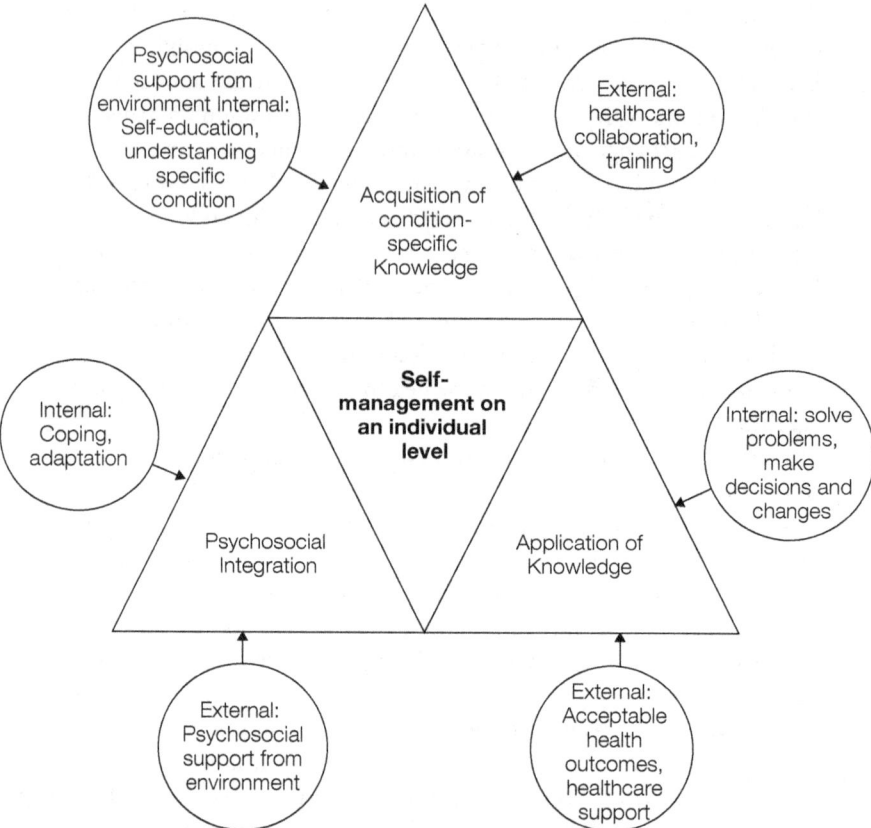

Figure 2.1 Expanded Tripartite Model of Self-Management for Individuals with Chronic Health Conditions.

health condition that needs daily management and adjusting his or her goals, roles, and priorities in life, given the existence of a chronic health condition.

External: If the individual finds that his or her coping strategies are not sufficient to deal with condition-related stress, he or she seeks psychosocial support from outside, whether it is from individual or group counseling or psychotherapy, peer-support groups, or other healthcare providers (e.g., health coaches). Further, individuals use socially oriented skills, such as accessing social support, in order to seek help for a range of psychosocial issues.

In summary, the expanded tripartite model of self-management (see Figure 2.1) includes condition-specific *knowledge* about the expected/typical symptoms and understanding the treatment plan and the possible options when those symptoms occur, *integration of that condition-specific knowledge,* and using *coping skills* to address the emotional components related to having a chronic health condition.

CONCLUSION

The need to understand how to promote self-management continues to grow in importance as the number of individuals who experience one or more chronic health conditions continues to expand as the science that treats acute-care health issues improves and as people age and live longer. This chapter covered a variety of definitions of the concept of self-management and distinguished it from related concepts. By understanding what self-management means, healthcare professionals who make the macro-decisions about healthcare (e.g., diagnoses and treatments) can better collaborate with individuals who have to make the micro-decisions about their own health.

Self-management signals a *shift of the locus of care* from the healthcare provider to the individual: the healthcare professional provides the information and education to help inform the minute-by-minute choices that individuals with chronic health conditions must make. The emergence of self-directed care and the explosion of free information (e.g., on the Internet) have provided more tools for individuals to take more control over their chronic health conditions. While individuals can be viewed as experts on their own conditions, healthcare professionals can be viewed as the experts on the best types of treatment interventions for specific conditions. By obtaining condition-specific knowledge and utilizing problem-solving, decision-making, and emotional management, individuals with chronic health conditions will have a greater understanding of how to manage their conditions, symptoms, and health-related stress. By empowering individuals to take responsibility for micro-managing their chronic health conditions, healthcare providers can encourage more active partnerships in dealing with chronic health conditions. Input from both parties is needed in order to facilitate beneficial outcomes in the self-management of chronic health conditions.

ACKNOWLEDGMENTS

Thanks go to Dr. Hanoch Livneh and Ms. Joan Martz for providing feedback on this chapter.

REFERENCES

Audulv, Å., Packer, T., Hutchinson, S., Roger, K. S., & Kephart, G. (2016). Coping, adapting or self-managing-what is the difference? A concept review based on the neurological literature. *Journal of Advanced Nursing, 72*(11), 2629–2643.

Barlow, J., Wright, C., Sheasby, J., Turner, A., & Hainsworth, J. (2002). Self-management approaches for people with chronic illness: A review. *Patient Education and Counseling, 48*(2), 177–187.

Bodenheimer, T., Lorig, K., Holman, H., & Grumbach, K. (2002). Patient self-management of chronic disease in primary care. *JAMA, 288*(19), 2469–2475.

Butler, M., Kane, R. L., McAlpine, D., Kathol, R. G., Fu, S. S., Hagedorn, H., & Wilt, T. J. (2008). *Integration of mental health/substance abuse and primary care.* Evidence Report/Technology Assessment 173. Rockville, MD: Agency for Healthcare Research and Quality.

Clark, N. M., Becker, M. H., Janz, N. K., Lorig, K., Rakowski, W., & Anderson, L. (1991). Self- management of chronic disease by older adults: A review and questions for research. *Journal of Aging and Health, 3*(1), 3–27.

Corbin, J. M., & Strauss, A. (1988). *Unending work and care: Managing chronic illness at home.* San Fransicso, CA: Jossey-Bass.

Costa, P. T. Jr., Somerfield, M. R., & McCrae, R. R. (1996). Personality and coping: A reconceptualization. In M. Zeidner & S. Norman (Eds.), *Handbook of coping: Theory, research, applications.* New York: John Wiley.

Department of Health. (2001). *The expert patient: A new approach to chronic disease management for the 21st century.* London: Department of Health. Retrieved on from https://www.gov.uk/government/uploads/system/uploads/attachment_data/file/265576/4386.pdf

Department of Health and Human Services. (2012). *A framework to support self-management.* Retrieved from https://www.dhhs.tas.gov.au/__data/assets/pdf_file/0019/133480/19122012_FINAL_Self_Management_Framework.pdf

Edwards, A., & Elwyn, G. (2009). *Shared decision-making in health care: Achieving evidence-based patient choice.* Oxford: Oxford University Press.

Engel, G. L. (1977). The need for a new medical model: A challenge for biomedicine. *Science, 196*(4286), 129–136.

Folkman, S., & Moskowitz, J. T. (2004). Coping: pitfalls and promise. *Annual Review of Psychology, 55*, 745–774.

Foster, G., Taylor, S., Eldridge, S., Ramsay, J., & Griffiths, C. (2009). Self-management education programmes by lay leaders for people with chronic conditions. *Cochrane Database Systems Review, 4*, CD005108.

Grady, P. A., & Gough, L. L. (2014). Self-management: A comprehensive approach to management of chronic conditions. *American Journal of Public Health, 104*(8), e25–e31.

Health Council of Canada. (2012). *Self-management support for Canadians with chronic health conditions.* Toronto: Author.

Holman, H., & Lorig, K. (2000). Patients as partners in managing chronic disease: Partnership is a prerequisite for effective and efficient health care. *BMJ, 320*(7234), 526–527.

Holroyd, K. A., & Creer, T. L. (1986). *Self-management of chronic disease: Handbook of clinical interventions and research.* New York: Academic Press.

Jerant, A. F., von Friederichs-Fitzwater, M. M., & Moore, M. (2005). Patients' perceived barriers to active self-management of chronic conditions. *Patient Education and Counseling, 57*(3), 300–307.

Lazarus, R., & Folkman, S. (1984). *Stress, coping and adaptation.* New York: Springer.

Livneh, H. (2001). Psychosocial adaptation to chronic illness and disability: A conceptual framework. *Rehabilitation Counseling Bulletin, 44*(3), 151–160.

Livneh, H., & Antonak, R. F. (1990). Reactions to disability: An empirical investigation of their nature and structure. *Journal of Applied Rehabilitation Counseling, 21*(4), 13–21.

Livneh, H., & Antonak, R. F. (1991). Temporal structure of adaptation to disability. *Rehabilitation Counseling Bulletin, 34*(4), 298–319.

Livneh, H., & Antonak, R. F. (1997). *Psychosocial adaptation to chronic illness and disability.* Gaithersburg, MD: Aspen.

Livneh, H., & Parker, R. M. (2005). Psychological adaptation to disability perspectives from chaos and complexity theory. *Rehabilitation Counseling Bulletin, 49*(1), 17–28.

Lorig, K. R., & Holman, H. R. (2003). Self-management education: History, definition, outcomes, and mechanisms. *Annals of Behavioral Medicine, 26*(1), 1–7.

Martz, E., & Livneh, H. (Eds.). (2007). *Coping with chronic illnesses and disabilities: Theoretical, empirical, and clinical aspects.* New York: Springer.

Miller, W. R., Lasiter, S., Ellis, R. B., & Buelow, J. M. (2015). Chronic disease self-management: A hybrid concept analysis. *Nursing Outlook, 63*(2), 154–161.

Parsons, M. S., Bury, M., Carter, S., Hurst, P., Magee, H., & Taylor, D. (2010). *Self management support amongst older adults: The availability, impact and potential of locally based services and resources.* Retrieved from http://www.netscc.ac.uk/netscc/hsdr/files/project/SDO_FR_08-1715-161_V01.pdf.

Richard, A. A., & Shea, K. (2011). Delineation of self-care and associated concepts. *Journal of Nursing Scholarship, 43*(3), 255–264.

Ryan, P., & Sawin, K. J. (2009). The individual and family self-management theory: Background and perspectives on context, process, and outcomes. *Nursing Outlook, 57*(4), 217–225.

Sadler, E., Wolfe, C. D., & McKevitt, C. (2014). Lay and health care professional understandings of self-management: A systematic review and narrative synthesis. *SAGE Open Medicine, 2,* 1–18.

Schulman-Green, D., Jaser, S., Martin, F., Alonzo, A., Grey, M., McCorkle, R., . . . Whittemore, R. (2012). Processes of self-management in chronic illness. *Journal of Nursing Scholarship, 44*(2), 136–144.

Shontz, F. C. (1977). Six principles relating disability and psychological adjustment. *Rehabilitation Psychology, 24*(4), 207–210.

Taylor, S. J., Pinnock, H., Epiphaniou, E., Pearce, G., Parke, H. L., Schwappach, A., . . . Sheikh, A. (2014). A rapid synthesis of the evidence on interventions supporting self-management for people with long-term conditions: PRISMS–Practical systematic Review of Self-Management Support for long-term conditions. *Health Services and Delivery Research, 2*(53), 1–580.

Trappenburg, J., Jonkman, N., Jaarsma, T., van Os-Medendorp, H., Kort, H., de Wit, N., . . . Schuurmans, M. (2013). Self-management: One size does not fit all. *Patient Education and Counseling, 92*(1), 134–137.

Von Korff, M., Gruman, J., Schaefer, J., Curry, S. J., & Wagner, E. H. (1997). Collaborative management of chronic illness. *Annals of Internal Medicine, 127*(12), 1097–1102.

Wagner, E. H., Austin, B. T., Davis, C., Hindmarsh, M., Schaefer, J., & Bonomi, A. (2001). Improving chronic illness care: Translating evidence into action. *Health Affairs, 20*(6), 64–78.

Wagner, E. H., Bennett, S. M., Austin, B. T., Greene, S. M., Schaefer, J. K., & Vonkorff, M. (2005). Finding common ground: Patient-centeredness and evidence-based chronic illness care. *Journal of Alternative & Complementary Medicine, 11*(Suppl. 1), S7–S15.

Wilkinson, A., & Whitehead, L. (2009). Evolution of the concept of self-care and implications for nurses: A literature review. *International Journal of Nursing Studies, 46*(8), 1143–1147.

World Health Organization. (2001). *International classification of functioning, disability and health: ICF.* Geneva: Author.

Wright, B. A. (1983). *Physical disability: A psychosocial approach.* New York: HarperCollins.

PART I

Individual-Level Theories and Interventions to Promote Self-Management

3

Cognitive-Behavioral Therapy to Promote Self-Management

SHARON ELDAR, NORA M. ESSER, AND STEFAN G. HOFMANN ■

Individuals who cope with chronic conditions, such as physical impairments, chronic mental conditions, or chronic pain, need to adapt to a new lifestyle and adjust to the changes inherent in living with a chronic condition. In the past, individuals with impairments were more passive and less responsible for their health, which was often in the hands of the healthcare providers (e.g., doctors, nurses, psychiatrists, and psychologists). However, in recent years, responsibility for day-to-day management has gradually shifted from healthcare professionals toward the person in need. He or she is encouraged to monitor symptoms, be responsible for getting therapy, and pay attention to the physical and psychosocial consequences of having a chronic health condition. They are seen as experts on their healthcare needs (Barlow, Wright, Sheasby, Turner & Hainsworth, 2002) and in this role are expected to carry out the self-management tasks needed for their condition in the long term (Audulv, 2013). Efficacious self-management encompasses the ability to monitor one's condition and find the cognitive, behavioral, and emotional responses necessary to maintain a satisfactory quality of life (Barlow et al., 2002). Self-management includes some general skills and tasks, such as problem-solving, decision-making, resource utilization, forming a partnership between the person and the healthcare system, and taking action. Other skills and tasks are related to the type of health condition, for instance individuals with diabetes need to take insulin (Audulv, 2013). Healthcare providers can be seen as a guide to help increase people's self-management skills. However, when individuals lack this repertoire of effective coping skills to manage the psychological stressors and adaptive demands imposed by living with a chronic health condition, an emotional distress can arise and affect their psychological and physiological state (Devnis, Cameron, & Edworthy, 2000).

This chapter focuses on cognitive-behavioral therapy (CBT), which has been found to be one of the most efficient approaches for promoting self-management in all ages and across a variety of health conditions (Hofmann, 2011, 2014; Hofmann, Asnaani, Sawyer, & Fang, 2012). We begin with describing how CBT can promote self-management and review the main aspects of CBT. Subsequently, the main difficulties that accompany chronic health conditions are discussed, as well as how CBT techniques and skills can increase self-management for individuals with such conditions, followed by a description of the different formats in which CBT can be delivered to them.

WHY CBT CAN PROMOTE SELF-MANAGEMENT

CBT is probably the most extensively researched form of psychotherapy (Butler, Chapman, Forman, & Beck, 2006; Hofmann, 2014; Hofmann et al., 2012). It is an empirically supported, short-term therapy that presents a goal-oriented, systematic approach. CBT, originally developed to treat depression (Beck, 1967), has been successfully applied to the management of a variety of conditions including anxiety disorders (Beck, Emery, & Greenberg, 1985), substance-use disorders (Morgenstern, Morgan, McCrady, Keller, & Carroll, 2001), and schizophrenia (Pilling et al., 2002). It has also proven effective in the treatment of sleep problems and other health conditions. The cognitive-behavioral model emphasizes the inextricable link between cognitions, emotions, and behaviors. The aim is to help people with a chronic condition to identify and then challenge negative automatic thoughts and dysfunctional underlying core beliefs, as well as changing unhelpful behavioral patterns that are related to the problem that is targeted in the therapy (Cuijpers, van Straten, & Andersson, 2008; Williams, 2001). A more detailed description of CBT is presented in the next section.

The main reason to apply CBT to individuals with a chronic condition is the idea that although medical problems trigger physiological symptoms, there are cognitions, behaviors, and emotions that may prolong and maintain these symptoms over time (Spence & Moss-Morris, 2007). Targeting non-adaptive cognitions, behaviors, and emotions can reduce anxiety and depression and promote self-management skills and in turn improve the person's health condition. For example, changes in catastrophic thinking predict changes in activity level (Vlaeyen, & Linton, 2000), changes in managing activity and rest time are associated with decreased symptoms of chronic fatigue syndrome (Price, Mitchell, Tidy, & Hunot, 2008), and changes in the belief that pain signifies harm are associated with changes in depressive symptoms, physical functioning, and overall dysfunction (Turner, Holtzman, & Mancl, 2007).

Helping people with chronic health conditions to realize that they are experts on their own condition and not helpless or passive observers is another important aspect of CBT, which supports the self-management approach in this population. The ultimate goal of the therapy is to teach strategies to cope with non-adaptive cognitions, emotions, and behavior beyond the therapeutic setting. CBT therapists believe that their clients change because they learn how to think differently and act on that learning. Therefore, CBT therapists should focus on teaching rational self-counseling skills.

GENERAL DESCRIPTION OF CBT

As mentioned, the central notion in CBT is the idea that our behavioral and emotional responses are strongly moderated and influenced by our cognitions and perceptions. Effective CBT must target all of these aspects, including emotional experience, behaviors, and cognitions. CBT helps individuals to identify nonadaptive thoughts and behaviors and adopt more adaptive skills and habits. They learn how thoughts about a situation influence their actions, and how, in turn, actions can affect thoughts and feelings. The therapist and client work together to change the client's behaviors, or thinking patterns, or both. The focus on learning new ways of thinking and acting leads to long-term results. When people understand how and why they are doing well, they know what they need to do to continue doing well.

CBT is, by definition, a short-term therapy, and although different protocols work with a various number of sessions, they usually range from 8 to 24 sessions. Cognitive-behavioral therapists have a specific agenda for each session that includes teaching specific concepts and techniques, which are always guided by the client's goals. Therapists do not tell clients what to do; rather, they teach them how to think and behave in ways more likely to help them to obtain what they want.

CBT begins with psychoeducation. Individuals are informed about the formulation of their case and the rationale for the therapy. Furthermore, they are taught to understand the relationship between cognitions, behaviors, and emotions. This knowledge is usually delivered by explaining the three-component model (see next paragraph). This part of therapy is meant to provide the foundation for the remainder of the treatment. During this phase, it is important that the therapist elicit information about the person's current difficulties and incorporates it into the discussion of the model.

The three-component model consists of cognitive, behavioral, and physiological modules (Barlow et al., 2011). The cognitive component involves the negative thoughts that people have when they feel depressed, anxious, or angry. The behavioral component consists of behaviors a person engages in or avoids when having those feelings (e.g., avoiding joyful situations, avoiding dealing with problems, withdrawing from activities). Last, the physiological component involves the physical sensations that accompany those feelings (e.g., low energy, fatigue, sleep/concentration problems, physical tension, irritability; Safern, Gonzalez, & Soroudi, 2008).

The model is described as interactive: each of the three components impacts the other two. When people feel anxious or depressed, these three components tend to affect one another negatively, often exacerbating distress and leading to an inability to function, which in turn leads to feeling more anxious or depressed. For example, an uncomfortable situation (e.g. chronic health condition or disability) may cause physiological discomfort (e.g., pain, tension), which increases negative thinking (e.g., "It will just get worse and worse") and non-adaptive behavior (e.g., withdrawal from activities) that in turn worsens the situation (e.g., more physiological symptoms). As a result, instead of using coping self-statements to alleviate the negative feelings and sensations (e.g., "I can manage the situation"), the intensity of the non-adaptive cognitions and behaviors increases (e.g., "My life is worthless; there is nothing I can do.").

After explaining the negative influence the three components can have on each other, clients are told that these three components can also exert a positive influence. Using rational thinking and encouraging self-talk can prevent an exacerbation of physical symptoms and disrupted functioning.

Presenting this information at the beginning of therapy is important, as it is the first step to developing a solid therapeutic alliance. It is therefore crucial that the therapist and client reach a consensus regarding the goals of therapy, including identifying the type of interventions that will be used to reach these goals and delineating concrete, observable outcomes that will indicate whether each goal has been achieved.

Following the psychoeducation phase and the definition of problems and goals, the therapy starts to focus on each of the three components, usually starting with cognitions.

The Cognitive Component

Cognitions are usually classified into dysfunctional or irrational core beliefs and negative automatic thoughts (Hofmann, 2014; Hofmann et al., 2012). Dysfunctional, irrational, or non-adaptive core beliefs are assumptions that individuals have about the world, the future, and themselves. These more global, overarching beliefs provide a schema, which determines how a person may interpret a specific situation, and they are based on automatic thoughts. Those include both thoughts and imaginations of situations that involuntarily pop into our consciousness, and hence they determine how we perceive and interpret the situation. Individuals with high levels of depression and anxiety usually have disturbance cognitions, and they tend to internalize a negative valence of their automatic thoughts (e.g., Beck, 1967; Hofmann, 2011).

At the beginning of therapy, clients usually find it difficult to identify their core beliefs and automatic thoughts, because they can occur very rapidly without the person being consciously aware of them. Monitoring forms have been found to be very helpful with identifying non-adaptive cognitions and irrational thoughts (Buhrman, Fältenhag, Ström, & Andersson, 2004; Mattila et al., 2010). In order to identify their underlying automatic thoughts, individuals are instructed to "dig a little deeper" and to ask themselves questions such as: "What would happen if I wasn't be able to continue with my previous job?", "What would be the worst case scenario?", or "What does this mean to me?" (Radnitz, 2000).

After clients become more aware of their negative thinking, they learn how to treat these cognitions as hypotheses and challenge their way of thinking. This is the cognitive restructuring process, which is the main skill to be learned and practice in cognitive therapy. This can be done by using information from the person's past experiences (e.g., "What is the probability based on your past experience?"), by delivering more adequate information (e.g., "What are the risk factors of physical deterioration?"), and by reevaluating the outcome of a situation (e.g., "What is the worst thing that could happen?"). Clients need to ask themselves: "What are alternative ways of interpreting this particular event?" or "How would other people interpret this event?" They are also encouraged to observe the evidence for and against a particular assumption in a debate. The goal is to test their hypotheses and, if these hypotheses are invalid, to modify them in order to gain a more realistic perspective of the real world.

The Behavioral Component

Another way to challenge thoughts is to test the person's hypotheses by exposing him or her to feared and/or avoided activities, sensations, images, or situations. This confrontation provides the opportunity to conduct field experiments to examine the validity of the assumptions. Thus developing exercises that are relevant to the individual's condition need to be taken into careful consideration (Barlow, 2008; Hofmann & Reinecke, 2010; Vorstenbosch, Newman, & Antony, 2014). Engaging in these behavioral exposures emphasizes the reciprocal relationship between cognitions and behaviors. Another aim of behavioral exposures is to give patients the opportunity to experience the situations they avoid and teach them useful coping strategies.

Other behavioral proficiencies, some of which are taken from the behavioral therapy approach, can be assimilated into CBT. For example, behavioral activation began as a behavior therapy treatment condition in a component analysis study of cognitive therapy for depression (Beck, Rush, Shaw, & Emery, 1979). Since then, it has become a popular treatment approach, specifically for depression (Jacobson, Martell, & Dimidjian, 2001). Behavioral activation has been shown to be effective as a stand-alone treatment or in combination with CBT (Martell, Dimidjian, & Herman-Dunn, 2013). It attempts to help depressed people reengage their lives through focused activation strategies, such as increasing engagement in adaptive and pleasurable activities or giving self-rewards when achieving behavioral goals (Dimidjian, Barrera, Martell, Munoz, & Lewinsohn, 2011; Lejuez, Hopko, & Hopko, 2001). Behavioral activation is designed to help individuals to approach and access sources of positive reinforcement in their life (Jacobson, et al., 2001).

Problem-solving is another important skill that is addressed in CBT protocols (Beck et al., 1979; Leahy, Holland, & McGinn, 2012, Nezu & Nezu, 2014) and combines cognitive and behavioral aspects. The reason for practicing it is that people tend to be very stressed out, anxious, or depressed when experiencing difficulties in facing problems that arise. Their reactions make it harder to solve problems.

Someone who feels depressed might have trouble concentrating or thinking about solutions, someone who is worrying in spirals might have trouble weighing various alternatives and making a choice, and someone who is angry might have difficulties thinking calmly about the situation (Bilsker, Samra, & Goldner, 2009). Therapists work with people to help them build an outline of the behaviors they should or should not practice in order to solve the problem they are dealing with. Such an outline may include writing down the problem and possible solutions to solve it. This is followed by ranking these solutions and deciding on the plan of action that is needed to carry out each solution. The final step can be starting with the most reasonable solution and moving along the list until the problem is resolved. The problem-solving technique is helpful when individuals are facing problems that can be solved by changing one's behavior and when the person has an influence on the situation. In cases where the situation is ambiguous or uncontrollable (e.g., death of a loved one, low chances to recover from an illness), different strategies, with more focus on emotion regulation and relaxation, should be addressed (Livneh & Antonak, 1997).

The Physiological Component

The physiological part within CBT provides guidelines on how to relax in situation that may cause stress or pain. Progressive muscle relaxation (PMR) and breathing retraining are both ways to manage anxiety and reduce distress (Barlow, 2008; Day, Eyer, & Thorn, 2014). PMR is a skill that helps with tension and stress. It involves tensing and relaxing various muscle groups, one at a time, which results in a whole-body relaxation. Once the person is relaxed, he or she is asked to take note of what relaxation feels like, so it can be applied to stressful situations.

The objective of breathing retraining is to teach the client to use calm, slow breathing, through the diaphragm, in order to achieve a relaxed state. The opposite, overbreathing and chest-breathing (filling the lungs with air and taking shallow breaths), which people tend to do when feeling anxious, can actually exacerbate anxiety symptoms. Diaphragmatic breathing keeps the chest relaxed and enables deeper, healthier breaths. Both of these techniques are developed and improved through practice so that they can eventually be applied to real-life situations and ultimately to stress-provoking events (Safren et al., 2008).

Homework Practice

As therapy progresses, clients learn to combine the cognitive, behavioral, and physiological skills and techniques that they have acquired. One of the most significant ways to enhance their learning is by completing homework between sessions. This is essential to enable the person to apply the acquired skills to various situations that arise in everyday life. It also encourages individuals to practice the skills by themselves, thus promoting their independence, which is a crucial determinant of their long-term emotional health. Studies show that individuals who complete homework assignments have significantly better outcomes than those who fail to do homework (Kazantzis, Deane, & Ronan, 2000). It has also been shown that CBT that includes homework has better outcomes than CBT that focuses only on work during each session (Beutler et al., 2004) and that people who complete the most homework show the best outcomes (Burns & Spangler, 2000).

Termination of Therapy

The last session/s of therapy should review the concepts and skills that were learned. This should also include an evaluation of the person's progress—what has changed in his or her life, and what he or she is doing now to overcome a difficult situation. Clients should return to the list of therapy goals that they identified at the beginning of therapy and evaluate which goals were accomplished and which still need to be worked on. This can be a guideline for the objectives they still want to achieve; thus therapists should encourage them to use all the skills they have practiced in order to maintain their progress. The aim is to promote continued practice and generalization outside of the therapeutic setting.

In summary, CBT is an empirically based, short-term treatment that has been shown to be highly effective in therapies for many clinical problems. It involves helping individuals to think more realistically and practically about the situations they face. The overall goal is to modify one's thoughts, beliefs, and perceptions and to change one's usual behavioral patterns. Modifying thoughts can facilitate both emotional and behavioral change, and altering behaviors can result in cognitive and emotional change. With respect to a person's condition, therapy is tailored individually, and, also depending on individual goals, interventions are created to address specific and concrete problems to reduce harmful symptoms. Clients play an active role in the therapy: they are asked to complete homework between sessions and to adapt and practice the techniques they learned in sessions in real-life situations.

THE VICIOUS CYCLE OF DEALING WITH CHRONIC CONDITIONS

Chronic health problems can have a troubling impact on a person's life through pain, physical symptoms, and limitations on day-to-day activities. Individuals with a chronic health condition may need to undergo tests or treatments, take medications according to a schedule, change their diet, or make other adjustments. These demands can increase the general stress level and influence other aspects of life. On the cognitive side, for example, people with chronic conditions sometimes struggle with unwanted thoughts, such as catastrophic thoughts or assuming the worst (e.g., "My pain will never stop") (Kristjánsdóttir et al., 2011). These problematic thought patterns contribute to increased pain intensity, distress, and failure to utilize adaptive coping techniques. Non-adaptive or passive coping behavior strategies can manifest as depending on interventions provided by physicians and avoiding activities, people, or self-management behavior (Lau, Leung, & Wong, 2002). The person's close relationships can also be negatively affected, because a chronic condition can cause the social support network to grow weary of the daily involvement and the person's distress. Their tendency to feel irritable may harm relationships and result in avoidance and isolation (Thorn, 2004).

Living with these misunderstood cognitions and behaviors increases the probability of developing other emotional disorders. Thus these individuals sometimes experience co-occurring depression, anxiety, and anger, which may be expressed through feelings of hopelessness, frustration, excessive worry, muscle tension, and loss of control over their situation (Lau et al., 2002). Research on various illnesses, including diabetes (Bruce, Davis, & Davis, 2005) and chronic pain (Hoffman, Papas, Chatkoff, & Kerns, 2007), showed higher prevalence rates of depression and anxiety among this population.

These negative emotions cause an extra burden of suffering and impair peoples' ability to maintain usual activities and goals in life. Depression and anxiety may further worsen the health symptoms, due to the difficulty they cause in managing the impairment, attending medical appointments, and keeping up with self-management (Bilsker et al., 2009). This formulates a vicious cycle (see Figure 3.1), in which the individual becomes more sensitive and anxious, which in turn aggravates the general health state (Rhudy & Meagher, 2000). For example, people with diabetes have roughly twice the risk of depression as those without diabetes, and, by some estimates, major depression occurs in approximately 11% to 15% of individuals with diabetes (Anderson, Freedland, Clouse, & Lustman, 2001;

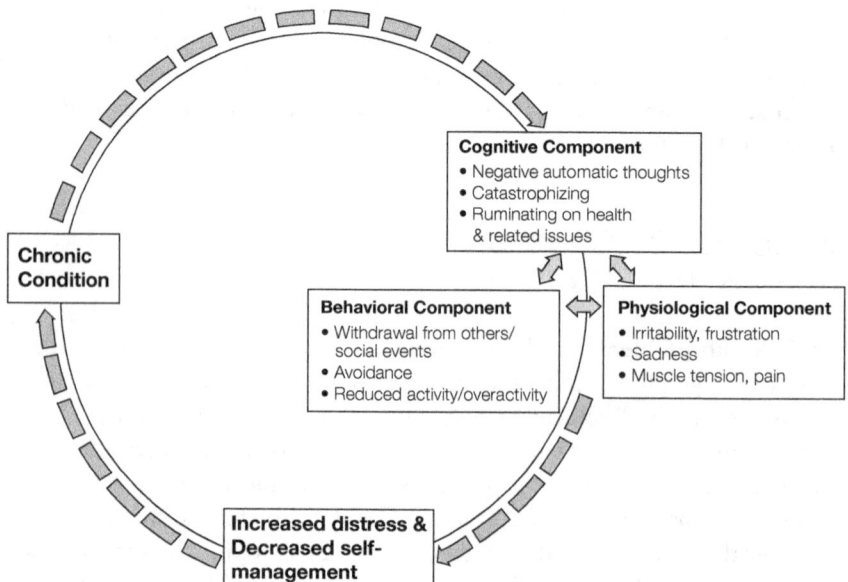

Figure 3.1 The vicious cycle of chronic conditions.

Katon et al., 2004). Depression, in turn, may worsen diabetes control, because the depressed person is less likely to stay active and to take all the steps necessary to ensure good blood glucose control (Anderson et al., 2001). Another example of this vicious cycle regards people with irritable bowel syndrome, who tend to be overactive in the face of their symptoms until they can no longer carry on (all-or-nothing behavior; Spence & Moss-Moris, 2007). They are also less likely to initially rest or reduce activity in response to their acute impairment (limiting behavior). If this behavior is repetitive, people may start to believe that they have a chronic incurable condition and become increasingly distressed by their ongoing symptoms. Distress, in turn, fuels these symptoms (Spence & Moss-Moris, 2007).

In sum, many people who are affected by chronic disabling conditions experience significant stress-related adjustment problems after the onset of the condition (Devins, Cameron, & Edworthy, 2002). Having a chronic health condition can affect peoples' cognitions, emotions, and behaviors, which in turn affect their daily life and the health condition they are struggling with. Denial, avoidance, anxiety, depression, anger, and hostility are all common reactions when starting to deal with a chronic health condition. It takes time for people to step out of this vicious cycle and start to adjust to their new life. Some people find adjusting to be a very hard process to accomplish. In order to stop the cycle, they need to work on acknowledging and accepting their chronic condition, which mainly means reappraising the way they view their situation and changing their non-adaptive responses to it (Livneh & Antonak, 1997). Breaking this cycle can be a long and nonlinear process; during its progress individuals experience normal ups and downs (Safren et al., 2008). With the use of CBT, which targets the impaired three components, clients can change their view about their chronic condition and adopt more helpful self-management and coping strategies.

HOW CBT CAN PROMOTE SELF-MANAGEMENT FOR CHRONIC HEALTH CONDITIONS

CBT-guided self-management can be seen as a key strategy to both decrease stress sensations and develop helpful, positive coping skills. The goals of CBT are to reduce symptoms and psychological distress and to improve role function. This can be accomplished by identifying and correcting non-adaptive thoughts and beliefs, as well as helping individuals to decrease non-adaptive behaviors and increase adaptive behavior to enhance self-efficacy for self-management (Turner & Romano, 2001). CBT protocols exist for a variety of chronic health conditions. Each health condition requires its own kind of self-management activities that reduce limitations (e.g., some conditions might require the ability to manage pain or limitations of physical activity; others may require the use of medications or assistance from others in daily activities). Nevertheless, respective intervention strategies can be adapted to address a long list of chronic health conditions and a wide range of medical management behaviors. Currently, CBT is the prevailing psychological therapy for individuals with chronic pain conditions, such as lower back pain, neck pain, headaches, arthritis, orofacial pain, and fibromyalgia (Bernardy, Klose, Busch, Choy, & Häuser, 2013; Glombiewski et al., 2010; Monticone et al., 2015), but CBT is also used for other chronic health conditions, such as diabetes (e.g., Kanton et al., 2004; Williams et al., 2004), fatigue (Price et al., 2008), and HIV (Safren et al., 2008).

CBT for chronic conditions, as conducted in research and clinical practice, varies in the setting, the number of sessions, and the specific techniques that are utilized (Ehde, Dillworth, & Turner, 2014). It can be delivered in one-on-one sessions or through self-management groups that teach people more about their condition and support them by giving them the opportunity to share their experiences with others who are facing similar challenges. CBT can also be delivered through respective workbooks, which may be helpful for individuals with a chronic condition who want to improve their self-management skills, as well as for health providers, peer counselors, and family members who are seeking better understanding, guidance, and support. They can be found in libraries, bookstores, and online (e.g., Bilsker et al., 2009; Safren et al., 2008). Despite these different settings, all the self-management manuals more or less consist of the same content: psychoeducation, goal-setting, daily diaries for self-monitoring, thought records and activity logs, exposures, relaxation training and sleep improvement, weekly homework sheets, and practice in real-life situations. The following section presents a general framework of CBT for individuals with chronic conditions, providing specific examples for this population.

Assessment

As all CBT protocols recommend, CBT for individuals with chronic health conditions should also start with a clinical interview and assessment before leading into psychoeducation about chronic conditions in general and about the person's specific impairment. This assessment typically involves an overview of the person's medical history and a clinical interview, in which people share their chronic health condition history and discuss how it has affected their lives. Asking for a detailed description of a typical day allows the therapist to capture the impact the chronic condition has on the person's life, including mood, physical and social activities, mobility, or sleep. This interview helps to build a therapist–client alliance, and the information therapists receive helps them to develop hypotheses about the client's core beliefs and patterns of thinking. However, therapists should also consider a discussion with the client's physician in order to receive more medical information about the present condition and prognosis.

Often therapists use self-reported measures to help them know their clients better. These measurements are used throughout the therapy in order to follow treatment progress and to identify areas that may need more clinical attention. Examples of measurements for individuals with chronic health conditions may include the Social Interaction Self Statement Test (Glass, Merluzzi, Biever, & Larsen, 1982), the Physical Dimension of the Sickness Impact Profile (Bergner,

Bobbitt, Carter, & Gilson, 1981), the Pain Catastrophizing Scale (Sullivan, Bishop, & Pivik, 1995), or the Illness Intrusiveness Scale (Devins et al., 1984).

Psychoeducation and Goal-Setting

After gathering all of this baseline information, the psychoeducation part can take place. As previously mentioned, this part of therapy helps people to understand the rationale behind the treatment and to increase their motivation to engage in it. It is important to make the explanations relevant to the particular individual emotional needs and physical condition. The person should feel that the therapist understands the specific situation—both medically and emotionally. They need the reassurance of their therapist that the therapist does recognize the real chronic problems they are facing. Nonetheless, therapists should emphasize the importance of focusing on ways to deal with these real problems more easily and adaptively.

This orientation should start with clients receiving information about the health condition they are dealing with. For example, for individuals with chronic pain this should include information about the definition of chronic pain, an explanation of the pain mechanisms, and a description of a variety of approaches to pain treatment. Then the therapist should explain the structure of the therapy. The goal is to provide the person with a roadmap of what can be expected during therapy and to establish clear expectations for both client and therapist. The three-component model and the interaction between chronic conditions and emotions like stress, tension, depression, and anxiety should be presented. People should receive the rationale for intervening with thoughts to affect attention, behavior, emotions, mood, and physical well-being (Carpenter, Stoner, Mundt, & Stoelb, 2012; Lau et al., 2002). For example, the way they interpret their chronic condition—as a challenge, a threat, or a loss—will affect their emotions, thoughts, and behaviors. Usually, at the beginning of the process, people appraise their chronic condition as a threatening condition or as a condition that caused them a great loss. It takes time to appraise their impairment as a challenge and to seek new meanings and goals (Livneh & Antonak, 1997). Directing their thinking toward accepting their condition can be given as an example of a cognitive change that can be facilitated through the therapy.

Affiliated with the three-component model, clients should also become familiar with the importance of self-management behaviors (Safren et al., 2008). It is useful to describe these behaviors as an important part of the therapy of all chronic health conditions and introduce it as a foundation for future sessions. The person should be told that being able to manage his or her chronic condition will help to reduce stress levels, and, in the long term, it will help to increase activities and social interactions. This will also facilitate medical and physiological management, which has the potential to result in reducing a range of symptoms.

Short self-management goals are usually being set in this early phase of therapy to give individuals with a chronic condition the sense of how to start changing their behavior and to take better care of themselves (e.g., "take medication on time every day" or "exercise three times a week"). Writing down reasons why to keep up with these goals, such as "I want to be able to do my artwork once again" or "I want to be alive for my daughter's graduation," might help them to accomplish the goals and increase their motivation for therapy.

As part of the psychoeducation, the therapist should also emphasize that relapses during and after therapy are normal and only become a problem when they lead to giving up on self-management behaviors. It should be explained that behavioral change, against most expectations, does not proceed steadily and consistently and that progress happens in the context of the normal ups and downs of life. Instead of seeing worsening of symptoms or a relapse as failure, it should be seen as an opportunity to gather information about what contributed to the negative change and to stimulate new learning. Successfully dealing with these short-term relapses will help clients in the long term to be able to maintain therapy outcomes.

The co-occurring depression and anxiety, which can develop following the onset of a chronic condition, should be discussed as well (Lau et al., 2002; Livneh & Antonak, 1997). Symptoms of depression and anxiety can have a strong impact on the motivation and skills needed to maintain strict self-management behaviors and should therefore be targeted also in the therapy.

Psychoeducation should also teach people how to monitor their own thoughts, emotions, behaviors, and overall health. This can be accomplished by using worksheets that are filled out between sessions. The monitoring increases the person's awareness about feelings and thoughts related to the symptoms. Self-monitoring, especially when performed on a regular basis, has been found to be efficient in behavioral change and its maintenance (Mattila et al., 2010).

In sum, much of managing a chronic health condition relies on what the individual who is struggling with it does or does not do; this responsibility can be stressful to a certain degree, but it also means that the management of the person's health is under his or her control. The common feeling of being overwhelmed with self-management behaviors is difficult for a lot of people, but, in time, these behaviors become more automatic. The education process continues throughout therapy, as clients learn how their chronic health conditions are influenced by the adoption of active coping strategies and by changes in physical or emotional functioning.

The Cognitive Component for Individuals with a Chronic Condition

As mentioned earlier, having a chronic health condition can lead, at the beginning, to various problems that may induce negative thoughts and appraisals and a considerable amount of worry and depressive thinking (Radnitz, 2000). For some people, accepting the fact that they have a chronic health condition is the first cognitive change that they need to achieve. Accepting the chronic condition does not mean "stashing it away" but rather removing one's own resistance and struggles against reality. To accept a chronic condition means to experience all the feelings that accompany it, including grief over lost dreams, the fear of never getting better, and the resulting isolation. Avoiding these feelings and not accepting them prevents the person from taking appropriate action, and it interferes with effective self-management (McCracken, Vowles, Gregg, & Almada, 2010). However, even after acceptance has been reached, the process of coping with and adjusting to the chronic health condition can still involve negative cognitions and emotions (Livneh & Antonak, 1997).

The presence of a chronic condition sets the stage for an increase in misinterpreted negative thinking, because an uncomfortable stimulus is always present. Many people have concerns or fear about the risks associated with their health condition. They worry whether the condition will worsen, whether they will be able to keep up their activity level, and whether the pain or discomfort will intensify. These problems are real; however, excessive worry and the tendency to "internalize" thoughts and beliefs about being a "sick person" can color the person's interpretation of situations and events and enhance the focus on negative thoughts and appraisals. People need to understand how negative thoughts affect their self-management behaviors and how this, in turn, affects their chronic condition.

CBT starts with interactively identifying the person's negative, automatic thoughts and core beliefs. Specific attention needs to be paid to emerging negative, automatic thoughts that trap individuals' perceptions and hold them back from making a change. Usually clients are being taught to pay attention and notice a change in their emotions in response to stressful situations, because this often occurs right after an automatic thought. With individuals dealing with a chronic condition, it is also important to help them focus on changes in their physical sensations and comfort level, because the physiological response to stress can trigger their chronic condition. For example, waiting at a doctor's office may increase irritability and frustration, and negative thoughts associated with that experience may impact the emotional response (e.g., "My pain is just getting worse the longer I sit here"). Once the person identifies a situation and a change in emotions or physical sensations, the therapist encourages him or her to become aware of the thought or image that just crossed his or her mind. This can be done in session, as well as with homework assignments using worksheets. The aim is for the person to identify and modify automatic thoughts and examine their authenticity, as well as to match them to identified cognitive distortions (Beck, 1979; Bilsker et al., 2009).

Recognizing common cognitive distortion or erroneous thought processes that arise from a chronic condition, as well as from depression and anxiety, can help people gain awareness about how their thoughts relate to their chronic condition or their negative mood. These distortions become visible when people use "all-or-nothing" phrases, such as "Having this chronic condition means I will never be able to play basketball with my friends again." The level of intensity, as well as the threat attributed to the chronic condition, can be misunderstood. For example, "This pain is unbearable, I can't live with it." Other misinterpreted automatic thoughts can include overestimating the likelihood that bad things will happen, as when people worry that they will become physically helpless and totally dependent on another person or several people, even after the individual has been told by the physician that only a tiny proportion of people with this condition becomes extremely impaired. Another, and presumably the most common example, is catastrophizing, or believing the worst regarding present and future events. It is characterized by the tendency to magnify the threat value of the chronic condition and to feel helpless in its context. Catastrophic thinking has been shown to be a robust predictor of pain and disability. People, who catastrophize more about their pain, function more poorly than individuals who do not catastrophize (Thorn, 2004). Some people with a heart condition, for example, think any physical exertion will trigger a heart attack or injure the heart muscles, even though physicians recommend mild physical exertion (Bilsker et al., 2009).

Addressing negative thought patterns and distortions can help people to view their experiences in a more balanced manner, which can contribute to improved mood. For them, some of these negative thoughts about their health condition might be true and should not be considered as misinterpreted (e.g., an individual may be indeed unable to return to play basketball but maybe can think about new hobbies or something similar as a replacement activity). It is recommended that these people try to access medical information and evidence regarding their condition so they can determine if and which part of their thought is misinterpreted.

Individuals with chronic conditions often develop a belief system in an attempt to make sense of their situation. For example, people with chronic pain have beliefs about the cause of pain, the meaning of pain, the amount of control they have over the pain, and the appropriate way of dealing with the pain. Because they are facing a stressful situation, their beliefs tend to be more negative, with a depressive or anxious component, such as helplessness ("The medications are my only hope and they don't help; I'm lost"), unlovability ("Nobody would want to be with me because I'm defective"), or self- degradation ("Because of my impairment, I am worthless"; Thorn, 2004).

In order to capture core beliefs, clients should first acknowledge their automatic thought and then ask themselves: "If the thought was true, what does it mean for me?" In addition, Bilsker and colleagues (2009) suggest that people with chronic pain also ask themselves, "Why me?" Usually these beliefs go together with phrases as "should" or "must" ("Because I smoked, I should suffer"; "I must support my family; otherwise I'm worthless"), and they promote dysfunction and disability.

Intermediate and core beliefs are difficult to challenge. But if they are being considered as ideas, not facts, they can be tested with questions similar to the ones used with automatic thoughts, which may result in the great value of thinking about alternative beliefs and changing them. Clients are encouraged to create alternative beliefs, test them, and try to adopt them ("I never chose to be in this condition"; "I am doing the best I can to support my family"). One of the ways to facilitate adopting these beliefs is to "act as if"—act as if the alternative belief was true—so changing the behavior will change the belief.

Another way to alter core beliefs is to try to adopt positive coping self-statements, which can be used to increase the sense of personal control over aspects of the impairment situation. This may also help with calming down during stressful situations. By phrasing them over and over again, people can start seeing them as realistic ("There's a high probability that I won't get worse; in fact I will probably get better, so why waste my time thinking about very unlikely outcomes?"; Bilsker et al., 2009). Individuals can integrate coping self-statement into their daily life by using coping cards—phrases in their calendar, on the fridge, or on their smart phone (Henriques, Beck, & Brown, 2003). This can be accomplished by writing down a coping self-statement relevant to the chronic health condition, such as "Carry on despite the pain," picking a place to display the card, and referring to it. Evidence suggests that those who use positive coping statements tolerate pain more effectively than those who use catastrophizing statements (Roditi, Robinson, & Litwins, 2009).

People can challenge their original thoughts using cognitive restructuring skills. This can be accomplished by asking themselves: "What would most people think in this situation? What would I say to a friend in the same situation? What will happen as a result of thinking that way? What is a more useful way of thinking?" People with a chronic health condition are encouraged to weigh the evidence that supports and does not support the cognition to recognize and reduce their belief in misinterpreted thoughts and increase their belief in realistic ones. This is particularly important for living with chronic conditions because many of the experienced stressors are real—and hence appraisals and cognitive restructuring techniques should involve realistic ways of thinking about situations that can objectively be negative and out of the person's control (i.e., for individuals with HIV, it can be thoughts about a worsening of the prognosis or the real threat that one might become resistant to medication). People need to practice these cognitive skills in order to promote a more realistic and healthy way of interpreting the world (Bilsker et al., 2009).

The Behavioral Component for Individuals with a Chronic Condition

Having a chronic health condition requires people to adapt their behavior to the new medical demands and physiological limits. These changes can be frustrating for individuals with chronic health conditions and might increase their depression and/or anxiety. Because medical treatments rely heavily on the person's self-management behaviors (i.e. self-managing medications, attending medical visits, making changes in diet, self-monitoring of symptoms, and balancing physical activity), these symptoms can have a strong impact on the motivation skills needed to maintain treatment devotion. Thus, as previously mentioned, therapy should start with setting up the goals of what clients should and want to accomplish in order to maintain their self-management behavior. These goals can be medical goals, such as making appointment or measuring symptoms, but also behavioral goals regarding what individuals want to include in their day-to-day activities.

One of the main behavioral goals when working with individuals with a chronic condition, especially those who have more depression and anxiety symptoms, is to help them "activate" themselves. Dimidjian and colleagues (2011) defined behavioral activation for depression as a structured brief approach that aims to increase engagement in adaptive activities (often connected to an experience of pleasure or mastery), decrease engagement in activities that maintain depression, and solve problems that limit access to reward or that maintain or increase aversive control. This goal is particularly important for prohibiting a vicious cycle because the chronic condition and poor sleep may leave one feeling too tired to participate in activities, which in turn can worsen the impairment and the motivation to be active. To achieve these goals, therapists may use a variety of behavioral strategies, such as self-monitoring of activities and mood, activity scheduling and structuring, social skills training, and rewards (Leahy et al., 2012).

Scheduling Pleasant Activities

Because individuals with recently occurring chronic health conditions are facing a new situation that they need to adapt to, it is essential to understand their health condition and their physiological limits. The goal should be to identify activities that make them feel more positive and that can be done in conjunction with the limitations of their chronic condition. It is important for these people to be engaged in and continue enjoyable activities. It may be helpful to brainstorm a list of events that the person no longer does but used to do before the onset of the chronic health condition (i.e., going to social events; engaging in hobbies like art, cooking, gardening, yoga; or going to a movie). Increasing these activities can help them to remember what was important to them in the past and can serve as a reward for their efforts in managing their condition. People need time to process their new disabilities and to think about alternative, regularly occurring activities they can participate in that involve pleasure on a daily basis. For example, an individual with asthma cannot engage in jogging but could go for short walks around the block.

Using a positive event checklist can help to identify activities that involve pleasure or mastery and can help individuals with chronic health conditions to start setting behavioral goals (Safren et al., 2008). The list can include activities that involve other people and self-management activities. People, especially those prone to black-and-white thinking, may not have considered more creative solutions for how to be involved in pleasurable activities. For example, if they report that they used to enjoy bowling but are now unable to bowl, one option might be to explore their willingness to teach bowling to children or adolescents.

Scheduling Physical Health Activities

As chronic conditions often come with depression and anxiety, self-management activities that target the person's psychological and physical health and well-being also are of high importance. This can include general basics, such as taking regular showers, eating healthy, and participating in moderate exercise, but also personal choices like going for a walk or taking a bath. Increasing activities in this area will help in stabilizing mood, and remind the person of his or her strengths and abilities. For example, someone with diabetes might set a goal of "meeting with a dietician to plan better eating," or someone with renal dysfunction might decide to "attend the renal clinic once a month." People who are limited in physical activities that they enjoyed in the past might enjoy interactive home-video games that include bowling, tennis, and more games that require a limited amount of physical activity with a realistic experience of the sport (Murphy et al., n.d.).

Regarding physical health, engaging in a moderate, safe level of activity on a regular basis is one way people can avoid an overactivity cycle (overactivity, increased pain/symptoms, increased rest). Clients should learn to pace their activity, which can be a helpful strategy that allows them to consistently engage in activities without causing detrimental consequences, and helps them plan realistic, balanced activities that can be scheduled ahead (e.g., painting a room for 45 minutes per day over a period of four days instead of working for three hours on a single day). One method, called "time-based pacing," suggests that activity breaks should be based on time intervals and not on how much of the job is completed (Otis, 2007).

SCHEDULING SOCIAL ACTIVITIES

Because activities sometimes include interacting with others, individuals with chronic health conditions might prefer to engage in avoidance because they do not want to talk about their health condition or they feel embarrassed about their limitations. This social avoidance contributes to decreased physical activity, as well as to lowered self-esteem and increased depressed mood, which can enhance alcohol and drug use (Radnitz, 2000). Thus it is important that therapists encourage people to expose themselves to social activities, so people will face their fear and concerns and realize that they can handle the consequences and that it might not be as bad as they expected. Engaging in social activities is also important because it helps with feeling connected and emotionally supported by others. Many times people with chronic health conditions withdraw from others, or they feel rejected by others because of their tension, irritability, or low mood. Going to family events, calling up friends, signing up for continuing education classes or volunteer organizations, and participating in support groups can all be helpful activity examples to integrate in therapy.

Another social behavior element that is usually targeted when treating people with chronic conditions is their assertiveness communication skills. People of this population, especially those who engage in a lot of catastrophic thinking, may have a high need for emotional support but insufficient communication skills to express themselves in a straightforward, unapologetic, and honest manner. Their distress may be very high, which can fuel the tendency to express oneself in a negative emotional manner, which can lead to overwhelming others and driving them away; this is the opposite of what was intended. Assertive communication helps people to meet their interpersonal needs, express them properly so as to stand up for themselves, and enrich and improve their relationships (Otis, 2007; Williams, 2001).

Monitoring Activities

Together with their therapist, clients can schedule the social and physical events to their day-to-day activities, including medical self-management activities. Scheduling should be as specific as possible, defining where, for how long, and how many times for each activity. The effect that engaging in these events has on one's mood and physical symptoms should be monitored, for example by using an activity log. This can help people to learn the association between mood and activities, to see that they are able to enjoy some parts of their days, and to make sure they engage in activities that are not harmful for them (Safren et al., 2008). If they find the activity to be too hard, a new goal should be defined with more realistic expectations. A good strategy is to start with easily achievable activities, in order to develop a sense of mastery, and move to more difficult tasks after some proficiency has been established. After completing the planned activity, the person may feel motivated to expand this activity schedule. Individuals with chronic conditions should congratulate and reward themselves after initial successes to improve their self-esteem and self-efficacy (Bilsker et al., 2009; Safren et al., 2008).

Problem-Solving

During therapy, while learning to prepare to and engage in the variant activities, different problems can arise. Dealing with such problems can seem overwhelming for people without proper problem-solving training. Several explanations are possible for why problem-solving declines in individuals with a chronic condition. First, solving a problem takes energy, and energy level declines as the impairment worsens. Second, everyday problems take a backseat to a bigger problem—the condition and the possible accompanying depression. Last, chronic conditions as well as depression can cause difficulties in concentration, memory, decision-making, and creativity, which are cognitive skills that problem-solving requires (Paterson & Bilsker, 2002).

Practice in problem-solving can help people to get started and select a plan of action, even if there is no ideal solution available. A problem-solving sheet may be helpful to reduce cognitive avoidance by encouraging clients to define the problem and break it down into manageable steps. Building on that, they can make a manageable, action-oriented, specific, time-limited action plan (e.g., "I will go on a half-hour walk with my best friend on Tuesday at 7 PM"). After trying to complete that plan, an evaluation process can take place, in which, as mentioned, the person decides whether to keep going, revise the goal and try again, or take a new approach. Effective problem-solving techniques and skills are of high importance for the management of a chronic health condition, because it helps respective individuals to feel competent enough to carry out adaptive self-management behaviors (Safren et al., 2008).

Expressive Writing

Another behavioral strategy that can be beneficial for people with chronic health conditions is expressive writing, primarily developed by James W. Pennebaker in the late 1980s (Pennebaker, Kiecolt-Glaser, & Glaser, 1988). In this exercise, one is encouraged to write about and express one's deepest thoughts and feelings regarding the chronic health impairment. Recognizing, honoring, and understanding strong thoughts and emotions are part of coping with the stress associated with a long-term and potentially debilitating chronic condition. Expressive writing can help individuals vent emotions without criticism and improve their overall psychological well-being. For example, Graham, Lobel, Glass, and Lokshina (2008) showed that participants assigned to write about their angry feelings related to pain had improvement in perceived control over pain and depressed mood following the intervention. These effects were explained by the amount of anger expressed in participant letters and not by expression of sadness or anxiety. Participants also experienced marginally greater improvement in pain and enhanced feelings of control over pain after the intervention.

The Physiological Component for Individuals with a Chronic Condition

Coping with the chronic nature of their condition, not feeling understood by others, reduced involvement in enjoyable activities, and negative thoughts may all increase the stress related to the impairment. Therefore, it is helpful for people with chronic health conditions to engage in relaxation training and improve their stress management. The rationale behind the use of relaxation techniques can be explained by focusing on the chronic health condition as a chronic stressor, both physically and psychologically. In addition to PMR and deep breathing, which has already been described in this chapter, guided imagery is another technique that is designed to train people to create mental images that support a relaxed state. The client chooses a peaceful and calm location to mentally visit during the exercise and fully engages by giving full attention to all the specific details of the scene (e.g., smelling fresh-baked cookies in the air, imagining the sweet and sour taste of cold lemonade, feeling warm sand in the hand, or picturing the vivid color of tree leaves and hearing them crush underfoot). It is crucial to involve all five senses to take the person away from stressful thoughts and bodily tension.

It is useful to emphasize that practicing relaxation at least once every day is very important so people can learn to use these skills in various situations. For example, practicing relaxation in response to side effects of medication may help in preparation for any painful medical procedures or with sleep difficulties (Safren et al., 2008). Some people may find it helpful to pair relaxation with a daily activity such as going to bed or having a meal. Selecting a phrase or mantra that serves as a cue (e.g., calm, peace, or positivity) and putting it on the fridge or in the bathroom might be as helpful as using a relaxation application on a smart phone to be reminded of relaxation during the day.

The last session/s of therapy provides a review of the concept of CBT and the skills acquired during the program. It includes an evaluation of the progress and the accomplished, as well as the still unreached, goals. Using an improvement graph might help people to visualize their progress, and the provided homework serves as a reference (Safren et al., 2008).

CBT to promote self-management aims to help individuals understand how to cope with the chronic condition they are facing and teach them skills that can help them manage their life in an adaptive way. The idea is to help them be active in the process of managing their impairment. Completing therapy does not mean the person will not face difficulties in the future. However, it does mean he or she will be more prepared for probable relapses, expect them, and see them as normal instead of fearing them. The key to maintaining therapy goals in the long term is to be ready for periods of increased difficulties. It is helpful to keep up the efforts that have been made to plan ahead for stress, to lighten up on ongoing responsibilities, and to keep up the skilled self-management behaviors. Creating an emergency action plan with topics such as increasing rewarding activities, reducing obligations, getting support, and managing one's lifestyle may help people with relapse prevention (Bilsker & Paterson, 2005).

DIFFERENT FORMATS OF DELIVERING CBT FOR INDIVIDUALS WITH A CHRONIC CONDITION

Traditionally, CBT is delivered through professionals in one-to-one or group formats. For example, the Stanford Arthritis Self-Management Program is a six-week program of peer-led group therapy that can be applied across chronic health conditions (Lorig, Gonzalez, & Laurent, 1997). It includes CBT techniques, such as psychoeducation, problem-solving, self-monitoring, and scheduling pleasant activities (Devins et al., 2000).

However, the healthcare system does not have sufficient resources to support personalized interventions to everyone. In addition, engaging in CBT usually requires a substantial time commitment, which can interfere with other commitments, such as work or childcare (Kennedy et al., 2005). For individuals with chronic conditions, it can be physically difficult to arrive on a regular basis to therapy delivered outside their home (Cuijpers et al., 2008). Thus, it is important that other formats of CBT are within reach and explored in present and future research.

These other formats of CBT for self-management can be delivered via workbooks, books, digital recordings, minimal-contact formats, and telephone. All of these strategies have been found effective to reduce pain, pain-related disability, depression, and anxiety in arthritis, lower back pain, headache, and temporomandibular joint disorder (Carpenter et al., 2012). Another idea is to combine the formats in order to reduce the number of sessions (Buhrman et al., 2004).

For example, Moss-Morris, McAlpine, Didsbury, and Spence (2010) found that a structured CBT-based self-management manual together with three one-hour therapy sessions (one face-to-face and two telephone sessions) provided significant and consistent relief from symptoms of people with chronic conditions up to six months after therapy.

The most popular CBT intervention for these individuals that is completed without a face-to-face meeting is an Internet-based self-help intervention (Kristjánsdóttir et al, 2011). Internet access is increasing all around the world, and the Web is a common source for most people to access health-related information (Andersson, Strömgren, Ström, & Lyttkens, 2002). It has also become an accepted medium for the communication between physicians and clients. In these interventions, people are being introduced and taught all the CBT elements that are being delivered in the face-to face format. They are provided with information, explanations, and worksheets that they can work through themselves. In some formats, this is also combined with texting the therapist or arranging telephone sessions in which clients ask questions and update the therapist with their progress and difficulties. In addition, several studies have investigated the impact of virtual communities as a stand-alone treatment for self-managing chronic health conditions. Research evaluated Web-based discussion forums (e.g., Hamman, 2000), a chat room (Lafusco, Ingenito, & Prisco, 2000), or a combination of a chat room and newsgroup (Lieberman et al., 2003) indicate that online communication is a useful tool to cope with a chronic health condition and increase self-management skills (e.g., Josefsson, 2005).

Internet-based interventions have several advantages. They may save the time of the therapist and the person receiving treatment, as well as reduce waiting lists, allow clients to work at their own pace, abolish the need to schedule appointments with a therapist, save travel time, reduce the stigma of going to a psychologist or therapist, and facilitate help for the hard-of-hearing as self-help treatments typically work with visual rather than auditory information (Marks, Cavanagh, & Gega, 2007). Furthermore, Internet-delivered self-management may be designed to enhance people's motivation by presenting a wide range of attractive audiovisual information with audio instructions in whichever gender, age, accent, language, and perhaps game format that the client prefers. It also quickly and automatically reports the client's progress and self-ratings (Cuijpers et al., 2008). Providing therapy via the Internet has advantages over self-help books in the sense that advice can be given on a continuous basis without delay (Andersson et al., 2002). It has also been shown that including interventions, such as mobile phone text messages and/or some personal online contact, can be more helpful in supporting behavioral change than online interventions without those features (Kristjánsdóttir et al., 2011).

Internet interventions have been shown to be effective for a number of pain conditions, including headache, non-headache chronic pain, and rheumatoid arthritis, osteoarthritis, or fibromyalgia (Buhrman et al., 2004; Carpenter et al., 2012) and also for children and adolescents with chronic headaches (Connelly et al., 2006). Besides pain, research papers include virtual community interventions for diabetes (Lafusco et al., 2000), cancer (Lieberman et al., 2003; Seale,

Ziebland, & Charteris-Black, 2006), Parkinson's disease (Lieberman et al., 2005), and depression (Breuer & Barker, 2015). Overall, the effectiveness of Internet-based CBT seems to be similar to that of face-to-face CBT (Kristjánsdóttir et al., 2011), but further research could provide more guidance on the effective components and provide more evidence of its efficacy.

CONCLUSION

Strengthening self-management is important for individuals with chronic health conditions and for their healthcare providers (Devnis et al., 2000). Promoting this skill and implementing it in the healthcare system is a goal for the future. CBT can help promote self-management and encourage people to establish a new lifestyle while coping with a chronic health condition. This therapy can support individuals and their close family members, friends, and caregivers, and it is also easy to combine with other treatments, whether they are physical, pharmacological, or emotional.

CBT is a short-term intervention that focuses on the interactive relationship between cognitive, behavioral, and physiological components. It helps people understand and learn the concepts and techniques to break vicious cycle of negative thoughts, difficult emotions, and non-adaptive behaviors. Acquired skills, such as cognitive restructuring, problem-solving, behavioral activation, and relaxation, can help individuals who have chronic health conditions with taking care of medical requirements, as well as increasing social interactions and positive coping skills. This therapy provides a framework to promote self-management on a daily basis outside the therapeutic setting.

Current research (Moss-Morris et al., 2010) suggests that CBT is equally effective in face-to-face sessions that are one-on-one or in a group setting and online interventions with minimal therapeutic contact. CBT can also be delivered using workbooks or digital recordings at home. In all of these different deliveries, individuals with chronic health conditions learn to accept their condition, to acknowledge their non-adaptive cognition and behaviors, to adopt new skills, to reward the short-term progress as a way to achieve long-term goals, and to expect possible relapses as normal occurrences. It is also important for people to acknowledge that it can take time for them to master the many diverse domains of knowledge and component skills that the therapy targets (Radnitz, 2000). Thus, using the different medias of treatment and combining them can be helpful.

The basic ideas of CBT can be given by the primary-care providers, in the hospitals or medical centers, where individuals are being initially diagnosed and treated. There, people can learn the basic psychoeducation component and can be provided with workbooks and referrals to Internet websites and therapists. The assumption should be that people, with guidance and support, can become their own therapist, who understands their medical conditions and can take care of their basic medical treatment and the psychological outcomes. It can be beneficial not to wait until the person's emotional condition is escalating but rather to have this information given as a default at the beginning of treatment, so that the difficulties in the adjustment process would be normalized and CBT would be more accessible. This can also be helpful in the adaptation process. If the notion about the importance of self-management and the advantages of CBT in promoting it are explained to people upfront, it can save time, effort, and distress for many of them.

REFERENCES

Anderson, R. J., Freedland, K. E., Clouse, R. E., & Lustman, P. J. (2001). The prevalence of comorbid depression in adults with diabetes a meta-analysis. *Diabetes Care, 24*(6), 1069–1078.

Andersson, G., Strömgren, T., Ström, L., & Lyttkens, L. (2002). Randomised controlled trial of Internet-based cognitive behavior therapy for distress associated with tinnitus. *Psychosomatic Medicine, 64*, 810–816.

Audulv, Å. (2013). The over time development of chronic illness self-management patterns: A longitudinal qualitative study. *BMC Public Health, 13*(1), 452.

Barlow, D. H. (2008). *Clinical handbook of psychological disorders: A step by step treatment manual* (4th ed.). New York. Guilford Press.

Barlow, D. H., Farchione, T. J., Fairholme, C. P., Ellard, K. K., Boisseau C. L., Allen, L. B., & Ehrenrich-May, J. (2011). *Unified protocol for transdiagnostic treatment of emotional disorders.* Oxford: Oxford University Press.

Barlow, J., Wright, C., Sheasby, J., Turner, A., & Hainsworth, J. (2002). Self-management approaches for people with chronic conditions: A review. *Patient Education and Counseling, 48*(2), 177–187.

Beck, A. T. (1967). *Depression: Clinical, experimental, and theoretical aspects:* Vol. 32. Philadelphia: University of Pennsylvania Press.

Beck, A. T., Emery, G., & Greenberg, R. L. (1985). *Anxiety disorders and phobias: A cognitive approach.* New York: Basic Books.

Beck, A. T., Rush, A. J., Shaw, B. F., & Emery, G. (1979). *Cognitive therapy of depression.* New York: Guilford.

Bergner, M., Bobbitt, R. A., Carter, W. B., & Gilson, B. S. (1981). The sickness impact profile: Development and final revision of a health status measure. *Medical Care, 19*, 787–805.

Bernardy, K., Klose, P., Busch, A. J., Choy, E. H. S., & Häuser, W. (2013). Cognitive behavioural therapies for fibromyalgia. *Cochrane Database of Systematic Reviews, 9*, CD009796. doi:10.1002/14651858.CD009796.pub2

Beutler, L. E., Malik, M., Alimohamed, S., Harwood, T. M., Talebi, H., Noble, S., & Wong, E. (2004). Therapist effects. In M. J. Lambert (Ed.), *Bergin and Garfield's handbook of psychotherapy and behavior change* (5th ed.). New York: Wiley.

Bilsker, D., & Paterson, R. (2005). *Anti-depressant skills workbook.* Vancouver: University of British Columbia.

Bilsker, D., Samra, J., & Goldner, E. M. (2009). *Positive coping with health conditions: A self-care workbook.* Consortium for Organizational Mental Healthcare. Retrieved from www.comh.ca/selfcare/

Breuer, L., & Barker, C. (2015). Online support groups for depression. *SAGE Open, 5*(2). doi:10.1177/2158244015574936

Bruce, D. G., Davis, W. A., & Davis, T. M. (2005). Longitudinal predictors of reduced mobility and physical disability in patients with type 2 diabetes: The Fremantle Diabetes Study. *Diabetes Care, 28*, 2441-2447.

Buhrman, M., Fältenhag, S., Ström, L., & Andersson, G. (2004). Controlled trial of Internet-based treatment with telephone support for chronic back pain. *Pain, 111*(3), 368-377.

Burns, D. D., & Spangler, D. L. (2000). Does psychotherapy homework lead to improvements in depression in cognitive-behavioral therapy or does improvement lead to increased homework compliance? *Journal of Consulting and Clinical Psychology, 68*(1), 46-56.

Butler, A. C., Chapman, J. E., Forman, E. M., & Beck, A. T. (2006). The empirical status of cognitive-behavioral therapy: A review of meta-analyses. *Clinical Psychology Review, 26*, 17-31.

Carpenter, K. M., Stoner, S. A., Mundt, J. M., & Stoelb, B. (2012). An online self-help CBT intervention for chronic lower back pain. *The Clinical Journal of Pain, 28*(1), 14-22.

Connelly, M., Rapoff, M. A., Thompson, N., & Connelly, W. (2006). Headstrong: A pilot study of a CD-ROM intervention for recurrent pediatric headache. *Journal of Pediatric Psychology, 31*(7), 737-747.

Cuijpers, P., van Straten, A., & Andersson, G. (2008). Internet-administered cognitive behavior therapy for health problems: A systematic review. *Journal of Behavioral Medicine, 31*(2), 169-177.

Day, M. A., Eyer, J. C., & Thorn, B. E. (2014). Therapeutic relaxation. In D. J. A. Dozois & S. G. Hofmann (Eds.), *Cognitive behavioral therapy* (pp. 243-273). Chichester, UK. Wiley-Blackwell.

Devins, G. M., Binik, Y. M., Hutchinson, T. A., Hollomby, D. J., Barré, P. E., & Guttmann, R. D. (1984). The emotional impact of end-stage renal disease: Importance of patients' perceptions of intrusiveness and control. *The International Journal of Psychiatry in Medicine, 13*(4), 327-343.

Devins, G. M., Cameron, J. I., & Edworthy, S. M. (2002). Chronic disabling disease. In C. L. Radnitz (Ed.), *Cognitive-behavioral therapy for persons with disabilities* (pp. 105-143). Northvale, NJ: Jason Aronson.

Dimidjian, S., Barrera, M. Jr., Martell, C., Muñoz, R. F., & Lewinsohn, P. M. (2011). The origins and current status of behavioral activation treatments for depression. *Annual Review of Clinical Psychology, 7*, 1-38.

Ehde, D. M., Dillworth, T. M., & Turner, J. A. (2014). Cognitive-behavioral therapy for individuals with chronic pain: Efficacy, innovations, and directions for research. *American Psychologist, 69*(2), 153-166.

Glass, C.R., Merluzzi, T. V., Biever, J. L., & Larsen, K. H. (1982). Cognitive assessment of social anxiety: Development and validation of self-statement questionnaire. *Cognitive Therapy and Research, 6*, 37-55.

Glombiewski, J. A., Sawyer, A. T., Glombiewski, J. A., Sawyer, A. T., Gutermann, J., Koenig, K., . . . Hofmann, S. G. (2010). Psychological treatments for fibromyalgia: A meta-analysis. *Pain, 151*, 280-295.

Graham, J. E., Lobel, M., Glass, P., & Lokshina, I. (2008). Effects of written anger expression in chronic pain patients: Making meaning from pain. *Journal of Behavioral Medicine, 31*(3), 201-212.

Hamman, C. J. (2000). *Effect of a nurse-managed support group via an Internet bulletin board on the perception of social support among adolescents with insulin dependent diabetes mellitus.* Master's thesis, Texas Tech University Health Sciences Center, Lubbock.

Henriques, G., Beck, A. T., & Brown, G. K. (2003). Cognitive therapy for adolescent and young adult suicide attempters. *American Behavioral Scientist, 46*(9), 1258–1268. doi:10.1177/0002764202250668

Hoffman, B. M., Papas, R. K., Chatkoff, D. K., & Kerns, R. D. (2007). Meta-analysis of psychological interventions for chronic low back pain. *Health Psychology, 26*(1), 1–9.

Hofmann, S. G. (2011). *An introduction to modern CBT: Psychological solutions to mental health problems.* Chichester, UK: Wiley-Blackwell.

Hofmann, S. G. (Ed.). (2014). *The Wiley handbook of cognitive behavioral therapy:* Vol. I–III. Chichester, UK: John Wiley.

Hofmann, S. G., Asnaani, A., Vonk, J. J., Sawyer, A. T., & Fang, A. (2012). The efficacy of cognitive behavioral therapy: A review of meta-analyses. *Cognitive Therapy and Research, 36,* 427–440.

Hofmann, S. G., & Reinecke, M. A. (2010). *Cognitive-behavioral therapy with adults: A guide to empirically informed assessment and intervention.* Cambridge, UK: Cambridge University Press.

Jacobson, N. S., Martell, C. R., & Dimidjian, S. (2001). Behavioral activation treatment for depression: Returning to contextual roots. *Clinical Psychology: Science and Practice, 8*(3), 255–270.

Josefsson, U. (2005). Coping with illness online: The case of patients' online communities. *The Information Society, 21*(2), 133–141.

Katon, W. J., Simon, G., Russo, J., Von Korff, M., Lin, E. H., Ludman, E., . . . Bush, T. (2004). Quality of depression care in a population-based sample of patients with diabetes and major depression. *Medical Care, 42*(12), 1222–1229.

Kazantzis, N., Deane, F. P., & Ronan, K. R. (2000). Homework assignments in cognitive and behavioral therapy: A meta-analysis. *Clinical Psychology: Science and Practice, 7*(2), 189–202.

Kennedy, T., Jones, R., Darnley, S., Seed, P., Wessely, S., Chalder, C. (2005). Cognitive behaviour therapy in addition to antispasmodic treatment for irritable bowel syndrome in primary care: Randomised controlled trial. *British Medical Journal, 331,* 435–437.

Kristjánsdóttir, Ó. B., Fors, E. A., Eide, E., Finset, A., van Dulmen, S., Wigers, S. H., & Eide, H. (2011). Written online situational feedback via mobile phone to support self-management of chronic widespread pain: A usability study of a web-based intervention. *BMC Musculoskeletal Disorders, 12*(1), 51.

Lafusco, D., Ingenito, N., & Prisco, F. (2000). The chatline as a communication and educational tool in adolescents with insulin-dependent diabetes. *Diabetes Care, 23*(12), 1853–1853.

Lau, O. W., Leung, L. N., & Wong, L. O. (2002). Cognitive behavioural techniques for changing the coping skills of patients with chronic pain. *Hong Kong Journal of Occupational Therapy, 12*(1), 13–20.

Leahy, R. L., Holland, S. J. F., & McGinn, L. K. (2012). *Treatment plans and interventions for depression and anxiety disorders.* New York: Guilford Press.

Lejuez, C. W., Hopko, D. R., & Hopko, S. D. (2001). A brief behavioral activation treatment for depression treatment manual. *Behavior Modification, 25*(2), 255–286.

Lieberman, M. A., Golant, M., Giese-Davis, J., Winzlenberg, A., Benjamin, H., Humphreys, K., . . . Spiegel, D. (2003). Electronic support groups for breast carcinoma. *Cancer, 97*(4), 920–925.

Lieberman, M. A., Wizlenberg, A., Golant, M., & Di Minno, M. (2005). The impact of group composition on Internet support groups: Homogeneous versus heterogeneous Parkinson's groups. *Group Dynamics: Theory, Research, and Practice, 9*(4), 239–250.

Livneh, H., & Antonak, R. F. (1997). *Psychological adaptation to chronic illness and disability.* Gaithersburg, MD: Aspen.

Lorig, K., Gonzalez, V., & Laurent, D. (1997). *The chronic disease self-management course: Leader's manual.* Palo Alto, CA: Stanford University.

Marks, I. M., Cavanagh, K., & Gega, L. (2007). *Hands-on help: Computer-aided psychotherapy.* Hove, UK: Psychology Press.

Martell, C. R., Dimidjian, S., & Herman-Dunn, R. (2013). *Behavioral activation for depression: A clinician's guide.* New York: Guilford Press.

Mattila, E., Korhonen, I., Salminen, J. H., Ahtinen, A., Koskinen, E., Sarela, A., . . . Lappalainen, R. (2010). Empowering citizens for well-being and chronic disease management with wellness diary. *IEEE Transactions on Information Technology in Biomedicine, 14*(2), 456–463.

McCracken, L. M., Vowles, K. E., Gregg, J., & Almada, P. (2010). Acceptance and mindfulness as processes of change in medical populations. In *Assessing mindfulness and acceptance processes in clients: Illuminating the theory and practice of change.* Edited by Ruth A. Baer, 251–270. Oakland, CA: New Harbinger.

Monticone, M., Cedraschi, C., Ambrosini, E., Rocca, B., Fiorentini, R., Restelli, M., . . . Moja, L. (2015). Cognitive-behavioural treatment for subacute and chronic neck pain. *Cochrane Database of Systematic Reviews, 5,* CD010664. doi:10.1002/14651858.CD010664.pub2

Morgenstern, J., Morgan, T. J., McCrady, B. S., Keller, D. S., & Carroll, K. M. (2001). Manual-guided cognitive-behavioral therapy training: A promising method for disseminating empirically supported substance abuse treatments to the practice community. *Psychology of Addictive Behaviors, 15*(2), 83–88.

Moss-Morris, R., McAlpine, L., Didsbury, L. P., & Spence, M. J. (2010). A randomized controlled trial of a cognitive behavioural therapy-based self-management intervention for irritable bowel syndrome in primary care. *Psychological Medicine, 40*(01), 85–94.

Murphy, J. L., McKellar, J. D., Raffa, S. D., Clark, M. E., Kerns, R. D., & Karlin, B. E. (n.d.). *Cognitive behavioral therapy for chronic pain among veterans: Therapist manual.* Washington, DC: US Department of Veterans Affairs.

Nezu, A. M., & Nezu, C. M. (2014). Problem solving strategies. In D. J. A. Dozois & S. G. Hofmann (Eds.). *Cognitive behavioral therapy* (pp. 243–273). Chichester, UK. Wiley-Blackwell.

Otis, J. D. (2007). *Managing chronic pain: A cognitive-behavioral therapy approach.* Oxford: Oxford University Press.

Paterson, R. J., & Bilsker, D. (2002). *Self-care depression program: Patient guide.* Vancouver: Mental Health Evaluation & Community Consultation Unit, Department of Psychiatry, Faculty of Medicine, University of British Columbia.

Pennebaker, J. W., Kiecolt-Glaser, J. K., & Glaser, R. (1988). Disclosure of traumas and immune function: Health implications for psychotherapy. *Journal of Consulting and Clinical Psychology, 56*(2), 239–245.

Pilling, S., Bebbington, P., Kuipers, E., Garety, P., Geddes, J., & Orbach, G. (2002). Psychological treatments in schizophrenia: I. Meta-analysis of family interventions and cognitive behaviour therapy. *Psychological Medicine, 32,* 763–782.

Price, J. R., Mitchell, E., Tidy, E., & Hunot, V. (2008). Cognitive behaviour therapy for chronic fatigue syndrome in adults. *Cochrane Database of Systematic Reviews, 3,* CD001027. doi:10.1002/14651858.CD001027.pub2

Radnitz, C. L. (2000). *Cognitive-behavioral interventions for persons with disabilities.* Northvale, NJ: Jason Aronson.

Rhudy, J. L., & Meagher, M. W. (2000). Fear and anxiety: Divergent effects on human pain thresholds. *Pain, 84*(1), 65–75.

Roditi, D., Robinson, M. E., & Litwins, N. (2009). Effects of coping statements on experimental pain in chronic pain patients. *Journal of Pain Research, 2,* 109–116.

Safren, S., Gonzalez, J., & Soroudi, N. (2008). *Coping with chronic illness: A cognitive-behavioral approach for adherence and depression client workbook.* Oxford: Oxford University Press.

Seale, C., Ziebland, S., & Charteris-Black, J. (2006). Gender, cancer experience and Internet use: A comparative keyword analysis of interviews and online cancer support groups. *Social Science & Medicine, 62*(10), 2577–2590.

Spence, J., & Moss-Morris, R. (2007). The cognitive behavioral model of irritable bowel syndrome: A prospective investigation of patients with gastroenteritis. *Gut, 56*(8), 1066–1071.

Sullivan, M. J. L., Bishop, S.R., & Pivik, J. (1995). The pain catastrophizing scale: Development and validation. *Psychological Assessment, 7,* 524–532.

Thorn, B. E. (2004). *Cognitive therapy for chronic pain: A step-by-step guide.* New York: Guilford Press.

Turner, J. A., Holtzman, S., & Mancl, L. (2007). Mediators, moderators, and predictors of therapeutic change in cognitive–behavioral therapy for chronic pain. *Pain, 127*(3), 276–286.

Turner, J. A., & Romano, J. M. (2001). Cognitive-behavioral therapy for chronic pain. In J. D. Loeser & J. J. Bonica (Eds.), *Bonica's management of pain* (3rd ed., pp. 1751–1758.). Philadelphia, PA: Lippincott Williams & Wilkins.

Vorstenbosch, V., Newman, L., & Antony, M. (2014). Exposure techniques. In D. J. A. Dozois & S. G. Hofmann (Eds.), *Cognitive behavioral therapy* (pp. 243–273). Chichester, UK. Wiley-Blackwell.

Vlaeyen, J. W., & Linton, S. J. (2000). Fear-avoidance and its consequences in chronic musculoskeletal pain: A state of the art. *Pain, 85*(3), 317–332.

Williams, C. (2001). Use of written cognitive–behavioural therapy self-help materials to treat depression. *Advances in Psychiatric Treatment, 7*(3), 233–240.

Williams, J. W., Katon, W., Lin, E. H., Noel, P. H., Worchel, J., Cornell, J., . . . Unützer, J. (2004). The effectiveness of depression care management on diabetes-related outcomes in older patients. *Annals of Internal Medicine, 140*(12), 1015–1024.

4

Spreading HOPE

The Development of a Hope-Based Self-Management Intervention

ANDY TURNER AND FAITH MARTIN ■

INTRODUCTION

This chapter describes the development and evaluation of an innovative self-management program, called "Help to Overcome Problems Effectively" (HOPE). It describes how the HOPE program is underpinned by positive psychology and cognitive-behavioral theory and research. It further describes the importance of hope in helping to overcome the challenges of living with a chronic health condition and presents preliminary evidence of how the HOPE self-management program has the potential to benefit people with physical and mental chronic health condition. Finally, the implications of positive psychology for self-management research are discussed and suggestions provided for future work.

Many people living with a chronic health condition want to participate more in their healthcare and would feel more confident with support and encouragement from their healthcare provider. However, the majority of individuals feel this support and encouragement is currently lacking (Department of Health, 2005). Confidence about the ability to self-care is crucial to self-management: individuals with lower confidence in their self-care abilities are less likely to seek help, follow guidance, and perform self-management behaviors (Hibbard & Gilburt, 2014). Nearly two-thirds of individuals believe that their confidence about self-care would increase with the provision of support from peers who had similar health concerns (Department of Health, 2005). In the UK, the push toward greater involvement of individuals in their own care reflects the pressure on the National Health Service (NHS) from the rising number of individuals with chronic health conditions. The NHS *5 Year Forward View* (2014) identified the important role technology can play in supporting individuals with long-term conditions to be able to better to self-manage their own health, stay healthy, make informed choices, manage their conditions, and avoid complications. The NHS plans to invest significantly in evidence-based approaches supported by *Realising the Value Programme* (2016), which aims to promote evidence-based person-centered approaches to health, such as self-management, peer support, health coaching, group activities, and asset-based approaches.

Clark et al. (1991) suggest that successful self-management requires sufficient knowledge of the condition and its treatment, performance of condition-related management activities, and application of the necessary skills to maintain adequate psychosocial functioning. Barlow defined self-management in the following way:

> Self-management refers to the individual's ability to manage the symptoms, treatment, physical and psychosocial consequences and life style changes inherent in living with a chronic health condition. Efficacious self-management encompasses ability to monitor one's condition and to effect the cognitive, behavioral, and emotional responses necessary to maintain a satisfactory quality of life. Thus a continuous and dynamic process of self-regulation is established. (2001, p. 546)

A broader definition was proposed by Wagner (1998) as articulated in the chronic care model, which reflected the importance of support provided by the clinician and health service. According to this model, one of the main objectives for health services is to support self-management, which needs to be embedded in a system that includes knowledgeable and confident individuals, prepared clinicians, and a responsive and flexible administrative structure (Wagner et al., 2001).

Dominant models of self-management interventions for individuals with chronic health conditions have tended to include five core components: education about the impairment, psychological strategies to support adjustment, treatment implementation strategies, practical support for daily living, and social support (Taylor et al., 2014). These are often delivered within the context of teaching participants how to manage the negative aspects of living with a condition using cognitive-behavioral therapy (CBT) techniques to break the negative, downward spiral of emotional, psychological, and physical despair, and feelings of hopelessness. The reasons are obvious and understandable, given that many chronic health conditions cause significant physical and psychological impairment. This mirrors the overwhelming focus of CBT and other forms of mental health interventions (e.g., counseling) on pathological and problematic patterns of functioning and behavior. The literature on self-management interventions often reflects this focus on negative pathology and functioning aspects.

Peter Lomas is a psychotherapist who has argued for a therapeutic approach that is more balanced toward recognizing an individual's strengths, courage, and potential for positive change:

> We consult a doctor, a psychiatrist, or a psychotherapist because we feel that something is wrong with us. Insofar as he is influenced by the traditional medical model the psychotherapist will, in his turn, also focus on what is

wrong; he may make a diagnosis or look for defensive mechanisms. But this is not necessarily the best thing to do to someone who is already ashamed of themselves. It may be more useful to dwell on what is right, to acknowledge and celebrate the courage and ingenuity by which the patient has managed to carve out a life in the face of innate limitations and adverse experience. Contemporary teaching of psychotherapy tends to fail the student by steering him towards the negative (Lomas, 1999, p. 107).

Self-management research and practice, like CBT, has similarly tended to focus more on a person's pathology and skills deficit. For example, Lorig's chronic health condition self-management course (Lorig et al., 1999), which is one of the most established and well-researched, peer-led interventions, is guided by breaking the "negative circle" of pain, fear, anxiety, depression, and fatigue.

Recent papers have called for more published research into the important concept of hope in self-management programs for individuals living with a chronic health condition (Brooks et al., 2015; Veres et al., 2014). In this chapter, the development and evaluation of an innovative self-management program, called "Help to Overcome Problems Effectively" (HOPE) is described. This program, which was co-produced by researchers and service users at Coventry University (Turner, 2010), encourages psychological and behavioral change by fostering positive emotional states such as joy, gratitude, and hope. This approach to self-management is to maintain a strengths-based and well-being focus by building skills in living with a chronic health condition. Uniquely in self-management research, the HOPE program draws on positive psychological and psychotherapeutic approaches including Snyder's (2000) hope theory. Neither a psychotherapeutic nor a positive psychological understanding and analysis of self-management have been well-articulated and developed. The similarity in outcomes and processes between self-management, group psychotherapy, and positive psychology suggests that these provide useful cannons of work with which to inform and improve self-management research, theory, and practice.

HOPE CONCEPT AND DEFINITION

In contemporary mental health practice, a recovery orientation has evolved in which hope is a central concept (Slade & Hayward, 2007). Hope is considered central to the concept of personal recovery from mental health difficulties, both as a trigger and as a maintaining factor, because hope helps individuals to find the courage to start their recovery journey and the motivation to keep working on recovery despite potential obstacles (Bonney & Stickley, 2008). According to Carr (2010), the recovery approach in mental health has significant parallels with the positive psychology approach to self-management. Both are about individuals determining their own purpose and meaning in life and being supported to be active member of their communities (Carr, 2010). A central concept of recovery is based on ideas of self-determination and self-management. It emphasizes the importance of hope in sustaining motivation and supporting expectations of an individually fulfilled life (Shepherd et al., 2008, p. 1).

Hope is also essential for resilience (Ong et al., 2006) and is consistently identified by both individuals and therapists in various settings as a key factor in psychotherapy (Schrank et al., 2008). Lambert et al. (2008) identified the following unique contribution of four factors which predict successful outcomes in psychotherapy:

- Extra-therapeutic factors (e.g., clients' existing strength and resources, such as level of education, income, support network): 40%
- Therapeutic relationship (therapist who shows understanding, empathy, respect): 30%
- Models/techniques (e.g., cognitive restructuring, negative thought-stopping): 15%
- Expectancy/placebo effects (hope, positive expectancy): 15%

It is interesting to see that the creation of a positive, hopeful environment is as important as specific therapeutic models and techniques to a successful outcome. Snyder and Taylor (2000) see hope as an important common factor for psychological improvement and believe hope theory offers a plausible framework for understanding how therapies can be effective.

Hope has been defined in several and wide-ranging ways, including a virtue (Barilan, 2012) and a positive goal-related state (Snyder, 2000). In describing hope as a virtue, Munday (2012) believes that "hope lies between despair and, where there is no hope at all, and extreme optimism, where hope does not have any grounding in reality" (p. 188). The former Rabbi Jonathon Sacks (2010), made a similar point in describing the difference between hope, which is an active, deliberate act to improve a situation, and optimism, which is a passive belief that things will get better, when he said:

> Optimism is the belief that things will get better. Hope is the belief, that if we work hard enough, we can make things better. . . . Optimism is a passive virtue, hope an active one. It needs no courage, only a certain naivety, to be an optimist. It needs a great deal of courage to have hope.

Sacks argues that living a fulfilled life is more than optimistically thinking that things will turn out okay if we simply believe that they will. He warns of the limits of positive thinking: although optimism and hope sound quite similar, they are in fact quite different. He describes how individuals who experience chronic health condition and adversity can be "agents of hope."

Munday (2012) believes that hope can be maintained even in the face of a terminal condition, such as cancer, through the striving for development and enrichment (a hope-promotion focus), rather than simply hoping to escape death (hope-prevention focus).

A systematic literature review (Schrank et al., 2008) that looked at definitions and measurement of hope has identified some key components of the concept.

Hope has been defined as primarily focused on the future, through the pursuit and attainment of valued goals, which are aided by personal activity and resources (e.g., courage, resilience) and external factors (e.g., resource availability). Snyder's (2000) hope theory underpins the HOPE program intervention. Although hope theory is similar to self-efficacy theory, which is the dominant theoretical model underpinning much of self-management research and practice, there are important differences (Snyder, 2000). Whereas self-efficacy theory focuses on specific goals and behaviors, hope theory recognizes enduring cross-situational goals and behaviors and is therefore highly relevant to the broader task of managing the diverse impact of living with a chronic health condition. Further, self-efficacy theory emphasises the role of agency beliefs, whereas hope theory proposes a broader cognitive set (Snyder, 2000). Hope has been conceptualized and defined as a "cognitive set that is based on a reciprocally derived sense of successful agency (goal-directed determination) and pathways (planning to meet goals)" (Snyder, 2000, p. 571). Pathway thoughts describe the perceived ability to produce plausible routes to goals, whereas agency thought is the motivational element, which focuses on commencing and persevering with goal pursuits. Pathway and agency thoughts are iterative and additive (Snyder, 2000).

POSITIVE PSYCHOLOGY

Our early evaluations of versions of Lorig et. al's (1999) chronic health condition self-management course identified a renewed and increased sense of hopeful thinking as one of the key improvements among some participants attending self-management programs (Barlow et al., 2005; Barlow et al., 2009; Turner et al., 2002). Our evaluation of Lorig's arthritis self-management program included the Positive and Negative Affect Scale (PANAS) as an outcome measure (Barlow et al., 2000). The PANAS contains 20 adjectives to describe positive and negative emotional states. High positive affect refers to a general tendency to experience a "state of high energy, full concentration, and pleasurable engagement." Both negative and positive affect improved at 4 months, but at a 12-month follow-up, only positive affect showed further improvement. In other research, we explored the important role that positive emotions have among participants attending self-management programs in helping participants cope with their long-term health condition (MaFarland, Barlow, & Turner, 2009). We also found participants expressed positive emotions and a renewed sense of hope and a striving to use personal strengths in the pursuit of living well with their condition (Barlow et al. 2005; Barlow et al. 2009, Turner et al. 2002), which are positive psychological techniques.

Fredrickson (1998, 2001) suggests that increasing positive emotions is an efficient and often preferable approach to reducing negative. Fredrickson's broaden and build theory (1998) suggests that positive emotions such as optimism, joy, and hope broaden an individual's attention, thinking, and action, thus enabling the building of new, creative thought and action pathways (i.e., expanding an individual's coping skills) and the building of personal and social resources.

Professor Martin Seligman is attributed as responsible for officially launching positive psychology as a scientific endeavor during his American Psychological Association Presidential Lecture in 1998. However, as many others have noted, applied positive psychology has a research tradition that spans decades. Linley and Joseph (2004) point out that cognitive-behavioral therapists have a long tradition of using positive psychological techniques. Lopez, Edwards, Magyar-Mor, Pedrotti, and Ryder (2003) have described the potential usefulness of positive psychology to complement CBT because of the shared focus on a strengths approach to adjustment and development of the two approaches. Karwoski et al., (2006) suggest that there is considerable conceptual and technical overlap between CBT and positive psychological approaches including developing a strong therapeutic relationship between client and therapist/coach, focusing on goals, cognitive reappraisal/mindfulness, scheduling pleasant activities, identifying and reviewing successes, monitoring mood, relaxation training, and problem-solving.

In contrast to dominant models in clinical psychology, which tend to focus on psychopathology, positive psychology is concerned with the full range of human functioning and has the dual aims of alleviating psychological distress and promoting positive well-being. Self-management research and practice has traditionally tended to focus on the former and hardly at all on the latter, with the exception of the inclusion of self-efficacy. One positive intervention (Seligman, Rashid, & Parks, 2006) asks clients to write three good things that went well today and also reflect upon why they went well. This activity helps clients to end their day remembering and savoring positive events rather than negative ones. Similarly, the gratitude letter and visit (Seligman et al., 2006) may shift memory away from the embittering aspects of past relationships to savoring the good things that friends and family have done for clients. A positive intervention does not deny distressing, unpleasant, or negative experiences but rather refocuses attention and memory on positive experiences. Positive interventions essentially are reeducation of attention and memory (Rashid, 2009).

There is a growing body of evidence that suggests that gratitude improves psychological well-being and increases positive emotions (e.g., McCullough et al., 2004; Wood et al., 2008). Simple interventions, which are less cognitively demanding, such as gratitude diaries, have been shown to be as effective as more complex CBT techniques, such as thought monitoring and cognitive restructuring, with the additional advantage of increasing retention rates (Geraghty et al., 2010).

In the next section, we describe how the HOPE program interventions were developed and evaluated using positive psychology theory, research, and practice.

HOPE PROGRAM DEVELOPMENT

Between 2006 and 2009, in response to the shortage of tailored self-management support programs for individuals living with and affected by cancer, dementia, multiple sclerosis, HIV, and parent caregivers of children with autism, Coventry University was commissioned by various charities and NHS organizations to develop group-based and Web-based self-management programs, which we named the HOPE program. Development of all versions of the HOPE intervention followed a similar process. The development of the HOPE program for cancer survivors, which was funded by Macmillan Cancer Support (the UK's leading cancer charity) is used as an example of the development work undertaken, as the HOPE program for cancer survivors has achieved the widest reach, impact, and implementation.

HOPE PROGRAM INTERVENTION FOR CANCER SURVIVORS

We (Martin et al., 2010) completed an extensive development phase of the HOPE program in line with step 1 of the Medical Research Council's framework for testing complex behavioral interventions (Craig et al., 2008). We used the Antecedent Target Measure (ATM) approach (Renger & Hurley, 2006) and "intervention mapping" (Bartholomew et al., 1998) to develop HOPE. This combined approach has the advantage of resulting in the mapping of intervention components and measures for success, based on both primary data from stakeholders (e.g., cancer clinicians and cancer survivors) and a supporting evidence base from existing research literature to develop the content of each program. The entire process is guided by stakeholders' perceptions of need and priorities, ensuring that perceptions of cancer survivors and experts in cancer treatment and self-management are prioritized. The resulting intervention has a clear logic underlying the inclusion of every component, rendering areas for refinements to the intervention during the development cycle easy to locate, as each component has a clear and specific purpose.

Using the ATM approach, stakeholders described their perceived "antecedents" (condition or event that logically precedes the problem) about why effective self-management could be problematic. Our data highlighted the importance of hope and confidence. For example, many participants made statements like "Self-confidence is generally low after [cancer] treatment" and "don't feel capable after illness experience," which they reported were reasons why it was hard to self-manage. Others talked about fear of death, destroying their hope for the future and leading some to "catastrophize" about what may happen (Martin et al., 2010).

The HOPE program reflects an innovative approach to self-management because it encourages positive psychological and behavioral change by fostering positive psychological emotional states and builds on participants' existing strengths and resiliencies, rather than focusing predominantly on skills' deficits. The HOPE program for cancer survivors is a six-week, group-based, self-management program, which aims to enhance physical and mental well-being. Each session follows a similar pattern. There is a combination of psychoeducation, CBT-based skills' practice, in-depth discussions, and setting and reviewing goals.

During the introductory session, for example, participants are invited to create a common identity (universality) and instill hope by sharing examples of positive and successful coping attempts, rather than sharing problems and failures. Another distinct feature of the first session in the HOPE program is the introduction of the upward spiral of positive emotions and experiences, which is intended to promote well-being, resilience, and adaptive coping skills.

The HOPE program intervention for cancer survivors includes key behavioral change techniques, including those that have a strong evidence base, such as person-centered goal-setting, action-planning, and problem-solving (Abraham & Michie, 2008; Michie, Fixsen, Grimshaw, & Eccles, 2009). Participants set personally relevant and meaningful weekly goals, as "homework" tasks, which they are invited to share with other group members and provide goal attainment or goal barrier feedback the following week. Goal-setting fosters a sense of pride and achievement, and, in the group setting, participants are inspired and instilled with hope when witnessing others work toward achieving their goals.

The HOPE program emphasizes the importance of *having* goals and *working toward* goals, as well as the *completion* of goals. Smail (1996) has described the challenges associated with initiating behavioral change and concludes that in many cases, there is no alternative to simply *"walking the plank"* of change, which he suggests is less challenging in the presence of encouragement from others. In current CBT approaches, behavioral activation, which rests on the idea of increasing positively reinforcing activities, uses terminology of "acting from the outside-in" (Kanter et al., 2011, p. 127) and the idea that doing precedes feeling—that to feel better, one first must make a behavioral change. Hope, and other positive emotional states, underpin the motivation to create this change (Corr, 2013).

Other activities include cognitive and behavioral self-management techniques, anxiety, depression and stress-management techniques, relaxation training, and pacing. The HOPE program also includes positive psychological evidence-based activities, such as identifying personal strengths, scheduling pleasant activities, mindfulness, gratitude diaries, relaxation training, and reviewing successes (Karwoski et al., 2006). All of these techniques are positive psychological interventions in their own right and have a growing research evidence base. Combined in the HOPE program, they build a positive experience for participants and tutors alike. See Table 4.1 for the weekly content of the HOPE program for cancer survivors.

Our qualitative evaluations of self-management programs (Barlow et al., 2005; Barlow et al., 2009; Turner et al., 2002), which included interviews with self-management participants and tutors, have consistently shown that instillation of hope, universality (realizing one is not alone), group cohesion, altruism, inspirational modeling, and imitative learning are key active ingredients of self-management programs, which Yalom and Leszcz (2005) have described as "therapeutic curative factors." The HOPE program also utilizes these curative factors. Participants observe each other and the facilitators successfully overcoming the challenges of living with cancer through achieving their weekly goals (instillation of hope), share common experiences (universality), and are

Table 4.1. THE HOPE PROGRAM FOR CANCER SURVIVORS

Week 1 Content

1. Welcome/Introductions
2. Responsibilities/Ground Rules
3. Instilling HOPE
4. Diaphragmatic Breathing
5. Gratitude Diary
6. Goal-Setting

Week 2 Content

1. Solution-Focused Goal Feedback
2. Gratitude Diary
3. Managing Stress
4. Mindfulness
5. Goal-Setting

Week 3 Content

1. Solution-Focused Goal Feedback
2. Gratitude Diary
3. Managing Fatigue
4. Sleeping Better
5. Guided Imagery
6. Goal-Setting

Week 4 Content

1. Solution-Focused Goal Feedback
2. Gratitude Diary
3. Body Changes, Sexuality, and Intimacy
4. Communication
5. Goal-Setting

Week 5 Content

1. Solution-Focused Goal Feedback
2. Gratitude Diary
3. Fear of Recurrence
4. Get Active, Feel Good
5. Goal-Setting

Week 6 Content

1. Solution-Focused Goal Feedback
2. Gratitude Diary
3. Character Strengths
4. Priorities (Rocks in a Jar)
5. Motivational Imagery
6. Open Space Forum
7. Sharing our Successes/Word Cloud

encouraged to support each other through the provision of informational and emotional support (altruism).

DELIVERY

The HOPE program for cancer survivors can be codelivered by NHS health and social care staff (e.g., clinical nurse specialists, benefits advisors) and cancer survivors. This co-creation approach to providing self-management support is innovative, as it brings together the clinical/specialist and experiential expertise of professionals and cancer survivors, respectively, to support cancer survivors. The co-creation approach is highly valued by self-management participants (Sharma et al., 2013).

The growth of online groups of individuals with chronic health conditions has resulted in more opportunities for gaining knowledge and social support, leading to improved health-related quality of life (Bennett & Glasgow, 2009). Older adults, in particular, are willing to share self-care information within selected social networks for the purpose of giving and receiving impairment-specific self-management information (Capel et al., 2007). In the UK, 42% of older adults (> 65 years old) use the Internet, and their use of tablets doubled and smartphones trebled between 2012 and 2014. In 2013, Macmillan Cancer Support commissioned Coventry University to develop a Web-based version of the HOPE program called iHOPE.

IMPROVEMENTS IN OUTCOMES ACROSS HOPE PROGRAM INTERVENTIONS

Several feasibility trials have shown that HOPE and iHOPE has the potential to improve important postcourse (six-week) quality of life outcomes (e.g., anxiety, depression, positive mental well-being, fatigue) for individuals living with and affected by a range of chronic health conditions, including cancer (Turner et al., 2012; Whiteman et al., 2015); HIV (Hergenrather et al., 2013, 2008); multiple sclerosis (MS; Kosmala-Anderson et al., 2016); and parent caregivers of children with autism (Joshi et al., 2013). Table 4.2 shows the range of outcome measures that have been used to evaluate the HOPE interventions. In keeping with the underpinning positive psychological theory, we have balanced the selection of outcome measures to reflect the positive and negative aspects of living with and being affected by a chronic health condition.

Across several HOPE interventions (cancer group and Web-based; MS, parent caregivers of children with autism), hope was measured using Snyder's Adult State Hope Scale (ASHS; Snyder et al., 1991). The ASHS measures hope defined as "a cognitive set that is based on a reciprocally derived sense of successful agency (goal-directed determination) and pathways (planning to meet goals)" (Snyder et al., 1991, p. 571). The scale comprises six statements, three of which

Table 4.2. HOPE Program Outcome Measures

Outcome Measure	F2F Cancer (*N* = 84)	iHOPE Cancer (*N* = 51)	F2F MS (*N* = 21)	F2F Parents of Children with Autism (*N* = 108)
Adult State Hope Scale	✓*	✓*	✓*	✓*
Quality of Life in Adult Cancer Survivors Scale.	✓**	✓**		
Patient Health Questionnaire–9		✓* †		
General Anxiety Disorder Scale–7		✓* †		
Warwick Edinburgh Mental Well-being Scale		✓*		✓*
Gratitude questionnaire				
Self-reported health		✓*		
Health Education and Impact Questionnaire	✓***			
Multiple Sclerosis Impact Scale			✓*	
Multiple Sclerosis Fatigue Scale			✓*	
Multiple Sclerosis Self-Efficacy Scale			✓*	
Hospital Anxiety and Depression Scale			✓*	✓* ‡‡
Positive and Negative Affect Scale			✓*	

NOTE: F2F = group-based face-to-face courses; MS = multiple sclerosis.

* Statistically significant improvement $p \leq 0.05$ (pretest, posttest). ** Statistically significant improvement for these subscales (negative feelings, positive feelings, cognitive problems, sexual problems, pain, fatigue, social avoidance, benefit finding, appearance concerns, fear of recurrence $p \leq 0.05$ (pretest, posttest). ** Statistically significant improvement for these subscales (fear of recurrence, fatigue, these were the only subscales included in the evaluation) $p \leq 0.05$ (pretest, posttest). *** Statistically significant improvement for these subscales (skill and acquisition technique) $p \leq 0.05$ (pretest, posttest). † >40% of individuals with cancer had clinical levels of depression and anxiety. ‡‡ >60% of parents had clinical levels of anxiety and >30% depression.

represent pathways (e.g., "There are lots of ways around any problem that I am facing now") and three agency beliefs (e.g., "At the present time, I am energetically pursuing my goals"). Participants indicate the extent to which they agree with each of the six statements, with higher scores indicating greater levels of hopeful thinking.

We combined the scores of the ASHS across four HOPE program evaluation studies. In total, 264 participants completed the AHSH before attending the HOPE programs and at postcourse (six weeks). Table 4.3 shows that there were statistically significant improvements in ASHS *total* scores and ASHS *subscores* (agency and pathways). The most significant improvements were reported by participants in the HOPE program for parents of children with autism. At baseline, these participants were the least hopeful and therefore had the greatest capacity to improve.

Qualitative evaluations indicated *how* the participants from each of the HOPE interventions became more hopeful. Participants stated that they were able to witness others doing well and thus gain confidence in their own abilities to achieve their goals. Additionally, they saw others who were perceived as doing not as well as themselves, thus instilling hope:

"It was helpful and inspiring to see someone that's worse off than you and sort of witness how they cope with it"

"I've met some lovely people that have inspired me to keep going and have learnt to try to do that in a more positive, hopeful frame of mind."

"Just purely being able to discuss issues with other group members gave me the courage."

"Gave me courage as well. Gave me the courage to go forward and do things. I have taken away from the program what it says on the packet, 'hope for the future' "

In Snyder's conceptualization of hope, goals are a fundamental aspect of hope theory. The weekly process of setting and reporting goals on the HOPE program was an important factor in initiating self-management strategies (e.g., relaxation), achieving positive behavioral change (e.g., scheduling pleasant events, meeting up with friends), and improving quality of life (fewer negative emotions). Participants described how being held "accountable" by the tutors and other participants provided the necessary motivation and commitment to undertake personal goals. The inclusion of informing the group about the outcome of weekly goal-setting meant that participants felt proud when goals were achieved and their success was relayed to the group. Participants described how they used goal-setting process to actively approach their challenges:

"It pushes you just that little bit further doesn't it. I found that really helpful as well and I still do it now it's there in the back of my mind and, you know, if I've got to do something then I will do it now rather than put it off."

Table 4.3. Adult State Hope Scores Across Four Samples

Outcome variable	Total Sample (N = 264) How many courses in total			F2F Cancer (N = 84) Courses			iHOPE[a] Cancer (N = 51) Courses			F2F MS (N = 21) Courses			F2F Parents of Children with Autism (N = 108) Courses		
	M (SD) Baseline	M (SD) Post-course	ES[b]	M(SD) Baseline	M (SD) Post-course	ES	M (SD) Baseline	M(SD) Post-course	ES	M (SD) Baseline	M (SD) Post course	ES	M(SD) Baseline	M (SD) Post course	ES
Hope Total score (6-48, ↑ = better)	27.5 (10.0)	35.3 (8.1)	0.8	30.2 (10.0)	34.2 (9.9)	0.4	28.0 (10.0)	35.3 (7.4)	0.7	23.3 (10.7)	32.2 (10.6)	0.8	26.0 (9.4)	36.9 (5.7)	1.15
Hope agency score (3–24, ↑ = better)	12.8 (5.7)	17.3 (4.4)	0.8	14.3 (5.6)	16.7 (5.4)	0.4	13.1 (5.4)	17.4 (4.0)	0.8	10.5 (5.7)	15.7 (6.2)	0.9	11.9 (5.6)	18.1 (3.1)	1.0
Hope pathways score (3–24, ↑ = better)	14.7 (4.8)	18. (4.0)	0.7	15.8 (4.9)	17.6 (4.7)	0.4	14.9 (4.9)	17.9 (3.8)	0.6	12.9 (6.0)	16.6 (5.0)	0.6	14.1 (4.4)	18.7 (3.0)	0.9

NOTE: F2F = group-based face-to-face courses. MS = multiple sclerosis.

[a] Web-based course.

[b] Effect sizes (Cohen's d) were calculated as follows: the mean score at six months minus the mean score at baseline divided by the standard deviation at baseline. Boundaries recommended by Cohen (1998) were used to determine small (0.2), moderate (0.5), and large (0.8) effect sizes.

"I told everybody I'm going to do this goal which actually made you do it, and then you felt brilliant because you accomplished it, and of course with little steps you went further and further and further, and I found it's just, like from being in a black tunnel you suddenly can see the light at the end of the tunnel, so for me it's been absolutely brilliant."

"I think because you don't feel as if you can do anything, you haven't got the energy or you can't be bothered or you think oh I'll put it off till tomorrow, but goal-setting just starting small, just something little and simple made you realize, oh I can do that after all. There's things you can do, you don't have to wait until you're fantastically healthy to do anything, so it gives you that sort of self-confidence, oh I can actually do something, instead of just sitting and go oh dear, you know."

DISCUSSION

There is growing interest in applied positive psychology promoting research and practice into factors that enables individuals, communities, and societies to flourish and achieve optimal functioning. The HOPE program has put this theorizing into practice.

Hope Springs Eternal

To the best of our knowledge, the HOPE program is a unique self-management intervention to as it draws on the theory and practice from clinical and health psychology, psychotherapy, and positive psychology. We have shown that the HOPE program has the potential to improve several important outcomes for individuals living with and affected by a chronic health condition (see Tables 4.2 and 4.3) and improvements were seen in different delivery formats (e.g., group-based and Web-based).

The HOPE program has the potential to reduce depression and anxiety, thereby helping to reduce the demand placed on psychological services and reduce chronic health condition care costs. Several studies based on hope therapy (Cheavens et al., 2006; Klausner et al., 2000), which involved older depressed adults in the United States, reported a statistically significant increase and large effect size improvement in hope and reduced feelings of hopelessness, anxiety, and depression.

The NHS in England transformed the delivery of psychological services through the introduction of the Improved Access to Psychological Therapies (IAPT). It was launched in 2008 to enable swift access to evidence-based CBT (Department of Health, 2008) for individuals experiencing common mental-health impairments of depression and anxiety utilizing a "stepped-care model." Despite its success and consequent growth, IAPT has created significant waiting times, the level of need remains high, and many individuals with mental health problems do not engage with formal psychological therapy services (Richards & Borglin, 2011). Some commentators have argued that the narrow focus on providing CBT, largely via one-to-one and/or computerized interventions, is not effective in building personally sustainable change and that the role of mutually supportive self-help and self-management interventions involving the voluntary sector should be explored to enable services to be sustainable (Gilbert, 2009).

There is encouraging work already being undertaken involving users of mental health service. In Australia (Lawn et al., 2007) and the United States (Druss et al., 2010; Lorig et al., 2013), research has shown that individuals with a range of severe mental health conditions including schizophrenia found a version of Lorig's intervention to be helpful. There is a need for self-management programs that alleviate distress and promote hope and other positive emotional states. The HOPE program has the potential to be a suitable therapy for use in stepped care for those with depression and anxiety in addition to a long-term physical condition. Further, some individuals living with depression may prefer attending the HOPE program because of the lack of stigma attached with something that promotes a strengths-based approach to coping and recovery, rather than a deficit-based approach.

There is a growing evidence base showing that trained peers can respond safely and therapeutically to distressing issues, which often arise on self-management programs (Barlow et al., 2005; Kennedy et al., 2009). Recent evaluations of peer-led self-management programs have reported improvements in depression and other health outcomes for individuals with serious mental health conditions (Druss et al., 2010; Lorig et al., 2013). Participants with poorer mental health and lower confidence benefit the most from attending self-management programs (Reeves et al., 2008; Ritter et al., 2014; Turner et al., 2014). Targeting individuals with a chronic health condition, who are experiencing poorer mental health and lower confidence, would ensure that that the HOPE program is offered to those who have the most to gain.

LIMITATIONS

Across our research (Joshi et al., 2013; Kosmala-Anderson et al., 2016; Turner et al., 2014; Whiteman et al., 2015), the differences in the hope total, agency, and pathways means between pre- and postcourse were generally high, which is promising, but these results need to be interpreted with caution for several reasons. The studies had no control group. Only baseline and post-intervention data were collected, so we are unable to say whether the improvements are maintained in the longer term. The samples were self-selected, highly motivated, and homogenous, with most participants being of White ethnic origin, and the majority were women. It is possible that this self-selected group has a natural inclination to respond favorably to a positive psychological approach for managing their chronic health conditions. Adequately powered, randomized controlled trials are needed to establish whether the HOPE program has the potential to provide longer term positive effects and whether it is acceptable and useful in the longer term (e.g., in a 6, 9, or 12-month follow-up).

IMPLICATIONS FOR SELF-MANAGEMENT RESEARCH AND PRACTICE

We are limited in our knowledge about the mechanisms of action on the outcomes of self-management interventions. Self-efficacy theory has been the defining model underpinning much of self-management research. Improvements in self-efficacy have been shown to mediate important self-management outcomes (Lorig et al., 1989). However, some self-management studies have found improvement in outcomes independent of an improvement in self-efficacy (Kendall et al., 2007). This suggests that there may be other theoretical explanations and other factors behind the improvements in self-management intervention outcomes. From the therapeutic perspective, hope has been put forward as a common factor that explains client improvement. Our research suggests that a self-management program based on a positive psychological perspective inherent in hope theory can lead to consistent improvements in hope and other important outcomes. Research is needed to explore the extent to which hope creates changes in behaviors and/or impacts on other important and relevant outcomes. Further research should explore to what extent self-management, both in terms of condition-specific health behaviors and more general well-being related behaviors, can improve if hope is low.

Our research suggests that a self-management intervention based on positive psychology, CBT, and psychotherapy has the potential to improve important outcomes for individuals living with and affected by a chronic health condition. Importantly, the HOPE intervention also appears to have the potential to assist individuals who are experiencing clinical and non-clinical levels of mental health problems, which means it can have a wide appeal to a broad range of individuals.

CONCLUSION

To our knowledge, no other studies (e.g. Barlow et al., 2000; Buszewicz et al., 2006; Kennedy et al., 2007; Lorig et al. 1999, 2013; Osborne et al., 2007) have evaluated the potential of self-management interventions to promote and improve hope. The HOPE program is an innovative self-management intervention combining positive psychology theory and practice and CBT. Our research suggests that the HOPE program has the potential to improve a range of important outcomes for individuals living with and affected by cancer and MS and for parents of children with autism. Improvements were seen across delivery formats that are group-based and Web-based. Further robust evidence of the impact of the HOPE program is needed.

In describing the "neglected importance of hope" in self-management theory and practice, Veres et al. (2014, (p. 79) call for more research into how to design and deliver programs to foster hope and the related concept of resilience. The role of self-management and hope in mental health recovery–focused services has also been described as important components for making services fit for the twenty-first century, which help service-users to lead a more fulfilling life (South London and Maudsley NHS Foundation Trust & South West London and St. George's Mental Health NHS Trust, 2010).

REFERENCES

Abraham, C., & Michie, S. (2008). A taxonomy of behavior change techniques used in interventions. *Health Psychology, 27*(3), 379–387.

Barilan, Y. M. (2012). From hope in palliative care to hope as a virtue and a life skill. *Philosophy, Psychiatry, & Psychology, 19*(3), 165–181.

Barlow, J. (2001). How to use education as an intervention in osteoarthritis. *Best Practice & Research Clinical Rheumatology, 15*(4), 545–558.

Barlow, J. H., Bancroft, G. V., & Turner, A. P. (2005). Self-management training for people with chronic disease: A shared learning experience. *Journal of Health Psychology, 10*(6), 863–872.

Barlow, J., Edwards. R., & Turner, A. (2009). The experience of attending a lay-led, chronic disease self-management intervention from the perspective of participants with multiple sclerosis. *Psychology and Health, 24*(10), 1167–1180.

Barlow, J. H., Turner, A. P. & Wright, C.C. (2000). A randomised controlled study of the arthritis self management programme in the UK. *Health Education Research, Theory & Practice, 15,* 665–680.

Bartholomew, L. K., Parcel, G. S., & Kok, G. (1998). Intervention mapping: A process for developing theory and evidence-based health education programs. *Health Education & Behavior, 25*(5), 545–563.

Bonney, S., & Stickley, T. (2008). Recovery and mental health: A review of the British Literature. *Journal of Psychiatric and Mental Health Nursing, 15,* 140–153.

Bennett, G. G., & Glasgow, R. E. (2009). The delivery of public health interventions via the Internet: Actualizing their potential. *Annual Review of Public Health, 30,* 273–292.

Brooks, H. L., Rogers, A., Sanders, C. & Pilgrim, D. (2015). Perceptions of recovery and prognosis from long-term conditions: The relevance of hope and imagined futures. *Chronic Illness, 11*(1), 3–20.

Buszewicz, M., Rait, G., Griffin, M., Nazareth, I., Patel, A., Atkinson, A., . . . Haines, A. (2006). Self management of arthritis in primary care: Randomised controlled trial. *BMJ, 333*(7574), 879. doi:10.1136/bmj.38965.375718.80

Capel, S., Childs, S., Banwell, L., & Heaford, S. (2007). Access to information and support for health: Some potential issues and solutions for an ageing population. *Health Informatics Journal, 13*(4), 243–253.

Carr S. (2010). Personalisation: An introduction for mental health social workers. In P. Gilbert (Ed.), *The value of everything: Social work and its importance in the field of mental health.* London: Jessica Kingsley.

Clark, N., Becker, M., Janz, N., Lorog, K., Rakowski, W., & Anderson, L. (1991). Self-management of chronic disease by older adults: A review and questions for research. *Journal of Aging Health, 3*(1), 3–27.

Craig, P., Dieppe, P., Mcintyre, S., Michie, S., Nazareth, I., & Petticrew, M. (2008). Developing and evaluating complex interventions: The new Medical Research Council guidance. *BMJ, 377,* 979–983.

Cheavens, J., Feldman, D., Gum, A., Michael, S., & Snyder, C. (2006). Hope therapy in a community sample: A pilot investigation. *Social Indicators Research, 77,* 61–78.

Cohen, J. (1998). *Statistical power analysis for the behavioral sciences.* Hillsdale, NJ: Lawrence Erlbaum.

Corr, P. J. (2013). Approach and avoidance behaviour: Multiple systems and their interactions. *Emotion Review, 5*(3), 285–290.

Department of Health. (2005). *Public attitudes to self-care: Baseline survey.* London: Author.

Department of Health. (2008). *The IAPT Pathfinders: Achievements and challenges.* London: Author.

Druss, B. G., Zhao, L., von Esenwein, S. A., Bona, J. R., Fricks, L., Jenkins-Tucker, S., . . . Lorig, K. (2010). The Health and Recovery Peer (HARP) program: A peer-led intervention to improve medical self-management for persons with serious mental illness. *Schizophrenia Research, 118*(1–3), 264–270.

Fredrickson, B. L. (2001). The role of positive emotions in positive psychology: The broaden-and-build theory of positive emotions. *American Psychologist, 56*(3), 218–226.

Geraghty, A. W., Wood, A., & Hyland, M. E. (2010). Attrition from self-directed interventions: Investigating the relationship between psychological predictors, intervention content and dropout from a body dissatisfaction intervention. *Social Science & Medicine, 71*(1), 30–37.

Gilbert, P. (2009). Moving beyond cognitive therapy. *The Psychologist, 22,* 400–401.

Hergenrather, K. C., Geishecker, S., Clark, G., & Rhodes, S. D. (2013). A pilot test of the HOPE intervention to explore employment and mental health among African American gay men living with HIV/AIDS: Results from a CBPR study. *AIDS Education and Prevention, 25*(5), 405–422.

Hergenrather, K., Rhodes, S., Turner, A., Barlow, J., Bardhoshi, G., & Cowan, C. (2008). Enhancing employment for persons with HIV/AIDS through self-management behavioral coaching. Paper presented at the European Health Psychology Conference and BPS Annual Health Psychology Conference, University of Bath.

Hibbard, J., & Gilburt, H. (2014). *Supporting individuals to manage their health: An introduction to patient activation.* London: The King's Fund.

Joshi, P., McHattie, D., Malin, C., Dingley, W., Edwards, R., & Turner, A. (2013, July). Evaluation of the HOPE Programme: Improving psychological well-being for parents of children with ASD/ADHD. Conference of the European Health Psychology Society, Bordeaux, France.

Kanter, J. W., Bowe, W. M., Baruch, D. E., & Busch, A. M. (2011). Behavioral activation for depression. In D. W. Springer, A. Rubin, & C. G. Beevers (Eds.), *Treatment of depression in adolescents and adults.* Clinician's Guide to Evidence-Based Practice 4 (pp. 113–182). Hoboken, NJ: John Wiley.

Karwoski, L., Garratt, G. M., & Ilardi, S. S. (2006). On the integration of cognitive-behavioral therapy for depression and positive psychology. *Journal of Cognitive Psychotherapy, 20*(2), 159–170.

Kendall, E., Catalanoa, T., Kuipersa, P., Posner, N., Buysa, N., & Charkera, J. (2007). Recovery following stroke: The role of self-management education. *Social Science & Medicine, 64*, 735–746.

Kennedy, A., Rogers, A., Sanders, C., Gately, C., & Lee V. (2009). Creating "good" self-managers? Facilitating and governing an online self care skills training course. *BMC Health Services Research, 9*, 93.

Kennedy, A., Reeves, D., Bower, P., Lee, V., Middleton, E., Richardson, G., . . . Rogers, A. (2007). The effectiveness and cost effectiveness of a national lay led self care support programme for patients with long-term conditions: A pragmatic randomised controlled trial. *Journal of Epidemiology and Community Health, 61*, 254–261.

Klausner, E., Snyder, C. R., and & Cheavens, J. (2000). A hope-based group treatment for depressed older adult outpatients. In G. M. Willimason, D. R. Shaffer, & P. A. Parmelee (Eds.), *Physical illness and depression in older adults: A handbook of theory, research and practice* (pp. 295–310). New York: Kluwer Academic/Plenum.

Kosmala-Anderson, J., Turner, A., & Clyne, W. (2016). Evaluation of the effectiveness of HOPE self-management programme for people living with multiple sclerosis. *Disability and Rehabilitation*. Advance online publication. doi:10.1080/09638288.2016.1181211

Lambert, M. J. (1992). Psychotherapy outcome research: Implications for integrative and eclectic therapists. In J. C. Norcross & M. R. Goldfried (Eds.), Handbook of Psychotherapy Integration (pp. 94–129). New York: Basic Books.

Lawn, S. J., Battersby, M. W., Pols, R. G., Lawrence, J. S., Parry, T., & Urukalo, M. (2007). The mental health expert patient: Findings from a pilot study of a generic chronic condition self-management programme for people with mental illness. *International Journal of Social Psychiatry, 53*(1), 63–74.

Linley, P. A., & Joseph, S. (Eds.). (2004). *Positive psychology in practice*. Hoboken, NJ: John Wiley.

Lomas, P. (1999). *Doing good? Psychotherapy out of its depth*. Oxford: Oxford University Press.

Lopez, S. J., Edwards, L. M., Magyar-Mor, J. L., Pedrotti, J. T., & Ryder, J. A. (2003). Fulfilling its PROMISE: Counseling psychology's efforts to understand and promote optimal human functioning. In W.B. Walsh (Ed.), *Counseling psychology and optimal human functioning* (pp. 297–307). Mahwah, NJ: Lawrence Erlbaum.

Lorig, K., Ritter, P. L., Pifer, C., & Werner, P. (2013). Effectiveness of the chronic disease self-management program for persons with a serious mental illness: A translation study. *Community Mental Health Journal, 50*(1), 96–103.

Lorig, K. R., Sobel, D. S., Stewart, A. L., Brown, J. B.W., Ritter, P. L., González, V. M., . . . Holman, H. R. (1999). Evidence suggesting that a chronic disease self-management program can improve health status while reducing utilization and costs: A randomized trial. *Medical Care, 37*, 5–14.

Lorig, K., Chastai, R. L., Ung, E., Shoor, S., & Holman, H. R. (1989). Development and evaluation of a scale to measure perceived self-efficacy in people with arthritis. *Arthritis Rheumatism, 32*(1), 37–44.

Martin, F., Turner, A., McHattie, D., & Surendranath, S. (2010, May). *Systematic development of a general self-management intervention for survivors of cancer.* Poster presented at the International Conference on Support for Self Management of Health, University of Stirling, Scotland.

McFarland, L., Barlow, J., & Turner, A. (2009). Understanding metaphor to facilitate emotional expression. *Patient Education & Counseling, 77*(2), 255–259.

McCullough, M. E., Tsang, J. A., & Emmons, R. A. (2004). Gratitude in intermediate affective terrain: Links of grateful moods to individual differences and daily emotional experience. *Journal of Personality and Social Psychology, 86,* 295–309.

Michie, S., Fixsen, D., Grimshaw, J. M., & Eccles, M. P. (2009). Specifying and reporting complex behavior change interventions: The need for a scientific method. *Implementation Science 4*(40), 1–6.

Munday, D. (2012). Hope as a virtue. *Philosophy, Psychiatry, and Psychology 19*(3), 187–190.

NHS England, Care Quality Commission, Health Education England, Monitor, Public Health England, Trust Development Authority. (2014). *NHS five year forward view.* London: Author. Retrieved from www.england.nhs.uk/ourwork/futurenhs/

Ong, A. D., Edwards, L. M., & Bergeman, C. S. (2006). Hope as a source of resilience in later adulthood. *Personality and Individual Differences, 41*(7), 1263–1273.

Osborne, R. H., Wilson, T., Lorig, K. R., & McColl, G. J. (2007). Does self-management lead to sustainable health benefits in people with arthritis? A 2-year transition study of 452 Australians. *The Journal of Rheumatology, 34,* 1112–1117.

Tayyab Rashid, T. (2009). Positive interventions in clinical practice. *Journal of Clinical Psychology: In Session, 65,* 461–466.

Renger, R., & Hurley, C. (2006). From theory to practice: Lessons learned in the application of the ATM approach to developing logic models. *Evaluation and Program Planning, 29*(2), 106–119.

Richards, D., & Borglin, G. (2011). Implementation of psychological therapies for anxiety and depression in routine practice: Two year prospective cohort. *Journal of Affective Disorders, 133,* 51–60.

Ritter, P. L., Ory, M. G., Laurent, D. D., & Lorig, K. (2014). Effects of chronic disease self-management programs for participants with higher depression scores: Secondary analyses of an on-line and a small-group program. *Translational Behavioral Medicine, 4*(4), 398–406.

Realising the Value Programme. (2016). *At the heart of health: Realising the value of people and communities.* Retrieved from http://www.nesta.org.uk/sites/default/files/at_the_heart_of_health_-_realising_the_value_of_people_and_communities.pdf

Reeves, D., Kennedy, A., Fullwood, C., Bower, P., Gardner, C., Gately, C., . . . Rogers, A. (2008). Predicting who will benefit from an Expert Patients Programme self-management course. *British Journal of General Practice, 58*(548), 198–203.

Sacks, J. (2010). *Optimism is all very well, but it takes courage to hope.* Retrieved from http://www.rabbisacks.org/credo-optimism-is-all-very-well-but-it-takes-courage-to-hope/

Schrank, B., Stanghellini, G., & Slade, M. (2008). Hope in psychiatry: A review of the literature. *Acta Psychiatrica Scandinavica, 118,* 421–433.

Seligman, M. E. P., Rashid, T., & Parks, A.C. (2006). Positive Psychotherapy. *American Psychologist, 61*(8), 774–788.

Slade, M., & Hayward, M. (2007). Recovery, psychosis and psychiatry: Research is better than rhetoric. *Acta Psychiatrica Scandinavica, 116*, 81–83.

Sharma, S., Wallace, L. M., Kosmala-Anderson, J., & Turner A. (2013). A process evaluation using a self-determination theory measure of the co-delivery of self-management training by clinicians and by lay tutors. *Patient Education and Counseling, 90*, 38–45.

Shepherd, G., Boardman, J., & Slade M. (2008). *Making recovery a reality*. Sainsbury, UK: Centre for Mental Health.

Smail, D. (1996). *How to survive without psychotherapy*. London. Constable.

Snyder, C. R., & Taylor, J.D. (2000). Hope as a common factor across psychotherapy approaches: A lesson from the dodo verdict. In C.R. Snyder (Ed.), *Handbook of hope: Theory, measures, and applications* (pp. 89–108). New York: Academic Press.

Snyder, C. R. (2000). Hypothesis: There is hope. In C.R. Snyder (Ed.), *Handbook of hope: Theory, measures and application* (pp. 3–18). New York: Academic Press.

Snyder, C. R., Harris, C., Anderson, J. R., Holleran, S. A., Irving, L. M., Sigmon, S., & Harney, P. (1991). The will and the ways: Development and validation of an individual-differences measure of hope. *Journal of Personality and Social Psychology, 60*(4), 570–585.

South London and Maudsley NHS Foundation Trust & South West London and St. George's Mental Health NHS Trust. (2010). *Recovery is for all: Hope, agency and opportunity in psychiatry: A position statement by consultant psychiatrists*. London: Authors.

Turner, A. (2010). The HOPE course. In F. R. Jones (Ed.), *Perspectives on lay led self-management courses for people with long-term conditions* (pp. 26–33). Oxford: Oxford University Press.

Turner A. (2014). Symposium: Using Groups in the Delivery of Healthcare. The role of hope in group-based chronic disease self-management programmes. 10th Annual Scientific Meeting of the UK Society for Behavioural Medicine, 3rd-4th December, East Midlands Conference Centre, Nottingham.

Taylor, S., Pinnock, H., Epiphanou, E., Pearce, G., Parke, H., Schwappach, A., . . . A. Sheikh. (2014). A rapid synthesis of the evidence on interventions supporting self-management for people with long-term conditions: PRISMS—Practical systematic Review of Self-Management Support for long-term conditions. *Health Service Delivery Research, 2*, 53.

Turner, A., Williams, B., & Barlow, J. (2002). The impact of an arthritis self-management program on psychosocial well-being. *Health Education, 102*(3), 95–105.

Turner, A., McHattie, D., Martin, F., Surendranath, S., & Cooper, L. (2012, December). *The HOPE group coaching and support programme for cancer survivors*. Paper presented at the UK Society of Behavioral Medicine 6th Annual Scientific Meeting. University of Leeds.

Turner, A., Anderson, J. K., Bourne, C., & Wallace, L. M. (2014). An evaluation of a self-management program for patients with long-term conditions. *Patient Education and Counseling, 98*(2), 213–219.

Veres, A., Bain, L., Tin, D., Thorne, C., & Ginsburg, L. R. (2014). The neglected importance of hope in self-management programs—a call for action. *Chronic Illness, 10*(2), 77–80.

Wagner, E. H., Austin, B. T., Davis, C., Hindmarsh, M., Schaefer, J., & Bonomi, A. (2001). Improving chronic illness care: Translating evidence into practice. *Health Affairs, 2*, 64–78.

Whiteman, B., Grant-Pearce, C., Cooper, L., & Turner, A. (2015). Surviving cancer: Pilot of a web-based self-management support programme, eHOPE. *The Lancet, 386*, S7.

Wagner, E. H. (1998). Chronic disease management: What will it take to improve care for chronic illness? *Effective Clinical Practice, 1*, 2–4.

Wood, A. M., Maltby, J., Gillett, R., Linley, P. A., & Joseph, S. (2008). The role of gratitude in the development of social support, stress, and depression: Two longitudinal studies. *Journal of Research in Personality, 42*, 854–871.

Yalom, I,. & Leszcz, M. (2005). *Theory and practice of group psychotherapy* (5th ed.). New York: Basic Books.

5

Illness Intrusiveness and Self-Management of Medical Conditions

GERALD M. DEVINS AND AMY DECKERT ■

Happiness, purpose, and satisfaction with life derive from the rewards that accrue when people engage in psychologically meaningful activity. These positive states suffer when a medical condition or its treatment interfere with such pursuits by rendering it difficult or impossible to remain actively involved (e.g., when fatigue renders it impossible to maintain physical activity levels, when complex treatments require substantial time commitments, or when treatment schedules conflict with work schedules and require people to relinquish their involvement in paid employment). We label this interference *illness intrusiveness* and propose that it is a major determinant of the negative psychosocial impact of chronic, disabling, and life-threatening medical conditions (Devins et al., 1983). Effective medical management minimizes symptoms, disability, and treatment side effects. As a result, it can be expected also to reduce illness intrusiveness. The illness intrusiveness theoretical framework (Devins, 1994) maintains that this is, in fact, the case. It also posits, however, that psychological, social, and contextual factors influence the extent to which a condition and its treatment produce illness intrusiveness and shape its psychosocial impact. Thus, interventions that aim to ameliorate disease or treatment factors, exclusively, cannot suffice to minimize illness intrusiveness (Devins, 1989; Devins & Binik, 1996a).

Effective self-management of a chronic health condition is predicated on the notion that healthcare outcomes can be maximized when recipients collaborate actively and effectively with service providers (Lorig, 1996). This can be achieved by acquiring relevant information, communicating skillfully with service providers, mastering requisite skills, and enacting them appropriately. The goals are to minimize progression of disease, preserve or restore function, and maintain comfort. Initially, self-management efforts were aimed to control underlying disease processes (e.g., minimizing joint damage in rheumatoid arthritis), manage symptoms (e.g., minimize pain, reduce disability), and facilitate effective communication with health-service providers (Lorig & Fries, 1980). Subsequent efforts added preserving quality of life (e.g., alleviating distress and/or maintaining happiness; Nolte & Osborne, 2013) and cultivating empowerment (Kuo, Lin, & Tsai, 2014) as important goals of self-management.

We categorize self-management treatment targets into primary (disease), secondary (symptoms and side effects), or tertiary outcomes (psychosocial states). *Primary* targets include disease outcomes that can be influenced directly through self-management efforts, such as minimizing joint damage that can arise due to inflammatory processes, optimizing blood-glucose levels in metabolic disorders, or controlling hypertension. *Secondary* targets include symptoms that are amenable to self-management (e.g., pain, disability, or fatigue) and treatment side effects (e.g., nausea, drowsiness, or pruritus). *Tertiary* targets involve psychosocial or other effects that arise in response to medical conditions, treatment, or side effects and can be expected to improve given effective self-management (e.g., lifestyle disruptions, subjective well-being, or empowerment). By helping people affected by chronic, disabling, and/or life-threatening medical conditions to minimize illness intrusiveness, self-management interventions can preserve subjective well-being, minimize distress, and inculcate feelings of mastery (i.e., empowerment).

ILLNESS INTRUSIVENESS AND SUBJECTIVE WELL-BEING IN DISABLING AND LIFE-THREATENING CONDITIONS

Illness intrusiveness results when lifestyle disruptions that are caused by a medical condition and/or its treatment interfere with participation in valued activities and interests (Devins et al., 1983). Disability, fatigue, and weakness, for example, compromise performance and can force people to reduce involvements in valued activities, such as employment or recreational pursuits (e.g., exercise or other physical activities, such as sports). Treatment schedules (e.g., for the delivery of chemotherapy, radiation treatment, or maintenance hemodialysis) can interfere by introducing conflicting commitments. Dietary and fluid-intake restrictions limit the range of things people can eat or drink, compromising freedom of choice and depriving people of variety. Illness intrusiveness compromises psychological well-being and contributes to increased emotional distress by reducing (a) positively reinforcing outcomes derived from participation in valued activities and (b) personal control by limiting the ability to secure valued outcomes or to avoid undesired ones (Devins, 1994; Devins, Seland, Klein, Edworthy, & Saary, 1993). Illness intrusiveness is measured using the Illness Intrusiveness Ratings Scale (IIRS) (Devins, 2010; Devins et al., 1983), a 13-item self-report instrument that asks respondents to rate how much their "illness and/or its treatment interfere" with each of 13 life domains that are central to quality of life (the measurement of illness intrusiveness, the IIRS, and the scientific evidence bearing on its psychometric properties are presented in the appendix). Although it is measured by self-report, illness intrusiveness is not a perception, an appraisal, or a characteristic of the affected person (i.e., a so-called person variable). It is intrinsic to the *situation* of disease and treatment (i.e., constraints that they impose on the individual).

Figure 5.1 illustrates the illness intrusiveness theoretical framework in relation to the sources, consequences, and moderators of its effects in chronic life-threatening and disabling conditions. As noted, the central hypothesis is that a medical condition and its treatment interfere with ongoing participation in valued activities and interests, which, in turn, compromises subjective well-being (i.e., illness intrusiveness is an *intervening variable* that provides a causal pathway through which a condition and its treatment influence subjective well-being). A secondary mechanism by which illness intrusiveness compromises subjective well-being is by reducing personal control (i.e., the ability to influence whether an outcome—desired or undesired—will occur). Personal control can be primary or secondary, actual or illusory, distinctions that offer important clinical implications (e.g., Alloy, 1992).

Psychological, social, and contextual factors play important roles by moderating the impact of a medical condition and its treatment on illness intrusiveness. The same chronic condition may result in different lifestyle disruptions, for example, for women as compared to men (Dancey, Hutton-Young, Moye, & Devins, 2002). Psychological, social, and contextual factors also moderate the impact of illness intrusiveness on psychosocial outcomes. For example, the emotional impact of illness intrusiveness is greater when people feel stigmatized

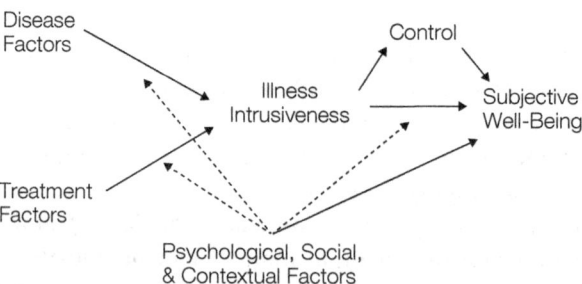

Figure 5.1 The Illness Intrusiveness Theoretical Framework.
Disease and treatment factors influence subjective well-being indirectly through their effects on illness intrusiveness. Illness intrusiveness influences subjective well-being directly by depriving people of the rewarding consequences of participation. It influences subjective well-being indirectly by reducing personal control. Psychological, social, and contextual factors influence subjective well-being directly, moderate the effects of disease and treatment on illness intrusiveness, and moderate the effects of illness intrusiveness on subjective well-being. Direct effects are signified by solid arrows. Moderating effects are indicated by dashed arrows.
Reprinted from Devins, G. M. (2010). Using the Illness Intrusiveness Ratings Scale to understand health-related quality of life in chronic disease. *Journal of Psychosomatic Research, 68*(6), 591–602.

by their condition, as in head and neck cancer (Devins, Stam, & Koopmans, 1994; Lebel et al., 2013) or irritable bowel syndrome (IBS; Dancey et al., 2002). Psychological (e.g., age or stage in the life cycle), social (e.g., culture, stigma), and contextual factors (e.g., stressful life events) establish the circumstances in which chronic medical conditions are experienced. Despite similarities in the objective circumstances, for example, illness intrusiveness is more distressing among younger as compared to older people, presumably because the two groups face different developmental challenges (Devins, Edworthy, Guthrie, & Martin, 1992; Devins et al., 1996). Moderating influences are depicted by dashed arrows in Figure 5.1.

The illness intrusiveness theoretical framework acknowledges that psychological, social, and contextual factors exert important influences on subjective well-being independently of the effects of illness intrusiveness (this hypothesis is represented by a solid arrow in Figure 5.1). A long tradition of theory and research addresses the interplay between stressful circumstances and the adaptive resources (e.g., defense mechanisms, coping skills, social supports) that are invoked to respond to them (e.g., Lazarus & Folkman, 1984; Pearlin & Schooler, 1978; Zeidner & Endler, 1996). The illness intrusiveness theoretical framework is conceptually situated within this broader context.

EMPIRICAL EVIDENCE FOR THE ILLNESS INTRUSIVENESS THEORETICAL FRAMEWORK

One might expect that disease and treatment influence subjective well-being directly by causing suffering and diminishing happiness, and, in fact, a number of findings are consistent with this notion. Statistically significant associations have been observed, for example, between (a) stage of disease and anxiety and depression in head and neck cancer (Aarstad, Aarstad, Heimdal, & Olofsson, 2005); (b) disease activity and depressive symptoms in systemic lupus erythematosus (Carr et al., 2011); (c) hypoglycemia and mental health-related quality of life in type 1 diabetes (Laiteerapong et al., 2011); (d) rates of immune-function decline and progression to AIDs and depression in HIV-infected people (Leserman, 2003); and (e) respiratory symptoms and hospitalizations and quality of life in chronic obstructive pulmonary disease (Monteagudo et al., 2013). Contradictory findings, too, have been reported. A number of studies fail to find evidence of a direct relation between disease or treatment factors and subjective well-being. Examples include reports of statistically non-significant associations between (a) neurological impairment and depressive symptoms in multiple sclerosis (Gilchrist & Creed, 1994); (b) disease severity and depressive symptoms or case-depression status in sickle-cell disease (Grant, Gil, Floyd, & Abrams, 2000); (c) recurrent headaches and several facets of subjective well-being (e.g., happiness and satisfaction, pessimism and illness-related concerns, or depression and distress) in end-stage renal disease (ESRD) treated by hemodialysis (Devins, Armstrong, et al., 1990); (d) transplant failure and subjective well-being (e.g., depressive symptoms, happiness, or self-esteem) in ESRD (Binik & Devins, 1986); and (e) diabetes complications and depressive symptoms (Talbot, Nouwen, Gingras, Belanger, & Audet, 1999). One study reported that severe limitations are "weakly related" to "emotional function" (i.e., embarrassment, depression, anxiety, and frustration; Guyatt, Townsend, Berman, & Pugsley, 1987). These inconsistencies imply that the relation between subjective well-being and a medical condition and its treatment is more complex than a simple, direct one. Rather, a third, intervening variable may mediate the effects of medical conditions and treatment on subjective well-being. The illness intrusiveness theoretical framework maintains that it is the disruption of lifestyles, activities, and interests caused by a medical condition and its treatment (i.e., illness intrusiveness) that is the pathway through which chronic, disabling, and life-threatening conditions compromise subjective well-being. In this section, we review empirical evidence that bears on the illness intrusiveness theoretical framework and elaborate on how it influences subjective well-being. The next sections address the following premises:

1. Disease and treatment factors induce illness intrusiveness by interfering with participation in lifestyles, valued activities, and interests (a corollary is that amelioration of disease and effective management of symptoms and side effects *reduces* illness intrusiveness).
2. Illness intrusiveness compromises subjective well-being (i.e., reducing psychological well-being and increasing emotional distress).
3. Illness intrusiveness influences subjective well-being indirectly by reducing personal control.
4. Psychological, social, and contextual factors modify (a) the effects of medical conditions and their treatment on illness intrusiveness and (b) the effects of illness intrusiveness on subjective well-being.

Medical Conditions and Treatment Induce Illness Intrusiveness

This premise has been tested extensively across chronic, disabling, and life-threatening conditions. Evidence from several populations of people affected by medical conditions substantiates that illness intrusiveness, as measured by the IIRS (Devins, 2010; Devins et al., 1983), correlates significantly with the *severity of disease* (i.e., illness intrusiveness rises with increasing severity of disease), including (a) intercurrent nonrenal conditions in ESRD (Devins et al., 1983; Devins, Mandin, et al., 1990); (b) advanced cancer (Sohl, Levine, Case, Danhauer, & Avis, 2014); (c) disease activity in systemic lupus erythematosus (Edworthy et al., 2003); (d) self-rated severity of disease in hyperhidrosis (Cinà & Clase, 1999); (e) neurologist-documented extent of disease in multiple sclerosis (Devins et al., 1993); (f) rheumatologist-documented severity of joint damage in rheumatoid arthritis (Devins, Edworthy, Guthrie, et al., 1992); (g) treatment-resistant seizure activity in epilepsy (Poochikian-Sarkissian, Sidani, Wennberg, & Devins, 2008b); and (h) "asthma severity" (Mullins, Chaney, Balderson, & Hommel, 2000).

Illness intrusiveness, as measured by the IIRS, is associated with increased severity and frequency of *symptoms* in many conditions. This includes (a) common symptoms associated with cancer (e.g., fatigue, pain, drowsiness, mouth sores, and nausea; Edelstein et al., 2016; Li et al., 2011; Mah, Bezjak, Loblaw, Gotowiec, & Devins, 2011b); (b) uremic symptoms in ESRD (Devins, Mandin, et al., 1990), intercurrent nonrenal medical conditions, sleep disorders, and daytime sleepiness (Mucsi et al., 2004), low self-rated health (Neri et al., 2011) and recurrent headaches and muscle cramps in people with ESRD treated by hemodialysis (Devins, Armstrong, et al., 1990); (c) severity of IBS symptoms (e.g., abdominal pain, constipation, diarrhea, bloating, and flatulence; Beata & Reka, 2012; Dancey et al., 2002); (d) severity of hyperhidrosis symptoms and the numbers of times affected people must change their clothing (Cinà & Clase, 1999); (e) heart failure symptoms (e.g., fatigue, dyspnea; LeMaire, Shahane, Dao, Kibler, & Cully, 2012); (f) postoperative pain associated with heart transplantation (Holtzman, Abbey, Stewart, & Ross, 2010); (g) symptom severity in type 1 and type 2 diabetes (DeCoster, Killian, & Rossler, 2013); (h) severity of symptoms in people with long-term asthma (Mullins et al., 2000); (i) fatigue and cognitive dysfunction (Goudsmit, Stouten, & Howes, 2009) and other symptoms (e.g., sore throat, sore glands, pain, and nonrestorative sleep; Dancey & Friend, 2008) in chronic fatigue syndrome; (j) restless sleep in ESRD, multiple sclerosis, and rheumatoid arthritis (Devins, Edworthy, Paul, et al., 1992); (k) vertigo, tinnitus, and dizziness in Ménière's disease (Arroll, Dancey, Attree, Smith, & James, 2012); (l) motion-perception problems and sensitivity to sound in mal de debarquement syndrome (Arroll, Attree, Cha, & Dancey, 2016); (m) fatigue and sleepiness in sleep disorders (Hossain et al., 2005); (n) symptom levels, number of positive symptoms, and symptom severity in schizophrenia (Bettazzoni, Zipursky, Friedland, & Devins, 2008); (o) occurrence of a depressive episode during the preceding year and current symptom levels in bipolar disorder (euthymic phase); and (p) sleep-related experiences (e.g., vivid or bizarre dreams, hypnagogic hallucinations, nightmares) in outpatient psychiatric patients with diverse diagnoses (Soffer-Dudek, Shalev, Shiber, & Shahar, 2011).

Several instruments have been developed to tap illness intrusiveness either by modifying the IIRS or by including very similar item content (these are reviewed in the appendix). In one study that tapped illness intrusiveness by examining "intrusions" into valued role identities (e.g., spouse, parent, homemaker, worker) among Latinas with diverse rheumatic diseases (e.g., rheumatoid arthritis, systemic lupus erythematosus, osteoarthritis), a significant association was evident between pain and illness intrusiveness (Abraido-Lanza, 1997). In another study that used a measure other than the IIRS, illness intrusiveness was significantly higher among transfusion recipients who received Hepatitis C–tainted blood products as compared to those who received untainted products (Hogg et al., 2003).

Disability attributable to disease processes has been identified as another determinant of illness intrusiveness. This has been demonstrated by significant associations between illness intrusiveness, as measured by the IIRS, and disability in rheumatoid arthritis (Devins, Edworthy, Guthrie, et al., 1992) and multiple sclerosis (Snyder et al., 2013). Illness intrusiveness correlates significantly with several facets of health-related quality of life (including cancer-related problems in physical, role, emotional, cognitive, and social function) in diverse cancer types (Li et al., 2011). Difficulty in conducting daily activities (e.g., walking, climbing stairs, doing housework, other household tasks, or working outside the home) correlates significantly with illness intrusiveness in ESRD (Devins, Mandin, et al., 1990). Studies employing alternative measures of illness intrusiveness, too, report consistent findings: Illness-induced intrusions into valued role identities correlated significantly with functional disability in Latinas with diverse rheumatic diseases (Abraido-Lanza, 1997; Abraido-Lanza & Revenson, 2006).

Contextual Factors

The illness intrusiveness theoretical framework posits that the context in which disease occurs exerts a moderating impact on the illness intrusiveness a person experiences. Although this aspect of the framework has not been tested extensively, some evidence bears on the role of context in relation to experienced illness intrusiveness. Exposure to disease-related stressors (e.g., lack of information about one's condition and treatment, difficulty communicating with treatment personnel) correlates significantly with illness intrusiveness. This has been demonstrated using the IIRS to tap illness intrusiveness in several cancer groups (e.g., gastrointestinal, prostate, breast, head and neck, lymphoma, and lung; Devins et al., 2013). Similarly, eventful stressors that are independent of disease or treatment (e.g., death of a loved one, children in trouble with the law) correlate consistently with illness intrusiveness (i.e., the occurrence of independent stressful life events is associated with increased illness intrusiveness; Devins, Bezjak, Mah, Loblaw, & Gotowiec, 2006; Edelstein et al., 2016). *Gender syntony* refers to the extent to which a care recipient's gender-based needs and preferences match the perceived social climate of the treatment setting (e.g., instrumental and action-oriented, as more often characterizes men, vs. nurturing and supportive, as more often characterizes women; Taylor et al., 2000). When the two conflict (i.e., the treatment setting emphasizes needs that conflict with gender-based needs and preferences), the resulting mismatch has been termed gender *dystony* (Woodend & Devins, 2005). In a study of people undergoing routine outpatient follow-up three months after their first myocardial infarction, gender dystony correlated positively and significantly with illness intrusiveness, indicating that treatment settings that emphasize needs and preferences that conflict with those of the care recipient are more likely to result in illness intrusiveness than those that are congruent (Woodend & Devins, 2005). Other contextual variables that relate systematically to illness intrusiveness include (low) income, (young) age, life domain (highest in relation to instrumental life, followed by intimacy and by relationships and personal development, respectively; Devins et al., 2006), and the centrality of affected life roles (Abraido-Lanza, 1997; Abraido-Lanza & Revenson, 2006; Bishop, Stenhoff, & Shepard, 2007; Devins et al., 2006).

Illness intrusiveness differs subtly across people affected by diverse types of cancer, presumably due to unique symptom profiles and treatment regimens (Mah et al., 2011b). Men with prostate cancer, in particular, report significantly higher illness intrusiveness into intimacy (relationship with spouse and sex life) than do people with gastrointestinal, lung, lymphoma, breast, or head and neck cancers, which is consistent with the fact that erectile failure is a much more common postsurgical complication in this group relative to the others (Mah et al., 2011b). A study of the trajectory with which illness intrusiveness evolves over the first two years of breast-cancer treatment and survivorship indicated that it is more likely to increase when women still have children at home, have comparatively advanced disease, and experience high symptom burden, but the three life domains tapped by IIRS subscales—relationships and personal development, intimacy, and instrumental life domains (Devins et al., 2001)—exhibit different patterns of change (Sohl et al., 2014). People who donate organs for transplantation, too, experience illness intrusiveness, and this appears to be shaped by several factors. A study of living liver donors indicated that they experienced high illness intrusiveness shortly after the organ donation occurred, when they were especially concerned about the donation process before it took place, when they earned a comparatively low income, and when they believed that the recipient was not taking proper care of the donated liver (Holtzman et al., 2009).

There is considerable evidence that *treatments* applied to manage medical conditions contribute to illness intrusiveness. When treatment interferes with ongoing, valued activities and interests, it is associated with increased illness intrusiveness. People affected by ESRD treated by hemodialysis (in which the blood must be circulated extracorporeally through an artificial kidney for three, weekly three- to four-hour sessions) or peritoneal dialysis (which can require either lengthy three times weekly in-hospital sessions or multiple daily exchanges of dialysate solution and is associated with the risk of peritonitis), for example, report significantly higher illness intrusiveness than do those treated by successful renal transplantation (which "merely" requires daily immunosuppression by oral medications and annual follow-up; Binik, Chowanec, & Devins, 1990; Devins et al., 1983; Devins, Mandin, et al., 1990). People with ESRD treated by dialysis also report significantly higher illness intrusiveness than those with progressive renal failure whose conditions have not yet reached the point at which they require renal replacement therapy (Binik et al., 1990). The amount of time required for treatment also contributes to illness intrusiveness in ESRD (Devins, Mandin, et al., 1990). In schizophrenia, the number of days of psychiatric hospitalization is associated with illness intrusiveness (Bettazzoni et al., 2008).

The corollary to the premise that treatment-related lifestyle disruptions contribute to increased illness intrusiveness is that it *decreases* when treatment effectively ameliorates such interference. Illness intrusiveness does decrease significantly, for example, among women treated successfully for anorexia nervosa (Carter, Bewell, & Devins, 2008). Significant reductions in illness intrusiveness into the intimacy life domain have been reported among women with systemic lupus erythematosus after participating in expressive-supportive group psychotherapy (Edworthy et al., 2003). Seizure freedom following successful surgical or pharmacological treatment for epilepsy is associated with decreased illness intrusiveness (Poochikian-Sarkissian, Sidani, Wennberg, & Devins, 2008a; Poochikian-Sarkissian et al., 2008b). Involvement in self-care and receiving education about one's condition and its treatment is associated with low illness intrusiveness in people living with diabetes (type 1 or type 2; DeCoster et al., 2013), although the study in which this was observed did not verify the effectiveness of these interventions. Similarly, the number of self-management strategies people employ and consider to be helpful in managing bipolar disorder correlates significantly and inversely with illness intrusiveness (Depp et al., 2009). A case study reporting the treatment of a middle-aged American Vietnam War veteran with sexual paraphilia (foot fetishism/sexual impulses) indicated that illness intrusiveness decreased reliably following effective treatment (behavioral activation and sensate focus; Sarver & Gros, 2014).

Not all findings have been supportive, however. This includes a randomized controlled trial that compared telemedicine versus in-person treatment for chronic pain. Results indicated that telemedicine produced lower overall costs and higher patient satisfaction than in-person treatment, but illness intrusiveness did not differ significantly between the two modes of delivery (Pronovost, Peng, & Kern, 2009). Because telemedicine did not demonstrate a differential impact on reported pain as compared to in-person treatment, the failure to detect a difference in reported illness intrusiveness is not surprising. An evaluation of the psychosocial impact of wait times for thyroid surgery found no association between the duration of wait times and illness intrusiveness, although anxiety did correlate significantly with wait-time durations (Eskander et al., 2013). This study examined the effect of a single time-limited intervention and, thus, may not have exerted a sufficiently substantial effect on lifestyles to influence illness intrusiveness.

Illness Intrusiveness Compromises Subjective Well-Being

The illness intrusiveness theoretical framework maintains that illness intrusiveness compromises subjective well-being by reducing the satisfaction and pleasure that result from participation in valued activities and interests. This is rooted Lewinsohn's (Lewinsohn, Shaffer, & Libet, 1969) theory of depression, which maintains that depression arises in response to and is maintained by the unavailability of response-contingent positive reinforcement. Evidence to support this premise has been observed in people affected by a number of chronic and life-threatening medical conditions. Depressive symptoms are the facet of subjective well-being that has been examined most commonly in this respect. Illness intrusiveness, as measured by the IIRS, is associated with depressive symptoms in (a) hematologic cancer treated by autologous bone marrow transplantation (Schimmer et al., 2001); (b) myalgic encephalomyelitis (chronic fatigue) (Goudsmit et al., 2009); (c) breast cancer (Avis et al., 2012; Avis et al., 2013); (d) glioblastoma (Edelstein et al., 2016); (e) systemic lupus erythematosus (Devins, Edworthy, & Group, 2000; Schattner, Shahar, Lerman, & Shakra, 2010); (f) ESRD treated by hemodialysis, continuous peritoneal dialysis, or renal transplantation (Devins et al., 1983; Devins, Mandin, et al., 1990); (g) head and neck cancer and lung cancer (Lebel et al., 2013); (h) juvenile rheumatic diseases (Fedele et al., 2012); (i) heart failure (Paukert, LeMaire, & Cully, 2009); (j) Ménière's disease (Arroll et al., 2012); and (k) mal de debarquement syndrome (Arroll et al., 2016). Illness intrusiveness, as measured by IIRS adaptations, too, correlates significantly with depressive symptoms. Controlling for duration of disease, physician-rated disability, and self-rated functional ability, children with juvenile rheumatic diseases showed a significant correlation between illness intrusiveness and depressive symptoms (Bonner et al., 2015). Controlling for physical limitations (e.g., difficulties in completing activities of daily living) attributable to heart failure, illness intrusiveness attributable to heart failure correlates significantly and uniquely with depressive symptoms in aged U.S. Veteran's Administration patients (Paukert et al., 2009). Among women living with systemic lupus erythematosus, illness intrusiveness predicts depressive symptoms significantly and uniquely (i.e., after controlling statistically for baseline depressive symptoms) over a period of one to three months (Schattner et al., 2010).

Some investigations have reported significant associations between facets of a medical condition (e.g., severity of disease) and depressive symptoms, such as the severity of disease in heart failure (LeMaire et al., 2012) and multiple sclerosis (Shawaryn, Schiaffino, LaRocca, & Johnston, 2002), and severity of complications in diabetes mellitus (Talbot et al., 1999). These studies also demonstrated, however, that the associations observed between disease variables and depressive symptoms were no longer statistically significant after adjusting for illness intrusiveness. This is consistent with the illness intrusiveness theoretical framework's position that disease and treatment variables influence subjective well-being indirectly through the disruption of lifestyles, activities, and interests.

The impact of illness intrusiveness has been examined in relation to positive psychological states too. Illness intrusiveness correlates significantly with (a) positive affect and psychological well-being in glioblastoma (Edelstein et al., 2016) and (b) self-esteem, positive affect, and life happiness in hematologic cancer treated by autologous bone marrow transplantation (Schimmer et al., 2001), ESRD treated by hemodialysis, continuous peritoneal dialysis, or renal transplantation (Devins et al., 1983; Devins, Mandin, et al., 1990), and in head and neck and lung cancers (Lebel et al., 2013).

Unlike the loss of positive reinforcement, which occurs under conditions of good physical health and about which Lewinsohn theorized, lifestyle disruptions attributable to serious medical conditions (i.e., illness intrusiveness) occur in the context of (often) painful symptoms, onerous treatments, and unpleasant side effects. These stressors introduce significant adaptive challenges in themselves, but the illness intrusiveness theoretical framework posits that the impact of such factors on subjective well-being occurs indirectly by disrupting lifestyles, activities, and interests. This has been tested by estimating the association between reported illness intrusiveness and indicators of subjective well-being after adjusting statistically for the effects of disease and/or treatment variables (e.g., partial correlation coefficients). Significant partial correlations between illness intrusiveness and subjective well-being are interpreted to signify that the effects of illness intrusiveness are incremental to those attributable to the effects of a medical condition and its treatment (Cohen, Cohen, West, & Aiken, 2003). A number of studies have employed the IIRS to test this hypothesis and have reported supportive evidence.

Among women affected by breast cancer, the incremental association between illness intrusiveness and depressive symptoms remains statistically significant after adjusting for co-occurring conditions, cancer stage, type of surgery, type of chemotherapy, duration of disease, symptom severity, and pain (Avis et al., 2012; Avis et al., 2013). Illness intrusiveness remains significantly correlated with depressive symptoms in children with rheumatic diseases after controlling statistically for duration of disease, physician-rated disability, and self-rated functional ability (Bonner et al., 2015). A similar finding has been reported in mal de debarquement syndrome (Arroll et al., 2016). Illness intrusiveness remains significantly and uniquely correlated with positive affect and depressive symptoms in people with glioblastoma after adjusting for physical-symptom burden and performance status (Edelstein et al., 2016). Controlling for co-occurring (i.e. intercurrent nonrenal) medical conditions, illness intrusiveness correlates significantly and uniquely with depressive symptoms, self-esteem, positive and negative affect, pessimism, and life happiness in ESRD (Devins et al., 1983). Controlling for disease activity, it correlates significantly and uniquely with psychological well-being and depressive symptoms in systemic lupus erythematosus, and these associations are evident in both White and Black people affected by the condition (Devins, Edworthy, et al., 2000). Controlling for seizure frequency, illness intrusiveness correlates significantly with depressive symptoms, positive affect, and self-esteem in people affected by epilepsy treated surgically and/or pharmacologically and with epilepsy-specific health-related quality of life, controlling for seizure frequency and treatment side effects (Poochikian-Sarkissian, 2005). Adjusting for course of illness (e.g., chronic-progressive vs. relapsing-remitting), severity of illness, fatigue, and disability, illness intrusiveness correlates significantly and uniquely with psychological well-being, life happiness, and emotional distress in multiple sclerosis (Devins et al., 1993; Shawaryn et al., 2002) and with health-related quality of life after adjusting for fatigue, severity of disability, and number of relapses (Turpin, Carroll, Cassidy, & Hader, 2007). Finally, illness intrusiveness correlates significantly and uniquely with psychological well-being and with emotional distress in people with head and neck cancer and with lung cancer after adjusting for age, education, stressful life events, and time since diagnosis (Lebel et al., 2013).

Not all findings have supported this central tenet of the illness intrusiveness theoretical framework. Illness intrusiveness did not correlate significantly with health-related quality of life in a sample of college students who self-identified as having childhood-onset asthma (Fedele et al., 2009). Unfortunately, the paper in which this finding was reported did not report the severity of respondents' conditions nor the extent to which their symptoms were under control. Thus the group, as a whole, may have been characterized by a comparatively low level of symptom burden and the resulting attenuation of ranges may have resulted in an inability to detect a statistically significant association (Anastasi, 1988). This study generated other counter-intuitive results (e.g., illness uncertainty correlated positively with health-related QOL and neither illness intrusiveness nor illness uncertainty correlated with the physical dimension of a widely used health-related quality of life instrument, the SF-36). The latter observation is noteworthy because this dimension taps problems in physical functioning attributable to one's medical condition, and thus the failure to detect significant associations with illness intrusiveness is especially puzzling.

Illness Intrusiveness and Personal Control

Personal control entails the ability to influence the occurrence of a given outcome (Devins et al., 1982). In relation to subjective well-being, it entails the ability to influence the occurrence of outcomes that are meaningful to and valued by a person. An extensive literature substantiates the premise that personal control is a powerful determinant of subjective well-being (Alloy, 1992; Grob, 2000; Helzer & Jayawickreme, 2015; Seligman, 1975). Personal control can enhance feelings of well-being through actual or perceived (e.g., illusory) effects (Alloy, 1992). In addition to influencing subjective well-being directly by interfering with continued involvements in psychologically meaningful activities, the illness intrusiveness theoretical framework posits that illness intrusiveness exerts an indirect influence by compromising personal control (Devins et al., 1983). Illness intrusiveness, as measured by the IIRS, correlates significantly and inversely with personal control in diabetes (type 1 and type 2; DeCoster et al., 2013), multiple sclerosis (Devins et al., 1993), and epilepsy (Poochikian-Sarkissian, 2005). It correlates significantly and inversely with perceived control over ESRD and over dialysis treatment (Devins et al., 1983). Illness intrusiveness attributable to type 2 diabetes, as tapped by the Multidimensional Diabetes Questionnaire (interference with daily activities, work and social and recreational activities), correlates significantly and inversely with perceived control (Talbot et al., 1999). Consistent with the premise that reducing personal control is only one of two mechanisms by which illness intrusiveness compromises subjective well-being, partial-correlation analyses demonstrate that both illness intrusiveness and personal control remain significantly and uniquely associated with subjective well-being after adjusting statistically for each other (i.e., illness intrusiveness correlates significantly with subjective well-being after controlling statistically for personal control and vice versa; Devins et al., 1983; Devins et al., 1993). Inasmuch as it may be easier to enhance perceived as compared to actual control in chronic, disabling, or life-threatening conditions, it would be helpful to determine whether the effects of illness intrusiveness on subjective well-being differ as a function of this distinction. Unfortunately, this has not yet been examined and represents a worthwhile direction for future research: for example, can we enhance illusory control to mitigate the negative psychosocial impact of illness intrusiveness in people affected by chronic disabling and life-threatening medical conditions without necessarily changing objective, or actual (i.e., primary), control as has been demonstrated in laboratory contexts (Alloy, 1992; Devins, 1989, 1991)?

Psychological, Social, and Contextual Variables Moderate Effects of Medical Conditions and Treatment on Illness Intrusiveness

The illness intrusiveness theoretical framework maintains that psychological, social, and contextual variables modify the effects of a medical condition and its treatment in determining illness intrusiveness. Evidence that supports this premise has been observed in diverse medical conditions. Illness intrusiveness differs, for example, as a function of age, education, income, recent stressful life events, and affected life domain in people affected by six common cancers (Devins et al., 2006). Figure 5.2 illustrates, for example, how illness intrusiveness differs across life domains among younger and older people affected by cancer (similar patterns are evident for stressful life events and income, with the upper curve indicating greater illness intrusiveness among people who have experienced recent stressful life events or people with comparatively low incomes).

Illness intrusiveness has been observed to differ as a function of race, but conflicting results have been reported across populations of people affected by or in treatment for chronic disabling and/or life-threatening conditions. Black American veterans with diverse diagnoses reported higher levels of illness intrusiveness, on average, than their White counterparts, a phenomenon that investigators attributed post hoc to differences in their use of adaptive versus non-adaptive coping tactics (DiNapoli, Cummings, Petersen, & Cully, 2015). White, aged people with ESRD undergoing maintenance hemodialysis, on the other hand, reported *higher* illness intrusiveness than their Black counterparts (Kutner & Devins, 1998). The latter two groups did not differ in disability or functional status, but more Blacks than Whites were diagnosed with diabetes. Whites on hemodialysis, on the other hand, reported more nausea, fatigue, and longer times to recover after dialysis treatments as compared to Blacks.

Sex and perceived social support appear to moderate the impact of medical conditions and their treatment on illness intrusiveness: One year after experiencing a cardiac event (myocardial infarction or unstable angina), men reported higher illness intrusiveness into the intimacy life domain than did women; men who felt more supported by their partners reported lower illness intrusiveness

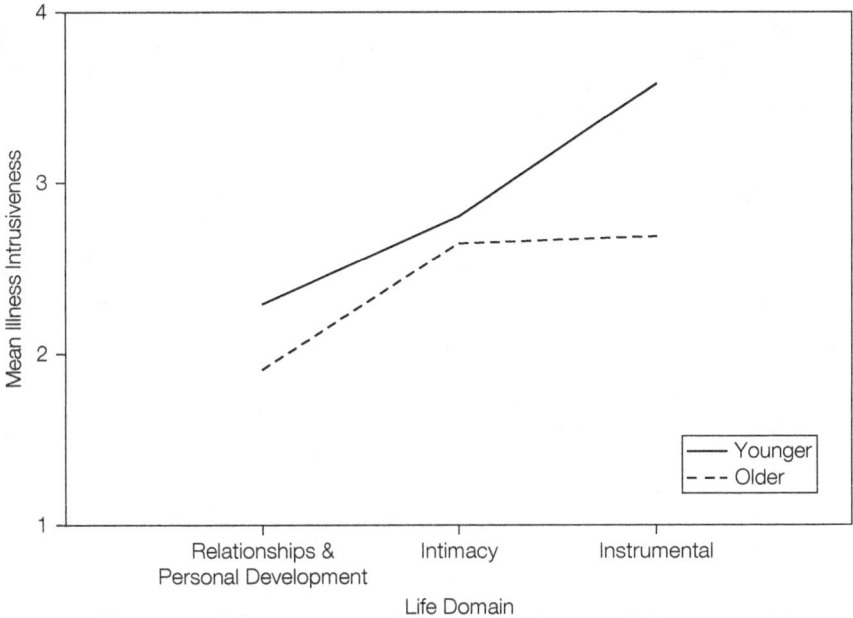

Figure 5.2 Age moderates the impact of illness intrusiveness across life domains. Young people affected by cancer report higher illness intrusiveness than their older counterparts. Illness intrusiveness is highest in the Instrumental life domain, intermediate in relation to Intimacy, and lowest in the domain of Relationships and Personal Development. A similar pattern is evident in relation to other demographic and contextual variables (e.g., income, recent stressful life events).
Reprinted from Devins, G. M., Bezjak, A., Mah, K., Loblaw, D. A., & Gotowiec, A. P. (Reprinted 2006). Context moderates illness-induced lifestyle disruptions across life domains: A test of the illness intrusiveness theoretical framework in six common cancers. *Psycho-Oncology, 15*(3), 221–233.

than those who felt less supported (Franche et al., 2004). In another study that investigated sex differences in illness intrusiveness three months after myocardial infarction, men reported significantly higher intrusiveness into intimacy than did women, a finding that was attributed to the fact that this domain entails disruptions to (a) the relationship with one's spouse, which is a more central source of social support for men than women (Harrison, Maguire, & Pitceathly, 1995), and (b) one's sex life (Woodend & Devins, 2005).

Psychological, Social, and Contextual Variables Moderate Effects of Illness Intrusiveness on Subjective Well-Being

A number of findings support the hypothesis that the impact of illness intrusiveness on subjective well-being is moderated by psychological, social, and contextual factors. Illness intrusiveness differs as a function of stage in the life cycle, as represented by chronological age. In general, the deleterious psychosocial impact of illness intrusiveness is greater among young as compared to old people.

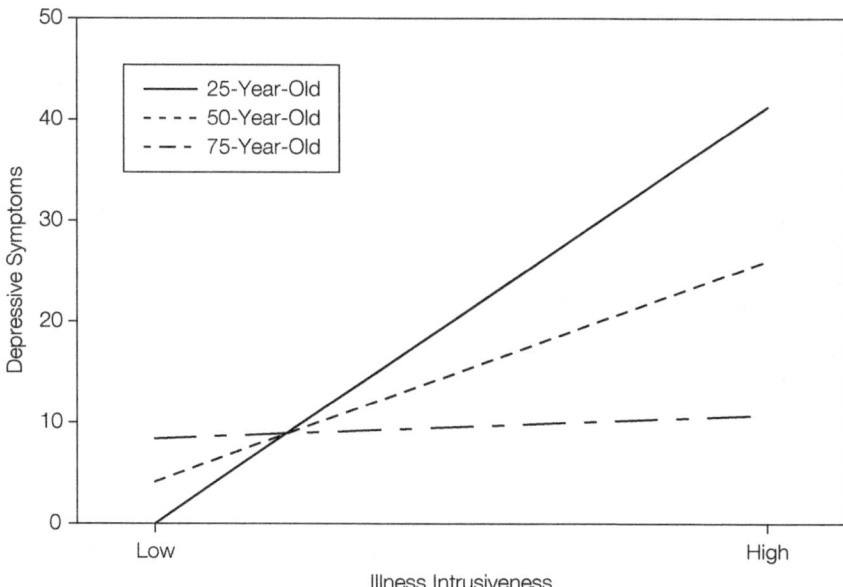

Figure 5.3 Age moderates the relation between illness intrusiveness and depressive symptoms.
Rising illness intrusiveness is associated with a dramatic increase in depressive symptoms in young people; the effect is increasingly muted as people age. This figure plots estimated regression lines for hypothetical 25-, 50-, and 75-year olds affected by rheumatoid arthritis. Reprinted with permission from Devins, G. M., Edworthy, S. M., Guthrie, N. G., & Martin, L. (1992). Illness intrusiveness in rheumatoid arthritis: Differential impact on depressive symptoms over the adult lifespan. *Journal of Rheumatology, 19*, 709–715.

Figure 5.3 illustrates this phenomenon in people affected by rheumatoid arthritis (Devins, Edworthy, Guthrie, et al., 1992). The finding has been replicated in an independent rheumatoid-arthritis sample (Devins et al., 2009) and in multiple sclerosis (Devins et al., 1996). Although a direct test of the mechanism that underlies this effect remains to be tested, a number of possibilities bear investigation: The fact that illness intrusiveness exerts a more powerful, negative effect on young, as compared to old people may reflect (a) the benefits of cumulative learning and mastery that arise due to a lifetime of effective coping (Gerstorf, Röcke, & Lachman, 2011); (b) the result of expectations that chronic medical conditions and disability are developmentally "on time" for older adults but not for younger ones (Nerenz & Leventhal, 1983); or (c) the effects of psychological disengagement (Neugarten, 1977). It may, of course, simply reflect a measurement artifact: For example, the life domains people value may change over the lifespan (Chen, 2003) and IIRS item content may not provide sufficient coverage of those most important to the aged. Future research should investigate these possibilities.

Sex, a proxy for gender, has been observed to moderate the psychosocial effect of illness intrusiveness. Health-related quality of life differs significantly as a function of illness intrusiveness between men and women with similar IBS symptoms (Dancey et al., 2002). The effect is subtle but reliable. Men with IBS reported higher health-related quality of life than affected women at low levels of illness intrusiveness. The men also demonstrated a more precipitous decline with increasing illness intrusiveness. The men and women who participated in this study did not differ in symptom severity, enhancing confidence in the interpretation that sex or gender shapes the psychosocial impact of illness intrusiveness. IBS is often construed as primarily a women's condition (Toner & Akman, 2000), which may render illness intrusiveness more normative for women and, thus, more stigmatizing—and, therefore, distressing—for men.

Indeed, stigma exerts a powerful moderating effect on the psychosocial impact of illness intrusiveness. Stigma moderates the impact of illness intrusiveness on emotional distress in long-term laryngeal cancer survivors after surgical treatment by laryngectomy (surgical removal of the larynx, resulting in visible disfigurement and the need to rely on artificial speech; Devins et al., 1994). As illustrated in Figure 5.4, long-term laryngeal cancer survivors who felt highly stigmatized by their disease and treatment demonstrated a dramatically steeper increase in depressive symptoms as compared to survivors who did not feel highly stigmatized. This effect was not evident, however, when the outcome of interest was psychological well-being (i.e., positive affect). Stigma may exacerbate the negative

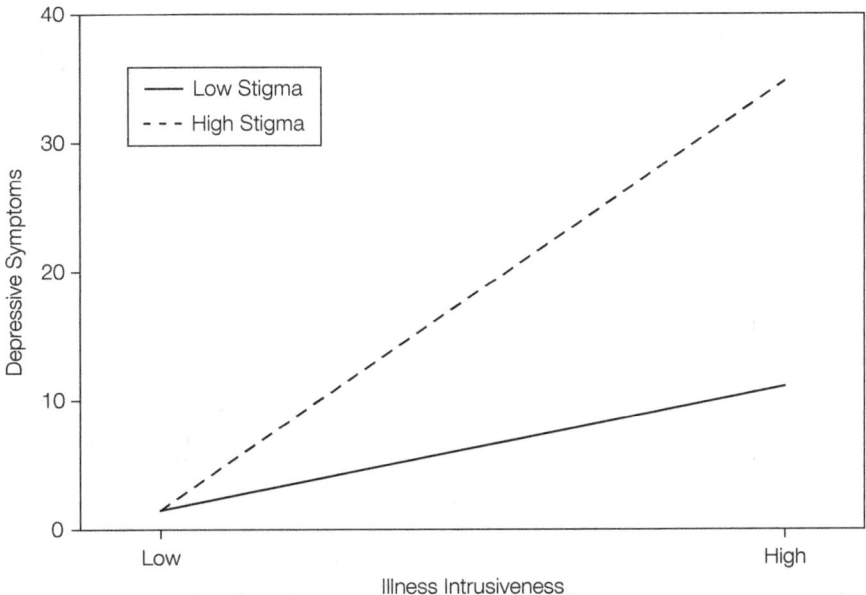

Figure 5.4 Stigma moderates the impact of illness intrusiveness on depressive symptoms. Among long-term survivors of laryngeal cancer treated by laryngectomy, people who feel highly stigmatized by their disease and treatment demonstrate a more rapid increase in depressive symptoms with rising illness intrusiveness than those who do not feel highly stigmatized.
Reprinted from Devins, G. M., Stam, H. J., & Koopmans, J. P. (1994). Psychosocial impact of laryngectomy mediated by perceived stigma and illness intrusiveness. *Canadian Journal of Psychiatry, 39*(10), 608–616.

effect of illness intrusiveness on depressive symptoms either by leading affected people to avoid social exchange and valued activities (Major & O'Brien, 2005) in which this plays a central role or by interfering with family relations (Badger et al., 2011), in particular, which was the life domain most highly related to depressive symptoms in this respondent group. Stigma exerts a similar, exacerbating effect in people affected by mal de debarquement syndrome (Arroll et al., 2016).

Self-concept can shape the experience and appraisal of stressors, threats, and adaptive demands. As a result, adopting a self-concept as a "chronic kidney patient" has been hypothesized to moderate the effect of illness intrusiveness on subjective well-being. A study in ESRD supported this assertion (Devins, Beanlands, Mandin, & Paul, 1997). Among people with ESRD treated by dialysis or transplantation, those who perceived themselves as similar to the stereotypic "chronic kidney patient" reported significantly rising severity of depressive symptoms as illness intrusiveness increased, but depressive symptoms did not differ among those who construed themselves as dissimilar (see Figure 5.5). This was interpreted as indicating that disease- and treatment-related constraints are more likely to limit the range and diversity of opportunities for rewarding experiences when people define themselves in terms of chronic life-threatening disease (Radley & Green, 1987); when

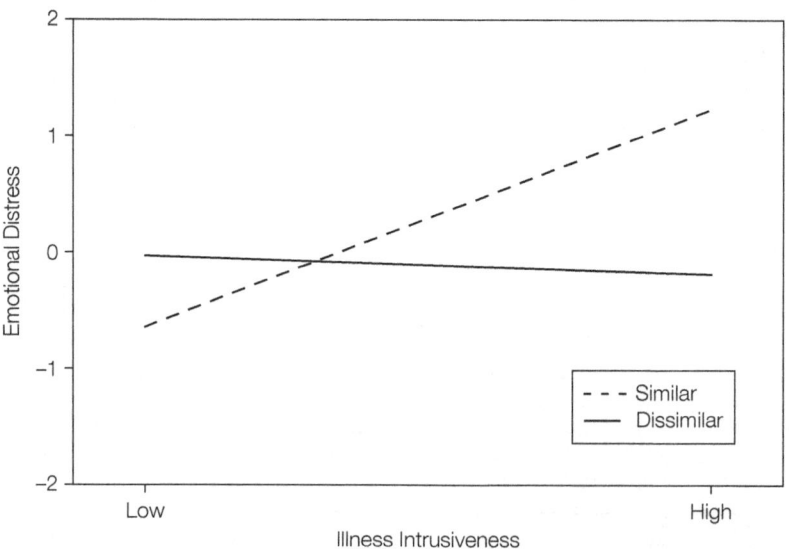

Figure 5.5 Self-concept as a "chronic patient" moderates the impact of illness intrusiveness on emotional distress.
People with end-stage renal disease treated by maintenance dialysis or renal transplantation who perceive themselves as similar to the "chronic kidney patient" report increasing depressive symptoms with rising illness intrusiveness; depressive symptoms demonstrate little change with increasing illness intrusiveness when they construe themselves as dissimilar. Reprinted from Devins, G. M., Beanlands, H., Mandin, H., & Paul, L. C. (1997). Psychosocial impact of illness intrusiveness moderated by self-concept and age in end-stage renal disease. *Health Psychology, 16*(6), 529–538.

people resist construing themselves as "patients," they may experience a protective, buffering effect that mitigates the deleterious psychosocial-impact of the constraints associated with their condition. A corresponding pattern was evident for psychological well-being (i.e., positive affect) among "older" (i.e., ≥ 57 years) people with ESRD (Figure 5.6a), but the effect was qualified by age: Among "younger" people with ESRD, the opposite pattern was evident (i.e., psychological well-being *increased* with increasing illness intrusiveness when people construed themselves as similar to the "chronic kidney patient"; Figure 5.6b). When chronic life-threatening medical conditions arise during the early adult years, people may experience increased motivation to restore their freedom to pursue valued life goals (Lieberman & Peskin, 1992) especially because the principal developmental tasks at this life stage involve establishing one's career and independence (Hurlock, 1980). At this developmental point, moreover, many people may still maintain fundamental assumptions of personal efficacy and optimism (Gutmann, 1995), enhancing persistence despite the barriers.

Self-concept as a "cancer patient," too, has been observed to moderate the psychosocial impact of illness intrusiveness (Devins, Wong, et al., 2015). As compared to those who construe themselves as comparatively dissimilar, people with head and neck cancer who perceive themselves as similar to the stereotypic "cancer patient" report more severe depressive symptoms, although their distress rises slightly less rapidly with increasing illness intrusiveness as compared to people who construe themselves as dissimilar. The psychosocial impact of illness intrusiveness is also moderated by the extent to which people with head and neck cancer maintain negative stereotypes of the "cancer patient": The severity of depressive symptoms increases with increasing illness intrusiveness when people do not hold negative stereotypes, but it actually *decreases* when they maintain highly negative stereotypes (Devins, Wong, et al., 2015). Increasing illness intrusiveness may lead people to attribute their distress to the effects of cancer and its treatment rather than reflecting negatively on themselves, as may be more likely when the obvious, "external" sources of their distress are less salient due to more subtle effects (i.e., low illness intrusiveness). Thus this counterintuitive phenomenon may reflect an esteem-preserving process whereby the deleterious self-relevant implications associated with negative stereotypes are reinterpreted as attributable to the more impersonal effects of life-threatening disease and the suffering associated with it (which are generally believed to be independent of an individual's status or actions). Evidence to support this interpretation includes the facts that illness intrusiveness correlates significantly with stigma (Arroll et al., 2016; Dancey et al., 2002; Devins et al., 1994; Lebel et al., 2013) and mediates the relation between stigma and distress in head and neck cancer (Lebel et al., 2013).

Cultural syndromes are global, multidimensional vectors that comprise diverse attitudes, beliefs, and values that characterize a given cultural group and have been identified as fundamental influences that shape perception, appraisal, coping, and subjective well-being (Triandis, 2000). Consistent with

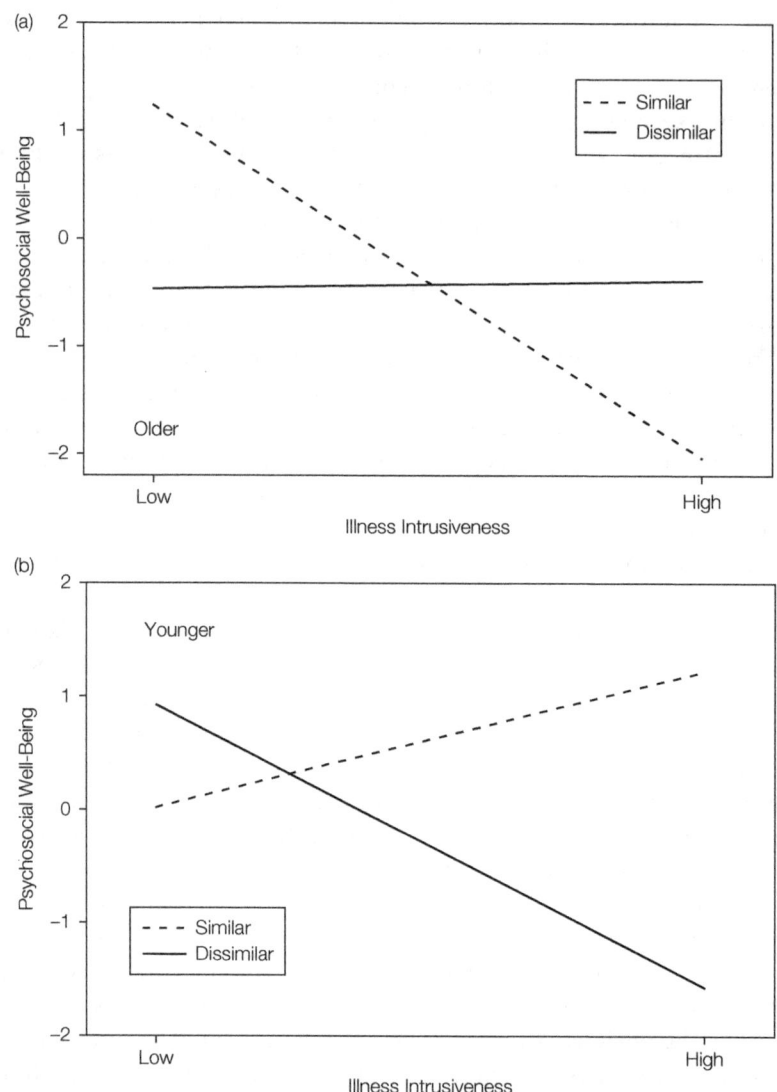

Figure 5.6 Self-concept as a "chronic patient" and age moderate the impact of illness intrusiveness on psychological well-being.

The moderating effect of self-concept as a "chronic patient" on psychological well-being differs as a function of the affected person's age. Figure 6a indicates that comparatively old people with end-stage renal disease treated by maintenance dialysis or renal transplantation who perceive themselves as similar to the "chronic kidney patient" report decreasing psychological well-being with rising illness intrusiveness; psychological well-being demonstrates little change with increasing illness intrusiveness when they construe themselves as dissimilar. Figure 6b illustrates a different pattern among comparatively young people: Psychological well-being decreases with increasing illness intrusiveness when people construe themselves as *dissimilar* to the "chronic kidney patient;" it increases when they construe themselves as similar.

Reprinted from Devins, G. M., Beanlands, H., Mandin, H., & Paul, L. C. (1997). Psychosocial impact of illness intrusiveness moderated by self-concept and age in end-stage renal disease. *Health Psychology, 16*(6), 529–538.

this conceptualization, cultural syndromes might be expected to entail social-contextual factors that moderate the psychosocial impact of illness intrusiveness. Evidence in rheumatoid arthritis has, in fact, supported this reasoning. Individualism-collectivism (Triandis, 1995), perhaps the most widely recognized cultural syndrome, moderates the impact of illness intrusiveness on emotional distress in people affected by rheumatoid arthritis (Devins et al., 2009). Figure 5.7 illustrates these effects. Horizontal individualism emphasizes interpersonal equality and autonomy and appears to exert a protective buffering effect of the impact of illness intrusiveness: Depressive symptoms decrease in intensity as illness intrusiveness into relationships and personal development increases among people who endorse this cultural syndrome highly, although the effect is moderated by age with comparatively young people exhibiting the most pronounced effect and comparatively old people showing a highly muted one (Figure 5.7). It may be that these values and beliefs allow for maximum flexibility in adapting lifestyles, activities, and interests to suit one's personal needs and circumstances without being bound by the constraints associated with obligations to other in-group members. Three other cultural syndromes appear to intensify the deleterious effects of increasing illness intrusiveness into intimacy (i.e., marital relationship and sexual relations) in particular. In each case, endorsement of these values, attitudes, and beliefs is associated with comparatively low distress as compared to non-endorsement, but distress increases significantly with increasing illness intrusiveness. Figures 8a-8c illustrate this phenomenon in relation to (a) vertical collectivism, which emphasizes hierarchical social relationships and the need to fulfill obligations to others; (b) vertical individualism, which emphasizes competitive relationships and the importance of excelling in comparison to others; and (c) horizontal collectivism, which emphasizes personal sacrifice to fulfill the needs and expectations of others in one's in-group. As compared to the freedom to adapt and change associated with horizontal individualism, adherence to any of the other cultural syndromes may exacerbate the negative emotional impact of illness intrusiveness into intimacy by constraining perceived personal freedom to substitute new activities that are compatible with the constraints associated with medical conditions and treatment for existing activities that may be incompatible.

Another social-contextual factor that appears to moderate the psychosocial impact of illness intrusiveness derives from the emotional reactions of family or close friends to a person's health problems. Illness intrusiveness correlated significantly with depressive symptoms in a sample of children with juvenile rheumatic diseases, and this was amplified significantly when their parents, too, were distressed (Wagner et al., 2003). The effect was most pronounced when children reported high levels of illness intrusiveness; it was more muted when they reported little illness intrusiveness (Bonner et al., 2015). This finding may reflect a special case of the cost-of-caring phenomenon (Kessler, McLeod, & Wethington, 1985), which may be the mechanism responsible for the effect.

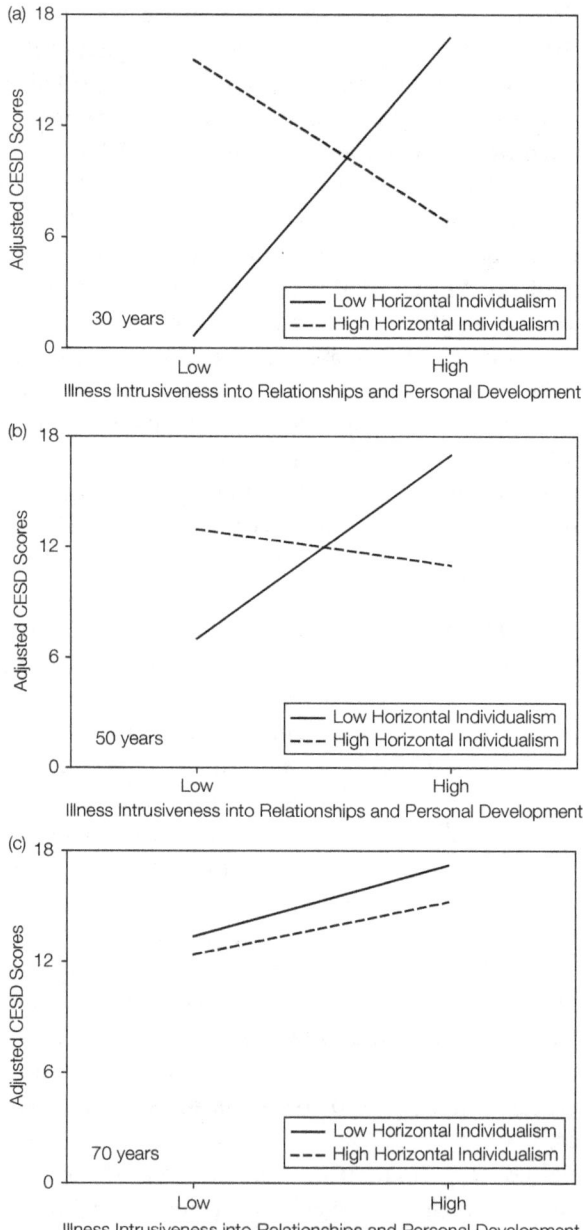

Figure 5.7 Cultural syndromes (horizontal individualism) and age moderate the impact of illness intrusiveness on emotional distress.

Horizontal individualism (emphasizing interpersonal equality and autonomy) buffers the effects of illness intrusiveness on emotional distress. This is evident in people affected by rheumatoid arthritis: The effect is most pronounced among the young (Figure 7a), is less marked in middle age (Figure 7b), and appears all but nonexistent among the aged (Figure 7c). Reprinted from Devins, G. M., Gupta, A., Cameron, J. I., Woodend, K., Mah, K., & Gladman, D. (2009). Cultural syndromes and age moderate the emotional impact of illness intrusiveness in rheumatoid arthritis. *Rehabilitation Psychology, 54*(1), 33–44.

Findings Not Predicted by the Illness Intrusiveness Theoretical Framework

Perhaps because it represents a variable that intervenes between the circumstances of medical conditions and their treatment on the one hand and subjective well-being on the other, some investigators have derived hypotheses involving illness intrusiveness that are not articulated by the illness intrusiveness theoretical framework. At least two studies have tested the notion that illness intrusiveness mediates the psychosocial impact of social and psychological stressors on subjective well-being. In a study of British men and women with IBS, results indicated that illness intrusiveness was a partial moderator of the effects of stigma on IBS-specific health-related quality of life (Dancey et al., 2002). Illness intrusiveness has been observed to function as a partial mediator of the relation between stigma and psychological well-being and emotional distress in people with head and neck or lung cancers (Lebel et al., 2013) and in mal de debarquement syndrome (Arroll et al., 2016).

Theoretical Refinements

The illness intrusiveness theoretical framework posits that the negative psychosocial impact of illness intrusiveness arises when medical conditions and their treatment interfere with valued activities and interests. As noted earlier, however, some have suggested that the intensity of distress produced by a given extent of illness intrusiveness may depend on the *degree* to which affected life domains are valued (Abraido-Lanza, 1997; Abraido-Lanza & Revenson, 2006; Bishop, 2005). There is some evidence to substantiate this. As noted earlier, among Latinas with rheumatoid arthritis, illness intrusiveness compromises psychological well-being (positive and negative affect) to the extent that affected roles are valued (Abraido-Lanza & Revenson, 2006). The Disability Centrality Model (Bishop et al., 2007), too, maintains that the deleterious psychosocial impact of illness intrusiveness is moderated by the extent to which people value the life domains affected by their medical conditions and treatment. It also posits that people are intrinsically motivated to optimize subjective well-being through the exercise of personal control when this is compromised. Although the evidence, to date, that bears on it specifically is limited, the Disability Centrality Model was derived from established psychological theory and research. Published findings are encouraging (Bishop, Frain, & Tschopp, 2008; Bishop et al., 2007). The model is entirely compatible with the illness intrusiveness theoretical framework and shares its clinical implications, including the enhancement of personal or perceived control to mitigate the deleterious effects of illness-induced lifestyle disruptions (e.g., Devins, 1989, 2006; Devins & Binik, 1996a; Devins, Cameron, & Edworthy, 2000; Devins et al., 2014; Devins, Mendelssohn, Barre, & Binik, 2003; Devins, Otto, Irish, & Rodin, 2015; Devins & Shnek, 2000; Devins et al., 2012; Edelstein et al., 2016; Edworthy, Devins, & Group, 1999; Edworthy et al., 2003; Poochikian-Sarkissian et al., 2008a, 2008b).

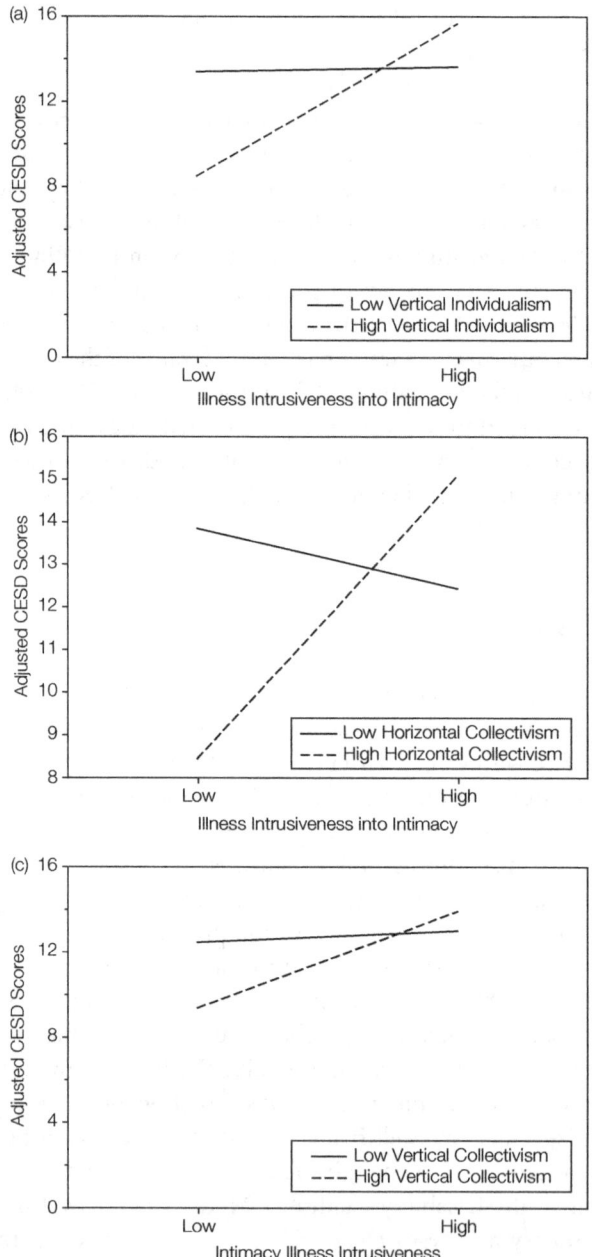

Figure 5.8 Cultural syndromes other than horizontal individualism moderate the impact of illness intrusiveness on emotional distress.
Maintaining cultural syndromes other than horizontal individualism appears to exacerbate the effects of illness intrusiveness on emotional distress. The effect is evident for vertical individualism, which emphasizes competitive relationships and the importance of excelling in comparison to others (Figure 8a); horizontal collectivism, which emphasizes personal sacrifice to fulfill the needs and expectations of others in one's in-group (Figure 8b), and vertical collectivisms, which emphasizes emphasizes hierarchical social relationships and

ILLNESS INTRUSIVENESS AND SELF-MANAGEMENT OF MEDICAL CONDITIONS

As an outcome that relates to the psychosocial consequences of medical conditions and/or their treatment and is amenable to change, we consider illness intrusiveness to be an ideal tertiary target for self-management interventions. Indeed, given its more proximal causal relation to the effects of a condition and its treatment, illness intrusiveness may be a more appropriate self-management target than other commonly identified tertiary targets that are influenced by a variety of additional factors (e.g., anxiety, depression, distress, psychological well-being, or empowerment). Self-management interventions targeting illness intrusiveness should (a) identify aspects of a given condition and its treatment that can interfere with lifestyles, valued activities, and interests; (b) educate affected people about the ways in which these effects arise; (c) assist affected people in mastering relevant strategies and behavioral tactics to minimize their disruptive effects; (d) facilitate the integration of self-management skills into everyday life; (e) help people to maintain active participation in the activities and interests that are important to them; and (f) enlist affected people as active collaborators with their healthcare providers to implement self-management insights and skills to maximize treatment benefits and minimize illness intrusiveness. Ideally, interventions should be introduced early in the trajectory of the condition and its treatment to socialize people into a self-management orientation (e.g., accepting responsibility for learning about and participating in treatment, acquiring relevant knowledge about one's condition and its treatment, and adopting an active-collaborative role in relation to service providers).

This approach has been applied to the self-management of "symptom interference," which entails "the degree to which a symptom limits or interferes in an individual's life" (Doorenbos et al., 2005, p. 575). An intervention grounded in cognitive-behavior therapy adopted this approach and demonstrated meaningful benefits. People recently diagnosed with a solid-tumor cancer and who had recently initiated chemotherapy reviewed 15 common cancer symptoms (e.g., pain, fatigue, nausea, vomiting, insomnia) and monitored them over the course of therapy. Participants and a study nurse collaboratively developed a care plan, which was invoked when symptom severity reached or exceeded a predetermined threshold. Based on a computer-guided protocol, symptoms were matched with problem-solving strategies intended to minimize symptom interference. These

---

Figure 5.8 (Continued)
the need to fulfill obligations to others (Figure 8c). In each case, people who endorse high levels of a cultural syndrome other than horizontal individualism demonstrate increasing emotional distress with increasing illness intrusiveness whereas those who do not endorse these cultural syndromes demonstrate less marked negative effects.
Reprinted from Devins, G. M., Gupta, A., Cameron, J. I., Woodend, K., Mah, K., & Gladman, D. (2009). Cultural syndromes and age moderate the emotional impact of illness intrusiveness in rheumatoid arthritis. *Rehabilitation Psychology, 54*(1), 33–44.

included self-care management, information and decision-making, counseling and support, and communication with providers (unfortunately, the publication does not describe intervention components in detail). The intervention comprised 10 sessions over a 20-week period, five face-to-face and five by telephone. Results indicated significant reductions in symptom interference for both the self-management and the usual-care control groups over the 20 weeks of the intervention, but the self-management group demonstrated significantly greater improvement as compared to the control group. Both groups displayed slight increases in symptom interference at the 12-week follow-up but remained significantly improved as compared to baseline (Doorenbos et al., 2005). This study is important because it establishes that self-management interventions that target illness intrusiveness directly can be effective. The study included a measure of depressive symptoms, too, but these results were not reported, and so it remains to be established that directly targeting and reducing illness intrusiveness (symptom interference) can ameliorate emotional distress.

MaxLife (Devins et al., 2014) is a newly developed self-management intervention that targets illness intrusiveness and was developed specifically for people affected by head and neck cancers. It entails core elements of the self-management approach outlined earlier. The intervention (a) educates people about illness intrusiveness, its psychosocial impact, and the ways in which these arise in head and neck cancers; (b) introduces relevant strategies and behavioral tactics to minimize illness intrusiveness and assists participants in mastering them; (c) facilitates the integration of the self-management skills into everyday life; and (d) encourages people to adopt an active-collaborative relationship with health-care providers to implement self-management insights and skills to minimize illness intrusiveness. *MaxLife* is initiated as soon possible after diagnosis. Four core sessions address (a) the illness intrusiveness theoretical framework as applied to head and neck cancer and its treatment, medical and treatment information, and communication with the treatment team; (b) speech and swallowing as affected by head and neck cancer and how to manage problems; (c) self-management of cancer-related pain, insomnia, and fatigue; and (d) stress and stress-management, including stress-inoculation. Three elective sessions can be added for those who are interested. These address (a) identifying and challenging unhelpful thoughts, (b) communication and social support, and (c) disfigurement and dealing with others' reactions. Each session includes a component that identifies cancer- or treatment-specific stressors that contribute to illness intrusiveness, which are mapped onto a schematic depiction of the illness intrusiveness theoretical framework using concrete examples from the participants' personal experience. In each session, the interventionist engages participants in a creative problem-solving task to explore how valued activities might be modified to render them more compatible with the constraints introduced by their condition and/or treatment (i.e., coping as compared to mastery modeling; Masters, Burish, Hollon, & Rimm, 1987)). Valued activities are scheduled for the coming week, and participants are expected to engage in them. Implementation of the intervention as intended is documented by self-monitoring forms, and these are reviewed with the interventionist at the subsequent session, when participant and interventionist consider how effective the strategy proved to be and, again, consider how the activity might be adapted further to accommodate the constraints and limitations imposed by one's condition and treatment. The intervention concludes with a one-month follow-up session. A patient workbook presents didactic content and provides worksheets to document completion of behavioral homework.

Because the *MaxLife* intervention requires considerable psychological insights and knowledge about head and neck cancer, it is ideal to involve a doctoral-level clinical psychologist with cancer- and treatment-relevant expertise (or someone with equivalent expertise and experience) to deliver it. A recently completed pilot study demonstrated the intervention's feasibility for people newly diagnosed with head and neck cancer, but the effectiveness of the intervention has not yet been evaluated.

FUTURE DIRECTIONS

We hope that the preceding discussion will have convinced the reader that illness intrusiveness is relevant and important in the self-management of medical conditions. The concept is anchored in an a priori theoretical framework that articulates a series of postulates about the ways in which a medical condition and its treatment influence subjective well-being in chronic disabling and life-threatening medical conditions. The notion is supported by a growing body of empirical evidence and has been useful in helping to explain these effects across a wide range of conditions. It offers practical, clinical implications. The IIRS provides a psychometrically sound means to assess illness intrusiveness and can be interpreted meaningfully (see appendix). Initial efforts to address illness intrusiveness directly as a target for self-management appear promising, but much remains to be done. A crucial first step is to evaluate existing interventions empirically and to revise them to enhance their effectiveness. Such work must verify that self-management efforts to minimize illness intrusiveness do, in fact, achieve this end and that doing so results in meaningful psychosocial benefits (e.g., reduced emotional distress and/or increased psychological well-being). Anticipating encouraging results, it will then be important to adapt existing interventions for people affected by other medical conditions.

Given its fundamental applicability across diagnostic groups, it seems reasonable to assert that illness intrusiveness is a relevant self-management target for most conditions. What remains to be done in adapting interventions, therefore, may largely involve tailoring them by developing relevant factual information about other conditions and their treatment. It will be important, of course, to tailor self-management tactics to render them congruent with sources of illness intrusiveness that may be specific to a given condition (e.g., acquiring artificial speech in the case of laryngeal cancer treated by laryngectomy, adapting sexual practices among couples affected by spinal-cord injury). Given increasing globalization, it will be important, too, to adapt interventions to render them culturally sensitive and appropriate for diverse cultural and gender groups (Bedi & Devins, 2016; Devins, 1999; Woodend & Devins, 2005). Inasmuch as family members and other informal caregivers contribute importantly to adaptation and rehabilitation (Ho, Horne, & Szer, 2002), it may prove valuable to modify self-management interventions to recruit their involvement or to assist affected individuals in negotiating the constraints associated with family life (e.g., participating in family outings or other activities, communicating about one's fears or desires, sharing meals).

Cognitive and motivational processes involved in the achievement of psychological adaptation must be acknowledged, but self-management of medical conditions is first and foremost anchored in behavior and behavioral theory (Bandura, 1986; Devins & Binik, 1996b; Kanfer & Karoly, 1972; Lorig & Fries, 1980). It will be crucial to retain an emphasis on the acquisition and effective implementation of self-management skills recognizing that underlying behavioral principles must be applied to achieve this. Thus the emphasis should be on helping people to acquire and implement self-management *behavior*. Relevant knowledge and insights are of central import, but effective outcomes cannot be achieved simply by (a) cultivating the confidence that one can engage in effective self-management (e.g., self-efficacy) or (b) describing the implementation of self-management strategies and tactics and instructing people to enact them. Effective self-management interventions must actually *help people to acquire* an effective behavioral repertoire (e.g., through education, modeling, and rehearsal) and must *facilitate mastery and uptake* (e.g., through iterative, consultation and supervised in-vivo implementation). It will be crucial to verify accurate understanding and implementation through direct behavioral observation and exchange between interventionists and people attempting to acquire and master relevant knowledge and skills if we are to succeed in facilitating effective self-management. As a facet of the environment introduced by medical conditions and their treatment, illness intrusiveness offers a self-management target that can be minimized to preserve subjective well-being and quality of life in chronic disabling and life-threatening conditions.

APPENDIX
MEASURING ILLNESS INTRUSIVENESS

The IIRS (Devins, 2010) is a self-report questionnaire that taps illness- and treatment-induced interference with valued activities and interests (the IIRS appears at the end of this appendix). Items ask respondents to use a 7-point rating scale (ranging from 1 = *not very much* to 7 = *very much*) to indicate the extent to which their "illness and/or its treatment interfere" with each of 13 life domains that are central to quality of life (Flanagan, 1978). These include health; diet (e.g., the things one eats and drinks); work; active recreation (e.g., sports); passive recreation (e.g., reading, listening to music); financial situation; relationship with spouse;

sex life; family relations; other social relations; self-expression/self-improvement; religious expression; and community and civic involvement. Total scores are generated by summing ratings across all 13 items and can range from 13 to 91, with high scores indicating high levels of illness intrusiveness. The IIRS can also be scored to generate three subscales: (a) *Relationships and Personal Development* (passive recreation, family relations, other social relations, self-expression/self-improvement, religious expression, and community and civic involvement); (b) *Intimacy* (relationship with spouse, sex life); and (c) *Instrumental* life domains (health, work, financial situation, and active recreation). Subscale scores are generated by calculating the mean rating reported for the items that comprise each subscale and, thus, range from 1 to 7. High subscale scores indicate high levels of illness intrusiveness into a given life domain.

There are no formal norms for the IIRS. Interpretation can be informed, however, by referring individual (or group) scores to those reported by people affected by diverse medical conditions or those undergoing various medical treatments. Data from 36 diverse patient populations have been collated for this purpose (Devins, 2010) and are reported in Table 5.1. Although IIRS scores cannot be interpreted absolutely, reference to the levels of illness intrusiveness characteristic of various medical conditions or treatment groups can provide insight into the extent to which a person or group has experienced illness-induced lifestyle disruptions.

Psychometric Properties

The IIRS boasts strong psychometric characteristics. *Reliability* of IIRS total and subscale scores is consistently above recommended thresholds (Nunnally, 1978) with very few exceptions. Internal consistency for IIRS total and subscale scores has been collated for 36 clinical groups, which substantiates this claim (Devins, 2010). Given that illness intrusiveness is conceptualized as a dynamic construct and, therefore, is subject to change with the circumstances of disease and treatment, it is crucial that IIRS scores be sensitive to change. The evidence is encouraging. IIRS scores decrease significantly following effective completion of a number of therapeutic procedures and interventions, including (a) surgery for hyperhidrosis (Cina, Robertson, Young, Cartier, & Clase, 2006); (b) hip replacement surgery (personal communication, S. M. Edworthy); (c) supportive-expressive group psychotherapy for women living with systemic lupus erythematosus (Edworthy et al., 2003) and for lesbians with primary breast cancer (Fobair et al., 2002); (d) patient education to increase self-management of chronic disease (Co, Jaramillo, Grimsley, Jacob, & Reich, 2004); (e) behavior therapy for acrophobia (i.e., fear of heights) and for pathological height vertigo (Whitney et al., 2005); (f) nurse coaching to promote adoption of health-promoting behavior in "older" adults (i.e., age >60 years) (Bennett et al., 2005); (g) nurse-assisted home care that emphasizes a collaborative patient-role in chronic obstructive pulmonary disease (Coultas, Frederick, Barnett, Singh, &

Table 5.1. Descriptive Statistics for 36 Chronic Disease Groups: Illness Intrusiveness Ratings Scale

Patient Population	N	Total Score	Subscale		
			Relationships and Personal Development	Intimacy	Instrumental
Antibiotic-Resistant-Infected Hospital Inpatients	69	43.0 (18.03) 38.6,47.3	3.2 (1.62) 2.8,3.6	1.9 (1.78) 1.5,2.4	4.2 (1.68) 3.8,4.6
Anxiety Disorders	135	55.3 (18.49) 52.2,59.0	4.2 (1.43) 3.9,4.4	3.9 (2.24) 3.6,4.3	4.6 (1.62) 4.3,4.8
Biliary Cirrhosis	88	32.2 (18.42) 28.3,36.1	2.3 (1.45) 2.0,2.6	2.3 (1.86) 1.9,2.7	2.8 (1.68) 2.4,3.1
Bipolar Depression	68	43.8 (19.81) 39.0,48.6	3.2 (1.46) 2.9,3.6	3.2 (2.17) 2.7,3.7	3.6 (1.90) 3.1,4.0
Cancer, Breast	111	31.1 (17.92) 27.7,34.5	2.0 (1.18) 1.8,2.2	2.3 (1.81) 2.0,2.7	3.0 (1.92) 2.6,3.3
Cancer, Cervical	45	36.5 (20.33) 30.4,42.6	2.3 (1.48) 1.9,2.8	2.5 (1.91) 2.0,3.1	3.6 (2.08) 3.0,4.2
Cancer, Gastrointestinal	107	39.6 (19.19) 35.9,43.3	2.5 (1.49) 2.2,2.8	3.1 (2.05) 2.7,3.5	3.8 (1.88) 3.4,4.1
Cancer, Head and Neck	336	25.9 (14.17) 24.4,27.4	1.6 (0.91) 1.5,1.7	1.7 (1.38) 1.6,1.9	2.5 (1.69) 2.3,2.7
Cancer, Hematologic Cancer (Bone Marrow Transplant)	177	43.4 (17.62) 40.8,46.1	2.6 (1.33) 2.4,2.8	3.1 (1.95) 2.8,3.3	4.5 (1.88) 4.2,4.8
Cancer, Lung	99	36.8 (18.54) 33.1,40.5	2.3 (1.36) 2.1,2.6	2.6 (1.82) 2.2,2.9	3.6 (2.01) 3.2,4.0
Cancer, Lymphoma	116	34.8 (17.68) 31.5,38.0	2.3 (1.40) 2.0,2.5	2.4 (1.75) 2.1,2.8	3.3 (1.91) 3.0,3.7

Table 5.1. CONTINUED

Patient Population	N	Total Score	Subscale		
			Relationships and Personal Development	Intimacy	Instrumental
Cancer, Prostate	120	26.4 (10.93) 24.4,28.3	1.5 (0.69) 1.4,1.6	3.3 (1.71) 3.0,3.6	2.2 (1.39) 1.9,2.4
Cardiac, Angioplasty	288	29.8 (14.18) 28.1,31.4	2.0 (1.25) 1.9,2.2	2.1 (1.57) 2.0,2.3	2.8 (1.35) 2.6,2.91
Cardiac, Atrial Fibrillation	288	29.8 (14.18) 28.1,31.4	2.0 (1.25) 1.9,2.2	2.1 (1.57) 2.0,2.3	2.8 (1.35) 2.6,2.9
Epilepsy	145	38.8 (19.66) 35.6,42.0	2.8 (1.53) 2.5,3.0	2.7 (1.99) 2.4,3.0	3.6 (2.01) 3.3,4.0
End-Stage Renal Disease Hemodialysis	178	41.8 (15.67) 39.5,44.1	2.2 (1.20) 2.0,2.4	3.1 (2.13) 2.8,3.4	4.4 (1.75) 4.2,4.7
Fibromyalgia	103	54.8 (17.44) 51.4,58.2	3.7 (1.44) 3.4,4.0	4.1 (2.24) 3.7,4.6	5.3 (1.49) 5.0,5.6
Hepatitis C-Infected (asymptomatic)	95	42.6 (20.65) 38.4,47.0	2.9 (1.51) 2.6,3.2	3.3 (2.02) 2.9,3.7	3.8 (2.00) 3.4,4.2
Human Immunodeficiency Virus-Infected	85	55.2 (18.26) 51.3,59.2	3.6 (1.51) 3.3,3.9	4.9 (2.16) 4.4,5.3	5.0 (1.57) 4.7,5.3
Hyperhydrosis	223	16.2 (24.05) 13.0,19.3	1.3 (1.98) 1.1,1.6	1.1 (1.84) 0.8,1.3	1.3 (2.02) 1.0,1.6
Insomnia	2,345	34.9 (17.63) 34.2,35.7	2.5 (1.39) 2.5,2.6	2.8 (1.85) 2.7,2.9	2.9 (1.59) 2.8,3.0
Irritable Bowel Syndrome	114	41.2 (18.59) 37.8,44.7	2.8 (1.45) 2.5,3.0	3.0 (2.11) 2.6,3.4	3.4 (1.63) 3.1,3.7
Multiple Sclerosis	174	44.8 (20.13) 41.8,47.9	3.2 (1.62) 3.0,3.5.	2.9 (2.66) 2.5,3.3	4.3 (1.79) 4.1,4.6

(continued)

Table 5.1. CONTINUED

Patient Population	N	Total Score	Subscale		
			Relationships and Personal Development	Intimacy	Instrumental
Non-Insulin-Dependent Diabetes Mellitus	178	27.3 (14.09) 25.2,29.4	1.7 (1.07) 1.5,1.8	1.8 (1.49) 1.6,2.0	2.4 (1.44) 2.2,2.6
Osteoarthritis	649	42.2 (18.75) 40.7,43.6	2.8 (1.56) 2.7,2.9	3.5 (2.81) 3.3,3.7	34.0 (1.65) 3.8,4.1
Progressive Renal Failure	289	30.5 (13.98) 28.9,32.1	1.7 (1.03) 1.6,1.8	2.2 (1.63) 2.0,2.3	3.0 (1.66) 2.8,3.2
Rheumatoid Arthritis	809	42.1 (16.83) 40.9,43.2	2.8 (1.42) 2.7,2.9	3.1 (2.33) 2.9,3.2	4.2 (1.58) 4.1,4.3
Schizophrenia	78	50.5 (16.68) 46.8,54.3	3.7 (1.46) 3.3,4.0	3.7 (2.26) 3.2,4.2	4.3 (1.62) 3.9,4.7
Sjögren's Syndrome	82	39.4 (17.24) 35.7,43.2	2.5 (1.41) 2.3,2.9	2.6 (1.96) 2.2,3.0	3.8 (1.77) 3.4,4.1
Spasmodic Dysphonia	42	35.2 (15.89) 30.3,40.2	3.0 (1.29) 2.6,3.4	1.9 (1.61) 1.4,2.4	2.8 (1.66) 2.3,3.3
Systemic Lupus Erythematosus	457	38.8 (19.88) 37.0,41.0	2.5 (1.50) 2.4,2.7	2.9 (2.00) 2.7,3.1	3.8 (1.92) 3.6,4.0
Transplant, Heart	54	43.5 (17.07) 39.0,48.1	2.8 (1.31) 2.5,3.2	3.4 (2.23) 2.8,4.0	4.0 (1.69) 3.5,4.5
Transplant, Liver	134	33.1 (15.58) 30.5,36.0	2.2 (1.22) 2.0,2.4	2.5 (1.66) 2.2,2.8	3.0 (1.76) 2.7,3.3
Transplant, Lung	74	35.3 (16.58) 31.6,39.3	2.2 (1.15) 2.0,2.5	2.7 (1.84) 2.3,3.1	3.0 (2.01) 3.0,4.0
Transplant, Renal	357	38.7 (18.42) 36.7,40.6	2.3 (1.39) 2.2,2.5	3.2 (2.01) 3.0,3.5	3.7 (1.87) 3.5,3.9

Table 5.1. CONTINUED

Patient Population	N	Total Score	Subscale		
			Relationships and Personal Development	Intimacy	Instrumental
Ulcerative Colitis	142	27.6 (16.62) 25.0,30.3	1.8 (1.14) 1.6,2.0	2.1 (1.63) 1.8,2.4	2.3 (1.54) 2.1,3.0

NOTE: Cell entries report group means, (standard deviations), and 95% confidence intervals (lower bound, upper bound).
SOURCE: Devins, G. M. (2010). Using the Illness Intrusiveness Ratings Scale to understand quality of life in chronic disease. *Journal of Psychosomatic Research, 68*, 591–602. Reprinted with permission from Elsevier.

Wludyka, 2005); (h) pelvic-floor muscle exercises and group support to reduce urinary incontinence following prostatectomy (Zhang, Strauss, & Siminoff, 2006); and (i) online (i.e., Internet-based) chronic disease self-management support for diverse conditions (including, arthritis, lung disease, mental-health conditions, hypertension, and type-2 diabetes; Lorig et al., 2008; Lorig, Ritter, Laurent, & Plant, 2006).

A large body of evidence supports the IIRS's *construct validity* across numerous medical conditions and treatment groups (i.e., scores behave as expected in relation to illness and treatment factors; scores conform to the other premises proposed by the illness intrusiveness theoretical framework). These findings are reviewed in the main body of this chapter in relation to the validity of the illness intrusiveness theoretical framework.

IIRS scores demonstrate considerable stability when the circumstances of the medical condition and treatment do not change. Total IIRS scores' *test–retest reliability* is high when illness and treatment remain stable: for example, $r_{tt} = .89$ over one day, .51 over one week, and .78 over one month in schizophrenia (Bettazzoni et al., 2008); .80 and .85 over 9-month intervals and .80 over 18 months in multiple sclerosis (Devins et al., 1993); and .79 over a three-month interval in ESRD (Devins, Mandin, et al., 1990). Coefficient kappa = .89 over four weeks in hyperhidrosis (Cina & Clase, 1999).

Evidence in support of the IIRS's *concurrent validity* includes observations that self-reported illness intrusiveness correlates significantly with ratings provided by others who are familiar with the affected person in diverse contexts, including nephrology health-service providers (Devins et al., 1983) and significant others (e.g., spouses) in ESRD (Devins et al., 1983) and in hyperhidrosis (Cina & Clase, 1999). People with heart failure who report physical limitations in work, hobbies, relationships with family and friends, and intimate relationships report significantly higher illness intrusiveness than those who do not (LeMaire et al., 2012). In spondyloarthritis, satisfaction with social-role participation is associated with illness intrusiveness (Davison et al., 2011).

Discriminant validity of the IIRS is supported by observations that it does not correlate significantly with defensive response styles as indicated by the Minnesota Multiphasic Personality Inventory *K* Scale (Binik et al., 1990; Devins et al., 1983; Devins, Mandin, et al., 1990), social-desirability responding, as indicated by the Marlow-Crowne Social Desirability Scale (Beanlands et al., 2003; Bettazzoni et al., 2008), or with cognitive impairment, as represented by the Mini-Mental State Exam (Devins et al., 1996). A Korean study of people undergoing treatment for coronary artery disease reported that IIRS scores were not systematically related to personality (type D personality; Son, 2009). Further evidence in support of discriminant validity is the fact that the IIRS correlates significantly but moderately with measures of perceived control in epilepsy (Poochikian-Sarkissian et al., 2008a), ESRD (Devins et al., 1983), and multiple sclerosis (Devins et al., 1993). Illness intrusiveness correlates moderately and inversely with perceived control over disease and treatment in ESRD (Devins et al., 1983) and in epilepsy (Poochikian-Sarkissian et al., 2008b).

Factor Structure and Factorial Invariance

The IIRS comprises three subscales: (a) *Relationships and Personal Development* (tapping passive recreation, family relations, other social relations, self-expression/self-improvement, religious expression, and community and civic involvement); (b) *Intimacy* (tapping relationship with spouse and sex life); and (c) *Instrumental life domains* (tapping health, work, financial situation, and active recreation). The subscales were derived by exploratory and confirmatory factor analyses based on the responses of 5,671 people sampled from eight patient groups: rheumatoid arthritis; osteoarthritis; systemic lupus erythematosus; multiple sclerosis; insomnia; ESRD (treated by maintenance dialysis); renal transplant recipients (i.e., ESRD); and heart, liver, and lung transplant recipients. The three subscales were initially extracted by exploratory factor (principal components) analysis applied to a random sample of 400 people (50 from each of the eight groups). A subsequent multisample confirmatory factor analysis applied to a random sample of 2,100 other respondents from seven of these groups (there was an insufficient number of people with multiple sclerosis) indicated an excellent fit to the hypothesized measurement model (Devins et al., 2001). Research in diverse cancer groups corroborated these findings: Multisample confirmatory factor analysis indicated that the hypothesized three-factor measurement model exhibited strong factorial invariance across four common cancer groups (gastrointestinal, head and neck, lymphoma, and lung cancer) and that this was true both for women and for men (Mah, Bezjak, Loblaw, Gotowiec, & Devins, 2011a). Confirmatory factor analysis replicated the three-factor solution in a sample of young adults with allergies and asthma (Molzon et al., 2013). The three-factor measurement model has been replicated by principal-components analysis in a Canadian sample of people with diverse anxiety disorders (e.g., panic disorder with or without agoraphobia, obsessive-compulsive disorder, social phobia, generalized anxiety, disorder, and others; Bieling, Rowa, Antony, Summerfeldt, & Swinson, 2001), aged people with heart failure (LeMaire et al., 2012), and a sample of Korean people affected by "diabetes, hypertension and/or arthritis" who completed a Korean translation of the IIRS (Chae, Kim, & Yoo, 2010).

Translations and Alternative Instruments

The IIRS has been translated into languages other than English. These include: Chinese (Li et al., 2011), French (Coutu-Wakulczyk, Woodend, & Devins, 2002), Hungarian (Novak et al., 2005), and Korean (Chae et al., 2010). Translated IIRS scales boast strong psychometric properties. Most, but not all (Li et al., 2011), demonstrate a good fit for the original three-factor measurement model. Unpublished translations are available in German and Spanish.

Some scales, developed in English, overlap considerably with the IIRS or address highly similar foci. These were developed for specific patient populations: for example, cancer (Eiser, Havermans, Craft, & Kernahan, 1995; Trask et al., 2001); cancer caregivers (Cameron, Franche, Cheung, & Stewart, 2002); multiple sclerosis (Osborne et al., 2006); chronic pain (Osborne et al., 2006; Tait, 1990); renal failure (Shidler, Peterson, & Kimmel, 1998; Tawney et al., 2000); rheumatoid arthritis (Katz, 1995; Katz & Yelin, 1994, 1995; Smith, Wallston, & Dwyer, 1995); type 2 diabetes (Talbot et al., 1999); systemic lupus erythematosus (Katz, Morris, Trupin, Yazdany, & Yelin, 2008); and children affected by juvenile rheumatic disease and their parents (Bonner et al., 2015; Fedele et al., 2012). The Physical Symptom Experience Tool (described by (Doorenbos et al., 2005)) taps the extent to which common cancer symptoms (e.g., vomiting, mouth sores, difficulty breathing, and pain) interfere with daily activities (this instrument also includes items that overlap with psychological problems, such as concentration problems, insomnia, and fatigue). The *Impact* subscale of the Disability Centrality Scale (Bishop et al., 2008) taps illness intrusiveness into 10 empirically identified, central life domains (all but one of which overlap with the IIRS) and employs a similar 7-point rating scale. The instrument includes three additional subscales that address the *importance* of each life domain, *satisfaction* with each domain, and the respondent's anticipated ability to exert *change* over each domain. A disadvantage, however, is that one (the non-IIRS) item involves "mental health (e.g., emotional well-being, happiness, enjoyment of life)," which overlaps with subjective well-being. Instruments (such as the Physical Symptom Experience Tool and the Disability Central Instrument) whose item content overlaps with subjective well-being, are compromised by the problem of measurement redundancy (Meehl, 1978), which threatens internal validity when they are employed to test hypotheses about illness intrusiveness as a determinant of subjective well-being. In general, findings based on alternative measures of illness intrusiveness have generated findings consistent with the illness intrusiveness theoretical framework.

ILLNESS INTRUSIVENESS RATINGS SCALE

The following items ask about how much your illness and/or its treatment interfere with different aspects of your life. *PLEASE CIRCLE THE ONE NUMBER THAT BEST DESCRIBES YOUR CURRENT LIFE SITUATION.* If an item is not applicable, please circle the number one (1) to indicate that this aspect of your life is not affected very much. Please do not leave any item unanswered. Thank you.

How much does your illness and/or its treatment interfere with your:

1. **HEALTH**
   Not Very Much   1   2   3   4   5   6   7   *Very Much*

2. **DIET** (i.e., the things you eat and drink)
   Not Very Much   1   2   3   4   5   6   7   *Very Much*

3. **WORK**
   Not Very Much   1   2   3   4   5   6   7   *Very Much*

4. **ACTIVE RECREATION** (e.g., sports)
   Not Very Much   1   2   3   4   5   6   7   *Very Much*

5. **PASSIVE RECREATION** (e.g., reading, listening to music)
   Not Very Much   1   2   3   4   5   6   7   *Very Much*

6. **FINANCIAL SITUATION**
   Not Very Much   1   2   3   4   5   6   7   *Very Much*

7. **RELATIONSHIP WITH YOUR SPOUSE** (girlfriend or boyfriend if not married)
   Not Very Much   1   2   3   4   5   6   7   *Very Much*

8. **SEX LIFE**
   Not Very Much   1   2   3   4   5   6   7   *Very Much*

9. **FAMILY RELATIONS**
   Not Very Much   1   2   3   4   5   6   7   *Very Much*

10. **OTHER SOCIAL RELATIONS**
    Not Very Much   1   2   3   4   5   6   7   *Very Much*

11. **SELF-EXPRESSION/SELF-IMPROVEMENT**
    Not Very Much   1   2   3   4   5   6   7   *Very Much*

12. **RELIGIOUS EXPRESSION**
    Not Very Much   1   2   3   4   5   6   7   *Very Much*

13. **COMMUNITY AND CIVIC INVOLVEMENT**
    Not Very Much   1   2   3   4   5   6   7   *Very Much*

REFERENCES

Aarstad, H. J., Aarstad, A. K., Heimdal, J. H., & Olofsson, J. (2005). Mood, anxiety and sense of humor in head and neck cancer patients in relation to disease stage, prognosis and quality of life. *Acta Oto-Laryngologica, 125*(5), 557–565.

Abraido-Lanza, A. F. (1997). Latinas with arthritis: Effects of illness, role identity, and competence on psychological well-being. *American Journal of Community Psychology, 25*(5), 601–627.

Abraido-Lanza, A. F., & Revenson, T. A. (2006). Illness intrusion and psychological adjustment to rheumatic diseases: A social identity framework. *Arthritis & Rheumatism, 55*(2), 224–232.

Alloy, L. B. (1992). Illusion of control: Invulnerability to negative affect and depressive symptoms after laboratory and natural stressors. *Journal of Abnormal Psychology, 101*, 234–245.

Anastasi, A. (1988). *Psychological testing* (6th ed.). New York: Macmillan.

Arroll, M. A., Attree, E. A., Cha, Y.-H., & Dancey, C. P. (2016). The relationship between symptom severity, stigma, illness intrusiveness and depression in Mal de Debarquement Syndrome. *Journal of Health Psychology, 21*(7), 1339–1350. doi:10.1177/1359105314553046

Arroll, M. A., Dancey, C. P., Attree, E. A., Smith, S., & James, T. (2012). People with symptoms of Ménière's disease: The relationship between illness intrusiveness, illness uncertainty, dizziness handicap, and depression. *Otology & Neurotology, 33*, 816–823.

Avis, N. E., Levine, B., Naughton, M. J., Case, D. L., Naftalis, E., & Zee, K. J. (2012). Explaining age-related differences in depression following breast cancer diagnosis and treatment. *Breast Cancer Research and Treatment, 136*(2), 581–591.

Avis, N. E., Levine, B., Naughton, M. J., Case, L. D., Naftalis, E., & Zee, K. J. (2013). Age-related longitudinal changes in depressive symptoms following breast cancer diagnosis and treatment. *Breast Cancer Research and Treatment, 139*(1), 199–206.

Badger, T., Segrin, C., Figueredo, A., Harrington, J., Sheppard, K., Passalacqua, S., . . . Bishop, M. (2011). Psychosocial interventions to improve quality of life in prostate cancer survivors and their intimate or family partners. *Quality of Life Research, 20*(6), 833–844. doi:10.1007/s11136-010-9822-2

Bandura, A. (1986). *Social foundations of thought and action: A social cognitive theory* (1st ed.). Englewood Cliffs, NJ: Prentice Hall.

Beanlands, H. J., Lipton, J. H., McCay, E. A., Schimmer, A. D., Elliott, M. E., Messner, H. A., & Devins, G. M. (2003). Self-concept as a "BMT patient," illness intrusiveness, and engulfment in allogeneic bone marrow transplant recipients. *Journal of Psychosomatic Research, 55*(5), 419–425.

Beata, N., & Reka, L. M. (2012). Specifikus eletminoseg-jellemzok egeszsegpszichologiai szempontu vizsgalata gyulladasos belbetegsegben szenvedo betegek koreben [Specific quality of life factors in patients with inflammatory bowel disease]. *Orvosi Hetilap, 153*(38), 1511–1519.

Bedi, M., & Devins, G. M. (2016). Cultural considerations for South Asian women with breast cancer. *Journal of Cancer Survivorship, 10*(1), 31–50.

Bennett, J. A., Perrin, N. A., Hanson, G., Bennett, D., Gaynor, W., Flaherty-Robb, M., . . . Potempa, K. (2005). Healthy aging demonstration project: Nurse coaching for behavior change in older adults. *Research in Nursing and Health, 28*, 187–197.

Bettazzoni, M., Zipursky, R. B., Friedland, J., & Devins, G. M. (2008). Illness intrusiveness and subjective well-being in schizophrenia. *Journal of Nervous and Mental Disease, 196*(11), 798–805.

Bieling, P. J., Rowa, K., Antony, M. M., Summerfeldt, L. J., & Swinson, R. P. (2001). Factor structure of the illness intrusiveness rating scale in patients diagnosed with anxiety disorders. *Journal of Psychopathology and Behavioral Assessment, 23*(4), 223–230.

Binik, Y. M., Chowanec, G. D., & Devins, G. M. (1990). Marital role strain, illness intrusiveness, and their impact on marital and individual adjustment in end-stage renal disease. *Psychology & Health, 4*, 245–257.

Binik, Y. M., & Devins, G. M. (1986). Transplant failure does not compromise quality of life in end-stage renal disease. *International Journal of Psychiatry in Medicine, 16*, 281–292.

Bishop, M. (2005). Quality of life and psychosocial adaptation to chronic illness and acquired disability: A conceptual and theoretical synthesis. *Journal of Rehabilitation, 71*(2), 5–13.

Bishop, M., Frain, M. P., & Tschopp, M. K. (2008). Self-management, perceived control, and subjective quality of life in multiple sclerosis: An exploratory study. *Rehabilitation Counseling Bulletin, 52*(1), 45–56.

Bishop, M., Stenhoff, D. M., & Shepard, L. (2007). Psychosocial adaptation and quality of life in multiple sclerosis: Assessment of the disability centrality model. *The Journal of Rehabilitation, 73*(1), 3–12.

Bonner, M. S., Ramsey, R. R., Ryan, J. L., Fedele, D. A., Mullins, L. L., Wagner, J. L., ... Chaney, J. M. (2015). Examination of parent–child adjustment in juvenile rheumatic diseases using depression-specific indices of parent and youth functioning. *Journal of Child Health Care, 19*(1), 63–72.

Cameron, J. I., Franche, R. L., Cheung, A. M., & Stewart, D. E. (2002). Lifestyle interference and emotional distress in family caregivers of advanced cancer patients. *Cancer, 94*, 521–527.

Carr, F. N., Nicassio, P. M., Ishimori, M. L., Moldovan, I., Katsaros, E., Torralba, K., ... Weisman, M. H. (2011). Depression predicts self-reported disease activity in systemic lupus erythematosus. *Lupus, 20*(1), 80–84. doi:10.1177/0961203310378672

Carter, J. C., Bewell, C., & Devins, G. M. (2008). Illness intrusiveness in anorexia nervosa. *Journal of Psychosomatic Research, 64*, 519–526.

Chae, S.-M., Kim, C.-J., & Yoo, H. (2010). Psychometric evaluation of the Korean version of the Adapted Illness Intrusiveness Rating Scale. *Asian Nursing Research, 4*(4), 194–204.

Chen, C. (2003). Revisiting the disengagement theory with differentials in the determinants of life satisfaction. *Social Indicators Research, 64*(2), 209–224.

Cina, C. S., & Clase, C. M. (1999). The Illness Intrusiveness Rating Scale: A measure of severity in individuals with hyperhidrosis. *Quality of Life Research, 8*(8), 693–698.

Cina, C. S., Robertson, S. G. W., Young, E. J. M., Cartier, B., & Clase, C. M. (2006). Effect of endoscopic sympathectomy for hyperhidrosis on quality of life using the Illness Intrusiveness Rating Scale. *Chirugia, 19*, 23–29.

Co, J., Jaramillo, B., Grimsley, S., Jacob, E. B., & Reich, L. (2004). Preliminary findings on the effectiveness of the "Healthy Living with Chronic Conditions" workshop in a managed care plan. *Managed Care Interface, 17*(6), 44–49.

Cohen, J., Cohen, P., West, S. G., & Aiken, L. S. (2003). *Applied multiple regression/correlation analysis for the behavioral sciences* (3rd ed.). Mahwah, NJ: Lawrence Erlbaum.

Coultas, D., Frederick, J., Barnett, B., Singh, G., & Wludyka, P. (2005). A randomized trial of two types of nurse-assisted home care for patients with COPD. *Chest, 128*(4), 2017–2024.

Coutu-Wakulczyk, G., Woodend, K., & Devins, G. M. (2002). Echelle d'evaluation de l'intrusion de la maladie: contribution a validation de la version francaise [Validation of a French-language version of the Illness Intrusiveness Ratings Scale]. *RSI: Recherche en Soins Infermiere, 68*, 42–49.

Dancey, C. P., & Friend, J. (2008). Symptoms, impairment and illness intrusiveness: Their relationship with depression in women with CFS/ME. *Psychology and Health, 23*(8), 983–999.

Dancey, C. P., Hutton-Young, S. A., Moye, S., & Devins, G. M. (2002). Perceived stigma, illness intrusiveness and quality of life in men and women with irritable bowel syndrome. *Psychology, Health & Medicine, 7*(4), 381–395.

Davison, A. M., Palaganas, M. P., Badley, E. M., Gladman, D. D., Inman, R. D., & Gignac, M. A. (2011). Measuring participation in people with spondyloarthritis using the social role participation questionnaire. *Annals of the Rheumatic Diseases, 70*(10), 1765–1769.

DeCoster, V. A., Killian, T., & Rossler, R. T. (2013). Diabetes intrusiveness and wellness among elders: A test of the illness intrusiveness model. *Educational Gerontology, 39*(6), 371–385.

Depp, C. A., Stricker, J. L., Zagorsky, D., Goodale, L. C., Eyler, L. T., Patterson, T. L., . . . Jeste, D. V. (2009). Disability and self-management practices of people with bipolar disorder: A web-based survey. *Community Mental Health Journal, 45*(3), 179–187.

Devins, G. M. (1989). Enhancing personal control and minimizing illness intrusiveness. In N. G. Kutner, D. D. Cardenas, & J. D. Bower (Eds.), *Maximizing rehabilitation in chronic renal disease* (1st ed., pp. 109–136). New York: PMA.

Devins, G. M. (1991). Illness intrusiveness and the psychosocial impact of end-stage renal disease. In M. A. Hardy, J. Kiernan, A. H. Kutscher, L. Cahill, & A. I. Bevenitsky (Eds.), *Psychosocial aspects of end-stage renal disease: Issues of our times* (pp. 83–102). New York: Haworth Press.

Devins, G. M. (1994). Illness intrusiveness and the psychosocial impact of lifestyle disruptions in chronic life-threatening disease. *Advances in Renal Replacement Therapy, 1*(3), 251–263.

Devins, G. M. (1999). Culturally informed psychosomatic research. *Journal of Psychosomatic Research, 46*(6), 519–524.

Devins, G. M. (2006). Psychologically meaningful activity, illness intrusiveness, and quality of life in rheumatic diseases. *Arthritis & Rheumatism, 55*(2), 172–174.

Devins, G. M. (2010). Using the Illness Intrusiveness Ratings Scale to understand health-related quality of life in chronic disease. *Journal of Psychosomatic Research, 68*(6), 591–602.

Devins, G. M., Armstrong, S. J., Mandin, H., Paul, L. C., Hons, R. B., Burgess, E. D., . . . Buckle, S. (1990). Recurrent pain, illness intrusiveness, and quality of life in end-stage renal disease. *Pain, 42*, 279–285.

Devins, G. M., Beanlands, H., Mandin, H., & Paul, L. C. (1997). Psychosocial impact of illness intrusiveness moderated by self-concept and age in end-stage renal disease. *Health Psychology, 16*(6), 529–538.

Devins, G. M., Bezjak, A., Mah, K., Loblaw, D. A., & Gotowiec, A. (2006). Context moderates illness-induced lifestyle disruptions across life domains: A test of the illness intrusiveness theoretical framework in six common cancers. *Psycho-Oncology, 15*(3), 221–233.

Devins, G. M., & Binik, Y. M. (1996a). Facilitating coping in chronic physical illness. In M. Zeidner & N. S. Endler (Eds.), *Handbook of coping* (pp. 640–696). New York: John Wiley.

Devins, G. M., & Binik, Y. M. (1996b). Predialysis psychoeducational interventions: Establishing collaborative relationships between health service providers and recipients. *Seminars in Dialysis, 9*(1), 51–55.

Devins, G. M., Binik, Y. M., Gorman, P., Dattel, M., McCloskey, B., Oscar, G., & Briggs, J. (1982). Perceived self-efficacy, outcome expectancies, and negative mood states in end-stage renal disease. *Journal of Abnormal Psychology, 91*, 241–244.

Devins, G. M., Binik, Y. M., Hutchinson, T. A., Hollomby, D. J., Barre, P. E., & Guttmann, R. D. (1983). The emotional impact of end-stage renal disease: Importance of patients' perceptions of intrusiveness and control. *International Journal of Psychiatry in Medicine, 13*(4), 327–343.

Devins, G. M., Cameron, J. I., & Edworthy, S. M. (2000). Chronic disabling disease. In C. L. Radnitz (Ed.), *Cognitive-behavioral interventions for persons with disabilities* (pp. 105–140). Northvale, NJ: Jason Aronson.

Devins, G. M., Dion, R., Pelletier, L. G., Shapiro, C. M., Abbey, S. E., Raiz, L., . . . Edworthy, S. M. (2001). The structure of lifestyle disruptions in chronic disease: A confirmatory factor analysis of the illness intrusiveness ratings scale. *Medical Care, 39*, 1097–1104.

Devins, G. M., Edworthy, S. M., & Group, A. L. S. M. R. (2000). Illness intrusiveness explains race-related quality-of-life differences among women with systemic lupus erythematosus. *Lupus, 9*(7), 534–541.

Devins, G. M., Edworthy, S. M., Guthrie, N. G., & Martin, L. (1992). Illness intrusiveness in rheumatoid arthritis: Differential impact on depressive symptoms over the adult lifespan. *Journal of Rheumatology, 19*, 709–715.

Devins, G. M., Edworthy, S. M., Paul, L. C., Mandin, H., Seland, T. P., Klein, G. M., & Shapiro, C. M. (1992). Restless sleep, illness intrusiveness, and depressive symptoms in three chronic illness conditions: Rheumatoid arthritis, end-stage renal disease, and multiple sclerosis. *Journal of Psychosomatic Research, 37*, 163–170.

Devins, G. M., Gupta, A., Cameron, J. I., Woodend, K., Mah, K., & Gladman, D. (2009). Cultural syndromes and age moderate the emotional impact of illness intrusiveness in rheumatoid arthritis. *Rehabilitation Psychology, 54*(1), 33–44.

Devins, G. M., Mandin, H., Hons, R. B., Burgess, E. D., Klassen, J., Taub, K., . . . Buckle, S. (1990). Illness intrusiveness and quality of life in end-stage renal disease: Comparison and stability across treatment modalities. *Health Psychology, 9*, 117–142.

Devins, G. M., Martino, R., Ringash, J., Haerle, S., Shaw, S. M., Gomes, A., . . . Irish, J. C. (2014). *MaxLife: Minimizing illness intrusiveness to get the most from life*. Unpublished manuscript, University of Toronto.

Devins, G. M., Mendelssohn, D. C., Barre, P. E., & Binik, Y. M. (2003). Predialysis psychoeductional intervention and coping styles influence time to dialysis in chronic kidney disease. *American Journal of Kidney Diseases, 42*(4), 693–703.

Devins, G. M., Otto, K. J., Irish, J. C., & Rodin, G. M. (2015). Head and neck cancer. In J. C. Holland, W. S. Breitbart, P. N. Butow, P. B. Jacobsen, M. J. Loscalzo, & R. McCorkle (Eds.), *Psycho-Oncology* (3rd ed., pp. 92–97). New York: Oxford University Press.

Devins, G. M., Payne, A. Y. M., Lebel, S., Mah, K., Lee, R. N. F., Irish, J. C., . . . Rodin, G. M. (2013). The burden of stress in head and neck cancer. *Psycho-Oncology, 22,* 668–676.

Devins, G. M., Seland, T. P., Klein, G. M., Edworthy, S. M., & Saary, M. J. (1993). Stability and determinants of psychosocial well-being in multiple sclerosis. *Rehabilitation Psychology, 38,* 11–26.

Devins, G. M., & Shnek, Z. M. (2000). Multiple sclerosis. In R. G. Frank & T. R. Elliot (Eds.), *Handbook of rehabilitation psychology* (pp. 163–184). Washington, DC: American Psychological Association.

Devins, G. M., Stam, H. J., & Koopmans, J. P. (1994). Psychosocial impact of laryngectomy mediated by perceived stigma and illness intrusiveness. *Canadian Journal of Psychiatry, 39*(10), 608–616.

Devins, G. M., Styra, R., O'Connor, P., Gray, T., Seland, T. P., Klein, G. M., & Shapiro, C. M. (1996). Psychosocial impact of illness intrusiveness moderated by age in multiple sclerosis. *Psychology Health & Medicine, 1*(2), 179–191.

Devins, G. M., Wong, J. C., Payne, A. Y. M., Lebel, S., Lee, R. N. F., Mah, K., . . . Rodin, G. (2015). Distancing, self-esteem, and subjective well-being in head and neck cancer. *Psycho-Oncology, 24*(11), 1506–1513. doi:10.1002/pon.3760

Devins, G. M., Wong, J. C., Payne, A. Y. M., Mah, K., Lebel, S., Lee, R. N. F., . . . Rodin, G. (2012). Disease specific self-concept, protective distancing, and subjective well-being in head and neck cancer. Manuscript submitted for publication. *Psycho-Oncology.*

DiNapoli, E. A., Cummings, J., Petersen, N. J., & Cully, J. A. (2015). Mediating role of maladaptive coping on race and illness intrusiveness in chronically ill older veterans. *Military Behavioral Health, 3*(4), 266–273.

Doorenbos, A., Given, B., Given, C., Verbitsky, N., Cimprich, B., & McCorkle, R. (2005). Reducing symptom limitations: A cognitive behavioral intervention randomized trial. *Pscho-Oncology, 14*(7), 574–584.

Edelstein, K., Coate, L., Massey, C., Jewitt, N. C., Mason, W. P., & Devins, G. M. (2016). Illness intrusiveness and subjective wellbeing in patients with glioblastoma. *Journal of Neuro-Oncology, 126*(1), 127–135.

Edworthy, S. M., Devins, G. M., & Group, P. E. S. (1999). Improving medication adherence through patient education distinguishing between appropriate and inappropriate utilization. *Journal of Rheumatology, 26,* 1793–1801.

Edworthy, S. M., Dobkin, P. L., Clarke, A. E., Da Costa, D., Dritsa, M., Fortin, P. R., . . . Devins, G. M. (2003). Group psychotherapy reduces illness intrusiveness in systemic lupus erythematosus. *Journal of Rheumatology, 30,* 1011–1016.

Eiser, C., Havermans, T., Craft, A., & Kernahan, J. (1995). Development of a measure to assess the perceived illness experience after treatment for cancer. *Archives of Disease in Childhood, 72,* 302–307.

Eskander, A., Devins, G. M., Freeman, J., Wei, A., Rotstein, L., Chauhan, N., . . . Goldstein, D. (2013). Waiting for thyroid surgery: A study of psychological morbidity and determinants of health associated with long wait times for thyroid surgery. *Laryngoscope, 123*(2), 541–547.

Fedele, D. A., Mullins, L. L., Eddington, A. R., Ryan, J. L., Junghans, A. N., & Hullmann, S. E. (2009). Health-related quality of life in college students with and without childhood-onset asthma. *Journal of Asthma, 46*(8), 835–840.

Fedele, D. A., Ryan, J. L., Ramsay, R. R., Grant, D. M., Bonner, M. S., Stermer, S. P., . . . Chaney, J. M. (2012). Utility of the Illness Intrusiveness Scale in parents of children diagnosed with juvenile rheumatic diseases. *Rehabilitation Psychology, 57*(1), 73–80.

Flanagan, J. C. (1978). A research approach to improving our quality of life. *American Psychologist, 33*, 138–147.

Fobair, P., Koopman, C., DiMiceli, S., O'Hanlan, K., Butler, L. D., Classen, C., . . . Spiegel, D. (2002). Psychosocial intervention for lesbians with primary breast cancer. *Psycho-Oncology, 11*(5), 427–438.

Franche, R. L., Abbey, S., Irvine, J., Shnek, Z. M., Grace, S. L., Devins, G. M., & Stewart, D. E. (2004). Sex differences in predictors of illness intrusiveness one year after a cardiac event. *Journal of Psychosomatic Research, 56*, 125–132.

Gerstorf, D., Röcke, C., & Lachman, M. E. (2011). Antecedent–consequent relations of perceived control to health and social support: Longitudinal evidence for between-domain associations across adulthood. *Journals of Gerontology Series B: Psychological Sciences and Social Sciences, 66B*(1), 61–71. doi:10.1093/geronb/gbq077

Gilchrist, A. C., & Creed, F. H. (1994). Depression, cognitive impairment and social stress in multiple sclerosis. *Journal of Psychosomatic Research, 38*(3), 193–201.

Goudsmit, E. M., Stouten, B., & Howes, S. (2009). Illness intrusiveness in myalgic encephalomyelitis: An exploratory study. *Journal of Health Psychology, 14*(2), 215–221.

Grant, M. M., Gil, K. M., Floyd, M. Y., & Abrams, M. (2000). Depression and functioning in relation to health care use in sickle cell disease. *Annals of Behavioral Medicine, 22*(2), 149–157.

Grob, A. (2000). Perceived control and subjective well-being across nations and across the life span. In E. Diener & E. M. Suh (Eds.), *Culture and subjective well-being* (pp. 319–339). Cambridge, MA: MIT Press.

Gutmann, D. (1995). Mastery types, development, and aging. In R. Kastenbaum (Ed.), *Encyclopedia of adult development* (pp. 311–316). Phoenix: Oryx Press.

Guyatt, G. H., Townsend, M., Berman, L. B., & Pugsley, S. O. (1987). Quality of life in patients with chronic airflow limitation. *British Journal of Diseases of the Chest, 81*(45), 45–54.

Harrison, J., Maguire, P., & Pitceathly, C. (1995). Confiding in crisis: Gender differences in pattern of confiding among cancer patients. *Social Science and Medicine, 41*(9), 1255–1260.

Helzer, E. G., & Jayawickreme, E. (2015). Control and the "Good Life." *Social Psychological and Personality Science, 6*(6), 653–660. doi:10.1177/1948550615576210

Ho, S. M., Horne, D. J., & Szer, J. (2002). The adaptation of patients during the hospitalization period of bone marrow transplantation. *Journal of Clinical Psychology in Medical Settings, 9*(2), 167–175.

Hogg, R. S., Craib, K. J., Pi, D., Lee, S. S., Minuk, G. Y., Shapiro, C. M., . . . O'Shaughnessy, M. V. (2003). Health and socioeconomic status differences among antibody hepatitis C positive and negative transfusion recipients: 1986–1990. *Canadian Journal of Public Health, 94*(2), 130–134.

Holtzman, S., Abbey, S. E., Stewart, D. E., & Ross, H. J. (2010). Pain after heart transplantation: Prevalence and implications for quality of life. *Psychosomatics, 51*(3), 230–236.

Holtzman, S., Adcock, L., Dubay, D. A., Therapondos, G., Kashfi, A., Greemwood, S., . . . Abbey, S. E. (2009). Financial, vocational, and interpersonal impact of living liver donation. *Liver Transplantation, 15*(11), 1435–1442.

Hossain, J., Ahmad, P., Reinish, L. W., Kayumov, L., Hossain, N. K., & Shapiro, C. M. (2005). Subjective fatigue and subjective sleepiness: Two independent consequences of sleep disorders? *Journal of Sleep Research, 14*(3), 245–253.

Hurlock, E. B. (1980). *Developmental psychology: A life-span approach* (5th ed.). New York: McGraw-Hill.

Kanfer, F. H., & Karoly, P. (1972). Self-control: A behavioristic excursion into the lion's den. *Behavior Therapy, 3*(3), 398–416.

Katz, P. P. (1995). The impact of rheumatoid arthritis on life activities. *Arthritis Care and Research, 8*(4), 272–278.

Katz, P. P., Morris, A., Trupin, L., Yazdany, J., & Yelin, E. (2008). Disability in valued life activities among individuals with systemic lupus erythematosus. *Arthritis & Rheumatism, 59*(4), 465–473.

Katz, P. P., & Yelin, E. H. (1994). Life activities of persons with rheumatoid arthritis with and without depressive symptoms. *Arthritis Care and Research, 7*(2), 69–77.

Katz, P. P., & Yelin, E. H. (1995). The development of depressive symptoms among women with rheumatoid arthritis. *Arthritis & Rheumatism, 38*(1), 49–56.

Kessler, R. C., McLeod, J. D., & Wethington, E. (1985). The costs of caring: A perspective on the relationship between sex and psychological distress. In I. G. Sarason & B. R. Sarason (Eds.), *Social support, theory, research and application* (pp. 491–506). Dordrecht: Martinus Nijhoff.

Kuo, C. C., Lin, C. C., & Tsai, F. M. (2014). Effectiveness of empowerment-based self-management interventions on patients with chronic metabolic diseases: A systematic review and meta-analysis. *Worldviews on Evidence-Based Nursing, 11*(5), 301–315.

Kutner, N. G., & Devins, G. M. (1998). A comparison of the quality of life reported by elderly whites and elderly blacks on dialysis. *Geriatric Nephrology and Urology, 8*(2), 77–83.

Laiteerapong, N., Karter, A. J., Liu, J. Y., Moffet, H. H., Sudore, R., Schillinger, D., . . . Huang, E. S. (2011). Correlates of quality of life in older adults with diabetes: The diabetes & aging study. *Diabetes Care, 34*, 1749–1753.

Lazarus, R. S., & Folkman, S. (1984). *Stress, appraisal, and coping*. New York: Springer.

Lebel, S., Castonguay, M., Mackness, G., Irish, J., Bezjak, A., & Devins, G. M. (2013). The psychosocial impact of stigma in people with head and neck or lung cancer. *Psycho-Oncology, 22*(1), 140–152.

LeMaire, A., Shahane, A., Dao, T. K., Kibler, J. L., & Cully, J. A. (2012). Illness intrusiveness mediates the relationship between heart failure severity and depression in older adults. *Journal of Applied Gerontology, 31*(5), 608–621.

Leserman, J. (2003). HIV disease progression: Depression, stress, and possible mechanisms. *Biological Psychiatry, 54*(3), 295–306. doi:10.1016/S0006-3223(03)00323-8

Lewinsohn, P. M., Shaffer, M., & Libet, J. (1969). *Depression: A clinical research approach*. Eugene: University of Oregon.

Li, H., Li, W., Chen, K., Halfyard, B., Qian, B., & Wang, P. P. (2011). Validation study of the Chinese version of the Illness Intrusiveness Ratings Scale. *Journal of Psychosomatic Research, 70*(1), 67–72.

Lieberman, M. A., & Peskin, H. (1992). Adult life crises. In J. Birren, R. B. Sloane, & G. D. Cohen (Eds.), *Handbook of mental health and aging* (2nd ed., pp. 119–143). San Diego: Academic Press.

Lorig, K. (1996). Chronic disease self-management: A model for tertiary prevention. *American Behavioral Scientist, 39*(6), 676–683.

Lorig, K., & Fries, J. F. (1980). *The arthritis helpbook*. Reading MA: Addison-Wesley.

Lorig, K., Ritter, P. L., Dost, A., Plant, K., Laurent, D. D., & McNeil, I. (2008). The expert patients programme online: A 1-year study of an Internet-based self-management programme for people with long-term conditions. *Chronic Illness, 4*(4), 247–256.

Lorig, K., Ritter, P. L., Laurent, D. D., & Plant, K. (2006). Internet-based chronic disease self-management: A randomized trial. *Medical Care, 44*(11), 964–971.

Mah, K., Bezjak, A., Loblaw, D. A., Gotowiec, A., & Devins, G. M. (2011a). Confirmatory factor analysis of the Illness Intrusiveness Ratings Scale's 3-factor structure in men and women with cancer: Measurement invariance in men and women with cancer. *Rehabilitation Psychology, 56*(1), 58–66.

Mah, K., Bezjak, A., Loblaw, D. A., Gotowiec, A., & Devins, G. M. (2011b). Do ongoing lifestyle disruptions differ across cancer types after the conclusion of cancer treatment? *Journal of Cancer Survivorship, 5*(1), 18–26.

Major, B., & O'Brien, L. T. (2005). The social psychology of stigma. *Annual Review of Psychology, 56*, 393–421.

Masters, J. C., Burish, T. G., Hollon, S. D., & Rimm, D. C. (1987). *Behavior therapy: Techniques and empirical findings* (3rd ed.). San Diego: Harcourt Brace Jovanovich.

Meehl, P. E. (1978). Theoretical risks and tabular asterisks: Sir Karl, Sir Ronald, and the slow progress of soft psychology. *Journal of Consulting and Clinical Psychology, 46*, 806–834.

Molzon, E. S., Ramsey, R. R., Suorsa, K. I., Bonner, M. S., Grant, D. M., Chaney, J. M., & Mullins, L. L. (2013). Factor structure of the illness intrusiveness ratings scale in young adults with allergies and asthma. *Journal of Asthma & Allergy Educators, 4*(2), 71–76.

Monteagudo, M., Rodriguez-Blanco, T., Llagostera, M., Valero, C., Bayona, X., Ferrer, M., & Miravitlles, M. (2013). Factors associated with changes in quality of life of COPD patients: A prospective study in primary care. *Respiratory Medicine, 107*(10), 1589–1597. doi:10.1016/j.rmed.2013.05.009

Mucsi, I., Molnar, M. Z., Rethelyi, J., Vamos, E., Csepanyi, G., Tompa, G., . . . Novak, M. (2004). Sleep disorders and illness intrusiveness in patients on chronic dialysis. *Nephrology Dialysis Transplantation, 19*(7), 1815–1822.

Mullins, L. L., Chaney, J. M., Balderson, B., & Hommel, K. A. (2000). The relationship of illness uncertainty, illness intrusiveness, and asthma severity to depression in young adults with long-standing asthma. *International Journal of Rehabilitation and Health, 5*(3), 177–186.

Nerenz, D. R., & Leventhal, H. (1983). Self-regulation theory in chronic illness. In T. G. Burish & L. A. Bradley (Eds.), *Coping with chronic disease: Research and applications* (1st ed., pp. 13–37). New York: Academic Press.

Neri, L., Brancaccio, D., Rey, L., Rossa, F., Martini, A., & Andreucci, V. E. (2011). Social support from health care providers is associated with reduced illness intrusiveness in hemodialysis patients. *Clinical Nephrology, 75*(2), 125–134.

Neugarten, B. L. (1977). Personality and aging. In J. E. Birren & K. W. Schaie (Eds.), *Handbook of the psychology of aging* (1st ed., pp. 626–649). New York: Van Nostrand Reinhold.

Nolte, S., & Osborne, R. H. (2013). A systematic review of outcomes of chronic disease self-management interventions. *Quality of Life Research, 22*(7), 1805–1816. doi:http://dx.doi.org/10.1007/s11136-012-0302-8

Novak, M., Mah, K., Molnar, M., Ambrus, C., Csepanyi, G., Kovacs, A., . . . Mucsi, I. (2005). Factor structure and reliability of the Hungarian version of the Illness Intrusiveness Scale: Invariance across North American and Hungarian dialysis patients. *Journal of Psychosomatic Research, 58*(1), 103–110.

Nunnally, J. C. (1978). *Psychometric theory* (2nd ed.). New York: McGraw-Hill.

Osborne, T. L., Turner, A. P., Williams, R. M., Bowen, J. D., Hatzakis, M., Rodriguez, A., & Haselkorn, J. K. (2006). Correlates of pain interference in multiple sclerosis. *Rehabilitation Psychology, 51*(2), 166–174.

Paukert, A. L., LeMaire, A., & Cully, J. A. (2009). Predictors of depressive symptoms in older veterans with heart failure. *Aging & Mental Health., 13*(4), 601–610.

Pearlin, L. I., & Schooler, C. (1978). The structure of coping. *Journal of Health and Social Behavior, 19*, 2–21.

Poochikian-Sarkissian, S. (2005). *Illness intrusiveness, quality of life, and self-concept in epilepsy*. Toronto: University of Toronto.

Poochikian-Sarkissian, S., Sidani, S., Wennberg, R. A., & Devins, G. M. (2008a). Psychological impact of illness intrusiveness in epilepsy—comparison of treatments. *Psychology, Health & Medicine, 13*(2), 129–145.

Poochikian-Sarkissian, S., Sidani, S., Wennberg, R. A., & Devins, G. M. (2008b). Seizure freedom reduces illness intrusiveness and improves quality of life in epilepsy. *Canadian Journal of Neurological Science, 35*(280), 286.

Pronovost, A., Peng, P., & Kern, R. (2009). Telemedicine in the management of chronic pain: A cost analysis study. *Canadian Journal of Anesthesia, 56*, 590–596.

Radley, A., & Green, R. (1987). Illness as adjustment: A methodology and conceptual framework. *Sociology of Health and Illness, 9*(2), 179–207.

Sarver, N. W., & Gros, D. F. (2014). A modern behavioral treatment to address fetishism and associated functional impairment. *Clinical Case Studies, 13*(4), 336–351.

Schattner, E., Shahar, G., Lerman, S., & Shakra, M. A. (2010). Depression in systemic lupus erythematosus: The key role of illness intrusiveness and concealment of symptoms. *Psychiatry, 73*(4), 329–340.

Schimmer, A. D., Elliott, M. E., Abbey, S. E., Raiz, L., Keating, A., Beanlands, H. J., . . . Devins, G. M. (2001). Illness intrusiveness in survivors of autologous bone and marrow transplantation. *Cancer, 92*(12), 3147–3154.

Seligman, M. E. P. (1975). *Helplessness: On depression, development, and death.* San Francisco: W. H. Freeman.

Shawaryn, M. A., Schiaffino, K. M., LaRocca, N. G., & Johnston, M. V. (2002). Determinants of health-related quality of life in multiple sclerosis: The role of illness intrusiveness. *Multiple Sclerosis, 8*(4), 310–318.

Shidler, N. R., Peterson, R. A., & Kimmel, P. L. (1998). Quality of life and psychosocial relationships in patients with chronic renal insufficiency. *American Journal of Kidney Diseases, 32*(4), 557–566.

Smith, C. A., Wallston, K. A., & Dwyer, K. A. (1995). On babies and bathwater: Disease impact and negative affectivity in the self-reports of persons with rheumatoid arthritis. *Health Psychology, 14*(1), 64–73.

Snyder, S., Foley, F. W., Farrell, E., Beler, M., & Zemon, V. (2013). Psychological and physical predictors of illness intrusiveness in patients with multiple sclerosis. *Journal of the Neurological Sciences, 332*(1-2), 41–44.

Soffer-Dudek, N., Shalev, H., Shiber, A., & Shahar, G. (2011). Role of severe psychopathology in sleep-related experiences: A pilot study. *Dreaming, 21*(2), 148–156.

Sohl, S. J., Levine, B., Case, L. D., Danhauer, S. C., & Avis, N. E. (2014). Trajectories of illness intrusiveness domains following a diagnosis of breast cancer. *Health Psychology, 33*(3), 232–241.

Son, H.-M. (2009). Quality of life and illness intrusiveness by TypetD personality in the patients with coronary artery disease. *Journal of Korean Academic Nursing, 39*(3), 349–356.

Tait, R. C. (1990). The pain disability index: Psychometric properties. *Pain, 40*, 171–182.

Talbot, F., Nouwen, A., Gingras, J., Belanger, A., & Audet, J. (1999). Relations of diabetes intrusiveness and personal control to symptoms of depression among adults with diabetes. *Health Psychology, 18*(5), 537–542.

Tawney, K. W., Tawney, P. J. W., Hladik, G., Hogan, S. L., Falk, R. J., Weaver, C., . . . Lee, M. Y. (2000). The life readiness program: A physical rehabilitation program for patients on hemodialysis. *American Journal of Kidney Diseases, 36*(3), 581–591.

Taylor, S. E., Klein, L. C., Lewis, B. P., Gruenewald, T. L., Gurung, R. A. R., & Updegraff, J. A. (2000). Biobehavioral responses to stress in females: Tend-and-befriend, not fight-or-flight. *Psychological Review, 107*(3), 411–429.

Toner, B. B., & Akman, D. (2000). Gender role and irritable bowel syndrome: Literature review and hypothesis. *The American Journal of Gastroenterology, 95*(1), 11–16. doi:10.1111/j.1572-0241.2000.01698.x

Trask, P. C., Paterson, A. G., Wang, C., Hayasaka, S., Milliron, K. J., Blumberg, L. R., . . . Merajver, S. D. (2001). Cancer-specific worry interference in women attending a breast and ovarian cancer risk evaluation program: Impact on emotional distress and health functioning. *Psycho-Oncology, 10*, 349–360.

Triandis, H. C. (1995). *Individualism and collectivism*. Boulder, CO: Westview Press.

Triandis, H. C. (2000). Cultural syndromes and subjective well-being. In E. Diener & E. M. Suh (Eds.), *Culture and subjective well-being* (pp. 13–36). Cambridge, MA: MIT Press.

Turpin, K. V., Carroll, L. J., Cassidy, J. D., & Hader, W. J. (2007). Deterioration in the health-related quality of life of persons with multiple sclerosis: The possible warning signs. *Multiple Sclerosis, 13*(8), 1038–1045.

Wagner, J. L., Chaney, J. M., Hommel, K. A., Page, M. C., Mullins, L. L., White, M. M., & Jarvis, J. N. (2003). The influence of parental distress on child depressive symptoms in juvenile rheumatic diseases: The moderating effect of illness intrusiveness. *Journal of Pediatric Psychology, 28*(7), 453–462.

Whitney, S. L., Jacob, R. G., Sparto, P. J., Olshansky, E. F., Detwiler-Shostak, G., Brown, E. L., & Furman, J. M. (2005). Acrophobia and pathological height vertigo: Indications for vestibular physical therapy? *Physical Therapy, 85*(5), 443–458.

Woodend, A. K., & Devins, G. M. (2005). Gender of the care environment: Influence on recovery in women with heart disease. *Canadian Journal of Cardiovascular Nursing*, *15*(3), 21–31.

Zeidner, M., & Endler, N. S. E. (1996). *Handbook of coping: Theory, research, applications.* Edited by M. Zeidner & N. S. Endler. New York: John Wiley.

Zhang, A. Y., Strauss, G. J., & Siminoff, L. A. (2006). Intervention of urinary incontinence and quality of life outcome in prostate cancer patients. *Journal of Psychosocial Oncology*, *24*(2), 17–30.

6

Motivational Interviewing to Promote Self-Management

REBECCA PHILLIPS, ANNE HOGDEN,
AND DAVID GREENFIELD ■

Motivational interviewing is a counseling-based approach for facilitating behavior change that focuses on goal-setting and building self-efficacy (Emmons & Rollnick, 2001; McCarley, 2009; Miller, 2010). Both clinicians working specifically in mental health and those working in the broader health sector can use this approach to guide individuals with chronic health conditions to identify behaviors they want to change, their motivations for this change, and how they can achieve their goals (Emmons & Rollnick, 2001; Hettema, Steele, & Miller, 2005). Traditionally, clinicians have taken a didactic approach to educating individuals with chronic health conditions about the actions they should take, for example, exercising more and eating less (Emmons & Rollnick, 2001). The didactic approach is often met by resistance and as a result is not always effective in achieving behavior change and self-management (Emmons & Rollnick, 2001). Instead, clinicians can use motivational interviewing to engage the individual's own motivation and commitment and by doing so support individuals to recognize how self-management may help them to achieve their goals (Dellasega, Anel-Tiangco, & Gabbay, 2012).

This chapter provides an overview of motivational interviewing, highlighting how it can be used with individuals to promote self-management. The first part of the chapter provides a brief overview of what motivational interviewing is and presents evidence for its effectiveness. The chapter then discusses how motivational interviewing can be used in practice, covering the training that clinicians need, adapting it for use in healthcare settings, and using it to promote self-management in individuals with chronic health conditions. The chapter concludes with a summary of the key considerations for using motivational interviewing to promote self-management in individuals with chronic health conditions.

MOTIVATIONAL INTERVIEWING: A BRIEF OVERVIEW

William Miller developed motivational interviewing in 1983 as a style of therapy for addiction, rather than a set of treatment techniques (Miller, 1983). Instead of being based on theory, motivational interviewing stemmed from Miller's clinical experience in the field of alcohol treatment (Miller, 1996). His research found that the more a therapist confronted an individual about the need to change his or her behavior, through argument, disagreement, and emphasizing the problem, the less likely it was that behavior change would occur (Miller, 1996).

Motivational interviewing addresses ambivalence by prompting individuals to explore conflict between their current behavior and where they would like to be, including reasons for concern and arguments for change (Rollnick, Heather, & Bell, 1992). Confrontation is side-stepped to continue exploration. The goal is for the individual to identify a difference between their present behavior and desired goals (Miller, 1996). Non-directive approaches, such as reflective listening, are used to explore the individual's wants and experiences (Britt, Hudson, & Blampied, 2004; Elwyn et al., 2014). Nevertheless, motivational interviewing is directive in that it aims to explore ambivalence and barriers, so that individuals are more likely to change their behavior (Britt et al., 2004; Elwyn et al., 2014).

Guiding Principles

Motivational interviewing is described as a "collaborative, person-centered form of guiding to elicit and strengthen motivation for change" (Miller & Rollnick, 2009, p. 137). It is based on collaboration, evocation (i.e., eliciting information rather than advising and educating), and autonomy (i.e., the individual has responsibility for change; Miller & Rollnick, 2002). The clinician prompts the individual to discuss reasons for concern and change, and reinforces these in a supportive environment (Miller, 1996). Motivational interviewing has four guiding principles (Miller & Rollnick, 2002):

- *Express empathy*
  Reflective listening is the foundation of motivational interviewing. The clinician seeks to understand and accept the individual's feelings and perspectives without judgment.
- *Develop discrepancy*
  The clinician directs the person to identify a discrepancy between his or her current behavior and his or her goals. It is important that

clinicians do not pressure individuals and impose their own goals. The individual needs to articulate the argument for change.
- *Roll with resistance*
  The clinician involves the individual in active problem-solving and should not oppose resistance.
- *Support self-efficacy*
  The clinician encourages the individual's confidence in his or her ability to change.

Strategies for Using Motivational Interviewing in Practice

"Brief motivational interviewing" was developed for use by clinicians who had reported time constraints and skill inadequacies when using motivational interviewing (Britt et al., 2004; Rollnick et al., 1992). It contains a suite of eight concrete strategies (see Box 6.1), each taking 5 to 15 minutes (Rollnick et al., 1992). Clinicians select between one and three strategies to use each session, based on the individual's readiness for change. Nevertheless, doubts about the perceived usefulness of brief motivational interviewing persist. Specialists in motivational interviewing believe that this brief motivational interviewing approach is too simplistic and prescriptive, while clinicians report that it is too complex (Rollnick et al., 1992).

Clarifying the Focus of Motivational Interviewing

Motivational interviewing spread quickly across the world and disciplines, with adaptations deviating from the described overarching intent, or, as it is referred to in the literature, the motivational interviewing "spirit" (Miller & Rollnick, 2009). To assist understanding of the focus and scope of the approach, Miller and Rollnick (2009) have described 10 things that motivational interviewing is not (see Box 6.2).

THE EFFECTIVENESS OF MOTIVATIONAL INTERVIEWING

The evidence for the effectiveness of motivational interviewing is inconclusive (see Table 6.1 for a summary of recent reviews). Some studies have supportive findings, while others reveal no positive effects. The variation in findings might be due to the challenges associated with evaluating the effectiveness of motivational interviewing. Motivational interviewing is designed to be individualized, which is at odds with research protocols for evaluating efficacy that require standardized and replicable intervention protocols (Emmons & Rollnick, 2001). Also, sufficient information is not always provided on the type of intervention or how motivational interviewing has been modified for the target population (Britt et al., 2004).

Box 6.1

Brief Motivational Interviewing

Brief motivational interviewing includes the following eight strategies, ordered from those that require the lowest readiness to change to those needing the highest readiness to change (Rollnick, Heather, & Bell, 1992):

- *Opening strategy: lifestyle, stresses, and substance abuse*
  The clinician talks to the individual about his or her current lifestyle and then raises the subject of concern with an open-ended question about where the concern (e.g., substance abuse) fits in.
- *Opening strategy: health and substance abuse*
  The clinician asks an open-ended question to find out how the individual thinks the area of concern (e.g., substance abuse) affects his or her health.
- *A typical day*
  The clinician asks the individual to spend 5 to 10 minutes talking through a typical day from beginning to end. This builds rapport and helps the clinician to understand the individual's readiness for change, as well as the context of his or her behavior. The clinician avoids using terms such as "problem" or "concern."
- *The good things and the less good things*
  Similar to the previous activity, this activity builds rapport and helps assess readiness for change. The clinician prompts the individual to identify the good things and the less good things about his or her behavior without labeling them as problematic.
- *Providing information*
  At the appropriate time, the clinician asks permission to provide information (e.g., "Would you be interested in knowing more about . . .?"). After the information is provided in a neutral manner, the clinician can ask what the individual thinks about the information and how it fits with his or her current behavior.
- *The future and the present*
  The clinician asks the individual to describe how he or she would like things to be different in the future. After this is clarified, the clinician can ask the individual about what is stopping him or her from making these changes.
- *Exploring concerns*
  The clinician asks the individual to describe the concerns that he or she has about his or her current behavior.
- *Helping with decision-making*
  After identifying concerns in the previous activity, the clinician can ask the individual where this leaves him or her. In this activity, it is important that the clinician supports the individual's ability to problem-solve rather than do the problem-solving for the individual.

Box 6.2

10 Things That Motivational Interviewing Is Not

To increase clarity about the scope of motivational interviewing, Miller and Rollnick (2009) have described the following 10 things that motivational interviewing is not:

1. Motivational interviewing is not based on the transtheoretical model of change; however, they are complementary, with the transtheoretical model providing a conceptual framework for how and why change occurs and motivational interviewing offering a clinical method focused on increasing motivation.
2. Motivational interviewing is not a way to coerce people into behavior change. Motivational interviewing is about personal autonomy, and people making their own behavioral choices.
3. Motivational interviewing is not a technique: it is a communication method that requires a high level of skill.
4. Motivational interviewing is not a decisional balance. The decisional balance technique (exploring the pros and cons of change) may sometimes be used within motivational interviewing.
5. It is not essential for clinicians to provide individuals with feedback on test results to initiate discussions. It can be a useful tool to highlight where behavior change may be beneficial but is not necessary.
6. Motivational interviewing is not a form of cognitive behavior therapy. Cognitive behavior therapy is about providing individuals with something that they are missing (e.g., additional information/ support, coping skills, or education about how behavior is learned), whereas motivational interviewing is about exploring what the individual already knows.
7. Motivational interviewing is not just client-centered counseling because it is goal-oriented, working toward change.
8. Motivational interviewing is not easy; it requires a complex skill-set that clinicians can be flexible in responding to what clients say. Clinicians need practice and feedback to develop these skills, not just training.
9. Motivational interviewing is not what clinicians are already doing.
10. Motivational interviewing is not a panacea and is not needed for individuals who are ready for change.

USING MOTIVATIONAL INTERVIEWING IN PRACTICE

The previous sections in this chapter have provided an overview of what motivational interviewing is and its effectiveness. This section describes how motivational interviewing can be used in practice. It begins by outlining the training that clinicians require to successfully use motivational interviewing and is followed

Table 6.1. Effectiveness of Motivational Interviewing in Improving Outcomes

	Health Risk Factors	Self-Management	Addiction
Studies indicating that motivational interviewing is effective for improving these outcomes	• Oral health~a • Cholesterol level~a • Blood pressure~a • Body weight~a • Physical strength~a • Quality of life~a • Sedentary behavior~a	• Self-monitoring~a • Individuals' confidence and engagement in treatment~a • Self-management of medication in adults over 65 with chronic health conditions*b • Self-management of medication for chronic pain~f • Diet control, regular exercise, glucose monitoring, foot care, and prevention and treatment of hyperglycemia and hypoglycemia for individuals with Type 2 diabetes*e • Health behaviors supporting self-management of rheumatoid arthritis~g	• Smoking cessation*a,c • Substance abuse^~#a,d,h • Gambling#^~a,d • Alcohol consumption~a
Studies indicating that motivational interviewing is not effective for improving these outcomes	• Safe sex behaviors~a • Heart rate~a • Blood glucose~a • Injury prevention~a	• Healthy eating~a • Self-management of medication~a • Self-care~a	• Substance abuse*h

NOTE: Type of comparison group: *Usual care. #No treatment or waitlist. ^ Alternative active treatment such as cognitive behavioral therapy. ~A combination of the previous types of comparison groups.

[a]Lundahl et al., 2013, [b]Moral et al., 2015, [c]Lindson-Hawley, Thompson, & Begh, 2015, [d]Lundahl & Burke, 2009, [e]Song, Xu, & Sun, 2014, [f]Alperstein & Sharpe, 2016, [g]Georgopoulou, Prothero, Lempp, Galloway, & Sturt, 2015, [h]Smedslund et al., 2011.

by discussion about considerations for adapting motivational interviewing—first for promoting health in general and then more specifically in promoting self-management for individuals with chronic health conditions.

Training

The importance of formal training and supervision for developing skills in motivational interviewing has been emphasized within the self-management research literature (McGowan, 2013; Mullin, Forsberg, Savageau, & Saver, 2015). Miller and Moyers (2006) propose eight skills (see Box 6.3) that clinicians should attain in sequential order to develop their expertise in motivational interviewing.

To be effective, training needs to be followed by practice, supervision, and benchmarking of competency to consolidate skills and achieve proficiency (Emmons & Rollnick, 2001; Hall, Staiger, Simpson, Best, & Lubman, 2015; Madson, Loignon, & Lane, 2009; Miller, Yahne, Moyers, Martinez, & Pirritano, 2004; Rollnick et al., 1992). One single training is not sufficient to achieve changes to practice (Emmons & Rollnick, 2001; Miller & Mount, 2001). Therefore, considerable resources,

---

Box 6.3

Eight Sequential Steps for Developing Expertise in Motivational Interviewing

Miller and Moyers (2006) describe eight steps for developing expertise in motivational interviewing. Clinicians should develop skills in each of the following steps before moving on to the next one.

Skill 1: The spirit of motivational interviewing (an understanding of and willingness to work in this spirit).

Skill 2: OARS client-centered counseling skills (skills in empathy/ reflective listening and asking open questions [O], affirming [A], reflecting [R], and summarizing [S]).

Skill 3: Recognizing and reinforcing change talk.

Skill 4: Eliciting and strengthening change talk.

Skill 5: Rolling with resistance. Rather than challenging resistance, use simple, amplified, or double-sided reflections. Double-sided reflections involve the clinician reflecting both the individual's current resistant statement as well as a previous contradictory statement.

Skill 6: Developing a change plan (knowing when to transition to development of a change plan; timing is key).

Skill 7: Consolidating the individual's commitment (waiting to hear and consolidating commitment language from the individual).

Skill 8: Switching between motivational interviewing and other counseling methods.

which are often unavailable in healthcare settings, are required to train clinicians in motivational interviewing (Hall et al., 2015; Resnicow, DiIorio, et al., 2002).

Scales have been developed to assess the fidelity of motivational interviewing (see Box 6.4; Martino et al., 2011; Miller, Moyers, Ernst, & Amrhein, 2008; Moyers, Martin, Manuel, Hendrickson, & Miller, 2005). These scales can be used in clinical practice and research studies to examine the proficiency of clinicians in delivering motivational interviewing. A systematic review of studies using these scales reported low levels of proficiency in motivational interviewing at follow-up post-training, with only 2 out of 11 studies reporting at least 75% of clinicians being proficient (Hall et al., 2015). In these two studies, clinicians received ongoing training and supervision (Hall et al., 2015). Meta-analysis has indicated that three to four feedback/coaching sessions are needed over a six-month period to sustain skill development from motivational interviewing training workshops (Schwalbe, Oh, & Zweben, 2014).

The intensity of training and follow-up required may vary depending on profession. Clinicians from counseling-based professions, such as psychologists, social workers, or counselors, may only require a moderate refinement of skills (Resnicow, DiIorio, et al., 2002). In comparison, clinicians who do not have a

---

Box 6.4

Assessing Motivational Interviewing Fidelity

Several scales have been developed to assess the fidelity of motivational interviewing including the Motivational Interviewing Treatment Integrity (MITI) scale (Moyers, Martin, Manuel, Hendrickson, & Miller, 2005), the Motivational Interviewing Skills Code (Miller, Moyers, Ernst, & Amrhein, 2008), and the Independent Tape Rater Scale (Martino et al., 2011). The MITI is the most frequently used scale (Moyers, Rowell, Manuel, Ernst, & Houck, 2016). Development of the MITI stemmed from the observation that people purporting to use motivational interviewing were actually displaying behaviors contradictory to this approach (Miller, 2010; Moyers et al., 2005). Over the years revisions have continued to be made to this scale, and MITI 4.0 has recently been developed (Moyers et al., 2016.). The MITI 4.0 consists of two components: global ratings and behavioral counts. Global ratings are given on a 5-point Likert scale ranging from 1 (low) to 5 (high) for four items—cultivating change talk, softening sustain talk, partnership, and empathy (Britt, Hudson, & Blampied, 2004; Moyers et al., 2016; Riegel et al., 2006). Behavioral counts are tallies of how often a behavior is observed for the following 10 categories: questions, simple reflections, complex reflections, persuade with permission, giving information, affirmations, emphasize autonomy, seeking collaboration, persuade, and confront (Moyers et al., 2016). Interrater reliability of the MITI 4.0 was estimated (using intraclass correlation coefficient for four coders) to be between 0.87 and 0.91 for the global ratings and between 0.82 and 0.97 for the behavior counts (Moyers et al., 2016).

---

counseling background, such as nurses (Ostlund, Kristofferzon, Haggstrom, & Wadensten, 2015), dieticians, physical therapists, or physicians, may tend to provide information to individuals with chronic health conditions in a more prescriptive way and therefore may need to reorient their approach to use motivational interviewing (Resnicow, DiIorio, et al., 2002).

When using motivational interviewing, the focus is on *asking individuals what behavior change means to them*, rather than interpreting information on their behalf (Resnicow, DiIorio, et al., 2002). This can be challenging for some clinicians, who may be able to develop competence in the technical skills of motivational interviewing but not in conveying the empathy necessary to the approach (Resnicow, DiIorio, et al., 2002).

Using Motivational Interviewing in Healthcare

Motivational interviewing is often used in healthcare when behavior change is needed around lifestyle choices or the self-management of medication (Elwyn et al., 2014) and has successfully been used to promote the self-management of mental health conditions (Docherty, Sheridan, & Kenealy, 2015; Tan, Lee, Lim, Leong, & Lee, 2015). When adapting motivational interviewing to other areas of healthcare, it is important to consider the differences between them and those of the addictions field where it originated (Resnicow, DiIorio, et al., 2002). First, in the addictions field, individuals often seek help and intervention programs, but in healthcare settings, clinicians may be the first to raise concerns about health behaviors (Emmons & Rollnick, 2001; Resnicow, DiIorio, et al., 2002). For example, an individual may be seeing a clinician for an acute injury or illness when the clinician raises concerns about health behaviors related to smoking, exercise, or diet. Second, individuals with other healthcare concerns often have shorter encounters with clinicians. For example, individuals with acute problems see clinicians in focused, time-limited encounters, while individuals in rehabilitation see counselors for extended periods. The acute setting restricts the opportunity to fully explore the individual's ambivalence (Emmons & Rollnick, 2001; Resnicow, DiIorio, et al., 2002). In these settings, it is also difficult for clinicians to develop their skills in motivational interviewing (Miller & Rollnick, 2002). To address these constraints, techniques such as brief motivational interviewing have been developed that are not reliant on counseling skills (Miller & Rollnick, 2002).

Using Motivational Interviewing to Promote Chronic Health Condition Self-Management

Individuals with chronic health conditions often have good intentions to change health behaviors, but this often is not translated into action or maintained (Christie & Channon, 2014). Clinicians use motivational interviewing to support individuals with chronic health conditions to reshape their thinking about the burden of long-term change in terms of what is gained versus what is lost (Resnicow, Dilorio, et al., 2002). It may also increase individual's performance of self-management tasks by tailoring them to the individual's life and increasing his or her confidence (Riegel et al., 2006). In the context of chronic health conditions, motivational interviewing may be focused on the modification of behaviors rather than their elimination and may be incorporated as part of a broader treatment program (Hogden et al., 2012; Resnicow, Dilorio, et al., 2002). Similarly, changes for improved management of diabetes, such as increasing exercise, healthy eating, and self-monitoring behaviors, may seem simple, but there is a gap between knowledge and behavior resulting from competing motivations and pressures (Christie & Channon, 2014). Motivational interviewing seeks to bridge this divide in order to engage individuals to improve their health goals.

The practical application of motivational interviewing to chronic health condition self-management hinges on a range of strengths and limitations, acknowledged in the chronic health condition research literature (Hogden et al., 2012; Lawn & Schoo, 2010). The following sections explore the perspectives of users of the approach, that is, both clinicians and individual with chronic health conditions, so as to provide a clearer understanding of how well motivational interviewing has transferred from the addictions field to self-management of chronic health conditions.

Clinician Perspectives of Using Motivational Interviewing to Promote Chronic Health Condition Self-Management

To demonstrate clinician views on the applicability of motivational interviewing as an approach to promote chronic health condition self-management, we report on a study conducted by the authors that explored the perspectives of Australian clinicians on their use of motivational interviewing (Hogden et al., 2012). The participants were 17 clinicians with extensive experience in working with individuals with chronic health conditions.

Although devised as a stand-alone method, motivational interviewing is frequently used alongside other approaches to promote chronic health condition self-management. Our findings reiterated this point, when participants indicated that motivational interviewing was utilized as part of a "toolbox" approach to the self-management of chronic health conditions. This toolbox incorporated motivational interviewing, health coaching, mindfulness techniques, and education programs for individuals with chronic health conditions. Clinicians viewed motivational interviewing as complementary to other approaches to promote chronic health condition self-management, which allowed them to use motivational interviewing in combination with other approaches available to them. In particular, health-coaching models that contained motivational interviewing were favored to tailor care to the needs of individuals with chronic health conditions.

The Perspectives of Individuals with chronic health conditions on Participating in Motivational Interviewing

Investigations of the views of individuals with chronic health conditions about motivational interviewing are rare. Two studies have explored individual's perspectives of motivational interviewing in diabetes management. They reveal that individuals with chronic health conditions hold mixed views of motivational interviewing as an approach to support chronic health condition self-management (Dellasega et al., 2012; Miller, 2010). The views articulated in these two studies align with evaluations of individuals' perceptions of chronic health condition self-management more broadly (Dwarswaard, Bakker, van Staa, & Boeije, 2015; Rogers, Kennedy, Nelson, & Robinson, 2005).

Miller (2010) asked rural, female, African American individuals to give their opinions of a motivational interviewing–based consultation. On the one hand, individuals perceived that motivational interviewing promoted better levels of communication between them and clinicians. This was valued as improving the individuals' engagement in the consultation, by facilitating an environment in which individuals felt comfortable to talk about managing their condition. On the other hand, many disliked the client-centric approach of motivational interviewing as they had previously experienced a directed style of care delivery. They expected to receive greater direction from their clinicians than motivational interviewing offered.

Dellasega's (2012) study of 19 American individuals with chronic health conditions revealed more positive attitudes toward motivational interviewing. Participants viewed motivational interviewing as enabling client empowerment and aiding in the development of care partnerships between individuals with chronic health conditions and clinicians. This led to expression of dissatisfaction with the clinician-directed style of care that they had previously received.

Strengths of Chronic Health Condition Self-Management in Clinical Practice

Lawn and Schoo (2010) identified numerous advantages of motivational interviewing as an approach to promote chronic health condition self-management. These included the availability of motivational interviewing training for practitioners, a flexible approach applicable to many health settings and care models, applicability to various chronic conditions, utility in long or short consultations, suitability to ongoing self-management and behavior change, and demonstrated effectiveness of motivational interviewing in diverse populations.

Clinician perceptions of the strengths and benefits of motivational interviewing as an approach to promote chronic health condition self-management reflect its practical application (Hogden et al., 2012). The strength of motivational interviewing is in facilitating behavior change. In Hogden et al.'s study, motivational interviewing was considered the best of available approaches to prepare individuals with chronic health conditions for active engagement and participation in chronic health condition self-management. As such, motivational interviewing was valued for managing the co-occurring conditions (Hogden et al., 2012). This allowed clinicians to assist individuals to holistically manage multiple complex health and lifestyle issues, such as the management of diabetes and depression (Kaltman et al., 2016). Motivational interviewing is also viewed by clinicians as an approach to promote healthier lifestyle choices (Efraimsson et al., 2015; O'Halloran, Sheilds, Blackstock, Wintle, & Taylor, 2015), including increased physical activity (Karnes, Meyer, Berger, & Brondino, 2015; Knittle, De Gucht, Hurkmans, Vliet Vlieland, & Maes, 2016).

The benefits of motivational interviewing to the care of individuals with chronic health conditions are multifaceted (Hogden et al., 2012). First, motivational interviewing facilitates preparation for behavior change by helping individuals to identify reasons to make change, the benefits of these changes, and their readiness to make change. Delivered over time, motivational interviewing has the capacity to assist individuals with chronic health conditions to improve their self-efficacy, with long-term benefits realized as the chronic health conditions persist (Rosenbek Minet, Lonvig, Henriksen, & Wagner, 2011).

Second, motivational interviewing takes a client-centered approach, evidenced by deeper engagement with clinicians through enhanced communication and development of trusting relationships between the individual and their clinician. Motivational interviewing is viewed as a person-centered approach that is easy for an individual to understand (Hogden et al., 2012). With its non-judgmental and non-confrontational approach, motivational interviewing supports the individual's choice and control. The focus on client-centered care is enhanced by treatment plans based on the individual's nominated priorities (Elwyn et al., 2014; Zoffmann et al., 2015).

Third, evidence suggests that motivational interviewing is a practical approach with a high success rate. Individuals with chronic health conditions have seen rapid results, with change sometimes reported on a daily basis (Hogden et al., 2012). Individuals are able to build trusting relationships with clinicians as their self-confidence improves and they perceive change occurring in their lives. Motivational interviewing addresses both the physical and emotional aspects of chronic health condition. The benefits to clinicians and individuals are described as rewarding and are found to promote the clinician's sense of job satisfaction (Hogden et al., 2012). In practical terms, there is also flexibility in how motivational interviewing approaches can be provided to individuals with chronic health condition. Successful delivery may incorporate technological or phone-based interventions (Landry et al., 2015; Lee et al., 2015; Shingleton & Palfai, 2016).

Barriers to Implementation in Clinical Practice

Several disadvantages to motivational interviewing as an approach to promote self-management for people with chronic health conditions have also been reported

(Hogden et al., 2012; Lawn & Schoo, 2010). These relate to clinician skills, experience, and training.

As motivational interviewing lacks a formal structure in the consultation, the skills of the clinician are key components for ensuring that the approach is delivered as designed. Practitioners, who received counseling training as part of their profession, are already experienced in counseling-based models of care, while extensive training is required for clinicians who were not. Moreover, the long-term effectiveness of motivational interviewing is dependent on practitioners receiving ongoing training and supervision (Hogden et al., 2012). Inexperienced clinicians may underestimate the complexity of motivational interviewing and thus may rely on superficial training and not seek ongoing support and supervision.

Barriers to using motivational interviewing in clinical practice are also reflective of barriers to using client-centered care and chronic health condition self-management approaches more generally. For example, clinicians are concerned that not all individuals are able to self-manage (Phillips, Short, Dugdale, Nugus, & Greenfield, 2014). Fear of change needs to be overcome before individuals with chronic health conditions are able to participate in self-management (Hogden et al., 2012; Miller & Rose, 2015).

In our research (Hogden et al., 2012), clinicians raised potential pitfalls with the implementation of motivational interviewing. First, it requires longer consultation time than clinician-directed care, to allow individuals with chronic health conditions and clinicians adequate time to explore the individual's issues. Additionally, time is needed to guide and monitor individuals with chronic health conditions as they progress. Second, the success of the approach relies on the individual's awareness, confidence, and willingness to change. Third, adequate training and ongoing supervision for clinicians to use motivational interviewing is necessary for the program to be conducted effectively (Efraimsson et al., 2015; Mullin et al., 2015; Ostlund et al., 2015). Moreover, clinicians require adequate support from health services to allow them to attend training sessions. The type of support includes time, clinical backfill, or financial support for training costs.

KEY CONSIDERATIONS FOR USING MOTIVATIONAL INTERVIEWING TO PROMOTE SELF-MANAGEMENT

The preceding review and discussion highlights a range of issues for consideration prior to an individual, or organization, deciding to implement motivational interviewing in a practice setting. We recommend that decision-makers consider three interrelated categories of issues: clinician skills and capacity, the organizational context, and suitability of motivational interviewing for individuals with chronic health conditions' expectations and needs (see Table 6.2).

A clinician, prior to implementing motivational interviewing in practice, needs to reflect on whether his or her personal attitudes and skills align with the "spirit" and approach of motivational interviewing, respectively. Additionally, suitability of the immediate setting and broader organizational context should

Table 6.2. KEY CONSIDERATIONS FOR USING MOTIVATIONAL INTERVIEWING TO PROMOTE SELF-MANAGEMENT

Category	Issues
Clinician skills and capacity	• Has the clinician made a realistic assessment that their attitude and beliefs suit the spirit of motivational interviewing? • Does a clinician have the clinical and counseling skills and capacity for motivational interviewing? • Training and supervision: Are there appropriate resources and opportunities for the development of expertise, ongoing benchmarking of competence, and evaluation of motivational interviewing practice? • Has the clinician carefully matched motivational interviewing and its various techniques to the needs of the individual? • What kind of documentation requirements does the use of motivational interviewing place on the clinician? • Are the necessary time and physical environment appropriate for motivational interviewing available?
Organizational context	• Are there resources for training, supervision, and evaluation of practice? • What documentation requirements are there for clinicians? • Are there appropriate clinical workload expectations, including time and physical space for sessions?
Individual with chronic health conditions	• Does the motivational interviewing approach match the individual's expectations and readiness for change? • Is the motivational interviewing approach suitable for the individual's clinical needs?

be determined. Is the clinical practice environment equipped to enable application of motivation interviewing? A clinician should realistically assess if he or she has the resources, time, workload support of the organization, and a suitable environment to undertake motivational interviewing. Opportunities for clinician training, supervision, and ongoing evaluation of practice are necessary to realize effective outcomes. The final component is identifying appropriate individuals for use of the approach to promote self-management. Matching the motivational interviewing approach to individuals with compatible expectations and health needs is required to ensure their engagement and maximize their capacity for change.

CONCLUSION

This chapter has provided an overview of motivational interviewing to promote individuals' self-management. A brief overview of motivational interviewing and evidence for its effectiveness was presented, followed by discussion of how motivational interviewing can be used in practice, including clinician training, adaptation for use in healthcare settings, and promotion of self-management among individuals with cchronic health conditions. Finally, the key considerations for using motivational interviewing with individuals with chronic health conditions demonstrate that, while motivational interviewing is demanding on clinician time, skills, and resources, the result is individuals equipped with lifelong self-management skills. Implemented effectively, motivational interviewing will continue to underpin user-centric and collaborative approaches of self-management that empower individuals living with chronic health conditions.

REFERENCES

Alperstein, D., & Sharpe, L. (2016). The efficacy of motivational interviewing in adults with chronic pain: A meta-analysis and systematic review. *Journal of Pain*, 17(4). Advance online publication. doi:10.1016/j.jpain.2015.10.021

Britt, E., Hudson, S.M., & Blampied, N.M. (2004). Motivational interviewing in health settings: A review. *Patient Education and Counseling*, 53(2), 147–155. doi:10.1016/S0738-3991(03)00141-1

Christie, D., & Channon, S. (2014). The potential for motivational interviewing to improve outcomes in the management of diabetes and obesity in paediatric and adult patients: A clinical review. *Diabetes, Obesity and Metabolism*, 16(5), 381–387. doi:10.1111/dom.12195

Dellasega, C., Anel-Tiangco, R. M., & Gabbay, R. A. (2012). How patients with type 2 diabetes mellitus respond to motivational interviewing. *Diabetes Research and Clinical Practice*, 95(1), 37–41. doi:10.1016/j.diabres.2011.08.011

Docherty, B., Sheridan, N., & Kenealy, T. (2015). Developing brief opportunistic interactions: Practitioners facilitate patients to identify and change health risk behaviours at an early preventive stage. *Primary Health Care Research and Development*. Advance online publication. doi:10.1017/s1463423615000511

Dwarswaard, J., Bakker, E. J., van Staa, A., & Boeije, H. R. (2015). Self-management support from the perspective of patients with a chronic condition: A thematic synthesis of qualitative studies. *Health Expectations*. Advance online publication. doi:10.1111/hex.12346

Efraimsson, E. O., Klang, B., Ehrenberg, A., Larsson, K., Fossum, B., & Olai, L. (2015). Nurses' and patients' communication in smoking cessation at nurse-led COPD clinics in primary health care. *European Clinical Respiratory Journal*, 2, 27915. doi:10.3402/ecrj.v2.27915

Elwyn, G., Dehlendorf, C., Epstein, R. M., Marrin, K., White, J., & Frosch, D. L. (2014). Shared decision making and motivational interviewing: Achieving patient-centered care across the spectrum of health care problems. *Annals of Family Medicine*, 12(3), 270–275. doi:10.1370/afm.1615

Emmons, K.M., & Rollnick, S. (2001). Motivational interviewing in health care settings. *American Journal of Preventive Medicine*, 20(1), 68–74.

Georgopoulou, S., Prothero, L., Lempp, H., Galloway, J., & Sturt, J. (2015). Motivational interviewing: Relevance in the treatment of rheumatoid arthritis? *Rheumatology*. Advance online publication. doi:10.1093/rheumatology/kev379

Hall, K., Staiger, P.K., Simpson, A., Best, D., & Lubman, D.I. (2015). After 30 years of dissemination, have we achieved sustained practice change in motivational interviewing? *Addiction*. Advance online publication. doi:10.1111/add.13014

Hettema, J., Steele, J., & Miller, W.R. (2005). Motivational interviewing. *Annual Review of Clinical Psychology, 1*, 91–111. doi:10.1146/annurev.clinpsy.1.102803.143833

Hogden, A., Short, A., Taylor, R., Dugdale, P., Nugus, P., & Greenfield, D. (2012). Health coaching and motivational interviewing: Evaluating the chronic disease self-management toolbox as a resource for person-centred care. *The International Journal of Person Centered Medicine, 2*(3), 520–530.

Kaltman, S., Serrano, A., Talisman, N., Magee, M. F., Cabassa, L. J., Pulgar-Vidal, O., & Peraza, D. (2016). Type 2 diabetes and depression: A pilot trial of an integrated self-management intervention for Latino immigrants. *The Diabetes Educator, 42*(1), 87–95. doi:10.1177/0145721715617536

Karnes, S. L., Meyer, B. B., Berger, L. M., & Brondino, M. J. (2015). Changes in physical activity and psychological variables following a web-based motivational interviewing intervention: Pilot study. *JMIR Research Protocols, 4*(4), e129. doi:10.2196/resprot.4623

Knittle, K., De Gucht, V., Hurkmans, E., Vliet Vlieland, T., & Maes, S. (2016). Explaining physical activity maintenance after a theory-based intervention among patients with rheumatoid arthritis: Process evaluation of a randomized controlled trial. *Arthritis Care and Research, 68*(2), 203–210. doi:10.1002/acr.22647

Landry, A., Madson, M., Thomson, J., Zoellner, J., Connell, C., & Yadrick, K. (2015). A randomized trial using motivational interviewing for maintenance of blood pressure improvements in a community-engaged lifestyle intervention: HUB city steps. *Health Education Research, 30*(6), 910–922. doi:10.1093/her/cyv058

Lawn, S., & Schoo, A. (2010). Supporting self-management of chronic health conditions: Common approaches. *Patient Education and Counseling, 80*(2), 205–211. doi:10.1016/j.pec.2009.10.006

Lee, C. S., Longabaugh, R., Baird, J., Streszak, V., Nirenberg, T., & Mello, M. (2015). Participant report of therapist-delivered active ingredients in a telephone-delivered brief motivational intervention predicts taking steps towards change. *Addiction Research and Theory, 23*(5), 421–428. doi:10.3109/16066359.2015.1025062

Lindson-Hawley, N., Thompson, T.P., & Begh, R. (2015). Motivational interviewing for smoking cessation. *Cochrane Database of Systematic Reviews, 3*. doi:10.1002/14651858.CD006936.pub3

Lundahl, B., & Burke, B.L. (2009). The effectiveness and applicability of motivational interviewing: A practice-friendly review of four meta-analyses. *Journal of Clinical Psychology, 65*(11), 1232–1245. doi:10.1002/jclp.20638

Lundahl, B., Moleni, T., Burke, B.L., Butters, R., Tollefson, D., Butler, C., & Rollnick, S. (2013). Motivational interviewing in medical care settings: A systematic review and meta-analysis of randomized controlled trials. *Patient Education and Counseling, 93*(2), 157–168. doi:10.1016/j.pec.2013.07.012

Madson, M.B., Loignon, A.C., & Lane, C. (2009). Training in motivational interviewing: A systematic review. *Journal of Substance Abuse Treatment, 36*(1), 101–109. doi:10.1016/j.jsat.2008.05.005

Martino, S., Ball, S.B., Nich, C., Canning-Ball, M., Rounsaville, B.J., & Carroll, K.M. (2011). Teaching community program clinicians motivational interviewing using expert and train-the-trainer strategies. *Addiction, 106*(2), 428–441. doi:10.1111/j.1360-0443.2010.03135.x

McCarley, P. (2009). Patient empowerment and motivational interviewing: Engaging patients to self-manage thier own care. *Nephrology Nursing Journal, 36*(4), 409–413.

McGowan, P. (2013). The challenge of integrating self-management support into clinical settings. *Canadian Journal of Diabetes, 37*(1), 45–50. doi:10.1016/j.jcjd.2013.01.004

Miller, N. H. (2010). Motivational interviewing as a prelude to coaching in healthcare settings. *Journal of Cardiovascular Nursing, 25*(3), 247–251. doi:10.1097/JCN.0b013e3181cec6e7

Miller, W., & Rose, G.S. (2015). Motivational interviewing and decisional balance: Contrasting responses to client ambivalence. *Behavioural and Cognitive Psychotherapy, 43*(2), 129–141. doi:10.1017/S1352465813000878

Miller, W.R. (1996). Motivational interviewing: Research, practice, and puzzles. *Addictive Behaviors, 21*(6), 835–842.

Miller, W.R, & Mount, K.A. (2001). A small study of training in motivational interviewing: Does one workshop change clinician and client behavior? *Behavioural and Cognitive Psychotherapy, 29*(4), 457–471. doi:10.1017/S1352465801004064

Miller, W.R, & Moyers, T.B. (2006). Eight stages in learning motivational interviewing. *Journal of Teaching in the Addictions, 5*(1), 3–17. doi:10.1300/J188v05n01_02

Miller, W.R, Moyers, T.B., Ernst, D., & Amrhein, P. (2008). *Manual for the Motivational Interviewing Skill Code (MISC)*. Albuqerque: Center on Alcoholism, Substance Abuse and Addictions, University of New Mexico.

Miller, W.R, & Rollnick, S. (2002). *Motivational interviewing: Preparing people for change* (2nd ed.). New York: Guilford Press.

Miller, W.R, & Rollnick, S. (2009). Ten things that motivational interviewing is not. *Behavioural and Cognitive Psychotherapy, 37*(2), 129–140. doi:10.1017/S1352465809005128

Miller, W.R, Yahne, C.E., Moyers, T.B., Martinez, J., & Pirritano, M. (2004). A randomized trial of methods to help clinicians learn motivational interviewing. *Journal of Consulting and Clinical Psychology, 72*(6), 1050–1062.

Miller, W.R. (1983). Motivational interviewing with problem drinkers. *Behavioural Psychotherapy, 11*(2), 147–172.

Moral, R.R., de Torres, L.A.P., Ortega, L.P., Larumbe, M.C., Villalobos, A.R., Garcia, J.A.F., . . . Collaborative Group ATEM-AP Study. (2015). Effectiveness of motivational interviewing to improve therapeutic adherence in patients over 65 years old with chronic diseases: A cluster randomized clinical trial in primary care. *Patient Education and Counseling, 98*(8), 977–983. doi:10.1016/j.pec.2015.03.008

Moyers, T. B., Martin, T., Manuel, J. K., Hendrickson, S. M. L., & Miller, W. R. (2005). Assessing competence in the use of motivational interviewing. *Journal of Substance Abuse Treatment, 28*(1), 19–26.

Moyers, T. B., Rowell, L. N., Manuel, J. K., Ernst, D., & Houck, J. M. (2016). The Motivational Interviewing Treatment Integrity Code (MITI 4): Rationale, preliminary reliability and validity. *Journal of Substance Abuse Treatment*. Advance online publication. doi:10.1016/j.jsat.2016.01.001

Mullin, D. J., Forsberg, L., Savageau, J. A., & Saver, B. (2015). Challenges in developing primary care physicians' motivational interviewing skills. *Families, Systems and Health, 33*(4), 330–338. doi:10.1037/fsh0000145

O'Halloran, P. D., Sheilds, N., Blackstock, F., Wintle, E., & Taylor, N. F. (2015). Motivational interviewing increases physical activity and self-efficacy in people living in the community after hip fracture: A randomized controlled trial. *Clinical Rehabilitation*. Advance online publication. doi:10.1177/0269215515617814

Ostlund, A. S., Kristofferzon, M. L., Haggstrom, E., & Wadensten, B. (2015). Primary care nurses' performance in motivational interviewing: A quantitative descriptive study. *BMC Family Practice*, *16*, 89. doi:10.1186/s12875-015-0304-z

Phillips, R., Short, A., Dugdale, P., Nugus, P., & Greenfield, D. (2014). Supporting patients to self-manage chronic disease: Clinicians' perspectives and current practices. *Australian Journal of Primary Health*, *20*(3), 257–265. doi:10.1071/PY13002

Resnicow, K., DiIorio, C., Soet, J. E., Borrelli, B., Ernst, D., Hecht, J., & Thevos, A. K. (2002). Motivational interviewing in medical and public health settings. In W. R. Miller & S. Rollnick (Eds.), *Motivational interviewing: Preparing people for change* (251–269). New York: Guilford Press.

Resnicow, K., DiIorio, C., Soet, J. E., Borrelli, B., Hecht, J., & Ernst, D. (2002). Motivational interviewing in health promotion: It sounds like something is changing. *Health Psychology*, *21*(5), 444–451. doi:10.1037/0278-6133.21.5.444

Riegel, B., Dickson, V. V., Hoke, L., McMahon, J. P., Reis, B. F., & Sayers, S. (2006). A motivational counseling approach to improving heart failure self-care: Mechanisms of effectiveness. *Journal of Cardiovascular Nursing*, *21*(3), 232–241.

Rogers, A., Kennedy, A., Nelson, E., & Robinson, A. (2005). Uncovering the limits of patient-centeredness: Implementing a self-management trial for chronic illness. *Qualitative Health Research*, *15*(2), 224–239. doi:10.1177/1049732304272048

Rollnick, S., Heather, N., & Bell, A. (1992). Negotiating behaviour change in medical settings: The development of brief motivational interviewing. *Journal of Mental Health*, *1*(1), 25–37.

Rosenbek Minet, L. K., Lonvig, E. M., Henriksen, J. E., & Wagner, L. (2011). The experience of living with diabetes following a self-management program based on motivational interviewing. *Qualitative Health Research*, *21*(8), 1115–1126. doi:10.1177/1049732311405066

Schwalbe, C. S., Oh, H. Y., & Zweben, A. (2014). Sustaining motivational interviewing: A meta-analysis of training studies. *Addiction*, *109*(8), 1287–1294. doi:10.1111/add.12558

Shingleton, R. M., & Palfai, T. P. (2016). Technology-delivered adaptations of motivational interviewing for health-related behaviors: A systematic review of the current research. *Patient Education and Counseling*, *99*(1), 17–35. doi:10.1016/j.pec.2015.08.005

Smedslund, G., Berg, R. C., Hammerstrøm, K. T., Steiro, A., Leiknes, K. A., Dahl, H. M., & Karlsen, K. (2011). Motivational interviewing for substance abuse. *Cochrane Database of Systematic Reviews*, *5*. doi:10.1002/14651858.CD008063.pub2

Song, D., Xu, T., & Sun, Q. (2014). Effect of motivational interviewing on self-management in patients with type 2 diabetes mellitus: A meta-analysis. *International Journal of Nursing Sciences*, *1*(3), 291–297.

Tan, S. C., Lee, M. W., Lim, G. T., Leong, J. J., & Lee, C. (2015). Motivational interviewing approach used by a community mental health team. *Journal of Psychosocial Nursing and Mental Health Services*, *53*(12), 28–37. doi:10.3928/02793695-20151020-03

Zoffmann, V., Hornsten, A., Storbaekken, S., Graue, M., Rasmussen, B., Wahl, A., & Kirkevold, M. (2015). Translating person-centered care into practice: A comparative analysis of motivational interviewing, illness-integration support, and guided self-determination. *Patient Education and Counseling*. Advance online publication. doi:10.1016/j.pec.2015.10.015

PART II

Research about Specific Chronic Health Conditions

7
Self-Management of Addictive Behaviors

VANJA RADONCIC, BETTY MARCOUX, AND DENISE HIEN ■

FUNCTIONAL LIMITATIONS OF ADDICTIVE BEHAVIORS

According to the *Diagnostic and Statistical Manual of Mental Disorders* (5th ed.; *DSM-5*; American Psychiatric Association [APA], 2013), addiction describes a problematic pattern of using alcohol and/or other substance that results in impairments in daily life and/or noticeable distress. Addiction occurs when the recurrent use of alcohol and/or drugs causes clinically and functionally significant impairment, such as health problems, disability, and failure to meet major responsibilities at work, school, or home. A diagnosis of addiction is based on evidence of impaired control, social impairment, risky use, and pharmacological criteria (APA, 2013).

Impaired control over substance use refers to spending a great deal of time obtaining the substance, using the substance, or recovering from its effects. Social impairments refer to a failure to fulfill major obligations at work, school, or home. The individuals continue substance use despite having or recurrent social or interpersonal problems caused by substance use. The individuals may also withdraw from family activities in order to use the substance (APA, 2013). Individuals who engage in risky behaviors related to substance use are often aware that their persistent problems are likely to have been caused or exacerbated by the substance (APA, 2013). According to the *DSM-5*, pharmacological criteria include symptoms of tolerance and withdrawal. Tolerance is characterized by requiring a markedly increased dose of the substance to achieve the desired effect or a significantly reduced effect when the usual dose is consumed. Withdrawal is a syndrome that occurs when blood or tissue concentrations of a substance decline in an individual who had maintained prolonged heavy use of the substance. In order to relieve the withdrawal symptoms, the individuals often relapse and continue to use the substance (APA, 2013).

EVIDENCE-BASED PRACTICES ON INTERVENTIONS THAT IMPROVE HEALTH OUTCOMES

Evidence-based practices of interventions that improve health outcomes incorporate different treatment modalities that address and foster changes in individual's behaviors and attitudes, executive functioning, thought processes, emotion regulation, and social functioning.

Assessing Addiction: Concepts and Instruments

Efficient assessment of addiction is essential for treatment planning, referral to treatment services, and clinical research. Screening for alcohol and/or drug misuse is critical to the prevention of or early intervention in addiction. For those at risk of developing a serious problem with drinking or drugs, the identification of early warning signs can be enough to change negative drinking or drug-use habits. For others, these assessments are important first steps toward treatment of and recovery from addiction.

The appropriate way to assess a substance-use disorder depends on the objective. For example, semistructured instruments (e.g., Addiction Severity Index [ASI]; McLellan, Luborsky, O'Brien, & Woody, 1980) assist treatment planning by providing a standardized comparison of an individual's characteristics with those of individuals who have benefitted from interventions in clinical trials (Samet et al., 2007). Clinicians also obtain a comprehensive, objective picture of the auxiliary services the individual may need to benefit maximally from treatment. For instance, the ASI is a semistructured interview designed to address seven potential problem areas in substance-abusing individuals: medical status, employment and support, drug use, alcohol use, legal status, family/social status, and psychiatric status. In one hour, a skilled interviewer can gather information on recent (past 30 days) and lifetime problems in all of the problem areas. The ASI provides an overview of problems related to substance, rather than focusing on any single area. Individuals with identified problems related to their substance use receive referral to specialty treatments of addiction. A number of effective evidence-based psychosocial treatment approaches to treat people with addiction problems has significantly increased in the past three decades.

Psychosocial Treatments for Addiction

Psychosocial treatments for addiction focus on counteracting compulsive substance use by bringing about changes in individual's behaviors, thought processes, affect regulation, and social functioning (Practice Guideline for the Treatment of Patients with Substance Use; APA, 2006). The techniques and theories of therapeutic action vary across different therapeutic approaches for addiction, but they all address one or more of a set of common tasks that include the following: enhancing motivation to reduce and/or stop substance use, teaching coping skills, changing reinforcement contingencies, improving emotion regulation, and enhancing social support and interpersonal functioning (Rounsaville, Carroll, & Onken, 2001). Treatment for impairments related to addiction takes place within a care continuum that include motivational interventions, cognitive-behavioral, behavioral, psychodynamic/interpersonal, recovery-oriented therapies, and pharmacotherapy approaches (Carroll, & Onken, 2005; Silva, & Serra, 2004).

MOTIVATIONAL ENHANCEMENT INTERVENTIONS

These are based on different techniques employed to help people explore and resolve ambivalence about behavioral change. In this section, we discuss two motivational interventions: motivational interviewing (MI) and the "Stages of Change" model.

Motivational Interviewing

MI suggests that people approach change with varying levels of readiness; thus the role of health professionals is to assist clients to become more aware of the implications of change and/or of not changing through a series of interviews (Lundahl et al., 2010; McHugh et al., 2010; Rollnick, Miller, & Butler, 2008). MI interventions are collaborative in nature and are based on a strong working alliance/rapport between the therapist and the client. A working alliance is established when clients perceive the therapist as trustworthy and capable of helping them with their problems (Teyber, 2006). MI principles are used to evoke an internally motivated rather than externally initiated change. MI postulates that certain therapeutic conditions in themselves promote positive change. Accurate empathy appears to be a major predictor of such positive change. For example, through collaborative exploration, the therapist links what the clients has said to what might be meaningful rather than offering well-intended but vague reassurances (Teyber, 2011). Therapist empathy during treatment predicted a two-thirds of the variance in client drinking six months later ($r = .82, p < .0001$; Miller & Rose, 2010). Even 12 and 24 months after treatment, the therapist's empathy continued to account for one-half ($r = .71$) and one-quarter ($r = .51$) of the variance in behavioral outcomes, respectively.

"Stages of Change" Model

This model, developed by Prochaska and DiClemente (1992), proposes that indicators of readiness to change are important dimensions of positive change of different non-adaptive behaviors, especially non-adaptive behaviors related to substance use. Intervening on individual's motivation facilitates engagement, implementation of treatment, and behavior change. Prochanska and DiClemente designed their model after studying the structure of change that underlies both self-mediated and treatment-facilitated modification of addictive and other problem behaviors (Prochaska, DiClemente, & Narcross, 2010; Prochaska, Norcross, & DiClemente, 2013). They focused on the phenomenon of intentional change as opposed to societal, developmental, or imposed change and postulated that the fundamental, common principles can reveal the structure of change occurring with and without psychotherapy. Those common principles incorporate several stages of change. For example, pre-action stages (e.g., focusing on the tasks needed to prepare for taking action) include precontemplation, contemplation, and preparation stages (DiClemente et al., 2008). On the other hand, action-oriented stages focus on practicing new behaviors (e.g., improving self-efficacy for dealing with obstacles), continuing commitment to sustaining new behaviors (e.g., reinforcing internal rewards for going to therapy), and increasing awareness about relapse (e.g., evaluating triggers for relapse, improving coping strategies). Stage-specific tasks play an important role in facilitating motivation to change a behavior and successful integration of new behaviors. Individuals often cycle through the stages multiple times to accomplish this (DiClemente et al., 2008).

Motivational enhancement interventions help individuals move through these stages and accomplish stage-relevant tasks. Brief motivational interventions prior to treatment often improve treatment engagement and therapy outcomes. A small number of studies have assessed behavioral outcomes related to the "stages of change" model. The paucity of data on the treatment outcomes is explained by structural difficulties, such as assessing ultimate changes in behavior (Whitelaw et al., 2000). The small number of studies, however, managed to indicate a degree of evidence to suggest that stage-matched interventions result in significantly higher levels of ultimate behavior change than those that are non-stage-matched (Evers et al., 2006; Prochaska et al., 1993; Prochaska et al., 2001).

Cognitive-Behavioral Therapies

Cognitive-behavioral therapy (CBT) refers to a group of therapeutic techniques that can be categorized broadly as psychoeducation, cognitive restructuring, and behavioral exposure (Kushner, 2007). CBTs for the treatment of addictive behaviors are based on three perspectives: behavioral theory (e.g., classical conditioning and operant learning), cognitive social learning theory (e.g., observational learning, modeling, and the role of cognitive expectancies in determining behavior), and cognitive theory (e.g., thoughts, cognitive schema, beliefs, attitudes, and attributions that influence one's feelings and mediate the relationship between antecedents and behavior; SAMHSA, 2016). CBTs posit that learning processes play a crucial role in the development of addiction. These learning processes include dysfunctional thinking, such as the beliefs that the use of substances is completely uncontrollable, and attitudes and non-adaptive behaviors, such as acceptance of offers to use drugs (Carroll, 1998).

CBT for substance-use disorders captures a broad range of treatments including those targeting operant learning processes, cognitive and motivational barriers to improvement, and interventions that build coping skills. A focus of CBTs is on learning cognitive and coping strategies as an alternative to substance use. The cognitive strategies include exploring positive and negative consequences of continued use, identifying dysfunctional thoughts about substance use, and recognizing attitudes, decisions, and behaviors that result in high-risk situations (Carroll, 1998; Magill et al., 2009; Marlatt & Donovan, 2005). These treatments target cognitive, affective, and situational triggers for substance use and provide skills training specific to coping alternatives. CBT treatment for addiction include the following strategies: (a) identifying intrapersonal and interpersonal triggers for relapse, (b) coping-skills training, (c) drug-refusal skills training, (d) functional analysis of substance use, and (e) increasing nonuse-related activities (Magill et al., 2009). These models have been manualized (e.g., Carroll, 1998; Kadden et al., 1992) and adapted for implementation in a variety of clinical capacities.

During assessment and early treatment sessions, case conceptualization requires consideration of a variety of factors (e.g., affective and social/environmental factors) contributing to impairments related to substance use. CBT models for treatment for substance use rely on a structure that incorporates agenda-setting, identification of goals, and the assignment and review of homework (McHugh et al., 2010). This is especially important for individuals who may struggle with from cognitive deficits, difficulty concentrating, or organizational and problem-solving skills deficits. CBTs are comprised of several components/approaches like functional analysis and relapse prevention.

Functional Analysis

Functional analysis is a component of CBT treatment that focuses on the identification of antecedents or triggers for use and helps determine situations and behaviors to target (e.g., avoiding liquor stores or areas where drugs are commonly sold in the neighborhood; McHugh et al., 2010). Functional analyses help identify patterns and reason for alcohol and/or drug use, such as a nature of motives and its association to particular triggers like depressed mood. For example, according to NIDA (2016), the functional analysis plays an important role in helping the individual and therapist assess high-risk situations, especially early in the treatment, that are likely to lead to drug use and provides insights into some of the reasons the individual may be using (e.g., to cope with interpersonal difficulties, to experience risk or euphoria not otherwise available in the individual's life).

Relapse Prevention

Relapse prevention (RP) therapy (Marlatt and Gordon, 1985) is the approach with demonstrated effectiveness in reducing risk of relapse to substance use (Brandon et al., 2007; Lancaster et al., 2006). The theory of change underlying relapse prevention is that interactions between the individual and the environment can increase the risk of relapse, such as social influences, greater access to substances, and an individual's inability to cope with craving (Range & Marlatt, 2008; Witkiewitz and Marlatt, 2004). With this framework in mind, practitioners delivering relapse prevention therapy help the client to identify situations that trigger relapse and teach clients cognitive and behavioral skills to reduce the risk of relapse (Brandon et al., 2007). The RP approach promotes functional analysis of cues for alcohol and/or drug use and learning about alternative responses to these cues. RP focuses on the identification and prevention of high-risk situations (e.g., frequenting a bar after work with colleagues who drink) to help individuals develop greater self-control to avoid relapse. RP strategies include discussing the individual's ambivalence about the substance-use disorder, identifying emotional and environmental triggers of craving and substance use, developing and reviewing specific coping strategies to deal with internal or external stressors, exploring the factors leading to relapse, embracing and learning from relapse episodes about triggers leading to relapse, and developing effective techniques for intervention and providing psychoeducation to help the individual make a more informed choice in the threatening situation (Hendershot et al., 2011).

MINDFULNESS-BASED RELAPSE PREVENTION

Mindfulness-based relapse prevention (MBRP) is a specific relapse treatment approach that incorporates mindfulness-based meditations with relapse-prevention techniques for individuals in recovery from substance use behaviors (Bowen, Chawla, & Marlatt, 2011) with the goal of decreasing the risk and severity of relapse to substance use following treatment. MBRP involves identifying individual risk factors or common precursors to relapse; recognizing underlying reasons for non-adaptive substance use; teaching meditation practices to increase awareness of and change one's relation to challenging emotional, cognitive, and physical states arising from craving or withdrawal from substance use; and providing skills to tolerate these states (Bowen, Chawla, & Marlatt, 2011; Bowen, Chawla, & Witkiewitz, 2014; Witkiewitz et al., 2013).

Behavioral Therapies

Behavioral therapies are based on basic principles of learning theory, which deals with the role of externally applied positive or negative reinforcement on modifying individuals' attitudes and behaviors related to drug abuse. Reinforcement provides incentives to remain abstinent and to increase skills to handle stressful circumstances and environmental cues that may trigger intense craving for drugs and prompt another cycle of compulsive abuse (Petry et al., 2000). Behavioral therapies are broadly based on two classes of learning theory: classical conditioning (e.g., focus on antecedent stimuli, such as cue exposure therapy) and operant conditioning (e.g., focus on consequences, such as community reinforcement therapy). Behavioral therapies based on classical conditioning include the following techniques.

CUE EXPOSURE AND RELAXATION TRAINING

Cue exposure approaches expose the individual to the cues related to substance use (e.g., the sight or smell of alcohol), thereby allowing the individual to practice responses to such cues in real-life situations. In addition, this approach teaches a variety of coping skills for dealing with urges caused by such cues (Monti & Rohsenow, 1999). Relaxation training can be paired with the cue exposure to facilitate the extinction of classically conditioned craving, or it can be used alone as a technique helpful to regulate emotions of anxiety (Klajner, Hartman, & Sobell, 1984).

Behavioral therapies based on operant conditioning include the following two techniques.

Contingency Management

The treatment approaches using contingency management principles involve giving clients tangible rewards to reinforce positive behaviors, such as abstinence, and decreasing undesirable approaches by optimizing the implementation of treatment plan that is right for each person. Research data shows that incentive-based interventions are highly effective in increasing treatment retention and promoting abstinence from drugs (Principles of Drug Addiction Treatment, 2012).

Community Reinforcement Approach

The community reinforcement approach (CRA) is based on the belief that environmental contingencies can play a powerful role in supporting or discouraging drinking or drug-using behaviors. It utilizes familial, social, recreational, and occupational reinforcers to aid clients in the recovery process (Smith et al., 2009).

The CRA is a treatment approach promoting positive reinforcement for both drug and alcohol sobriety. CRA integrates several treatment components, including building the client's motivation to quit using substances, helping the client initiate sobriety, analyzing the client's drug using pattern, increasing positive reinforcement, learning new coping behaviors, and involving significant others in the recovery process (Milford et al., 2007; Smith et al., 2001). These components can be adjusted to the individual client's needs to achieve optimal treatment outcome. In addition, treatment outcome can be influenced by different factors, such as therapist style and working alliance between the therapist and client (Miller, Meyers, & Tonigan, 1999).

Psychodynamic Therapies

Contemporary psychodynamic perspective of addiction places greater emphasis on painful or confusing affects (e.g., emotions) that make addictive drugs compelling (Khantzian, 2014). Psychodynamic approaches consider addictive behaviors as (a) a special adaptation, (b) an attempt to self-medicate painful or confusing emotions, (c) an overarching problem in self-regulation, and (d) a reflection of disorder in personality organization (Khantzian & Weegmann, 2009, 2014). This evolving perspective complements and resonates with other treatment perspectives for addiction.

Psychodynamic perspectives incorporate interventions that address deficits in regulating affects and behaviors. The goals of psychodynamic therapy are increasing self-awareness and understanding of the influence of the past on present behaviors. Psychodynamic approach enables the individuals to examine unresolved conflicts and symptoms that arise from past dysfunctional relationships and manifest themselves in the need and desire to abuse substances. Psychodynamic psychotherapies generally examine how trauma exposure attributes to symptoms, personality characteristics, and deficits contribute to the development of unconscious psychological conflict, faulty learning, and distortions of intrapsychic structures (Khantzian, 2009).

Group Therapy

Group therapy is viewed as an integral and valuable part of the treatment regimen for many individuals with substance-use disorders. Different types of evidence-based therapies have been used in a group format with this population (SAMHSA, 2016). Aspects of group therapy may make this approach more effective than individual treatment for individuals with a substance-use disorder. Group members offer continued support inside and outside of group sessions in a way that therapists do not.

Pharmacotherapy

According to the *Principles of Drug Addiction Treatment* by the National Institute on Drug Abuse (2014), pharmacotherapy refers to drug treatment intended to help individuals to stop seeking and using drugs. For example, this treatment can be used alone or in a combination with other treatments such as CBT. Specific type of pharmacotherapy depends on the individual's needs and the types of drugs that the individual used (NIDA, 2014). Treatment medications, such as methadone, buprenorphine, and naltrexone, are available for individuals addicted to opioids, while combining medications such as vareniclene and bupropion for tobacco-dependence treatment may increase smoking abstinence (Ebbert et al., 2014).

Treatments for prescription drug abuse tend to be similar to those for illicit drugs that affect the same brain systems. For example, buprenorphine, used to treat heroin addiction, can also be used to treat addiction to opioid pain medications. Addiction to prescription stimulants, which affect the same brain systems as illicit stimulants like cocaine, can be treated with behavioral therapies, as there are not yet medications for treating addiction to these types of drugs (NIDA, 2014).

Self-Help Movements: Alcoholics Anonymous and Narcotics Anonymous Programs

When considering self-management of co-occurring conditions, recovery can be achieved through a combination of peer support, "self-help" activities, combined treatment (e.g., treatment approaches addressing both the substance use and mental health problems), and integration of relapse episodes as part of the recovery process (Laudet, Stanick, & Sands, 2007). Self-help groups, such as Alcoholics Anonymous (AA) and Narcotics Anonymous (NA) programs, are characterized with a sense of belonging and family. Often individuals with addictions have experienced their family of origin giving up on them, due to the difficulties of living with someone with an addiction or due to the problems that happened as a consequence of addictive, disinhibited behavior or impaired judgment. Therefore, AA can become a community providing a sense of hope and result in a sense of renewal and family reconnection. AA can be a place to reflect upon past actions, with no judgment from like-minded people, which helps individuals cope with their pain. In the context of the AA program, people use their experience to relate to others struggling with addiction. In this sense, a former addict can be a positive force.

KNOWLEDGE ABOUT THE IMPAIRMENT THAT AN INDIVIDUAL NEEDS FOR SELF-MANAGEMENT

Self-management refers to an active engagement of the mental health care consumer in dealing with problems related to substance use; this means that the person has an active role in treatment as opposed to someone who passively follows recommendations and instructions (Bilsker, 2003; Lorig & Holman, 2003). One critically important component of self-management for addictions is psychoeducation.

Psychoeducational Interventions

Individuals with substance-use problems are often unaware of the neurological and psychological factors that drive their addiction. The focus of psychoeducational approach is to teach individuals about the nature of addiction, addiction-related problems, and relapse (SAMHSA, 2015). Family members and significant others may also take part in educational sessions. The more that individuals understand about an etiology and different components of their addictions, the better they can take charge of their recovery process. Thus an exposure to some of the scientific underpinnings (e.g., genetics/neurobiological influence) and other psychoeducational intervention make a productive component for the addiction treatment approaches. Providing psychoeducation may help raise individuals' awareness of their own behavioral and emotional difficulties and how those difficulties impact them and others. This awareness may, in turn, help the individuals in making informed decisions about seeking and receiving help for problems.

Posttraumatic Growth

While there are many negative emotions involved in the recovery process that can present barriers for recovery, there are also striking and positive aspects of the recovery process. Posttraumatic growth (PTG) facilitates the individual's recovery process. PTG is the subjective experience of positive psychological change reported by an individual as a result of the struggle with trauma (Prati, & Pietrantoni, 2009). There are five areas of PTG, which involve (a) a greater appreciation of life, (b) closer relationships, (c) identification of new possibilities, (d) increased personal strength, and (e) positive spiritual change (Tedeschi and Calhoun, 1996; Calhoun, 2006).

Individuals with addiction problems, who lack in-depth knowledge of the recovery process and understanding of how dimensions of the self are affected, may neglect their emotional needs, which ultimately contributes to negative long-term effects on their recovery (Turner & Cox, 2004). In contrast, PTG includes a changed sense in one's relationships, a changed sense of self, and a changed philosophy of life. Personal perceptions constitute the experience of recovery and may determine the efficacy of rehabilitation programs and the speed and success of recovery (Turner & Cox, 2004). PTG involves an experience of deepening of relationships, increased compassion and sympathy for others, and greater ease at expressing emotions. Thus the change in self-perception in individuals working on their recovery from addiction may include an increased sense of vulnerability but an increased experience of oneself as capable and self-reliant (Calhoun & Tedeschi, 2013). Because of the changes in self-perception, individuals report a greater appreciation for life, a changed set of life priorities, and positive changes in spiritual or existential matters (Calhoun & Tedeschi, 2013).

Understanding Internal and External Triggers

As individuals who suffer from substance-use disorders learn more about the associations between specific emotional states and stimulant cues, they become increasingly sophisticated about identifying and avoiding or defusing potential triggers. Increased capacity to recognize and understand conditions contributing to the impairment is essential for improving self-management. An individual's ability to identify cues and triggers changes over time. Many individuals who suffer from substance use lose their sense of self and their ability to care for their own personal needs and the needs of others. Urges and/or cravings to use substances are quite common for clients to experience when cutting back or quitting substance use. It is important that individuals understand that urges are predictable and controllable and that they can learn to manage them (NIDA, 2000; Boston Center for Treatment Development and Training [BCTDT], 2007).

The more clients understand about their experiences with urges and what triggers an urge, the more skillful they become at identifying them. As a result, urges become more predictable, rather than random, unpredictable events that are difficult to control. This enables the client to learn specific skills to manage urges (Otto, 2003).Individuals learn to recognize that experiencing craving is a normal phase in a recovery process and that experiencing craving does not mean something is wrong or that the individual wants to resume drug use (NIDA, 2000; BCTDT, 2007).

Talking about urges improves an individual's capacity to recognize, identify, and appropriately respond before urges becomes overwhelming and too difficult to control. Learning about different aspects of the experience associated with the urge helps to label the experience and prevent automatic responses to urges (e.g., reaching out to alcohol or drug use). Cravings or urges are experienced in a variety of ways (Otto et al., 2007). These experiences can be primarily somatic (e.g., "I just get a feeling in my stomach"). Sometimes, cravings are experienced more cognitively (e.g., "I can't get it out of my head"). Furthermore, urges can also be experienced affectively (e.g., "I get nervous"). It is important that the individual obtain a clear understanding of how, when, and where the craving is experienced. Individuals should practice self-monitoring of craving, so they can begin to identify new and more complex cues.

Developing an ability to recognize urges is closely related to implementing successful coping strategies, discussed elsewhere, and timely identification of triggers for having urges. Common triggers include being around people with whom one used drugs, having money or getting paid, drinking alcohol, social situations, and certain affective states, such as anxiety, depression, or joy.

Substance use becomes strongly associated with certain people, places, activities, behaviors, and feelings, resulting in a daily life of individuals who use substances filled with numerous reminders or cues that can trigger cravings and continuous substance use (Laberg et al., 1992; NIDA, 2002). The goal is that the clients learn how cues are developed and how these cues can trigger drug craving and use and to encourage them to actively identify their cues and triggers.

An action plan should be developed to find and eliminate all substances and drug-related paraphernalia. In addition, materials associated with drug use should be discarded including phone numbers of dealers, containers used to hold drug supplies, mirrors used to cut stimulants, and weighing scales (NIDA, 2002). Furthermore, the clients should learn how to avoid high-risk places. This involves identifying places strongly associated with substance use and making specific plans to avoid them. This may include taking different routes home from work or going to certain locations at times different than normal (NIDA, 2002; SAMHSA, 2016).

Coping Strategies for External Triggers

Clients learn to manage urges by identifying specific strategies for coping with these triggers. It is important to emphasize how different strategies may be more appropriate for different types of triggers (Caroll, 1997; SAMHSA, 2006). Multiple strategies for all triggers should be considered, and clients should be encouraged to try new ones to manage urges across situations.

Escape is a strategy that focuses on finding a safe way out of situations in which an urge might occur. This may involve an unexpected situation (e.g., a dealer pays a sudden visit) or a situation that the client sees as unavoidable (e.g., social setting). The client should have a plan for getting out of these situations. *Distraction* is a strategy involving a shift in attention away from thoughts about using alcohol or drugs. There are numerous distracting activities that can take a client's mind off urges to use alcohol or drugs, such as going to a movie, calling someone, reading a book, or exercising. Urges tend to pass more quickly when a person becomes involved with an alternative activity. *Endurance* is a strategy that forces the individual to face the urge and cope with it directly (e.g., talking it through with someone who is supportive; Otto et al., 2007; Powell et al., 1993).

Coping Strategies for Internal Triggers

Clients can use many of the same strategies for internal triggers that are used using for external triggers. *Self-talk* is a strategy that involves the use of inner voice aiming at enhancing performance through the activation of appropriate responses, which can have a significant impact on one's ability to handle an urge. For example, "The urge feels overwhelming right now but I know if I just hang in there it will pass." *Thinking about the benefits and consequences* is a strategy that involves a tendency to focus only on the positive effects of alcohol or drug use (e.g., feeling less depressed, feeling more social) and that minimizes the negative consequences of their use. While experiencing an urge, it is helpful to review the benefits of not drinking or using drugs and/or the negative consequences of resuming these behaviors. As previously mentioned, *distraction* is a strategy helping the individual to shift one's attention to something else can decrease the intensity of an urge related to a though or feeling. *Endurance* encompasses strategies that focus on going through the experience rather than around it (SAMHSA, 2006).

BARRIERS TO SELF-MANAGEMENT

Self-management involves active engagement of the mental health care consumers in managing their own substance-use related problems. Increasing emotional awareness, positive affect, and one's ability to identify different emotional states can be particularly difficult to achieve when taken into consideration stigma associated with impairments related to substance use.

Stigma of Being "an Addict"

The stigma of being "an addict," as a deviant, antisocial, and inherently morally weak person, is often used to separate and segregate those whose symptoms and/ or characteristics that individuals fear, either because those characteristics are very different from the social norms or because those characteristics are perceived to be very destructive (Gillett, 2009; Gunn et al., 2015; Semple et al., 2005; Woll, 2005). Stereotypes and myths are components of stigma, and they are used to "reduce" individuals to a set of simple and negative characteristics, giving people a sense of psychological distance and manageability. One of the central myths about substance use is that individuals engage in addictive behaviors because those individuals are perceived to be weak-willed or morally inferior. Related to this myth, individuals are often labeled as "Once a junkie, always a junkie." Further, the following may be said about them: "They could quit if they wanted to" or "Treatment doesn't work, and nobody ever recovers."

There can be many explanations of disapproval. For example, disapproval may serve to separate the person holding the stigma from the object of that stigma (Woll, 2005; White, Evans, & Lamb, 2009). In addition, discrimination is often employed in order to further separate the one perceiving from the one being perceived and so gives the perceiver a feeling of greater emotional distance and psychological safety. Discrimination, on the other hand, can be employed as an instrument of redirecting, limiting, or controlling resources. Discrimination is another agent of separation, creating more distance from people whose circumstances are challenging and disturbing (Gillett, 2009; Goffman, 2001Woll, 2005). Thus dealing with the stigma of being "an addict" incorporates a number of complex aspects, which need to be better understood and addressed in treatment, recovery, and healing processes related to family and community.

Affect and Substance Use

An abundance of research conducted on the impact of addiction and chronic health condition of emotions, focusing on both positive and negative affect, is evident in the literature. Negative emotions among individuals with substance-use problems commonly include depression and anxiety that can be crippling to overcome without strategies, techniques, and support. According to the American Society of Addiction Medicine (2016) "addiction" often encompasses dysphoria that can include emotional pain and suffering. In fact, the self-medication model has been used to understand the linkages between emotional states and emotion regulation and its role in the development and maintenance of addictive behaviors (Murphy et al., 2012).

Most individuals with substance-use problems report the idea that substance use will help manage their negative emotions and stress. Yet research indicates that the use of substances does just the opposite: it increases stress (American Society of Addiction, 2016). Under the influence of substances, individuals may temporarily forget their troubles, seeking temporary pleasure, such as the elimination of inhibitions and negative emotions. Moreover, many with a chronic health condition of addiction will look for other solutions to their problems, rather than acknowledging that the impairment itself has created many of them. The chronic health condition approach promotes clients' realization that having an addiction is another part of their life and that being in recovery is not a deficit but rather a process of taking care of one's self. Individuals should be taught how to manage symptoms, urges, and stress, especially in the absence of available treatments. A clinician's most powerful role, therefore, might be to ensure that clients are given all the tools they may need to sustain healthy lives with as little formal intervention as possible.

Executive Functioning and Self-Regulation

Recovery is made more challenging given that addictive behaviors trigger neurochemical reactions that are temporarily satisfying. According to Bradley (2015):

> When one engages non-pathologically in potentially addictive behaviors such as gambling or eating, one may experience a "high," felt as a "positive" emotional state associated with increased dopamine and opioid peptide activity in reward circuits. After such an experience, there is a neurochemical rebound, in which the reward function does not simply revert to baseline, but often drops below the original levels. This is usually not consciously perceptible by the individual and is not necessarily associated with functional impairments (p. 30).

Brain functions can be altered through substance abuse, and, as a consequence, both executive functioning and individual's capacity to self-regulate can be significantly impaired in individuals with substance-use problems, either before the addiction started or as a result of chronic use of certain substances. Executive functioning refers to neuropsychological processes needed to sustain problem-solving toward a goal (Barkley, 2001; Duijkers et al., 2016). When individuals have a barrier of some executive function problems, they may have difficulty with problem-solving, coping, and goal-oriented decision making.

Self-regulation, or the capacity by which individuals manage themselves in order to attain their goals, involves actions that individuals direct at themselves so as to result in a change in their behavior (from what they might otherwise have done), in order to change the likelihood of a future consequence or attainment of a goal (Rothman et al., 2004). Deficits in both executive functioning and self-regulation in individuals with addiction problems result in an inability to efficiently involve with goal-directed, future-oriented actions, to sustain actions over time to achieve one's goals, and to problem-solve as part of those goal-directed actions.

OTHER BARRIERS TO SELF-MANAGEMENT

Socioeconomic issues, race/ethnic issues, and family dynamics play important contextual roles in self-management and need to be taken into account and understood when a person is involved in self-management of addictive behaviors.

Class, status, and power influence the availability of resources and level of support in the individual's life. Those with higher socioeconomic status have access to resources affecting the type of mental health and addiction care received, regardless of race or ethnicity (Acevedo et al., 2012; Acevedo et al., 2015). Those with lower socioeconomic status often struggle with limited access to care, availability of treatments, and medications. In addition, many individuals from racial/ethnic minority backgrounds may be reluctant to seek out help for mental health or addictions providers due to stigmatization and feelings of marginalization or culturally unacceptability.

Another barrier to self-management is co-occurring impairments. Co-occurrence of mental health diagnoses with addictions are common (NIDA, 2010) and provide another significant barrier to recovery and self-management. Dual diagnosis has been a major focus in mental health care in recent years. Substance abuse occurring with any other psychological diagnosis qualifies as a dual (or multiple) diagnoses. Individuals with dual diagnoses tend to have more severe addictions and health outcomes (Saisan, Smith, & Segal, 2015). According to NIDA (2010), drug-use disorders commonly occur with other mental health disorders, but this does not mean that one caused the other, even if it is apparent which disorder appeared first. In fact, establishing which came first or why can be difficult. Research findings (Dixon, 1999; Flynn et al., 2008; McGovern et al., 2014; Moore et al., 2007; Wilson, 2010) suggest that the drug use may elicit symptoms of another mental health issue, as is the case in vulnerable users of marijuana, who are at increased risk to develop psychosis. Mental health issues can lead to drug abuse, possibly as a means of "self-medication." That is, according to NIDA (2010), individuals suffering from anxiety, depression, or other related psychiatric conditions may rely on drugs (e.g., marijuana, alcohol) to temporarily alleviate their symptoms.

The relationship between drug dependencies and mental health conditions is often not properly recognized or diagnosed. An ability to identify other mental health conditions provides self-managers with the opportunity to recognize that there are other factors influencing their use of substances and they may need to address them separately in their efforts to self-manage their addictions. Recovering from co-occurring disorders takes commitment, courage, and time, often months or even years, but people with substance-use and mental health problems can and do get better (Saisan, Smith, & Segal, 2015).

It is also important to note that treatment may also complicated by denial, which is common among individuals who abuse substances (SAMHSA, 2005). These individuals may find it difficult to admit how dependent they have become on alcohol or drugs or how much it may be affecting their relationships and work lives. Denial frequently occurs in mental health issues as well (Ross et al., 1992; Rapp et al., 2006). The symptoms of depression or anxiety can be frightening, so clients may ignore them and hope they will go away on their own. Or they may be ashamed or afraid of being viewed as weak if they admit a problem (McKenzie et al., 2011).

COPING STRATEGIES OR SKILLS TAUGHT FOR IMPAIRMENT

What are some coping strategies and what can be done for those with chronic health conditions? There are many coping strategies in regards to affect, emotion, social, and even management of interactions. The self-management idea is to learn to be self-sufficient, because an individual cannot always depend on a doctor, a therapist, another person, or any outside support.

There are different approaches used to promote coping. For example, emotion-focused coping may be of extreme importance when it comes to learning problem-solving and other coping skills. A person suffering from addiction must find different ways to manage the feelings and recognize the triggers that led to use in the past. Using relaxation techniques such as yoga, meditation and breathing exercises can be a source of coping (Khanna & Greeson, 2014; Zgierska et al., 2009). The skills, insights, and self-awareness learned through yoga and mindfulness practice can target multiple psychological, neural, physiological, and behavioral processes implicated in addiction and relapse (Khanna & Greeson, 2013). Exercise is also a great way to eliminate stress and can be a distraction from one's problems.

TESTED TECHNIQUES TO FACILITATE SELF-MANAGEMENT

Self-management allows individuals who suffer from substance-use problems to take an active role in their recovery. Applying self-management principles to substance-use problems suggests improved overall health, reduced use, stabilized living situations, improved employment situation, and other improvements that contribute to the individual's stabilization and reintegration into society (Lorig & Holman, 2003; Bilsker, 2003; Dive, 2003; Griffin et al., 2009). Self-management encourages individuals to participate in creating their own goals and determining the type of intervention that is best suited for them. This approach supports a variety of goals, meaning that the same goals are not appropriate for everyone (Dive, 2003; Griffin et al., 2009). The treatment approaches created to facilitate self-management include harm reduction, community reinforcement, self-help approaches, and couples and family treatments (Kelly & White, 2012).

Harm-Reduction Approach

Changing addictive, self-defeating behavior is often related to healing self-regulation deficits through the acquisition of a set of self-management skills (represented by indicators of decision-making, problem-solving, self-reinforcement, and self-control skills; Griffin et al., 2009). These skills are necessary for implementing tasks of integrative harm-reduction approach. Harm reduction seeks to reduce the harmful consequences of substance use and other risky behaviors without requiring abstinence (Tatarsky & Kellogg, 2010).

The Community Reinforcement Approach and Community Reinforcement Approach and Family Training

CRA is a comprehensive behavioral program for treating substance-abuse problems. It is based on the belief that environmental contingencies can play a significant role in promoting or demoting substance use. It utilizes social, recreational, familial, and vocational reinforces to assist consumers in the recovery process (Smith, Campos-Melady & Meyers, 2009).

Community reinforcement approach and family training (CRAFT) proposes that concerned family members, called "concerned significant others" (CSOs) have significant influence in treatment of the individuals dealing with substance use–related problems. This method was developed with the belief that since family members can and do make important contributions in other areas of addiction treatment (e.g., family and couples therapy), the CSO can play a powerful role in helping to engage the individual, who abuses substances and who is in denial about their abuse, to submit to treatment. In addition, individuals with substance-use problems often report that family pressure or influence is the reason they sought treatment. Also, CSOs who attend the CRAFT program benefit by becoming more independent and reducing their depression, anxiety, and anger symptoms, even if their family member does not enter treatment (Smith et al., 2009).

Self-Help Movements: AA and NA

Many communities have support groups and self-help groups to help individuals break their addiction and provide support throughout recovery. When considering self-management of co-occurring conditions, recovery can be achieved through a combination of peer support, "self-help" activities, combined treatment (e.g., treatment approaches addressing both the substance use and mental-health problems), and through integration of relapse episodes as part of the recovery process (Donovan, Ingalsbe, Benbow, & Daley, 2013; Vederhus & Kristensen, 2006). As mentioned, self-help groups, such as AA and NA programs, are characterized by a sense of belonging and family.

According to the AA 12-step philosophy (Alcoholics Anonymous, 2015), addiction is a lifelong disease that must be dealt with for the remainder of the person's life; life-long abstinence is the goal achieved through sobriety, one day at a time; and problems can be solved through spiritual change. The AA philosophy is strongly tied to religious/spiritual beliefs (e.g., "higher power"). The philosophy of AA has been applied to form the structure of other self-help groups to aid individuals with addiction (SAMHSA, 2006).

Couples and Family Treatments

The defining feature of couples and family treatments is that they treat drug-using individuals in the context of family and social systems. Thus, they include treatment of the environment in which substance use may develop or be maintained. The engagement of the individual's social networks in treatment can be a powerful predictor of change, and thus the inclusion of family members in treatment may be helpful in reducing attrition and addressing multiple problems (Carrol et al., 2005).

Many family-based approaches combine a variety of techniques, including family and individual therapies, skills training, and communication training. Behavioral couples' therapy and family counseling approaches combine abstinence contracts and behavioral principles to reinforce abstinence from drugs. These approaches require the participation of a non-substance-abusing spouse or cohabitating partners (McHugh et al., 2010; Kumpfer et al., 2014).

CONCLUSION

Substance use is a chronic condition for which multiple episodes of treatment, remission, relapse, and retreatment frequently occur before achieving stable recovery. In this chapter, challenges related to substance use and recovery processes, in addition to the available treatment options, are discussed. Different models of addiction emphasize different approaches to treatment and overall understanding of this condition. The chronic health condition approach promotes clients' beliefs and behaviors that recovery is the process that facilitates change and that being in recovery is not a deficit but rather a client's process of taking care of one's self. Self-management is an approach that allows individuals who struggle with addiction to take more active role in their recovery. Implementation of self-management principles is associated with better treatment outcomes, improved overall health, and quality of life.

REFERENCES

Acevedo, A., Garnick, D., Lee, M., Horgan, M., Ritter, G., Panas, L., . . . Reynolds, M. (2012). Racial/ethnic differences in substance abuse treatment initiation and engagement. *Journal of Ethnicity in Substance Abuse, 11*(1), 1–21. doi:10.1080/15332640.2012.652516.

Acevedo, A., Garnick, D., Ritter, G., Horgan, C., & Lundgren, L. (2015). Race/ethnicity and quality indicators for outpatient treatment for substance-use disorders. *American Journal of Addiction, 24*(6): 523–531. doi:10.1111/ajad.12256.

American Psychiatric Association. (2013). *Diagnostic and statistical manual of mental disorders* (5th ed.) Washington, DC: Author.

American Society of Addiction Medicine. (2016). Quality and Practice: Definition of Addiction.

Barkley R. A. (2001). The executive functions and self-regulation: an evolutionary neuropsychological perspective. Neuropsychology Review, *11*, 1–29. doi:10.1023/A:1009085417776

Bilsker, D. (2003). Self-Management in the Mental Health Field. *Visions, CMHA BC Division, 18*(1), 4–5.

Boston Center for Treatment Development and Training (BCTDT). (2007). Comprehensive Addiction Treatment: A cognitive-behavioral approach to treating substance use disorders.

Bowen, S., Chawla, N., & Marlatt, G. A. (2011). *Mindfulness-Based Relapse Prevention: A Clinician's Guide.* New York: Guilford.

Bowen, S., Witkiewitz, K., Clifasefi, S. L., Grow, J., Chawla, N., Hsu, S. H., ... Larimer, M. E. (2014). Relative Efficacy of Mindfulness-Based Relapse Prevention, Standard Relapse Prevention, and Treatment as Usual for Substance Use Disorders: A Randomized Clinical Trial. *JAMA Psychiatry, 71*(5), 547–556. doi.org/10.1001/jamapsychiatry.2013.4546

Brandon, T. H., Vidrine, J. I., & Litvin, E. B. (2007). Relapse and Relapse Prevention. *Annual Review of Clinical Psychology, 3*, 257–284. doi:10.1146/annurev.clinpsy.3.022806.091455

Calhoun, L. G., & Tedeschi, R. G. (2006). The foundations of posttraumatic growth: An expanded framework. In L. G. Calhoun & R. G. Tedeschi (Eds.), *Handbook of posttraumatic growth: Research and practice* (pp. 1–23). Mahwah, NJ: Lawrence Erlbaum.

Calhoun, L. G., & Tedeschi, R. G. (2013). *Posttraumatic growth in clinical practice.* New York: Brunner Routledge.

Carroll, K. M. (1997). *Cognitive-Behavioral Coping Skills Treatment for Cocaine Dependence.* Yale University Psychotherapy Development Center Substance Abuse Center.

Carroll, K. M. (1998). *A Cognitive Behavioral Approach: Treating Cocaine Addiction.* NIH PublicationNumber: 984308. Rockville, MD: National Institute on Drug Abuse.

Caroll, K. M., & Onken, L. S. (2005). Behavioral Therapies for Drug Abuse. *American Journal of Psychiatry, 162*(8), 1452–1460. doi:10.1176/appi.ajp.162.8.1452

Counselor's Treatment Manual Matrix Intensive Outpatient Treatment for People With Stimulant Use Disorders (2006). U.S. Department of Health and Humna Services Administration Center for Substance Abuse Treatment. Rockville, MD 20857.

Dennis, M., & Scott, C. K. (2007). Managing Addiction as a Chronic Condition. *Addiction Science & Clinical Practice, 4*(1), 45–55.

DiClemente, C. C., Nidecker, M., & Bellack, A. S. (2008). Motivation and the stages of change among individuals with severe mental illness and substance abuse disorders. *Journal of Substance Abuse Treatment, 34*, 25–35.

Dive, L. (2003). Self-Management and Addictions. From *"Self-Management" Issues of Visions Journal, 1*(18), 12–13.

Dixon, L. (1999). Dual diagnosis of substance abuse in schizophrenia: prevalence and impact on outcomes. *Schizophrenia Research, 35*(Supplement 1), S93–S100. http://doi.org/10.1016/S0920-9964(98)00161-3

Donovan, D. M., Ingalsbe, M. H., Benbow, J., & Daley, D. C. (2013). 12-Step Interventions and Mutual Support Programs for Substance Use Disorders: An Overview. *Social Work in Public Health, 28*(0), 313–332. http://doi.org/10.1080/19371918.2013.774663

Duijkers, J. C. L. M., Vissers, C. T. W. M., & Egger, J. I. M. (2016). Unraveling Executive Functioning in Dual Diagnosis. *Frontiers in Psychology, 7*, 979. http://doi.org/10.3389/fpsyg.2016.00979

Ebbert, J. O., Hatsukami, D. K., Croghan, I. T., Schroeder, D. R., & Allen, S. S. (2014). Combination varenicline and bupropion SR for tobacco-dependence treatment in cigarette smokers: A randomized trial. *JAMA*, *311*(2), 155–163. doi:10.1001/jama.2013.283185.

Evers, K. E., Prochaska, J. O., Johnson, J. L., Mauriello, L. M., Padula, J. A., Prochaska, J. M. (2006). A randomized clinical trial of a population- and transtheoretical model-based stress-management intervention. *Health Psychology*, *25*(4), 521–529.

Flynn, P., & Brown, B. (2008). Co-occurring disorders in substance abuse treatment: Issues and prospects. *Journal of Substance Abuse Treatment*, *34*(1), 36–47.

Gillett, G. (2009). The subjective brain, identity, and neuroethics. *American Journal of Bioethics-Neuroscience*, *9*(9), 5–13.

Goffman, E. (2001). *Stigma: Notes on the management of spoiled identity*. London: Pelican Books.

Griffin, K. W., Scheier, L. M., & Botvin, G. J. (2009). Developmental trajectories of self-management skills and adolescent substance use. *Health and Addictions*, *9*, 15–37.

Gunn, A. J., & Canada, K. E. (2015). Intra-group stigma: Examining peer relationships among women in recovery for addictions. *Drugs*, *22*(3), 281–292.

Hendershot, C. S., Witkiewitz, E., George, W. H., & Marlatt, G. A. (2011). Relapse prevention for addictive behaviors. *Substance Abuse Treatment, Prevention, and Policy*, *6*, 17. doi:10.1186/1747-597X-6-17

Kadden, R. M., Carroll, K., Donovan, D., Cooney, N., Monti, P., Abrams, D., Litt, M., & Hester, R. (Eds.) (1992). *Cognitive-Behavioral Coping Skills Therapy Manual: A Clinical Research Guide for Therapists Treating Individuals with Alcohol Abuse and Dependence*. Volume 4, Project MATCH Monograph Series. Rockville, MD: National Institute on Alcohol Abuse and Alcoholism.

Kelly, J., & White, W. (2012) Broadening the base of addiction recovery mutual aid. *Journal of Groups in Addiction & Recovery*, *7*(2-4), 82–101.

Klajner, F., Hartman, L. M., & Sobell, M. B. (1984). Treatment of substance abuse by relaxation training: A review of its rationale, efficacy and mechanisms. *Addictive Behaviors*, *9*(1), 41–55.

Khanna, S., & Greeson, J. M. (2013). A narrative review of yoga and mindfulness as complementary therapies for addiction. *Complementary Therapies in Medicine*, *21*(3), 244–252. doi:10.1016/j.ctim.2013.01.008

Khantzian, E. J. (2014). A Psychodynamic Perspective on the Efficacy of 12-Step Programs. *Alcoholism Treatment Quarterly*, *32*(2-3). Alcoholics Anonymous: New Directions in Research on Spirituality and Recovery; 225–236. http://dx.doi.org/10.1080/07347324.2014.907027

Khantzian, E. J., & Weegmann, M. W. (2009). Questions of substance: Psychodynamic reflections on addictive vulnerability and treatment. *Psychodynamic Practice*, *15*(4), 365–380. doi:10.1080/14753630903230484

Kumpfer, K. L. (2014). Family-Based Interventions for the Prevention of Substance Abuse and Other Impulse Control Disorders in Girls. *ISRN Addiction*, *2014*, Article ID 308789, 23 pages. doi:10.1155/2014/308789

Kushner, M. G. (2007). The use of cognitive-behavioral therapy in the University of Minnesota's outpatient psychiatry clinic. *Minnesota Medicine*, *90*(1), 31–33.

Laberg, J. C., Hugdahl, K., Stormark, K. M., Nordby, H., & Aas, H. (1992). Effects of visual alcohol cues on alcoholics's autonomic arousal. *Psychology of Addictive Behaviors*, *6*, 181–187.

Lancaster, T., Hajek, P., Stead, L. F., West, R., & Jarvis, M. J. (2006). Prevention of Relapse After Quitting SmokingA Systematic Review of Trials. *Archives of Internal Medicine, 166*(8), 828–835. doi:10.1001/archinte.166.8.828

Laudet, A., Stanick, V., & Sands, B. (2007). An exploration of the effect of onsite 12-step meetings on post-treatment outcomes among polysubstance-dependent outpatient clients. *Evaluation Review, 31*(6), 613–646. http://doi.org/10.1177/0193841X07306745

Link, B., & Phelan, J. (2001). Conceptualizing stigma. *Annual Reviews in Sociology, 27*, 363–385.

Lorig, K., & Holman, H. (2000). Self-management education: Context, definition, outcomes and mechanisms. *First Chronic Disease Self-Management Conference*, Australia.

Lorig, K. R., & Holman, H. (2003). Self-management education: history, definition, outcomes, and mechanisms. *Annals of Behavioral Medicine, 26*(1), 1–7.

Lundahl, B. W., Kunz, C., Brownell, C., Tollefson, D., & Burke, B. L. (2010). A Meta-Analysis of Motivational Interviewing: Twenty-Five Years of Empirical Studies. *Research on Social Work Practice, 20*(2), 137–160.

Magill, M., & Ray., L. A. (2009). Cognitive-behavioral treatment with adult alcohol and illicit drug users: A meta-analysis of randomized controlled trials. *Journal of Studies on Alcohol and Drugs, 70*(4), 516–527.

Marlatt, G. A., & Donovan, D. M. (Eds.). (2005). *Relapse Prevention: Maintenance strategies in the treatment of addictive behaviors* (2nd Ed). New York, NY: Guilford Press.

McGovern, M. P., Lambert-Harris, C., Gotham, H. J., Claus, R. E., & Xie, H. (2014). Dual diagnosis capability in mental health and addiction treatment services: An assessment of programs across multiple state systems. *Administration and Policy in Mental Health, 41*(2), 205–214. http://doi.org/10.1007/s10488-012-0449-1

McHugh, R. K., Hearon, B. A., & Otto, M. W. (2010). Cognitive behavioral therapy for substance use disorders. *Psychiatric Clinics of North America, 33*(3), 511–525. http://dx.doi.org/10.1016/j.psc.2010.04.012

McKenzie, M., Jorm., A. F., Romaniuk, H., Olsson, C. A., & Patton, G. C. (2011). Association of adolescent symptoms of depression and anxiety with alcohol use disorders in young adulthood: findings from the Victorian Adolescent Health Cohort Study. *The Medical Journal of Australia, 195*(3), 27.

McLellan, A. T., Luborsky, L., O'Brien, C. P., & Woody, G. E. (1980). An improved diagnostic instrument for substance abuse patients: The Addiction Severity Index. *Journal of Nervous & Mental Diseases, 168*, 26–33.

Milford, J. L., Austin. J. L., & Smith, J. E. (2007). Community reinforcement and the dissemination of evidence-based practice: Implications for public policy. *International Journal of Behavioral Consultation and Therapy, 3*(1), 77–87.

Miller, W. R., & Rose, G. S. (2010). Toward a theory of motivational interviewing. *American Psychologist, 64*(6), 527–537. doi:10.1037/a0016830.

Miller, W. R., Meyers, R. J., & Tonigan, J. S. (1999). Engaging the unmotivated in treatment for alcohol problems: a comparison of three strategies for intervention through family members. *Journal of Consulting and Clinical Psychology, 67*, 688–697.

Monti, P. M., & Rohsenow, D. J. (1999). Coping-Skills Training and Cue-Exposure Therapy in the Treatment of Alcoholism. *Alcohol Research & Health, 23*(2), 107–115.

Moore, T., Zammit, S., Lingford-Hughes, A., Barnes, T., Jones, P., Burke, M., & Lewis, G. (2007). Cannabis use and risk of psychotic or affective mental health outcomes: a systematic review. *The Lancet, 370*(9584), 319-328. doi:http://dx.doi.org/10.1016/S0140-6736(07)61162-3

Murphy, A., Taylor, E., & Elliot, R. (2012). The detrimental effects of emotional process dysregulation on decision-making in substance dependence. *Frontiers in Integrative Neuroscience, 6,* 101.

National Institute on Drug Abuse. (2000). *Principles of drug addiction treatment: A research-based guide.* Bethesda, MD: National Institutes of Health. Retrieved from www.nida.nih.gov/PODAT/PODATindex.html

National Institute on Drug Abuse (NIDA). (2010). Comorbidity: Addiction and other mental illnesses. Research Report Series, NIH publication #10 -5771. Bethesda, MD: NIDA. https://www.drugabuse.gov/publications/research-reports/comorbidity-addiction-other-mental-illnesses

National Institute on Drug Abuse, NIDA (2014). Drugs, Brains, and Behavior: The Science of Addiction. From https://www.drugabuse.gov/publications/drugs-brains-behavior-science-addiction

National Institute on Drug Abuse, NIDA (2016). Treatment. https://www.drugabuse.gov/related-topics/treatment

Prati, G., & Pietrantoni, L. (2009). Optimism, social support, and coping strategies as factors contributing to posttraumatic growth: A meta-analysis. *Journal of Loss and Trauma, 14,* 364-388.

Otto, M. W. (2003). *Therapist manual for cognitive-behavior therapy for interoceptive cues (CBT-IC).* Unpublished manuscript, Massachusetts General Hospital, Boston.

Otto, M. W., O'Cleirigh, C. M., & Pollack, M. H. (2007). Attending to emotional cues for drug abuse: Bridging the gap between clinic and home behaviors. *Science & Practice Perspectives, 3*(2), 48-55.

Petry, N. M., Martin, B., Cooney, J. L., & Kranzler, H. R. (2000). Give them prizes and they will come: Contingency management for treatment of alcohol dependence. *Journal of Consulting and Clinical Psychology, 68*(2), 250-257. http://dx.doi.org/10.1037/0022-006X.68.2.250

Powell, J., Gray, J., & Bradley, B. P. (1993). Subjective craving for opiates: Evaluation of a cue exposure protocol for use with detoxified opiate addicts. *British Journal of Clinical Psychology, 32,* 39-53.

Prochaska, J. O., DiClemente, C. C., & Norcross, J. C. (1992). In search of how people change: Applications to addictive behaviors. *American Psychologist, 47*(9), 1102-1114. doi.10.1037/0003-066X.47.9.1102

Prochaska, J. O., DiClemente, C. C., Velicer, W. F., & Rossi, J. S. (1993). Standardized, individualized, interactive, and personalized self-help programs for smoking cessation. *Health Psychology, 12*(5), 399-405.

Prochaska, J. O., DiClemente, C. C., & Norcross, J. C. (2010). In search of how people change: Applications to addictive behaviors. South Kingston: Cancer Prevention Research Consortium, University of Rhode Island.

Prochaska, J. O., Norcross, J. C., & DiClemente, C. C. (2013). Applying the stages of change. *Psychotherapy in Austrailia, 19*(2), 10-15. PMID: 9155212.

Prochaska, J. O., Velicer, W. F., Fava, J. L., Rossi, J. S., & Tsoh, J. Y. (2001). Evaluating a population-based recruitment approach and a stage-based expert system intervention for smoking cessation. *Addictive Behaviors, 26*(4), 583-602.

Rangé, B. P., & Marlatt, G. A. (2008). Cognitive-behavioral therapy for alcohol and drug use disorders. *Revista Brasileira de Psiquiatria, 30*(Suppl. 2), 88–95. doi.org/10.1590/S1516-44462008000600006

Rapp, R. C., Xu, J., Carr, C. A., Lane, D. T., Wang, J., & Carlson, R. (2006). Treatment barriers identified by substance abusers assessed at a centralized intake unit. *Journal of Substance Abuse Treatment, 30*(3), 227–235. http://doi.org/10.1016/j.jsat.2006.01.002

Rollnick, S., Miller, W. R., Butler, C. C., & Aloia, M. S. (2008). Motivational Interviewing in Health Care: Helping Patients Change Behavior. *COPD: Journal of Chronic Obstructive Pulmonary Disease. 5*(3), 5–203. doi.org/10.1080/15412550802093108

Ross, M. W., & Darke, S. (1992). Mad, bad, and dangerous to know: Dimensions and measurements of attitudes toward injecting drug users. *Drug and Alcohol Dependence, 30*(1), 71–74.

Rothman, A. J., Baldwin, A. S., & Hertel, A. W. (2004). Self-regulation and behavior change: Disentangling behavioral initiation and behavioral maintenance. In R. Baumeister & K. Vohs (Eds.), *Handbook of self-regulation: Research, theory, and applications* (pp. 130–148). New York: Guilford Press.

Rounsaville, B. J., Carroll, K. M., & Onken, L. S. (2001). A stage model of behavioral therapies research: Getting started and moving on from stage I. *Clinical Psychology: Science & Practice, 8*, 133–142.

Saisan, J., Smith, M., & Segal, J. (2015). Substance Abuse and Mental Health: Substance Abuse and Co-Occurring Disorders. HELPGUIDE.org. Retrieved from: http://www.helpguide.org/articles/addiction/substance-abuse-and-mental-health.htm

Samet, S., Hatzenbuehler, M., & Hasin, D. S. (2007). Assessing addiction: Concepts and instruments. *Addiction Science and Clinical Practice, 4*(1), 19–31.

Semple, S. J., Grant, I., & Patterson, T. L. (2005). Utilization of drug treatment programs by methamphetamine users: The role of social stigma. *American Journal on Addictions, 14*(4), 367–380.

Silva, C. J., & Serra, A. M. (2004). Cognitive and Cognitive-Behavioral Therapy for substance abuse disorders. *Rev. Bras. Psiquiatr*, Suppl 1, S33–9.

Smith, J. E., Campos-Melady, M., & Meyers, R. J. (2009). CRA and CRAFT. *Journal of Behavior Analysis in Health, Sports, Fitness and Medicine, 2*(1), 4–31. http://dx.doi.org/10.1037/h0100371

Smith, J. E., Meyers, R. J., & Miller, W. R. (2001). The Community Reinforcement Approach to the Treatment of Substance Use Disorders. *The American Journal on Addictions. American Academy of Addiction Psychiatry, 10*(Suppl.), 51–59.

Substance Abuse and Mental Health Services Administration (2016). Treatments for Substance Use Disorders.

Tatarsky, A., & Kellogg, S. (2010). Integrative harm reduction psychotherapy: a case of substance use, multiple trauma, and suicidality. *Journal of Clinical Psychology, 66*, 123–135. doi:10.1002/jclp.20666

Tedeschi, R. G., & Calhoun, L. G. (1996). The Posttraumatic Growth Inventory: Measuring the positive legacy of trauma. *Journal of Traumatic Stress, 9*(3), 455–471.

Teyber, E. (2006). *Interpersonal process in therapy: An integrative model (5th ed.)*. Belmont, CA: Brooks/Cole Publishing.

Turner, de S., & Cox, H. (2004). Facilitating post traumatic growth. *Health and Quality of Life Outcomes, 2*, 34. http://doi.org/10.1186/1477-7525-2-34

U.S. Department of Health and Human Services National Institutes of Health National Institute on Drug Abuse. (2002). Therapy Manuals for Drug Addiction Drug Counseling for Cocaine Addiction: The Collaborative Cocaine Treatment Study Mode.

Vederhus, J. K., & Kristensen, Ø. (2006). High effectiveness of self-help programs after drug addiction therapy. *BMC Psychiatry, 6*, 35. http://doi.org/10.1186/1471-244X-6-35

White, W. L., Evans, A. C., & Lamb, R. (2009). Reducing addiction-related social stigma. *Counselor, 10*(6), 52–58.

Whitelaw, S., Baldwin, S., Bunton, R., & Flynn, D. (2000). The status of evidence and outcomes in Stages of Change research. *Health Education Research: Theory and Practice, 15*(5), 707–718.

Wilson, G. T. (2010), Eating disorders, obesity and addiction. *European Eating Disorders Review, 18*, 341–351. doi:10.1002/erv.1048.

Witkiewitz, K., Bowen, S., Douglas, H., & Hsu, S. H. (2013). Mindfulness-Based Relapse Prevention for Substance Craving. *Addictive Behaviors, 38*(2), 1563–1571.

Witkiewitz, K., & Marlatt, G. A. (2004). Relapse Prevention for Alcohol and Drug Problems: That Was Zen, This Is Tao. *American Psychologist, 59*(4), 224–235. http://dx.doi.org/10.1037/0003-066X.59.4.224

Woll, P. (2005). Healing the stigma of addiction: A guide for treatment professionals. Chicago, IL: Great Lakes Addiction Technology Transfer Center.

Zgierska, A., Rabago, D., Chawla, N, Kushner, K., Koehler, R., & Marlatt, A. (2009). Mindfulness meditation for substance use disorders: A systematic review. *Substance Abuse, 30*(4), 266–294.

8
Self-Management of Arthritis

JESSICA M. BROOKS, KANAKO IWANAGA, AND FONG CHAN ■

Arthritis is one of the most prevalent chronic conditions in middle-aged to late adulthood and is ranked among the top 10 causes of disability worldwide (Centers for Disease Control and Prevention [CDC], 2015b). In the United States, medical doctors have diagnosed nearly 52.5 million (22.7%) adults. More women than men are diagnosed at any point in time, with prevalence rates increasing steadily with age (Barbour et al., 2016; CDC, 2009, 2010). Adults first manifest signs and symptoms between 30 and 50 years and by 65 years of age over half of older adults are diagnosed (CDC, 2016). Arthritis is projected to impact as many as 67 million American adults by 2030 due to the rapidly growing baby boomer population (Hootman & Helmick, 2006).

Arthritis refers to "over 100 musculoskeletal conditions of varying etiologies that cause pain, aching, or stiffness in or around the joint" (Hootman, Helmick, & Brady, 2012, p. 426). The most common types of arthritis diagnosed are osteoarthritis (OA) and rheumatoid arthritis (RA), with OA being more pervasive than RA (Pendleton et al., 2000). These pain conditions are significantly associated with fatigue, sleep problems, social isolation, and loss of employment, resulting in functional disability, complex medical needs, and lost productivity (Backman, 2006; CDC, 2015a; Kahvecioglu, Moore, Michaelides, Ruiz, & Bertrand, 2010; Kobelt, Eberhardt, Jonsson, & Jönsson, 1999; Riemsma, Kirwan, Taal, & Rasker, 2003; Ryan, 2014). With total national health expenditures exceeding $3 trillion dollars per year, expenditures for arthritis care will continue to rise and account for a high percentage of healthcare costs and annual gross domestic product in the next several decades (Centers for Medicare and Medicaid Services, 2016).

Despite recent improvements in medications and medical treatment, there is no known cure for arthritis. Arthritis has physical, psychological, and social components (Stone & Baker, 2014), and it is common for people with arthritis to have secondary health consequences including multiple co-occurring physical conditions (CDC, 2015a). Anxiety and depression are also well-documented co-occurring conditions. Physical and psychological conditions often interact and negatively influence one another--worsening arthritis-related symptoms and increasing the risk for other co-occurring conditions and early mortality (Furner, Hootman, Helmick, Bolen, & Zack, 2011; Hootman et al., 2012). Providing evidence-based psychoeducation and counseling services to adults with arthritis on how to cope with and manage pain and associated disability will lessen the impact of arthritis on the individual and society (Dures et al., 2016).

The purpose of this chapter is to provide an overview of the most common arthritic conditions, co-occurring physical conditions, and psychosocial factors associated with arthritis. Barriers to self-management and existing self-management programs are discussed along with the current state of scientific evidence.

ARTHRITIC CONDITIONS

Because OA is more pervasive than RA (Pendleton et al., 2000), OA is typically what many people think of as "arthritis" (Allaire, Keysor, & AlHeresh, 2013). It affects nearly 27 million Americans, with 12 million people with OA age 65 years old or older (Lawrence et al., 2008). For older adults age 75 years and older, the prevalence rates for OA escalate to between 70% and 90% (Hunter & Eckstein, 2009).

Osteoarthritis

Historically, OA was considered a "wear and tear" disease--caused by increased pressure on specific joints or from fragile or weakened cartilage--leading to a loss of cartilage, boney outgrowth, and joint damage (Bedson, Mottram, Thomas, & Peat, 2007; Berenbaum, 2013). However, it is now known that OA has a more complicated process involving inflammatory properties released by cartilage, bone, and synovial membrane. Common symptoms include pain, limited range of motion, and morning stiffness (Kraus, 1997; Lefevre-Colau et al., 2014; Parkinson & Harris, 2010; Wittenauer, Smith, & Aden, 2013). The etiology for OA is unknown, but the pathogenesis is characterized by the gradual deterioration of cartilage providing support and "cushioning" to the bones in joints. When a person's cartilage is healthy, it replaces itself--yet this process is disrupted when a person is experiencing symptoms of OA. While there is no known antidote for OA, knowledge of risk factors provides the opportunity to prevent arthritis or at least to better manage impairment and slow down the progression (Brennan & Turrell, 2012). Risk factors associated with the onset and progression of OA are multifactorial and include genetics, age, sex, obesity, physical trauma, rural residency, and low bone density (Krasnokutsky, Samuels, & Abramson, 2007; Lutfiyya et al., 2013; Pearson-Ceol, 2007).

OA is rated 11th in the world for major causes of disability (Vos et al., 2013). The long-term implications of OA for working-age and older adults involve pain and stiffness as well as permanent damage to joints that bear weight--most often knees, hips, spine, and hands (Bedson et al., 2007; Hubertsson, Petersson, Thorstensson, & Englund, 2012). Consequently, people with OA frequently experience functional impairment resulting in an altered range of motion and limitations in activities of daily living, such as walking, extended sitting and standing, opening jars and doors, and writing or typing (Allaire, Keysor, & AlHeresh, 2013).

There is also evidence that older adults experience more issues related to physical disability than younger-aged peers. Out of adults with arthritis age 65 years and older, almost half report activity limitations that can be attributed to arthritis (Hootman, Helmick, & Schappert, 2002) and approximately one out of four report severe pain (Bolen et al., 2010). On the other hand, younger or preretirement age adults affected by arthritis may experience more psychological distress related to work impairment, financial problems, and other disruptions to normal day-to-day functioning (Weinberger, Tierney, Booher, & Hiner, 1990). Work disability impacts one-third to over 50% of younger to middle-aged individuals who report functional limitations related to arthritis (Gignac, Jetha, Bowring, Beaton, & Badley, 2012; Sharif et al., 2016; Theis, Murphy, Hootman, Helmick, & Yelin, 2007). These arthritis-related impairments are linked to physical inactivity, obesity, and depression (CDC, 2011), leading to poor health-related quality of life (Furner et al., 2011; Hootman & Cheng, 2009; Strine et al., 2004). People with OA can also have significant workplace restrictions on the type or amount of work that they can do (Sharif et al., 2016; Theis et al., 2007), with frequent absenteeism, limited productivity, or the inability to retain employment.

Rheumatoid Arthritis

The other common type of arthritis is RA, which is a systemic autoimmune disorder where the immune system reacts to a person's own tissues. RA affects 0.5% to 1% of the general population and approximately 1.3 million adults in the United States (Widdifield et al., 2014). RA appears to be universal as there are no countries or racial or ethnic groups in which RA is not found. While the exact cause for RA is unclear (Cross et al., 2014; Kourilovitch, Galarza-Maldonado, & Ortiz-Prado, 2014), its prevalence and incidence can differ according to various biological, personal, and environmental factors, including genetics, geographic location or birthplace, sex, birth weight, socioeconomic status, age, and calendar time (Alamanos, Voulgari, & Drosos, 2006; Kourilovitch et al., 2014; Liao, Alredsson, & Karlson, 2009). There are also behavioral risk factors, such as smoking, obesity, and alcohol intake, that can significantly increase susceptibility to RA—increasing the risk up to 40 times compared with people who are not exposed to these factors.

Similar to OA, RA often develops gradually over time in middle-aged adults. Early symptoms manifest as pain and stiffness primarily in multiple joints in the hands and feet. Pain, multiple joint tenderness, swelling, and other symptoms such as fatigue eventually become chronic, although RA is characterized by phases of remission and flares unique to each individual (Rouse et al., 2015). The painful effects of RA usually progress from distal to more proximal joints and can lead to permanent structural joint damage, erosion, and deformity (Lee & Weinblatt, 2001). Recurrent flares can also result in functional decline and long-term disability (Bertin et al., 2015; McInnes & Schett, 2011). Other complications may interfere with the organ systems, such as the heart, lungs, and blood vessels (Lee & Weinblatt, 2001).

Even with improved medical care, RA is often debilitating and diminishes health-related quality of life, with nearly 30% to 50% of adults with RA stopped working five years after initial diagnosis (Young et al., 2002). Research evidence indicates older age, poor health status, functional limitations, and lower educational attainment are associated with employment problems such as absenteeism, leaving the labor force, and difficulties with managers and co-workers (Bansback et al., 2012; Gignac, Cao, Tang, & Beaton, 2011; Lacaille, White, Backman, & Gignac, 2007; Verstappen et al., 2004). Functional impairment is often invisible in the early stages, and the flare and remission pattern of symptoms can be difficult for others to understand, which can lead to disbelief and lack of support from co-workers and others. Job context is also critical to understanding employment participation, as jobs with high physical demands and where there are few workplace adaptations or accommodations available are associated with greater employment difficulties (Geuskens, Hazes, Barendregt, & Burdorf, 2008; Verstappen et al., 2004; Yelin, 2007). Job activities requiring repetitive activities, energy, and stamina may also be impaired.

CO-OCCURRING PHYSICAL CONDITIONS

The burden of arthritis extends well beyond the joint (Cutolo, Kitas, Piet, & van Riel, 2014). Arthritis is associated with a number of physical co-occurring conditions, such as cardiovascular disease (CVD), diabetes, respiratory illness, chronic fatigue, sleep disturbances, and cognitive dysfunction. Among US adults with at least two chronic conditions, arthritis is the most common chronic condition in all age groups (CDC, 2015a). Of those reporting arthritis, at least 88% have one other co-occurring physical condition (Gadermann, Alonso, Vilagut, Zaslavsky, & Kessler, 2012). The presence of multiple conditions is linked to a number of functional limitations, such as physical and work-related disability (Nicassio et al., 2012; Schofield, Callander, Shrestha, Passey, Percival, & Kelly, 2014; Verstappen, 2015). The significance of the auxiliary treatment and management of arthritis and multiple chronic conditions cannot be overlooked, given its impact on pain severity, functional limitations, and ability to work. Three of the most prevalent and disabling co-occurring physical conditions for people with arthritis include CVD, respiratory illness, and diabetes (CDC, 2016).

Cardiovascular Disease

The prevalence of CVD including heart attacks and strokes in people with RA has been found to be as high as or even higher than those with a primary diagnosis of type 2 diabetes (Van Halm et al., 2009). Nearly 30% of people with arthritis also have heart disease or are stroke survivors (Murphy, Bolen, Helmick, & Brady, 2009). Out of adults age 18 years and older with CVD, 50% of these individuals also have arthritis (Barbour et al., 2013). Several studies have shown an underdiagnosis and undertreatment of classical CVD risk factors, such as obesity, smoking, dyslipidaemia, high cholesterol, and hypertension in RA, which likely contributes to the higher likelihood of CVD and poorer health outcomes (Panoulas et al., 2010; Toms, Panoulas, & Kitas, 2011).

The course of RA and other forms of arthritis has improved following the introduction of effective medications and regular adjustment of treatment to the targets of recurring symptoms or remission, yet co-occurring conditions like CVD may cause complications and early mortality (Dougados et al., 2013). For instance, Panoulas et al. (2010) indicated that 32% of people with RA with organ damage also had undiagnosed hypertension. Individuals with RA, therefore, should be routinely screened for CVD risk factors and receive CVD-related treatment (Van Breukelen-van der Stoep, Klop, van Zeben, Hazes, & Cabezas, 2013).

Respiratory Illness

About one in five of US adults with arthritis are current smokers (Murphy et al., 2009). Smoking can cause respiratory illness, which is the second most common physical co-occurring condition among adults with arthritis. Smoking is an environmental risk factor and accounts for about 25% of the risk to develop RA (Lahiri, Morgan, Symmons, & Bruce, 2011). A recent meta-analysis showed that the prevalence of ever, current, and past smokers in RA was as high as 50.6%, 26.5%, and 26.3%, respectively (Sugiyama, et al., 2010).

Although smoking is a shared risk factor for arthritis, respiratory illness, and other co-occurring conditions, there is heterogeneity in smoking advice provided by healthcare providers. In one study, approximately two-thirds of rheumatologists recommended smoking cessation to individuals with RA, but only one in five departments had a specific protocol for smoking cessation (Naranjo et al., 2014). Compared to nonsmoking groups, current smokers with arthritis are at an increased risk for all-cause mortality (Joseph, Movahedi, Dixon, & Symmons, 2016). In a pilot study of a tailored smoking-cessation intervention, people with RA showed decreased rates of smoking (Aimer et al., 2016). More research is needed to evaluate whether smoking-cessation programs tailored to people with RA may have the potential to reduce the prevalence of co-occurring conditions.

Diabetes

Obesity is an important and widespread risk and maintenance factor in all arthritic conditions and type 2 diabetes (Anandacoomarasamy, Caterson, Sambrook, Fransen, & March, 2008). About 47% of adults age 18 years and older with diabetes also have arthritis, and 31% of obese adults also have arthritis (Barbour et al., 2013). Obesity and diabetes place an extra burden on individuals with arthritis with regard to pain severity, functional status, work disability, medical costs, and mortality (Ajeganova, Andersson, & Hafstrom, 2013; Tunceli, Li, & Williams, 2006; Wolfe & Michaud, 2012). In a longitudinal study of 24,535 people with RA, obesity was found in approximately 63% to 68% of people with RA. This cohort was also significantly more likely to have type 2 diabetes mellitus, hypertension, myocardial infarction, joint replacement, and work disability over their normal-weight counterparts (Wolfe & Michaud, 2012).

Because excess weight adds pressure to joints, it is not a surprise that modest weight loss has been shown to improve symptoms of arthritis in people with arthritis, particularly in those with arthritis, obesity, and diabetes (Bolen et al., 2010; Hootman et al., 2012). While physical activity and exercise can reduce pain-related symptoms, obesity, and diabetes risk for arthritis populations (Cooney et al., 2011), only about 50% of people with arthritis are sufficiently active, and many people with arthritis are sedentary (Wallis, Webster, Levinger, & Taylor, 2013). Clinical practice guidelines recommend that overweight and obese individuals with arthritis be encouraged to lose weight to prevent diabetes and reduce the risks for other chronic conditions (Zhang et al., 2008).

PSYCHOLOGICAL AND SOCIAL FACTORS

Although medical advances have stalled the progression of arthritic symptoms and improved quality of life in some arthritis cases, there remains a large proportion of people with arthritis suffering from symptoms and disability. Consequently, more comprehensive models of pain and disability are needed to better understand arthritis. The biopsychosocial model of chronic pain conceptualizes the effects of physical factors as well as psychological and social factors related to arthritis. Over the past few decades, there has been a growing body of literature on psychosocial factors affecting severity, both physical and psychological co-occurring conditions, trajectory, and outcomes of people living with arthritis (Gatchel, Peng, Peters, Fuchs, & Turk, 2007).

Rates of anxiety and depression may be as high as 18% to 33% among people with arthritis (Murphy, Sacks, Brady, Hootman, & Chapman, 2012). Studies have shown that the use of passive psychosocial coping strategies (e.g., avoiding situations or giving up control) increases the risks of developing a co-occurring psychological condition such as depression (Treharne, Lyons, Booth, & Kitas, 2007). In one study, only half of the individuals with arthritis with anxiety and/or depression had sought help in the past year, suggesting there is an unmet need for mental health treatment. Consistent with biopsychosocial models of pain and disability (Keefe et al., 2002), mental health problems can worsen pain, co-occurring conditions, and functional disability and, in turn, affect health status, health-related quality of life, and community integration and participation (Matcham et al., 2014; Wolfe & Michaud, 2009).

The coexistence of various psychological and social issues may lead to further issues with underregulation or misregulation of arthritis. For instance, depression is often associated with barriers to self-care, reduced self-management skills, and non-adherence to treatment in people with arthritis (Harrison et al., 2012). Other psychosocial factors, such as job stress, perceived work-health conflict, and passive coping among people with arthritis, are also linked to functional limitations and negative employment outcomes (Gignac et al., 2012; Lacaille et al., 2007). People living with arthritis with low social participation have been reported to experience more pain and fatigue, poorer mental health, and lower mastery (Benka et al., 2016). Unsurprisingly, life satisfaction in people with arthritis is negatively affected by limited social support, negative affect, depressive symptoms, functional disability, and restricted home, social, and work participation (Coty & Wallston, 2010; Katz & Morris, 2007). Life satisfaction also seems to be lower in individuals with RA in comparison to the general population, with only 22% of all individuals with RA reporting feeling satisfied with their life (Hewlett, Smith, & Kirwan, 2002; Karlsson, Berglin, & Wållberg-Jonsson, 2006).

Despite such life dissatisfaction, psychological distress, and social problems (Rouse et al., 2015), many people report experiencing personal growth (Dirik & Karanci, 2008) and finding benefits (Danoff-Burg & Revenson, 2005) from living with arthritis. Psychological thriving is a result of continued growth and is related to coping efficacy, expectations for future growth, and reduced depression in people with arthritis (Sirois & Hirsch, 2013). Learning to "thrive" may help to address psychosocial issues associated with arthritis. Those with arthritis who use active coping strategies (e.g., exercise, meditation, social support) to manage daily tasks, personal standards, and life goals have more favorable outcomes and higher subjective well-being than those who use passive coping strategies (Evers, Kraaimaat, Geenen, Jacobs, & Bijlsma, 2003). Learning to adapt to one's long-term condition, social or role expectations, and external stressors play an important role in how people with arthritis prioritize self-management (Sanderson, Hewlett, Richards, Morris, & Calnan, 2012). Maintaining employment is also a vital source of support and livelihood for adults with arthritis and their families. Studies have also found that actively engaging in employment is also associated with improved self-esteem, social support, life satisfaction, health status, and reduced depression and pain in individuals with RA (Hoving, van Zwieten, van der Meer, Sluiter, & Frings-Dresen, 2013).

BARRIERS TO ARTHRITIS SELF-MANAGEMENT

Managing or keeping life as it was before diagnosis is often difficult for people with chronic pain such as arthritis. Adults with arthritis need to balance impairment-related symptoms together with life responsibilities, such as employment, parenting, housework, leisure, and social activities, which can contribute to actual and perceived stress (Coty, Salt, Myers, & Abusalem, 2015; Katz & Morris, 2007). Self-management programs can help people living with arthritis to learn to find balance and reengage in activities that protect and promote health. Monitoring and managing the arthritis-related symptoms and signs affect the impact of arthritis on a wide range of functioning and improves treatment engagement.

There are several empirically validated self-management intervention programs that are endorsed by the CDC, including the Arthritis Self-Management Program (ASMP) developed by Kate Lorig of Stanford University beginning in 1979. However, several person and environment (P × E) contextual factors are often reported as facilitators or barriers to arthritis self-management and warrant consideration in self-management interventions. These P × E contextual factors are discussed in the following sections.

Personal Factors

Personal factors are defined as coping style, age, gender, race/ethnicity, or other personal characteristics (Mpofu & Oakland, 2010). These characteristics are important to consider in arthritis rehabilitation because empirical studies have demonstrated that they can facilitate or impede the ability to engage in health promoting behaviors and activities in people with arthritis and other disabilities. For example, people with adaptive features, such as hope beliefs and reduced depression, have better disability adjustment (Chan, Cardoso, & Chronister, 2009; Chan, Chan, Ditchman, Phillips, & Chou, 2013; Elliott, Witty, Herrick, & Hoffman, 1991; Wilson, et al., 2013). On the other hand, people with non-adaptive coping strategies, such as avoidance behaviors, tend to have poorer outcomes in rehabilitation (Hill & Kennedy, 2002).

Cognitive Vulnerabilities

It is common for people with arthritis to maintain negative, distorted interpretations of pain, such as catastrophizing. Pain catastrophizing is described as exaggerated negative orientation toward pain or anticipated pain (Backman, 2006; Mann, LeFort, & VanDenKerkhof, 2013; Sullivan, Bishop, & Pivik, 1995). Extensive literature reviews and longitudinal research studies have consistently found that pain catastrophizing is associated with increased psychological distress, pain intensity, and functional disability (Edwards, Cahalan, Mensing, Smith, & Haythornthwaite, 2011; Smeets, Vlaeyen, Kester, & Knottnerus, 2006). People who catastrophize also report higher rates of healthcare usage and use pain medications more than those who do not catastrophize (Keefe, Rumble, Scipio, Giordano, & Perri, 2004). Another non-adaptive cognitive belief and behavior--also related to anxiety--is referred to as fear avoidance. Experimental and cross-sectional research have demonstrated the relevance of pain-related avoidance factors, which are shown to be associated with pain intensity and functional disability (Gatchel et al., 2007; Keefe et al., 2002; Lööf, et al., 2015). Due to the overwhelming evidence on the roles of pain non-adaptive beliefs and related behaviors, rehabilitation and healthcare professionals should aim to address these barriers to self-management.

Self-Efficacy

Decades of research studies have demonstrated that self-efficacy is a facilitator of psychosocial rehabilitation, health-behavior change, and health maintenance in people with and without chronic conditions. Self-efficacy is defined as a person's expectation that he or she can successfully initiate and complete an activity. The pain literature is replete with studies that indicate that higher perceived self-efficacy is linked to pain reduction, physical functioning, psychological adjustment, and treatment outcomes (Keefe et al., 2004). Certainly, for those with chronic pain like arthritis who are dealing with inadequate pharmacological and non-pharmacological treatment, lifelong self-management is essential for coping with arthritis. A sense of regulatory efficacy is important as the fluctuating course of arthritis and uncertain functional capacity may threaten autonomy and subjective well-being (Taal, Rasker, & Wiegman, 1996; Van Liew et al., 2013). Results from cross-sectional research and longitudinal studies demonstrate that higher self-efficacy is linked to decreased pain, less fatigue, increased physical ability, improved mood, and improved treatment engagement (Barlow, Cullen, & Rowe, 2002; Lefevre-Colau et al., 2014). In a recent study, positive physical activity experiences, confidence, social support, and intentions were predictors of increased physical activity among people with arthritis (Peeters, Brown, & Burton, 2014).

Closely related to self-efficacy, health literacy, or the degree to which people process, comprehend, and obtain health information and services, is also found to be low in individuals with arthritis (Field, Ziebland, McPherson, & Lehman, 2006; Parker, Ratzan, & Lurie, 2003). Nearly one-third of people with arthritis have been reported to be unaware of their specific type of arthritis, and many others have little understanding of the medications they are taking, especially men and those with lower educational attainment, suggesting that even basic knowledge related to diagnosis and treatment is an important health issue (Ling et al., 2000; Sacks, Luo, & Helmick, 2010). In a national study of more than 6,000 people with arthritis, low health literacy was found to be more negatively associated with functional status than medication use or smoking history (Caplan, Wolfe, Michaud, Quinzanos, & Hirsh, 2014). A narrative review of the RA literature on the barriers, benefits, and facilitators of self-management strategies, namely physical activity and exercise, found perceived similarities between barriers and benefits. For instance, both increased and reduced pain and fatigue were frequently mentioned as perceived barriers and benefits to physical activity and exercise (Van Zanten et al., 2015). Out of the people who did not regularly exercise, these individuals reported difficulties with learning how to overcome initial barriers to achieve long-lasting benefits from physical activity and exercise.

Pain Acceptance

Several empirical studies have found that the construct of pain acceptance is associated with lower pain, improved functioning, and better disability adjustment (McCracken & Eccleston, 2003). Pain acceptance is described as when a person responds to the painful experience without attempting to control or avoid the pain (Fish, McGuire, Hogan, Morrison, & Stewart, 2010). Pain acceptance involves participating in important activities of daily functioning and self-management programs that may exacerbate or cause pain. It may also require discontinuing avoidance or passive behaviors, such as sedentary activity, in order to prevent pain. A recent meta-analysis of 66 experimental studies of acceptance- and mindfulness-related processes concluded that these factors are supportive of positive rehabilitation outcomes in the context of pain (Levin, Hildebrandt, Lillis, & Hayes, 2012).

Environmental Factors

Personal and environmental factors are not easily disentangled; however, environmental variables are described as primarily influences external to an individual (Mpofu & Oakland, 2010). These factors can include physical environment factors, as well as social, family, provider, community, work, or cultural environmental variables. It is invaluable to consider these contextual variables because they can have a significant impact on pain-related disability and arthritis rehabilitation. For example, individuals with disabilities reporting strong social support have been shown to have lower mortality rates and better overall health outcomes (Chronister, 2009). In contrast, individuals with disabilities in acute rehabilitation settings with lower levels of family support tend to endure longer recovery times (Mpofu & Oakland, 2010). There are also studies that show that people with significant health conditions like chronic pain may be faced with negative stereotypes within a given context like healthcare settings, which ultimately discourages self-management, limits participation, and reduces quality of life (Brown, DeLeon, Loftis, & Scherer, 2008; Corrigan & Penn, 1999; Molina, Choi, Cella & Rao, 2013).

One environmental factor that may have a substantial impact on pain self-management is the social environment. Often, people learn to respond to and experience painful situations by observing people within their environment, including family members, friends, healthcare professionals, or other social influences (Gatchel et al., 2007; Turk & Monarch, 2002). Another source of social pressure occurs through the mechanism of operant conditioning, which posits that individuals who receive no external reinforcement (or punishment) will decrease or extinguish pain-related behaviors, while people who receive positive reinforcers will adopt pain behaviors (Turk & Monarch, 2002). For example, Mann et al. (2013) showed that support from family and friends helped to facilitate engagement in health self-management activities.

Likewise, support from healthcare providers is also an important factor for self-management. However, professionals often lack knowledge of appropriate health information and services, which contributes to the underutilization of health promotion interventions, such as structured exercise (Hootman, Helmick, & Brady, 2012). Healthy People 2010 (US Department of Health and Human Services, 2000) and Healthy People 2020 (US Department of Health and Human Services, 2010) encouraged healthcare providers to recommend weight loss and regular physical activity to overweight and obese adults with arthritis, but, unfortunately, there has only been a marginal improvement in self-reported rates of weight management counseling (Hootman, Helmick, & Brady, 2012).

SELF-MANAGEMENT EDUCATION PROGRAMS

Self-management education support is recognized as a core component of person-centered services for health care and rehabilitation and is recommended in guidelines for people with arthritis (Do et al., 2011). Self-management is defined as the ability to manage the symptoms, treatment, physical and psychosocial consequences, and lifestyle changes inherent in living with a chronic condition (Barlow, Turner, & Wright, 2000). Self-management education programs are used to improve self-efficacy, motivation, coping and problem-solving behaviors (Lorig, Mazonson, & Holman, 1993; Lorig, Ritter, & Plant, 2005). Most self-management education programs are based on Bandura's (1997, 2000) self-efficacy theory, which emphasizes the mastery of skills, modeling, the reinterpretation of symptoms, and social persuasion. These self-management education programs differ from other educational or skills-training programs because of their focus on initiation and self-motivation.

Self-management education programs vary in content domains used to educate people about their chronic health conditions. Some educational programs may opt to focus on managing only the chronic condition itself, while other programs may take a holistic approach to managing the overall health and well-being of the individual. Other variations in self-management interventions include the mode of delivery (face-to-face, Internet, telephone), intervention approaches (psychotherapeutic techniques or strategies used), the audience (group, individual), the duration (single session, several months, ongoing), the frequency (once a week, once every two months), and the personnel (healthcare professionals, peers; Kroon et al., 2014).

Exemplary Self-Management Education Programs

One of the most recognized arthritis self-management intervention programs is ASMP-endorsed and recommended by CDC, the Arthritis Foundation, and the American College of Rheumatology. It was developed by Dr. Kate Lorig and her research team at Stanford University. It was designed to help people with different types of rheumatic diseases (e.g., OA, RA, fibromyalgia, and lupus) learn to adapt to their condition and gain confidence and control over their lives. It is a six-week course facilitated by two trained leaders, one or both of whom are non-health professionals with arthritis themselves. The workshops are held in community settings such as senior centers, churches, libraries, and hospitals. There is also an Internet-based version of the ASMP (Lorig, Ritter, Laurent, & Plant, 2008).

For ASMPs, participants meet weekly for two hours to learn and practice techniques for building an arthritis self-management program tailored to their own needs. Workshops include educational sessions covering eight topics: (a) techniques to deal with problems such as pain, fatigue, frustration and isolation; (b) appropriate exercise for maintaining and improving strength, flexibility, and endurance; (c) appropriate use of medications; (d)) communicating effectively with family, friends, and health professionals; (e) healthy eating; (f) making informed treatment decisions; (g) arthritis-related problem-solving; and (h) getting a good night's sleep. Participants engage in group discussions to obtain feedback and suggestions from their peers. Participants are expected to practice suggested approaches at home and report their progress in group discussion. Each participant also receives the *Arthritis Helpbook* (6th ed.), which contains all of the program content.

Expected benefits of the ASMP include reduced fatigue and health distress, ability to exercise more frequently, decreased depression and anxiety, better communication with physicians, and increased confidence in managing arthritis. Despite the advantages of AMSP, there are some critiques of the program, which include concerns related to potential language barriers for non-native English speakers or participants with limited health literacy, the program's restrictive time frame, and the workshop itself being overly strenuous and requiring considerable resources. In addition, group dynamics could also have a negative impact on the participants due to social comparisons (Corbin & Strauss, 1985; Haslbeck et al., 2015).

Another self-management education program recommended by CDC is the Living Well with a Disability (LWWD) program, a self-management intervention developed by researchers at the University of Montana in partnership with the national network of Centers for Independent Living and with support from CDC's Disability and Health Branch (Ipsen, Ravesloot, Arnold, & Seekins, 2012; Ravesloot et al., 2007; Ravesloot, Seekins, & White, 2005; Seekins, Clay, & Ravesloot, 1994; Seekins et al., 1999). The LWWD program was developed to support individuals with disabilities, including people with arthritis, to manage their health (Ravesloot et al., 2007). The curriculum helps participants achieve early success in self-management of quality-of-life goals to build confidence for making health behavior changes. The program has been implemented by 279 community-based agencies in 46 states as of May 2015.

The LWWD program includes 11 chapters with an orientation session and 10 weekly, two-hour sessions. In the first chapter, an orientation session, participants explore potential obstacles to attendance, examine the potential benefits of participating in the program, and consider strategies they might use to overcome barriers. The next four sessions encourage peer support through a supportive, solution-focused group process; they help participants develop hope that they can achieve a more meaningful and healthy life while addressing the early challenges of pursuing new goals. These sessions build analytical and problem-solving skills (e.g., frustration management and self-monitoring for depression to identify needs that may need outside clinical attention). The last six sessions focus on specific self-management skills for improving health status, including strategies for effective communication with healthcare providers, strategies for information acquisition and use, strategies for increasing activity (through six levels—from sedentary to recommended levels of exercise), strategies for improving diet (based on US Department of Agriculture guidelines), strategies for advocating for both personal and healthcare systems improvements, and cognitive and behavioral strategies for maintaining health behavior changes over time. Expected benefits of participating in the LWWD program include reduced limitations from secondary conditions, fewer unhealthy days, and less healthcare utilization.

RESEARCH EVIDENCE

Over the past several decades, the evidence base has been emerging on arthritis self-management programs. Warsi, LaValley, Wang, Avorn, and Solomon (2003) conducted a meta-analytic study of the effect of arthritis self-management education programs on pain and disability. Of the 35 studies they found, 17 studies with 4,114 participants met their inclusion criteria. The average drop-out rate for these studies was 19%. Three reported using the ASMP. The overall effect size indicated a small effect of self-management education interventions on pain ($d = 0.12$; 95% confidence interval [CI] 0.00, 0.24) and an even smaller effect on disability ($d = 0.07$; 95% CI 0.00, 0.15). Subgroup analysis of the ASMP interventions also revealed a small, non-significant effect on pain ($d = 0.04$; 95% CI 0.19, 0.27) and on disability ($d = 0.10$; 95% CI 0.05, 0.24).

Foster, Taylor, Eldridge, Ramsay, and Griffiths (2007) conducted a systematic review of self-management education programs led by lay leaders for people with chronic conditions including arthritis. Seventeen randomized controlled trials (RCTs) involving 7,442 participants met the inclusion criteria for their study. Results of RCTs were pooled using a random-effects model with standardized mean differences for continuous outcomes. They found that self-management programs led by lay leaders only had modest, short-term improvements in perceived confidence to manage arthritis and perceptions of health status. These interventions also increased the frequency that people with arthritis engaged in aerobic exercise. Foster et al. (2007) questioned the clinical significance of self-management programs due to only small improvements in pain, disability, fatigue, and depression. Moreover, the self-management programs did not improve quality of life and did not reduce the number of times people with arthritis visited their doctor or the amount of time spent in hospital.

Kroon and his associates (2014) examined 29 RCTs comprising 6,753 individuals with OA comparing self-management education programs to attention control

(5 studies), usual care (17 studies), information alone (4 studies), or another intervention (7 studies). Components of the self-management interventions were extracted using the eight domains of the Health Education Impact Questionnaire and contextual and participant characteristics using PROGRESS-Plus and the Health Literacy Questionnaire. Outcomes included self-management of OA, participant's positive and active engagement in life, pain, global symptom score, self-reported function, quality of life, and withdrawals (including dropouts and those lost to follow-up). The majority of the self-management programs included elements of skill and technique acquisition (94%), health-directed activity (85%), and self-monitoring and insight (79%). However, it should be noted that social integration and support were addressed in only 12% of the RCTs. The authors reported that low to moderate quality evidence indicates that self-management education programs result in no or small benefits in people with OA. Specifically, compared with attention control, self-management education programs do not appear to improve self-management skills, pain, OA symptoms, function or quality of life; and the effects of self-management education programs on positive and active engagement in life are unknown. Compared with usual care, self-management education programs appear to have a small effect on improving self-management skills, pain, function and symptoms.

To sort through the evidence specifically for the ASMP, researchers at the CDC (2011) conducted a meta-analysis to examine the effect of ASMP on multiple outcomes for people with arthritis in terms of physical and psychological health status (including self-efficacy), health behaviors, and healthcare utilization. A total of 24 studies with 6,812 participants were included in the CDC study. The analysis of heterogeneity by study design (RCT and longitudinal) indicated that it was acceptable to analyze the overall effect size for each outcome by combining the effects of RCTs and longitudinal studies. For RCTs only, the meta-analysis results indicated a small to moderate effect size for increased self-efficacy for pain and other symptom management (effect size [ES] = 0.340), increased communication with physician (ES = 0.277), decreased fatigue (ES = –0.210), decreased anxiety (ES = –0.200), and decreased depression (ES = –0.200). In terms of overall effects at 4 to 6 months and 9 to 12 months, self-efficacy increased moderately in the shorter term and persisted longer term (9 to 12 months). Psychological health status (health distress, depression, and anxiety) also showed consistent small to moderate improvements for both the RCTs and longitudinal studies. These small to moderate benefits were found to persist at 9- to 12-month follow-up. Changes in fatigue, pain, and functional disability were less consistent than the changes in psychological health status outcomes. There was a small effect size for reducing fatigue at 4 to 6 months and 9 to 12 months and no significant changes in functional disability and pain intensity. Health behaviors (exercise, cognitive symptom management, and communication with physician) all showed statistically significant moderate improvements at 4 to 6 months and persisted at 9 to 12 months for all variables except exercise behaviors. Healthcare utilization data were limited to physician visits and the results indicated a small and significant decrease (ES = –0.12) for the longitudinal studies only. Researchers in this CDC study concluded that even though the effects of self-management education are very modest, these findings have public health significance when the cumulative impact of small changes across a large population is considered. They contended that these changes in health behaviors if sustained could have a significant effect on health-related quality of life and the physical, psychological, and social impact of people with chronic health conditions.

There is limited research conducted on the LWWD self-management program. Seekins and his colleagues demonstrated in several pilot studies that participants who completed the Living Well intervention program rated themselves as less limited by secondary conditions than individuals who did not complete the intervention (Ravesloot, Seekins, & Young, 1998; Seekins et al., 1999). In 2005, Ravesloot et al. (1998) conducted a national study implemented by staff recruited from community-based agencies located in geographically diverse areas around the United States with 188 individuals with disabilities. They found that participants who completed the LWWD program had significant reductions in limitation from secondary conditions and that the intervention effect was maintained 2, 4, and 12 months after the conclusion of the intervention. Specifically, Ravesloot et al. (2005) concluded the LWWD intervention was successful in reducing the average degree of limitation people report due to secondary conditions, the number of symptom days they experience, and their healthcare costs ($807 per person due to reductions in healthcare utilization) while increasing their overall life satisfaction and the behaviors they used to improve health status. Importantly, they found that increased in physical activity is significantly related to improved health conditions.

Most recently, Ravesloot et al. (2016) summarized research findings for the LWWD program. They reported that the program has been implemented by 279 community-based agencies in 46 states and approximately 8,900 individuals have received LWWD training since 1995. Ravesloot et al. indicated these community-based LWWD programs may have incurred an estimated savings of $6.4 million to $28.8 million for healthcare payers. They also reported results from their 2007 study (Ravesloot et al., 2007) that participants in the LWWD treatment group were three times more likely than those in the control group to be below the median for secondary conditions (adjusted odds ratio [AOR]: 3.05; 95% CI: 1.33–7.01), after controlling for demographics and preintervention status with respect to the median of each variable (Ravesloot et al., 2007). In addition, people in the treatment group were significantly more likely to be below the median in terms of symptom days (AOR: 1.96; 95% CI: 0.91–4.26) and healthcare use (AOR: 1.94; 95% CI: 1.03–3.67).

CONCLUSION

Managing arthritis and life after diagnosis is difficult and complicated by arthritis-specific, physical, psychological, and social factors. There are also a number of personal and contextual barriers to arthritis management. Given the small to moderate effect sizes at best of ASMP and other self-management programs, there are several questions that remain. Should content in arthritis self-management programs include additional information on co-occurring conditions? Would a stronger emphasis on components of psychotherapeutic or behavioral interventions be more effective? What are the ideal delivery methods for implementation? Because self-efficacy is a well-established construct, program developers should also consider integrating features of other empirically supported health behavior theories, such as self-determination theory, or theories highly relevant to people with chronic pain like the fear-avoidance model (Crombez, Eccleston, Van Damme, Vlaeyen, & Karoly, 2012).

Arthritis is one of the most commonly occurring chronic conditions and is projected to increase in prevalence with the aging baby boomers. Arthritis self-management should be a priority area for intervention development and implementation in healthcare and rehabilitation services. Evidence-based modifications to existing self-management programs or the development of novel programs may better suit the unique needs of the arthritis population in the current era. With fast-paced advances in communication technology for healthcare delivery, the time may also be ripe to leverage technology to improve cost-effectiveness and have a wider reach and impact.

REFERENCES

Aimer, P., Stamp, L. K., Stebbings, S., Cameron, V., Kirby, S., Croft, S., & Treharne, G. J. (2016). Developing a tailored smoking cessation intervention for rheumatoid arthritis patients. *Musculoskeletal Care, 14*(1), 2–14.

Ajeganova, S., Andersson, M. L., & Hafström, I. (2013). Association of obesity with worse disease severity in rheumatoid arthritis as well as with co-occurring conditions: A long-term follow up from disease onset. *Arthritis Care & Research, 65*(1), 78–87.

Alamanos, Y., Voulgari, P. V., & Drosos, A. A. (2006). Incidence and prevalence of rheumatoid arthritis, based on the 1987 American College of Rheumatology criteria: A systematic review. *Seminars in Arthritis and Rheumatism, 36*, 182–188.

Allaire, S. J., Keysor, J. J., & AlHeresh, R. (2013). Effect of arthritis and other rheumatic conditions on employment. *Work, 45*(3), 417–420.

Anandacoomarasamy, A., Caterson, I., Sambrook, P., Fransen, M., & March, L. (2008). The impact of obesity on the musculoskeletal system. *International Journal of Obesity, 32*(2), 211–222.

Backman, C. L. (2006). Review: Arthritis and pain: Psychosocial aspects in the management of arthritis pain. Retrieved from http://arthritis-research.biomedcentral.com/articles/10.1186/ar2083

Bandura, A. (1977). Self-efficacy: Toward a unifying theory of behavioral change. *Psychological Review, 84*, 191–215.

Bandura, A. (2000). Health promotion from the perspective of social cognitive theory. In P. Norman, C. Abraham, & M. Conner (Eds.), *Understanding and changing health behaviour* (pp. 299–339). Reading, UK: Harwood.

Bansback, N., Zhang, W., Walsh, D., Kiely, P., Williams, R., Guh, D., . . . Young, A. (2012). Factors associated with absenteeism, presenteeism and activity impairment in patients in the first years of RA. *Rheumatology, 51*(2), 375–384.

Barbour, K. E., Helmick, C. G., Boring, M., Zhang, X., Lu, H., & Holt, J. B. (2016). Prevalence of doctor-diagnosed arthritis at state and county levels—United States, 2014. *Morbidity and Mortality Weekly Report, 65*, 489–494.

Barbour, K. E., Helmick, C. G., Theis, K. A., Murphy, L. B., Hootman, J. M., Brady, T. J., & Cheng, Y. J. (2013). Prevalence of doctor-diagnosed arthritis and arthritis-attributable activity limitation—United States, 2010–2012. *Morbidity and Mortality Weekly Report, 62*(44), 869–873.

Barlow, J. H., Cullen, L. A., & Rowe, I. F. (2002). Educational preferences, psychological well-being and self-efficacy among people with rheumatoid arthritis. *Patient Education and Counseling, 46*(1), 11–19.

Barlow, J. H., Turner, A. P., & Wright, C. C. (2000). A randomized controlled study of the Arthritis Self-Management Programme in the UK. *Health Education Research, 15*(6), 665–680.

Bedson, J., Mottram, S., Thomas, E., & Peat, G. (2007). Knee pain and osteoarthritis in the general population: What influences patients to consult? *Family Practice, 24*(5), 443–453.

Benka, J., Nagyova, I., Rosenberger, J., Macejova, Z., Lazurova, I., van der Klink, J. L., . . . van Dijk, J. P. (2016). Social participation in early and established rheumatoid arthritis patients. *Disability and Rehabilitation, 38*(12), 1172–1179.

Berenbaum, F. (2013). Osteoarthritis as an inflammatory disease (osteoarthritis is not osteoarthrosis!). *Osteoarthritis and Cartilage, 21*(1), 16–21.

Bertin, P., Fagnani, F., Duburcq, A., Woronoff, A. S., Chauvin, P., Cukierman, G., . . . Kobelt, G. (2015). Conséquences de la polyarthrite rhumatoïde sur la trajectoire professionnelle, la productivité et l'employabilité: étude PRET. *Revue du Rhumatisme, 82*(5), 306–311.

Bolen, J., Schieb, L., Hootman, J. M., Helmick, C. G., Theis, K., Murphy, L. B., & Langmaid, G. (2010). Differences in the prevalence and impact of arthritis among racial/ethnic groups in the United States, National Health Interview Survey, 2002, 2003, and 2006. *Preventing Chronic Disease, 7*(3), A64.

Brennan, S. L., & Turrell, G. (2012). Neighborhood disadvantage, individual-level socioeconomic position, and self-reported chronic arthritis: A cross-sectional multilevel study. *Arthritis Care & Research, 64*(5), 721–728.

Brown, K. S., DeLeon, P. H., Loftis, C. W., & Scherer, M. J. (2008). Rehabilitation psychology: Realizing the true potential. *Rehabilitation Psychology, 53*(2), 111–121.

Caplan, L., Wolfe, F., Michaud, K., Quinzanos, I., & Hirsh, J. M. (2014). Strong association of health literacy with functional status among rheumatoid arthritis patients: A cross-sectional study. *Arthritis Care & Research, 66*(4), 508–514.

Centers for Disease Control and Prevention. (2009). Recommended community strategies and measurements to prevent obesity in the United States. *Morbidity and Mortality Weekly Report, 58*, 1–26.

Centers for Disease Control and Prevention. (2010). *A national public health agenda for osteoarthritis 2010*. Retrieved from www.cdc.gov/arthritis/docs/OAagenda.pdf

Centers for Disease Control and Prevention. (2011). *Sorting through the evidence of the Arthritis Self-Management Program and the Chronic Disease Self-Management*

Program: Executive summary of the ASMP/CDSMP meta-analyses. Retrieved from http://www.cdc.gov/arthritis/docs/ASMP-executive-summary.pdf

Centers for Disease Control and Prevention. (2015a). *Comorbidities among people with arthritis.* Retrieved from http://www.cdc.gov/arthritis/data_statistics/comorbidities.htm

Centers for Disease Control and Prevention. (2015b). *Health, United States, 2015, with special feature on racial and ethnic health disparities.* Retrieved from http://www.cdc.gov/nchs/data/hus/hus15.pdf#019

Centers for Disease Control and Prevention. (2016). *National health expenditure fact sheet.* Retrieved from https://www.cms.gov/research-statistics-data-and-systems/statistics-trends-and-reports/nationalhealthexpenddata/nhe-fact-sheet.html

Centers for Medicare and Medicaid Services. (2016). *Arthritis-related statistics.* Retrieved from http://www.cdc.gov/arthritis/data_statistics/arthritis-related-stats.htm

Chan, F. E., Da Silva Cardoso, E. E., & Chronister, J. A. (2009). *Understanding psychosocial adjustment to chronic illness and disability: A handbook for evidence-based practitioners in rehabilitation.* Dordrecht: Springer.

Chan, J. Y. C., Chan, F., Ditchman, N., Phillips, B., & Chou, C. C. (2013). Evaluating Snyder's hope theory as a motivational model of participation and life satisfaction for individuals with spinal cord injury: A path analysis. *Rehabilitation Research, Policy, and Education, 27*(3), 171–185.

Chronister, J. (2009). Social support and rehabilitation: Theory, research and measurement. In F. Chan, E. Cardoso, & J. Chronister (Eds.), *Understanding psychosocial adjustment to chronic illness and disability: A handbook for evidence-based practitioners in rehabilitation* (pp. 149–183). New York: Springer.

Cooney, J. K., Law, R. J., Matschke, V., Lemmey, A. B., Moore, J. P., Ahmad, Y., . . . Thom, J. M. (2011). Benefits of exercise in rheumatoid arthritis. *Journal of Aging Research, 2011*, 1–25.

Corbin, J., & Strauss, A. (1985). Managing chronic illness at home: three lines of work. *Qualitative Sociology, 8*(3), 224–247.

Corrigan, P. W., & Penn, D. L. (1999). Lessons from social psychology on discrediting psychiatric stigma. *American Psychologist, 54*(9), 765–776.

Coty, M. B., & Wallston, K. A. (2010). Problematic social support, family functioning, and subjective well-being in women with rheumatoid arthritis. *Women & Health, 50*(1), 53–70.

Coty, M. B., Salt, E. G., Myers, J. A., & Abusalem, S. K. (2015). Factors affecting well-being in adults recently diagnosed with rheumatoid arthritis. *Journal of Health Psychology.* Advance online publication. doi/abs/10.1177/1359105315604887

Crombez, G., Eccleston, C., Van Damme, S., Vlaeyen, J. W., & Karoly, P. (2012). Fear-avoidance model of chronic pain: the next generation. *Clinical Journal of Pain, 28*(6), 475–483.

Cross, M., Smith, E., Hoy, D., Carmona, L., Wolfe, F., Vos, T., . . . Buchbinder, R. (2014). The global burden of rheumatoid arthritis: Estimates from the Global Burden of Disease 2010 study. *Annals of the Rheumatic Diseases, 73*, 1323–1330.

Cutolo, M., Kitas, G. D., & Van Riel, P. L. (2014). Burden of disease in treated rheumatoid arthritis patients: Going beyond the joint. *Seminars in Arthritis and Rheumatism, 43*, 479–488.

Danoff-Burg, S., & Revenson, T. A. (2005). Benefit-finding among patients with rheumatoid arthritis: Positive effects on interpersonal relationships. *Journal of Behavioral Medicine, 28*(1), 91–103.

Dirik, G., & Karanci, A. N. (2008). Variables related to posttraumatic growth in Turkish rheumatoid arthritis patients. *Journal of Clinical Psychology in Medical Settings*, *15*(3), 193–203.

Do, B. T., Hootman, J. M., Helmick, C. G., & Brady, T. J. (2011). Monitoring healthy people 2010 arthritis management objectives: Education and clinician counseling for weight loss and exercise. *Annals of Family Medicine*, *9*(2), 136–141.

Dougados, M., Soubrier, M., Antunez, A., Balint, P., Balsa, A., Buch, M., . . . Hajjaj-Hassouni, N. (2013). Prevalence of co-morbidities in rheumatoid arthritis (RA) and evaluation of their monitoring: Results of an international, cross-sectional study. *Annals of the Rheumatic Diseases*, *72*, 62–68.

Dures, E., Almeida, C., Caesley, J., Peterson, A., Ambler, N., Morris, M., Pollock, J., & Hewlett S. (2016). Patient preferences for psychological support in inflammatory arthritis: A multicentre survey. *Annals of the Rheumatic Diseases*, *75*,142–147.

Edwards, R. R., Cahalan, C., Mensing, G., Smith, M., & Haythornthwaite, J. A. (2011). Pain, catastrophizing, and depression in the rheumatic diseases. *Nature Reviews Rheumatology*, *7*(4), 216–224.

Elliott, T. R., Witty, T. E., Herrick, S. M., & Hoffman, J. T. (1991). Negotiating reality after physical loss: Hope, depression, and disability. *Journal of Personality and Social Psychology*, *61*(4), 608.

Evers, A. W., Kraaimaat, F. W., Geenen, R., Jacobs, J. W., & Bijlsma, J. W. (2003). Pain coping and social support as predictors of long-term functional disability and pain in early rheumatoid arthritis. *Behaviour Research and Therapy*, *41*(11), 1295–1310.

Field, K., Ziebland, S., McPherson, A., & Lehman, R. (2006). "Can I come off the tablets now?": A qualitative analysis of heart failure patients' understanding of their medication. *Family Practice*, *23*(6), 624–630.

Fish, R. A., McGuire, B., Hogan, M., Morrison, T. G., & Stewart, I. (2010). Validation of the Chronic Pain Acceptance Questionnaire (CPAQ) in an Internet sample and development and preliminary validation of the CPAQ-8. *Pain*, *149*(3), 435–443.

Foster, G., Taylor, S. J., Eldridge, S. E., Ramsay, J., & Griffiths, C. J. (2007). Self-management education programmes by lay leaders for people with chronic conditions. *Cochrane Database of Systematic Reviews*, *4*(4), CD005108.

Furner, S. E., Hootman, J. M., Helmick, C. G., Bolen, J., & Zack, M. M. (2011). Health-related quality of life of US adults with arthritis: Analysis of data from the behavioral risk factor surveillance system, 2003, 2005, and 2007. *Arthritis Care & Research*, *63*(6), 788–799.

Gadermann, A. M., Alonso, J., Vilagut, G., Zaslavsky, A. M., & Kessler, R. C. (2012). Co-occurring conditions and Disease burden in the national co-occurring conditions survey replication (NCS-R). *Depression and Anxiety*, *29*(9), 797–806.

Gatchel, R. J., Peng, Y. B., Peters, M. L., Fuchs, P. N., & Turk, D. C. (2007). The biopsychosocial approach to chronic pain: Scientific advances and future directions. *Psychological Bulletin*, *133*(4), 581–624.

Geuskens, G. A., Hazes, J. M., Barendregt, P. J., & Burdorf, A. (2008). Work and sick leave among patients with early inflammatory joint conditions. *Arthritis Care & Research*, *59*(10), 1458–1466.

Gignac, M. A., Cao, X., Tang, K., & Beaton, D. E. (2011). Examination of arthritis-related work place activity limitations and intermittent disability over four-and-a-half years and its relationship to job modifications and outcomes. *Arthritis Care & Research*, 63(7), 953–962.

Gignac, M. A., Jetha, A., Bowring, J., Beaton, D. E., & Badley, E. M. (2012). Management of work disability in rheumatic conditions: A review of non-pharmacological interventions. *Best Practice & Research Clinical Rheumatology*, 26(3), 369–386.

Harrison, M., Reeves, D., Harkness, E., Valderas, J., Kennedy, A., Rogers, A., . . . Bower, P. (2012). A secondary analysis of the moderating effects of depression and multimorbidity on the effectiveness of a chronic disease self-management programme. *Patient Education and Counseling*, 87(1), 67–73.

Haslbeck, J., Zanoni, S., Hartung, U., Klein, M., Gabriel, E., Eicher, M., & Schulz, P. J. (2015). Introducing the chronic disease self-management program in Switzerland and other German-speaking countries: findings of a cross-border adaptation using a multiple-methods approach. *BMC Health Services Research*, 15(1), 1–19.

Hewlett, S., Smith, A. P., & Kirwan, J. R. (2002). Measuring the meaning of disability in rheumatoid arthritis: The Personal Impact Health Assessment Questionnaire (PI HAQ). *Annals of the Rheumatic Diseases*, 61(11), 986–993.

Hill, L., & Kennedy, P. (2002). The role of coping strategies in mediating subjective disability in people who have psoriasis. *Psychology, Health & Medicine*, 7(3), 261–269.

Hootman, J. M., & Cheng, W. Y. (2009). Psychological distress and fair/poor health among adults with arthritis: State-specific prevalence and correlates of general health status, United States, 2007. *International Journal of Public Health*, 54(1), 75–83.

Hootman, J. M., & Helmick, C. G. (2006). Projections of US prevalence of arthritis and associated activity limitations. *Arthritis & Rheumatism*, 54(1), 226–229.

Hootman, J. M., Helmick, C. G., & Brady, T. J. (2012). A public health approach to addressing arthritis in older adults: The most common cause of disability. *American Journal of Public Health*, 102(3), 426–433.

Hootman, J. M., Helmick, C. G., & Schappert, S. M. (2002). Magnitude and characteristics of arthritis and other rheumatic conditions on ambulatory medical care visits, United States, 1997. *Arthritis Care & Research*, 47(6), 571–581.

Hoving, J. L., van Zwieten, M. C., van der Meer, M., Sluiter, J. K., & Frings-Dresen, M. H. (2013). Work participation and arthritis: A systematic overview of challenges, adaptations and opportunities for interventions. *Rheumatology*, 52(7), 1254–1264.

Hubertsson, J., Petersson, I. F., Thorstensson, C. A., & Englund, M. (2012). Risk of sick leave and disability pension in working-age women and men with knee osteoarthritis. *Annals of the Rheumatic Diseases*, 72(3), 401–405.

Hunter, D. J., & Eckstein, F. (2009). Exercise and osteoarthritis. *Journal of Anatomy*, 214(2), 197–207.

Ipsen, C., Ravesloot, C., Arnold, N., & Seekins, T. (2012). Working well with a disability: Health promotion as a means to employment. *Rehabilitation Psychology*, 57(3), 187–195.

Joseph, R. M., Movahedi, M., Dixon, W. G., & Symmons, D. P. (2016). Smoking-related mortality in patients with early rheumatoid arthritis—a retrospective cohort study using the Clinical Practice Research Datalink. *Arthritis Care & Research*, 68(11), 1598–1606.

Kahvecioglu, D., Moore, T., Michaelides, M., Ruiz, R., & Bertrand, R. (2010). *Agency for healthcare research and quality: Final evaluation report.* Retrieved from http://www.

ahrq.gov/sites/default/files/wysiwyg/research/findings/final-reports/aoa/aoachronic.pdf

Karlsson, B., Berglin, E., & Wållberg-Jonsson, S. (2006). Life satisfaction in early rheumatoid arthritis: A prospective study. *Scandinavian Journal of Occupational Therapy*, *13*(3), 193–199.

Katz, P., & Morris, A. (2007). Time use patterns among women with rheumatoid arthritis: association with functional limitations and psychological status. *Rheumatology*, *46*(3), 490–495.

Keefe, F. J., Rumble, M. E., Scipio, C. D., Giordano, L. A., & Perri, L. M. (2004). Psychological aspects of persistent pain: Current state of the science. *The Journal of Pain*, *5*(4), 195–211.

Keefe, F. J., Smith, S. J., Buffington, A. L., Gibson, J., Studts, J. L., & Caldwell, D. S. (2002). Recent advances and future directions in the biopsychosocial assessment and treatment of arthritis. *Journal of Consulting and Clinical Psychology*, *70*(3), 640–655.

Kobelt, G., Eberhardt, K., Joensson, L., & Jönsson, B. (1999). Economic consequences of the progression of rheumatoid arthritis in Sweden. *Arthritis & Rheumatism*, *42*(2), 347–356.

Kourilovitch, M., Galarza-Maldonado, C., & Ortiz-Prado, E. (2014). Diagnosis and classification of rheumatoid arthritis. *Journal of Autoimmunity*, *48*, 26–30.

Krasnokutsky, S., Samuels, J., & Abramson, S. B. (2007). Osteoarthritis in 2007. *Bulletin— Hospital for Joint Diseases New York*, *65*(3), 222–228.

Kraus, V. B. (1997). Pathogenesis and treatment of osteoarthritis. *Medical Clinics of North America*, *81*(1), 85–112.

Kroon, F. P. B., van der Burg, L. R. A., Buchbinder, R., Osborne, R. H., Johnston, R.V., & Pitt, V. (2014). Self-management education programmes for osteoarthritis. *Cochrane Database of Systematic Reviews*, *1*, CD008963.

Lacaille, D., White, M. A., Backman, C. L., & Gignac, M. A. (2007). Problems faced at work due to inflammatory arthritis: New insights gained from understanding patients' perspective. *Arthritis Care & Research*, *57*(7), 1269–1279.

Lahiri, M., Morgan, C., Symmons, D. P., & Bruce, I. N. (2011). Modifiable risk factors for RA: Prevention, better than cure? *Rheumatology*, *51*, 499–512.

Lawrence, R. C., Felson, D. T., Helmick, C. G., Arnold, L. M., Choi, H., Deyo, R. A., . . . Jordan, J. M. (2008). Estimates of the prevalence of arthritis and other rheumatic conditions in the United States: Part II. *Arthritis & Rheumatism*, *58*(1), 26–35.

Lee, D. M., & Weinblatt, M. E. (2001). Rheumatoid arthritis. *Lancet*, *358*, 903–911.

Lefevre-Colau, M. M., Buchbinder, R., Regnaux, J. P., Roren, A., Poiraudeau, S., & Boutron, I. (2014). Self-management education programmes for rheumatoid arthritis. *Cochrane Database of Systematic Reviews*. Advance online publication. doi:10.1002/14651858.CD011338

Levin, M. E., Hildebrandt, M. J., Lillis, J., & Hayes, S. C. (2012). The impact of treatment components suggested by the psychological flexibility model: A meta-analysis of laboratory-based component studies. *Behavior Therapy*, *43*(4), 741–756.

Liao, K. P., Alfredsson, L., & Karlson, E. W. (2009). Environmental influences on risk for rheumatoid arthritis. *Current Opinion in Rheumatology*, *21*(3), 279–283.

Ling, S. M., Fried, L. P., Garrett, E., Hirsch, R., Guralnik, J. M., & Hochberg, M. C. (2000). The accuracy of self-report of physician diagnosed rheumatoid arthritis in moderately to severely disabled older women. Women's Health and Aging Collaborative Research Group. *The Journal of Rheumatology, 27*(6), 1390–1394.

Lööf, H., Demmelmaier, I., Welin Henriksson, E., Lindblad, S., Nordgren, B., Opava, C. H., & Johansson, U. B. (2015). Fear-avoidance beliefs about physical activity in adults with rheumatoid arthritis. *Scandinavian Journal of Rheumatology, 44*(2), 93–99.

Lorig, K. R., Mazonson, P. D., & Holman, H. R. (1993). Evidence suggesting that health education for self-management in patients with chronic arthritis has sustained health benefits while reducing healthcare costs. *Arthritis Rheumatology, 36*, 439–446.

Lorig, K. R., Ritter, P. L., Laurent, D. D., & Plant, K. (2008). The Internet-based arthritis self management program: A one year randomized trial for patients with arthritis or fibromyalgia. *Arthritis & Rheumatology, 59*, 1009–1017.

Lorig, K., Ritter, P. L., & Plant, K. (2005). A disease-specific self-help program compared with a generalized chronic disease self-help program for arthritis patients. *Arthritis Care & Research, 53*(6), 950–957.

Lutfiyya, M. N., McCullough, J. E., Saman, D. M., Lemieux, A., Hendrickson, S., McGrath, C. A., ... Lipsky, M. S. (2013). Rural/urban differences in health services deficits among US adults with arthritis: A population-based study. *Journal of Nursing Education and Practice, 3*(11), 43–53.

Mann, E. G., LeFort, S., & VanDenKerkhof, E. G. (2013). Self-management interventions for chronic pain. *Pain Management, 3*(3), 211–222.

Matcham, F., Scott, I. C., Rayner, L., Hotopf, M., Kingsley, G. H., Norton, S., ... Steer, S. (2014). The impact of rheumatoid arthritis on quality-of-life assessed using the SF-36: A systematic review and meta-analysis. *Seminars in Arthritis and Rheumatism, 44*, 123–130.

McCracken, L. M., & Eccleston, C. (2003). Coping or acceptance: What to do about chronic pain?. *Pain, 105*(1), 197–204.

McInnes, I. B., & Schett, G. (2011). The pathogenesis of rheumatoid arthritis. *The New England Journal of Medicine, 365*(23), 2205–2219.

Molina, Y., Choi, S. W., Cella, D., & Rao, D. (2013). The Stigma Scale for Chronic Illnesses 8-item version (SSCI-8): Development, validation and use across neurological conditions. *International Journal of Behavioral Medicine, 20*(3), 450–460.

Mpofu, E., & Oakland, T. (2010). *Assessment in rehabilitation and health*. Upper Saddle River, NJ: Merrill.

Murphy, L. B., Sacks, J. J., Brady, T. J., Hootman, J. M., & Chapman, D. P. (2012). Anxiety and depression among US adults with arthritis: prevalence and correlates. *Arthritis Care & Research, 64*(7), 968–976.

Murphy, L., Bolen, J., Helmick, C. G., & Brady, T. J. (2009, February). Co-occurring conditions are very common among people with arthritis. Poster presented at the 20th National Conference on Chronic Disease Prevention and Control, Atlanta.

Naranjo, A., Bilbao, A., Erausquin, C., Ojeda, S., Francisco, F. M., Rúa-Figueroa, I., & Rodríguez-Lozano, C. (2014). Results of a specific smoking cessation program for patients with arthritis in a rheumatology clinic. *Rheumatology International, 34*(1), 93–99.

Nicassio, P. M., Ormseth, S. R., Kay, M., Custodio, M., Irwin, M. R., Olmstead, R., & Weisman, M. H. (2012). The contribution of pain and depression to self-reported sleep disturbance in patients with rheumatoid arthritis. *Pain, 153*(1), 107–112.

Panoulas, V. F., Toms, T. E., Metsios, G. S., Stavropoulos-Kalinoglou, A., Kosovitsas, A., Milionis, H. J., . . . Kitas, G. D. (2010). Target organ damage in patients with rheumatoid arthritis: The role of blood pressure and heart rate. *Atherosclerosis, 209*(1), 255–260.

Parker, R. M., Ratzan, S. C., & Lurie, N. (2003). Health literacy: A policy challenge for advancing high-quality health care. *Health Affairs, 22*(4), 147–153.

Parkinson, L., & Harris, M. (2010). *Effective population health interventions for the primary prevention of musculoskeletal conditions*. Melbourne: State of Victoria.

Pearson-Ceol, J. (2007). Literature review on the effects of obesity on knee osteoarthritis. *Orthopaedic Nursing, 26*(5), 289–292.

Peeters, G., Brown, W., & Burton, N. (2014). Physical activity context preferences in people with arthritis and osteoporosis. *Journal of Physical Activity & Health, 11*(3), 536–542.

Pendleton, A., Arden, N., Dougados, M., Doherty, M., Bannwarth, B., Bijlsma, J. W. J., . . . Hauselmann, H. J. (2000). EULAR recommendations for the management of knee osteoarthritis: report of a task force of the Standing Committee for International Clinical Studies Including Therapeutic Trials (ESCISIT). *Annals of the Rheumatic Diseases, 59*(12), 936–944.

Ravesloot, C. H., Seekins, T., Cahill, T., Lindgren, S., Nary, D. E., & White, G. (2007). Health promotion for people with disabilities: Development and evaluation of the Living Well with a Disability program. *Health Education Research, 22*(4), 522–531.

Ravesloot, C., Seekins, T., & White, G. (2005). Living Well with a Disability health promotion intervention: Improved health status for consumers and lower costs for healthcare policy makers. *Rehabilitation Psychology, 50*, 239–245.

Ravesloot, C., Seekins, T., & Young, Q. R. (1998). Health promotion for people with chronic illness and physical disabilities: The connection between health psychology and disability prevention. *Clinical Psychology & Psychotherapy, 5*(2), 76–85.

Ravesloot, C., Seekins, T., Traci, M, Boehm, T., White, G., Witten, M. H., Mayer, M., . . . Monson, J. (2016). Living Well with a Disability, a self-management program. *CDC Morbidity and Mortality Weekly Report Supplements, 65*(1), 61–67.

Riemsma, R. P., Kirwan, J. R., Taal, E., & Rasker, J. J. (2003). Patient education for adults with rheumatoid arthritis. *Cochrane Database of Systematic Reviews, 2*, CD003688.

Rouse, P. C., Van Zanten, J. J. V., Ntoumanis, N., Metsios, G. S., Yu, C. A., Kitas, G. D., & Duda, J. L. (2015). Measuring the positive psychological well-being of people with rheumatoid arthritis: A cross-sectional validation of the subjective vitality scale. *Arthritis Research & Therapy, 17*(1), 1–7.

Ryan, S. (2014). Psychological effects of living with rheumatoid arthritis. *Nursing Standard, 29*(13), 52–59.

Sacks, J. J., Luo, Y. H., & Helmick, C. G. (2010). Prevalence of specific types of arthritis and other rheumatic conditions in the ambulatory healthcare system in the United States, 2001–2005. *Arthritis Care & Research, 62*(4), 460–464.

Sanderson, T., Hewlett, S., Richards, P., Morris, M., & Calnan, M. (2012). Utilizing qualitative data from nominal groups: Exploring the influences on treatment outcome prioritization with rheumatoid arthritis patients. *Journal of Health Psychology, 17*(1), 132–142.

Schofield, D. J., Callander, E. J., Shrestha, R. N., Passey, M. E., Percival, R., & Kelly, S. J. (2014). How co-morbidities magnify the effect of arthritis on labour force participation and economic status: A costs of illness study in Australia. *Rheumatology International, 34*(4), 481–489.

Seekins, T., Clay, J., & Ravesloot, C. (1994). A descriptive study of secondary conditions reported by a population of adults with physical disabilities served by three independent living centers in a rural state. *Journal of Rehabilitation, 60*(2), 47–51.

Seekins, T., White, G. W., Ravesloot, C., Norris, K., Szalda-Petree, A., Lopez, J. C., Golden, K., & Young, Q. R. (1999). Developing and evaluating community-based health promotion programs for people with disabilities. In R. J. Simeonsson & L. N. McDevitt (Eds.), *Issues in disability & health: The role of secondary conditions & quality of life.* (pp. 221–238). Chapel Hill: University of North Carolina, FPG Child Development Center.

Sharif, B., Garner R., Sanmartin, C., Flanagan, W. M., Hennessy, D., & Marshall, D. A. (2016). Risk of work loss due to illness or disability in patients with osteoarthritis: a population-based cohort study. *Rheumatology*. Advance online publication. http://rheumatology.oxfordjournals.org/content/early/2016/01/11/rheumatology.kev428.full.pdf+html

Sirois, F. M., & Hirsch, J. K. (2013). Associations of psychological thriving with coping efficacy, expectations for future growth, and depressive symptoms over time in people with arthritis. *Journal of Psychosomatic Research, 75*(3), 279–286.

Smeets, R. J., Vlaeyen, J. W., Kester, A. D., & Knottnerus, J. A. (2006). Reduction of pain catastrophizing mediates the outcome of both physical and cognitive-behavioral treatment in chronic low back pain. *The Journal of Pain, 7*(4), 261–271.

Stone, R. C., & Baker, J. (2014). Physical activity, age, and arthritis: Exploring the relationships of major risk factors on biopsychosocial symptomology and disease status. *Journal of Aging & Physical Activity, 22*(3), 314–323.

Strine, T. W., Hootman, J. M., Okoro, C. A., Balluz, L., Moriarty, D. G., Owens, M., & Mokdad, A. (2004). Frequent mental distress status among adults with arthritis age 45 years and older. *Arthritis Care & Research, 51*(4), 533–537.

Sugiyama, D., Nishimura, K., Tamaki, K., Tsuji, G., Nakazawa, T., Morinobu, A., & Kumagai, S. (2010). Impact of smoking as a risk factor for developing rheumatoid arthritis: a meta-analysis of observational studies. *Annals of the Rheumatic Diseases, 69*(01), 70–81.

Sullivan, M. J., Bishop, S. R., & Pivik, J. (1995). The pain catastrophizing scale: Development and validation. *Psychological Assessment, 7*(4), 524–532.

Taal, E., Rasker, J. J., & Wiegman, O. (1996). Patient education and self-management in the rheumatic diseases: A self-efficacy approach. *Arthritis & Rheumatism, 9*(3), 229–238.

Theis, K. A., Murphy, L., Hootman, J. M., Helmick, C. G., & Yelin, E. (2007). Prevalence and correlates of arthritis-attributable work limitation in the US population among persons ages 18–64: 2002 National Health Interview Survey Data. *Arthritis Care & Research, 57*(3), 355–363.

Toms, T. E., Panoulas, V. F., & Kitas, G. D. (2011). Dyslipidaemia in rheumatological autoimmune diseases. *Open Cardiovascular Medicine Journal, 5*, 64–75.

Treharne, G. J., Lyons, A. C., Booth, D. A., & Kitas, G. D. (2007). Psychological well-being across 1 year with rheumatoid arthritis: Coping resources as buffers of perceived stress. *British Journal of Health Psychology, 12*(3), 323–345.

Tunceli, K., Li, K., & Williams, L. (2006). Long-term effects of obesity on employment and work limitations among US adults, 1986 to 1999. *Obesity, 14*(9), 1637–1646.

Turk, D. C., & Monarch, E. S. (2002). Biopsychosocial perspective on chronic pain. In D. C. Turk & R. J. Gatchel (Eds.), *Psychological approaches to pain management: A practitioner's handbook* (pp. 3–29). New York: Guilford Press.

US Department of Health and Human Services. (2000). *Healthy people 2010*. Washington, DC: Author. Retrieved from http://www.health.gov/healthypeople

US Department of Health and Human Services. (2010). *Healthy People 2020*. Washington, DC: Author. Retrieved from http://www.healthypeople.gov/2020/default.aspx

Van Breukelen-van der Stoep, D. F., Klop, B., van Zeben, D., Hazes, J. M. W., & Cabezas, M. C. (2013). Cardiovascular risk in rheumatoid arthritis: How to lower the risk? *Atherosclerosis, 231*(1), 163–172.

Van Halm, V. P., Peters, M. J. L., Voskuyl, A. E., Boers, M., Lems, W. F., Visser, M., . . . Heine, R. J. (2009). Rheumatoid arthritis versus diabetes as a risk factor for cardiovascular disease: A cross-sectional study, the CARRE Investigation. *Annals of the Rheumatic Diseases, 68*(9), 1395–1400.

Van Liew, C., Santoro, M. S., Chalfant, A. K., Gade, S., Casteel, D. L., Tomita, M., & Cronan, T. A. (2013). The good life: Assessing the relative importance of physical, psychological, and self-efficacy statuses on quality of well-being in osteoarthritis patients. *Arthritis, 2013*, 1–9.

Van Zanten, J. J. V., Rouse, P. C., Hale, E. D., Ntoumanis, N., Metsios, G. S., Duda, J. L., & Kitas, G. D. (2015). Perceived barriers, facilitators and benefits for regular physical activity and exercise in patients with rheumatoid arthritis: A review of the literature. *Sports Medicine, 45*(10), 1401–1412.

Verstappen, S. M. (2015). Rheumatoid arthritis and work: The impact of rheumatoid arthritis on absenteeism and presenteeism. *Best Practice & Research: Clinical Rheumatology, 29*(3), 495–511.

Verstappen, S. M. M., Bijlsma, J. W. J., Verkleij, H., Buskens, E., Blaauw, A. A. M., Ter . . . Jacobs, J. W. G. (2004). Overview of work disability in rheumatoid arthritis patients as observed in cross-sectional and longitudinal surveys. *Arthritis Care & Research, 51*(3), 488–497.

Vos, T., Flaxman, A. D., Naghavi, M., Lozano, R., Michaud, C., Ezzati, M., . . . Abraham, J. (2013). Years lived with disability (YLDs) for 1160 sequelae of 289 diseases and injuries 1990–2010: A systematic analysis for the Global Burden of Disease Study 2010. *The Lancet, 380*, 2163–2196.

Wallis, J. A., Webster, K. E., Levinger, P., & Taylor, N. F. (2013). What proportion of people with hip and knee osteoarthritis meet physical activity guidelines? A systematic review and meta-analysis. *Osteoarthritis and Cartilage, 21*(11), 1648–1659.

Warsi, A., LaValley, M. P., Wang, P. S., Avorn, J., & Solomon, D. H. (2003). Arthritis self-management education programs: A meta-analysis of the effect on pain and disability. *Arthritis & Rheumatism, 48*(8), 2207–2213.

Weinberger, M., Tierney, W. M., Booher, P., & Hiner, S. L. (1990). Social support, stress and functional status in patients with osteoarthritis. *Social Science & Medicine, 30*(4), 503–508.

Widdifield, J., Paterson, J. M., Bernatsky, S., Tu, K., Tomlinson, G., Kuriya, B., . . . Bombardier, C. (2014). The epidemiology of rheumatoid arthritis in Ontario, Canada. *Arthritis & Rheumatology, 66*(4), 786–793.

Wilson, L., Catalano, D., Sung, C., Phillips, B., Chou, C. C., Chan, J. Y. C., & Chan, F. (2013). Attachment style, social support, and coping as psychosocial correlates of happiness in persons with spinal cord injuries. *Rehabilitation Research, Policy, and Education, 27*(3), 186–205.

Wittenauer, R., Smith, L., & Aden, K. (2013). *Background paper 6.12: Osteoarthritis.* Geneva: World Health Organization.

Wolfe, F., & Michaud, K. (2009). Predicting depression in rheumatoid arthritis: The signal importance of pain extent and fatigue, and co-occurring conditions. *Arthritis Care & Research, 61*(5), 667–673.

Wolfe, F., & Michaud, K. (2012). Effect of body mass index on mortality and clinical status in rheumatoid arthritis. *Arthritis Care & Research, 64*(10), 1471–1479.

Yelin, E. (2007). Work disability in rheumatic diseases. *Current Opinion in Rheumatology, 19*(2), 91–96.

Young, A., Dixey, J., Kulinskaya, E., Cox, N., Davies, P., Devlin, J., . . . Williams, P. (2002). Which patients stop working because of rheumatoid arthritis? Results of five years' follow up in 732 patients from the Early RA Study (ERAS). *Annals of the Rheumatic Diseases, 61*(4), 335–340.

Zhang, W., Moskowitz, R. W., Nuki, G., Abramson, S., Altman, R. D., Arden, N., . . . Dougados, M. (2008). OARSI recommendations for the management of hip and knee osteoarthritis, Part II: OARSI evidence-based, expert consensus guidelines. *Osteoarthritis and Cartilage, 16*(2), 137–162.

9

Self-Management of Burn Injury

JAMES A. FAUERBACH AND CARISA PERRY-PARRISH ■

INTRODUCTION

Burn injuries present individuals with a range of physical, psychological, emotional, social, and behavioral challenges. Burn injuries are painful, as are the necessary medical treatments that typically follow. Burn injuries are the fourth most common injury worldwide and are more common in low- and middle-income countries than in high-income countries (World Health Organization, 2008). The American Burn Association (ABA; 2016) estimates that 450,000 people receive medical treatment for burn injuries annually, including emergency department and hospital treatment. The vast majority of burn injuries are unintentional (Forjuoh, 1998), equally likely to occur across settings, with a variety of injury mechanisms, including flame/fire injuries (44%) and scald injuries (33%; ABA, 2016). Significant medical treatments have contributed to survivor rates of severe burns exceeding 95% in high-income countries such as the United States (Peck, 2011; Saffle, Davis, & Williams, 1995). There are approximately 3,400 deaths attributed to burn injuries per year in the United States due primarily to residential fires and less frequently to vehicle crash fires and other sources (e.g., smoke inhalation, scalding, and electricity; ABA, 2016). Burn injuries may result in short-term and permanent changes that challenge one's adaptive coping and abilities to optimally engage in self-management. In this chapter, we review how burn injuries result in functional limitations and then discuss evidence-based strategies to address impairments across domains, emotional impact, and methods for optimal coping and to facilitate self-management.

Functional Limitations Associated with Burn Injuries

The severity of a burn injury is determined by the size of the total body surface area (TBSA) affected by wounds that are deep partial thickness (2nd degree—epidermis and outer dermis) and full thickness (3rd degree—epidermis, dermis, often to fat layer and fascia). The classification system for major burn injury requiring treatment at a verified burn center was established by the ABA (2016) includes: ≥20% TBSA deep partial burn (≥10% TBSA when age is >70 years); ≥5% TBSA full thickness burns, all burns involving face, genitalia, hands, or feet; or inhalation injury. Injuries meeting these ABA criteria have a prolonged healing time, require twice-daily complex wound care, necessitate autologous skin grafting for wound closure, and increase the risk of a host of acute events (e.g., infectious, metabolic, cardiopulmonary). These and other complications impair function across multiple domains from the level of dysfunctional organ systems (e.g., renal failure, acute respiratory distress syndrome), to cognitive tasks dependent on intact cortical function and structure (e.g., sepsis, pain medications, and complex pharmaco-kinetics may lead to delirium and impaired attention, memory, learning), to psychological (disrupted sleep and unavoidable pain and distress may lead to poor emotion regulation, problem-solving, executive function), and psychiatric (trauma and aversive treatments may lead to difficulty regulating emotions, regaining a sense of safety and meaning or purpose, and perceived social isolation). The core functional domains derailed by major burns must undergo prolonged healing and extensive rehabilitation as they are responsible for maintaining or reestablishing the individual's social participation in multiple complex domains such as social networks, occupational interactions, and the domestic/family structure.

Normally, healthy skin is tight but flexible, stretching and bending while remaining firmly against the underlying structures. When burned skin heals, it tightens, contracts, and stiffens and thus restricts movement. There is a tendency to form excessive skin cells that are laid down in random patterns rather than side by side as in healthy skin. This disorganized cell layering also contributes to the tendency for new skin to contract, thus leading to the development of hypertrophic scars. Hypertrophic scars limit range of motion in affected joints; appear random, rigid, and raised; are typically hypo- or hyperpigmented; and are prone to chronic neuropathic pain and pruritus. Burn-damaged skin, skin graft "donor" sites, and graft "recipient" areas often present additional functional impairments to skin including decreased tolerance for heat or cold, diminished work tolerance due to loss of sweat glands, and fragile skin subject to frequent small tears, abrasions, punctures, and bleeding (Oster et al., 2010).

Evidence-Based Practices to Improve Health Outcomes

A common concern among individuals with burn injuries and their circle of family and friends is the appearance of burned skin. A recent systematic review was conducted to evaluate the evidence base for commonly used, nonsurgical methods of preventing, treating, or reducing hypertrophic burn scars in adults (Anthonissen et al., 2016). The authors report on findings from 22 randomized controlled trials in which the intervention (n = number of studies examined) were massage (n = 5), pressure (n = 4), silicone (n = 6), combined pressure with silicone (n = 3), hydration (n = 3), and ultrasound (n = 1). All of these interventions rely on an individual's consistent use of the method; for example, massage therapy involves self-directed deep pressure applied to the burn injury site for 5 to 15 minutes, three times per day, in an effort to reduce hypertrophic scar formation. Pressure therapy and silicone were reported to be "evidence-based conservative treatments of hypertrophic scar formation after a burn producing clinically relevant improvement of scar thickness, redness and pliability" (Anthonissen et al., 2016, p. 508). The effect of massage therapy on improving scar pliability and reducing pain and pruritus was limited but encouraging, while the evidence for products targeting pruritus (e.g., moisturizers, lotions) was inconsistent, and the authors found no controlled trials of splinting, casting, physical activity, or early mobilization. A moderate-sized sample of individuals with burn-related hypertrophic scars (n = 146) were randomly assigned to standard burn rehabilitation for hypertrophic scars with and without massage therapy (Cho et al., 2014). The study revealed significantly greater improvement on pre- to posttreatment change scores in the massage group versus the standard burn rehabilitation group ($p \leq 0.05$) in scar-related pain and pruritus and hypertrophic scar thickness, elasticity, and distension (immediate and delayed). The lack of randomized controlled trials is indicative of the developmental state of the science in burn care and rehabilitation research and does not necessarily cast doubt on the methods reviewed.

Individuals with acute burn pain often report that it is the most distressing aspect of the initial wound and the treatment until wound closure. Research has shown that acute burn pain in-hospital is longitudinally associated two years later with increased suicidal ideation (Edwards, Magyar-Russell, et al., 2007) and acute symptoms of anxiety and depression predict chronic pain at two-year follow-up (Edwards, Smith, et al., 2007). Chronic pain (n = 492; 18% chronic burn pain; Browne, Andrews, Schug, & Wood, 2011) and chronic pruritus (at discharge = 93%, 6 months = 86%, 12 months = 83%, 24 months = 73%) are two prevalent conditions common in the first months and often for years after burn injury. One small recent study showed that hypertrophic scarring (43%), pruritus (40%), and psychiatric diagnoses (36%) are also frequently associated with chronic pain (Schneider, 2006). For most people with burns, these secondary complications begin to develop after the skin has healed, whether healed spontaneously or with skin graft. The sensory experience of chronic burn pain is quite different from acute burn pain in that chronic pain is typically intermittent and unpredictable and it is usually short-lasting (seconds to extended minutes) and discontinuous. Chronic pain is not controllable by the same class of medications that are predictably efficacious (e.g., opiate-based analgesic regimen) for acute pain (Retrouvey & Shahrokhi, 2015). Basic science in this area notes the close overlap in receptors processing the sensations of chronic pain and pruritus via peripheral nociception and central neural pathways (Chen et al., 2016).

KNOWLEDGE THAT PROMOTES SELF-MANAGEMENT

Self-management of burn injuries and sequelae involves numerous activities to address the range of impairments experienced by youth and adults with burn injuries. As described in detail in chapter 2 in this volume, self-management comprises many aspects of self-care.

Defining Self-Management of Burns

Self-care that improves independence and inclusion often incorporates self-monitoring and decision-making (Holroyd & Creer, 1986), management of behaviors, medical treatment, emotions (Corbin & Strauss, 1988), and education about one's chronic health conditions and needs (Clark et al., 1991). This definition is intentionally neutral to avoid confusion with the historical focus on "adherence" to medical recommendations and to acknowledge that self-management may function adaptively or non-adaptively. Core self-management tasks are categorized into medical tasks and activities, performance in typical or adapted roles, and routine use of means to promote emotion regulation. These tasks require adequate performance of key self-management skills applied across these task categories, including, for example, problem-solving, decision-making, resource utilization, partnerships with providers, action-planning, and self-tailoring of health recommendations (Lorig & Holman, 2003).

An important component of self-management for an acquired chronic health condition is regulating the emotions associated with them. For example, changes in appearance and functional ability impair body image, increase barriers to social inclusion, and diminish self-esteem (Fauerbach, Rios, Mason, & Milner, 2102). An important article by Thombs et al. (2008) indicated that survivors are concerned about physical appearance and function early after wound healing (rehabilitation phase) and then become more focused on social comfort and acceptance (social reintegration phase) during the first year after wound healing. The importance lies in prioritizing timing of resource allocation and self-management toward optimizing rehabilitation access early in recovery and then transitioning into an emphasis on social skills and social comfort. These, of course, are not mutually exclusive, and clinical observation suggests that incorporating social support into psychosocial education and social skills training early in the process may be associated with better long-term social reintegration.

Acute Phase Injury, Impairments, and Self-Management

Following the acute phase of burn care (e.g., seeking medical attention, debridement, excision, surgical procedures), self-management may direct efforts of wound healing (e.g., dressing changes, application of topical medications, bathing accommodations), preventing scars (e.g., scar massage, application of moisturizer, compression garments, physical/occupational therapy), and coping with emotional and social sequelae (e.g., changed appearance, emotional symptoms of anxiety/depression, return to normal social activities, psychotherapy participation). A recent systematic review of self-management among individuals with burn injuries summarized literature that highlighted the following empirically derived domains: self-management of dietary recommendations, use of pressure garments and silicone-gel sheeting, physical/occupational therapy, exercise regimens, and attendance at follow-up appointments (Szabo, Urich, Duncan, & Aballay, 2016). By adopting a developmental focus on the role of the family and other potential caregivers, the person with burn injury, family and the team may enhance and optimize understanding self-management in the case of burns. That is, as caregivers play a more or less central role in providing support; optimal self-management may include reaching out for task assistance, information, and emotional support by caregivers and medical staff.

Self-management treatment factors are relevant across the lifespan but may vary in important ways across individuals. A central idea to the promotion of optimal adjustment to burn injuries is engaging multiple sources of support. Clinician knowledge of these systems allows for greater opportunity to optimize treatments (see chapter 17 in this volume) to target a range of modifiable variables that could in turn improve self-management of the diverse range of long-term impairments associated with burn injuries. These include physical consequences (e.g., pain, itch, sleep disturbance, limited range of motion), psychological functioning (e.g., depression with appetite suppression, low energy, and social withdrawal; posttraumatic distress with aversive memories; hyperarousal), and social belonging (e.g., peer rejection/stigmatization; low body image/self-image, and reduced self-esteem; Modi et al., 2012).

EMOTIONAL IMPACT OF IMPAIRMENTS

Medical stress can be defined as responses to pain, injury, serious health conditions, medical procedures, and invasive medical treatments (Kazak et al., 2006). Stress responses are not presumed to equate to a diagnosis of formal stress-related psychiatric disorders, such as acute stress disorder (ASD) or posttraumatic stress disorder (PTSD). This model is relevant for understanding emotional impact of burn injuries in adults and potential targets for intervention. First, a range of normative reactions to medical events is expected. Such stress reactions are responses to medical stress and do not necessarily imply presence of a mental health diagnosis (Livneh & Antonak, 1997). Second, a social contextual approach is optimal for intervention. Adults are not simply individuals-in-isolation; rather, they exist within multiple social contexts (e.g., family, dyadic relationship, community).

Distressing life events, such as experiencing a burn injury, may affect a person's perception of uncontrollability and unpredictability, both in the cause of the event as well as in the emotional feelings that follow. Fauerbach, Bresnick, and Smith (2007) proposed a model based on coping processes for adults with burn injuries involving emotional expressivity and emotional suppression that likely affect cognitive appraisal processes. In this model, external stressors, such as intrusive re-experiencing memories of a traumatic burn injury event, elicit negative emotional states that activate particular self-regulation processes. Among potential choices for self-regulating emotion there are two, termed emotional avoidant and emotional approach coping, that are particularly relevant for individuals who have experienced a burn injury. In emotional avoidant coping, an individual strives to gain control over stressors through avoiding negative emotions by suppressing them and avoiding cues that elicit them. Emotional approach coping includes acknowledgement, understanding, and expression of emotions (Austenfeld & Stanton, 2004). In emotional approach coping, one is motivated to achieve predictability regarding emotional experience by accepting, processing and expressing emotions. These processes have been studied extensively among general adult populations, as well as among adults experiencing medical stress. Use of either approach/processing or avoidance/suppression as primary means of self-regulating negative emotions have been shown to be associated with lower levels of posttrauma distress, depression and body image dissatisfaction in adults with burn injuries, while the use of both processing and suppressing (i.e., approach-avoidance conflict) is associated with more intense and prolonged distress. One key factor implicated in these models is cognitive appraisal. Cognitive appraisal processes and links to emotion regulation are known to be relevant to understanding individual differences in responses to burn injuries and represent a worthwhile target for enhancing self management and intervention.

Individuals who experience a burn injury may benefit from recognizing the types of emotion management strategies available to them, and clinicians may improve outcomes among these individuals by increasing use of adaptive emotion regulation strategies. Although cognitive reappraisal is a core strategy in cognitive therapy, Gross and Thompson (2007) have experimentally observed that use of reappraisal is not common (Suri et al., 2015), occurring approximately 16% of the time in an emotional induction experiment. Thus therapeutic approaches that increase use of reappraisal may provide significant relief from potential distress.

Emotion regulation is defined as the means by which individuals manage the emotions they experience, how strong the emotions are, and how long they persist (Gross & Thompson, 2007). Emotion regulation is conceptualized as management of the temporal dynamics of emotion, a definition of emotion regulation that nicely parallels the clinical goals of the previous model of medical stress. In that model, as in this definition, the goal of interventions is to change the intensity, duration, and type of emotion experienced by individuals and their families following a burn injury. While most could agree that some level of distressing emotional reaction is normative in response to a medical stressor, negative emotions that are intense and prolonged increase risk for more severe levels of mental health issues (e.g., a mental health diagnosis) and other non-adaptive threats to self-management and optimal treatment outcomes. A functionalist perspective of emotion emphasizes that emotions provide adaptive benefits in regulating cognitive, behavioral, and social processes through interactions with the environment (e.g., Campos et al., 1989). Such adaptive benefits include optimizing one's felt sense of self-efficacy, belonging, and connectedness.

The similarities among these various models of emotion management highlight the importance of identifying an individual's approach to the experience and management of emotionally arousing and distressing events. Moreover, these approaches are rooted in a functionalist approach, thus highlighting the adaptive aspects of emotions rather than focusing exclusively on the proposed disruptive elements of emotional distress. Clinicians working with individuals who have experienced a burn injury can observe the emotional impact of negative life events and direct treatment efforts to support optimally healthy and adaptive forms of emotion regulation. Understanding the normative emotional and psychosocial impact of negative life events, including burn injuries, helps inform treatment approaches to optimize overall treatment through enhancing one's belief in the capacity to cope with the experience effectively. Coping self-efficacy, in relation to traumatic burn events, "reflects the perceived level of capability to effectively deal with the event and its consequences, and determines appraisal of the event and its consequences" (Bosmans et al., 2015, p. 642). Coping self-efficacy assessed at baseline in a large sample of burn survivors followed over 12 months was the strongest prospective predictor of early recovery from PTSD symptoms controlling for demographics, number of surgeries, trait coping style, and changes in quality of life (Bosmans et al., 2015).

Important avenues for self-management after burn injury include the cognitive (images, appraisals of event, expectancies for future), emotional (self efficacy versus self-doubting), behavioral (approach, avoid, approach-avoidance conflict), and contextual (locations similar to event) components of posttrauma distress. The aim is to establish the sense that memories, even horrific ones, can no longer harm us directly (the damage is done) and may, in the long term, be beneficial in that they are the primary way that we learn from the past and become better prepared for the future. The ability to plan for the future is itself a means of self-management by reducing the likelihood of recurrence and providing one the means for helping others to acquire this knowledge without having to go through a similar episode. This positive aspect of coping may be viewed in contrast to the development of a foreshortened sense of the future among individuals who display symptoms of PTSD.

Burn injuries are among the most painful events an individual can experience, and the physical pain is not limited to the initial injury but rather extends to the necessary medical treatments. The uncertainty related to understanding the nature of the injury, prospects for healing, threats to the individual's appearance and function, and the emotionally challenging aspects of the injury and subsequent treatment course presents a multifaceted source of anxiety and distress to manage. Domains of emotional and psychosocial impact include experiences of negative emotions (e.g., sadness, guilt, anger, fear), body image (e.g., self-perceived appearance, social and self acceptance of appearance), socially oriented thoughts and cognitive processes (e.g., social expectations, beliefs about stigma) and social outcomes (e.g., reintegrating postinjury, relationship formation, social comfort).

In a substantial minority, an individual's level of negative affect and co-occurring impairment could increase risk for psychiatric impairment (e.g., a diagnosis of anxiety, PTSD, depression).

Emotional difficulties may emerge at any point during or after an individual experiences a burn injury; moreover, preexisting emotional problems may influence the manifestation and severity of postburn distress. Emotional sequelae of burn injuries may involve emotional distress and behavioral difficulties that span from normative reactions to a major stressor to clinically significant disorders in need of treatment. Negative emotions and emotional symptoms may include fear/anxiety, sadness/depression, and other stress reactions (Perry, Sharp, Rosenberg, Rosenberg, & Meyer, 2012). Anxiety can be further differentiated into sleep disturbances, anticipatory and procedural fears, generalized worrying, and separation anxiety. Emotional difficulties are worthy of study in their own right, as they inform understanding and treatment of potential psychological detriments to self esteem and social integration. However, psychological variables may also predict physical difficulties in the course of postburn adjustment, such as pain, fatigue, and physical functioning (Edwards et al., 2007; Corry, Klick, Fauerbach, 2010), and thus understanding emotional reactions may inform improvements to medical treatment as well.

Normative reactions to stress and formal psychiatric diagnoses must be considered when supporting optimal treatment and self-management of individuals with burn injuries. A recent population-based prevalence study of adults found that adults with a history of burn injuries had similar rates of mental health problems as non-burned individuals, once preinjury rates were taken into account (Logsetty et al., 2016). Many studies would suggest that the majority of youth do not display increased incidence of psychopathology following a burn injury; however, as noted by one author, "this lack of observable psychopathology does not equate to a happy or easy adjustment" (DeSousa, 2010, p. 155). One well-designed study used structured interviews and a national comparison sample (National Comorbidity Sample) and observed that preinjury lifetime mood alcohol and substance-use disorders were significantly higher and anxiety disorder significantly less common among the burn participants relative to comparison group (Fauerbach, Lawrence, Haythornthwaite, et al., 1997). In addition, postburn follow-up revealed that the presence of a preburn mood, alcohol, or substance-use disorder increased risk of postburn psychiatric diagnosis, and preburn mood disorder significantly raised the risk of PTSD at 12 months postburn.

Prospective longitudinal research has shown that the level of distress that one reports experiencing during the acute hospitalization tends to persist across at least two-years follow-up. Analyses of two-year longitudinal data quite consistently identified three to four groups of survivors whose level of distress (e.g., posttraumatic distress, body-image dissatisfaction/social discomfort, generalized distress) formed trajectories characterized as (a) chronically severe, (b) moderately severe (hovering around cutoff for clinical disorder), (c) subclinical, and (d) essentially without symptoms (PTSD, McKibben et al., 2008; body-image disturbances, Thombs et al., 2008; generalized distress, Mason, 2010). The stability of these trajectories is illustrated in that, across the two-year follow-up, only 5% to 10% of participants reported a reliable and clinically significant change in post-trauma distress that moved them from one trajectory to another (cf. McKibben et al., 2008). Notably, of the 5% to 10% of participants who changed from one trajectory to another, about half reported less distress (improved) and half reported increased distress (worsened). The stability in distress trajectories among survivors of major burns is largely unique relative to other trauma-exposed samples. These other populations tend to show recovery trajectories of early recovery (~6 months), midterm recovery (~12-months), and a chronic trajectory, and some studies found a delayed onset trajectory with early low symptom severity followed by increasing symptoms beginning about six months out (reviewed in Southwick, 2016).

EVIDENCE-BASED PRACTICES AND INTERVENTIONS TO PROMOTE COPING

There are numerous studies that demonstrate the benefit of cognitive-behavioral and related psychosocial approaches for improving outcomes in individuals with a history of exposure to negative life events, such as burn injuries or other traumatic injuries. Evidence-based interventions have focused on a range of outcomes to support positive adjustment among adults who have experienced a burn injury. These outcomes include quality of life, optimization of medical treatment recommendations (e.g., wearing compression garments, completing scar massage, participation in physical and occupational therapy), social difficulties, and psychological symptoms. Health-related quality of life is affected most severely in the acute phase, but studies would suggest that this domain normalizes over time, with the most improvements occurring in the first few months postinjury (Van Loey et al., 2012).

Evidence-based psychological approaches that are often applicable in this population include cognitive-behavioral therapy (CBT), prolonged exposure, and trauma-focused CBT. CBT approaches typically target challenging the cognitions that foster negative emotional states and also focusing on changing behavioral patterns (e.g., avoidance) that may lead to negative perceptions concerning the self, future, or world. CBT builds on the work of behavioral modification and therapies as well as cognitive therapy (Beck, 2010). Current theory would suggest that there are reciprocal interactions among thoughts, feelings, and behaviors and that these associations can be strategically targeted through attention to and analysis of cognitions and actions during situations. CBT has been applied to a range of internalizing symptoms including anxiety (James et al., 2015; Watts et al., 2015), depression, adjustment problems, and PTSD, as well as medically related symptoms such as sleep (Ho, Chan, & Tang, 2016) and pain (Williams, Eccleston, & Morley, 2012). See chapter 3 in this volume for details about CBT and its application to self-management.

For individuals experiencing difficulties in motivation (e.g., ambivalence to change behaviors), motivational interviewing has been shown to be an effective intervention to increase openness to change (see chapter 6 in this volume). In a similar vein, mindfulness and acceptance-based approaches are theorized to enhance an individual's openness to experience pain and discomfort and promote self-care and improve functioning and quality of life. Mindfulness-based approaches represent another group of emerging treatments that may serve as a useful adjunct to optimizing outcomes with individuals with a history of burn injuries. While these treatments are not intended to be primary interventions for traumatic stress, mindfulness-based interventions may be able to address longer-term outcomes and coping processes, such as body image, rumination, and emotional acceptance.

TECHNIQUES TO FACILITATE SELF-MANAGEMENT

Examples of self-management tasks and related skills required in burn care and rehabilitation and placed within Jerant et al.'s (2005) framework include medical-physical tasks (e.g., positioning limbs, splints in place), emotional (e.g., empathy for the pain, attention to changes in care, memory for progress), and social aspects (e.g., assertive communication and problem-solving, acknowledging and accepting injury, pain, scarring). This framework is particularly fitting during the acute in-patient and early outpatient rehabilitation phases when the plethora of physical, emotional, and social challenges so thoroughly deplete the psychobiological resources of the injured person (e.g., vital exhaustion). As mentioned, this is the time period when the external advocate's becomes so important. The importance of research investigating acute phase self-management is illustrated by Smith et al.'s (2008) finding that insomnia symptoms during acute hospitalization and Edwards, Smith, et al.'s (2007) finding that in-hospital anxiety and depression each significantly and independently predicted chronic pain at two-year long-term follow-up (Smith, Klick, et al., 2008). Furthermore, acute phase pain is a prospective, independent predictor of suicidal ideation up to two years later (Edwards et al., 2007).

The following are some activities that increase the need and utility for these external advocates: rest and procedural pain, polypharmacy (background and procedural opiate analgesics, surgical anesthesia, antibiotics), hypermetabolic/catabolic responses, twice-daily unavoidable painful dressing changes and demanding rehabilitation regimens, disrupted sleep, removal from social network and daily routine, and worries about scarring and social impact.

Delirium and vital exhaustion are two possible consequences of prolonged exposure to these stressors. The University of California, San Francisco, Research Network on Socio-Economic Status and Health has described the Vital Exhaustion (VE) construct as including excessive fatigue and lack of energy, increased irritability, and hopelessness (http://www.macses.ucsf.edu/research/allostatic/vital.php). In the case of major burn injuries, VE may occur in response to the seemingly endless and painful wound-care sessions that can persist twice daily for months and the subsequent scar maturation process whereby the scars seemingly respond to rehabilitation activities with geologic speed and are physically depleting, painful, and emotionally draining. Therefore, VE is a psychobiological state that people develop when adapting to environmental, physical, and social stressors that exceed their reserves and restorative resources and their ability to adapt is critically overwhelmed with insufficient time for recovery.

Delirium and vital exhaustion further impair the ability to complete complex self-management tasks such as problem-solving, emotion regulation, and interpersonal interactions. The external advocates are embedded within the transactions among multiple systems, domains of influence, and levels of care. These include individual (e.g., age, cognitive/developmental status, emotions), family (e.g., family composition/structure, financial/insurance, emotional climate), community setting (e.g., neighborhood, peer/social supports, communal understanding of health condition), and healthcare system (e.g., available resources, relationship to medical provider, model of health care services; Modi et al., 2012). Family, friends, clergy, and others in the social network of child, adolescent, and adults with burn injuries routinely assist them with nursing and rehabilitation tasks that require skills that are now impaired.

OTHER BARRIERS TO SELF-MANAGEMENT

Posttraumatic distress has been found to be associated with greater lengths of acute hospitalization enhanced sense of distress and impaired adjustment to injury. In the population of individuals who survive severe burns, certain aspects of pretrauma adjustment (e.g. history of mood disorder), high level of symptoms in-hospital, coping by avoidance, and social support can influence the risk of developing PTSD and level of symptom severity (Sveen, Ekselius, Gerdin, & Willebrand, 2011). Individual factors (e.g., avoidance of reminders) and aspects of the injury (e.g., facial injury) have been associated with poorer outcome. Individuals with high levels of trait neuroticism were found to be at greater risk of developing PTSD following burn injury, while those with high levels of extraversion appear at reduced risk (Fauerbach et al., 2000).

It might be assumed that PTSD is related to greater initial injury; however, PTSD among burn survivors has not been found to be related to severity of injury. McKibben et al., (2008) found that ASD was a valid and reliable predictor of PTSD at 1, 6, 12, and 24 month follow-up even when TBSA; burns to the hand(s), head, or neck; and number of burn-related surgeries were included in the model. On the other hand, high levels of acute posttrauma distress are positively related to more intense pain perception among hospitalized burn individuals. High emotional distress and ASD symptoms during hospitalization are risk factors for PTSD two years post-burn. Although posttrauma distress and PTSD are prevalent, posttraumatic growth has also been commonly observed and was best predicted by active coping and social support in a sample of burn survivors (*n*= 149; Rosenbach & Renneberg, 2008).

Recently, resilience and social support were discussed from a neuroscience perspective (Southwick et al., 2016). The authors stated that, following trauma exposure,

> A significant minority develop chronic, debilitating psychological symptoms that markedly interfere with their capacity to function; others may initially develop symptoms and recover, or develop late or delayed symptoms over time. What explains these differences? The answer is complex and only partially understood. Resilience is generally defined as the ability of an individual to bend but not break, to bounce back, and "to adapt well in the face of adversity, trauma, tragedy, threats or even significant sources of stress." (p. 16)

However, as noted earlier, individuals exist in social contexts and systems, and thus resilience likely reflects affordances of one's psychobiological, social, family, economic, and communal resources. Resilient individuals may be more likely to exert adaptive self-management through strategic use of friends, family, and available resources; viewed this way, resilience may function as an approach that can be nurtured rather than a trait that either is or is not possessed.

Body Image, Stigmatization, and Social Integration

Body image is one's self-evaluation of one's physical appearance. Negative body image—body image dissatisfaction—is the belief that one is unattractive or "ugly." Body image is highly correlated with self-esteem particularly among adolescents and young adults. Negative body image is a component of, or is highly associated with, a number of psychiatric disorders including depression, social anxiety, eating disorders, and drug abuse. Due to the fact that burn survivors are permanently scarred by their injuries, it is commonly hypothesized that burn survivors are at high risk of developing a negative body image. Like disability, body image is formed through the interaction between a person and his or her social environment. In order to understand the challenge of adapting one's body image to having acquired burn scars, it is necessary to be familiar with the appearance norms of the burn survivor's culture and the importance that one attaches to appearance and to social norms. Sociocultural norms establish criteria for the importance of appearance, how one should appear, and the room for deviation from the norms.

In burn injury, there are many factors that may affect social adjustment including mood disorder, PTSD, shame/guilt, or other psychological factors such as emotion regulation based on avoidance and emotion suppression. Also, among the most challenging issues to achieving a healthy body-image satisfaction and social adjustment following burn injury are related to scarring. Burn scars affect appearance, limit range of motion, and are associated with chronic pain and pruritus. These effects often have secondary impact on sleep, mood, energy, and comfort in social situations where they may elicit stigmatizing reactions from others. The experience and expectation of stigmatization by others often enhance the discomfort one feels about one's altered appearance and may lead to self-stigmatization and avoidance of places (e.g., bathrooms, malls, etc.), objects (mirrors, store windows), and social interactions (e.g., strangers, friends, family). Body image and social adjustment has been validly and reliably quantified using a 14-item self-administered measure—the Satisfaction with Appearance Scale (SWAP; Lawrence et al., 1998), as well as the Derriford Appearance Scale (Carr, Harris, & James, 2000; Carr, Moss, & Harris, 2005).

There are four core dimensions of body image and social adjustment (BISA) identified through factor analytic study of the SWAP: (a) comfort with appearance of face/head/neck, (b) comfort with appearance of the rest of one's body, (c) comfort in social situations, and (d) perceived comfort of others with one's appearance. These core dimensions remain fairly stable across two years postinjury (Mason et al., 2011). The trajectory of body-image satisfaction and social adjustment scores measured at discharge and at 6, 12, and 24 months postdischarge is, in essence, characterized by two groups with low BISA distress (which lessens over time) and a third group with high BISA distress that increases over time (Mason et al., 2011).

Predictors of Body-Image Dissatisfaction and Poor Social Adjustment

Psychosocial variables (e.g., higher depression symptom severity, lower levels of social support) predict body-image dissatisfaction and poor social adjustment better than scar visibility or severity of burn scars (Lawrence, Fauerbach, Heinberg, & Doctor, 2004). Similarly, body-image esteem, body-image dissatisfaction, and poor social adjustment are only weakly related to scar severity and more strongly related to comfort in social situations and depression (Lawrence, Fauerbach, & Thombs, 2006). The importance of one's appearance to one's self esteem mediated the relationship between burn-scar severity and body-image dissatisfaction and poor social adjustment among long-term burn survivors (Lawrence et al., 2006). Notably, the same in-hospital approach-avoidance conflict between two emotion regulation strategies (suppression and expression) that is predictive of higher PTSD symptom severity, also predicted greater body-image dissatisfaction and poorer social adjustment (specifically regarding non-facial aspects, and social impact) at two-month follow-up (Fauerbach et al., 2002).

Impact of Body-Image Dissatisfaction and Poor Social Adjustment on Outcomes

Severity of body-image dissatisfaction and poor social adjustment distress is greater in burn survivors who place high value on their appearance and worsens over time for females and individuals with larger burns (Thombs et al., 2008). Body-image dissatisfaction and poor social adjustment partially mediate the effects of gender, importance of appearance, size of burn, and level of psychosocial function prior to the injury on postburn psychosocial function (SF-36 Mental Composite Scale; Ware et al., 1993).

In-hospital body image and social anxiety predict short- and midterm health and function outcomes. Body-image dissatisfaction and poor social adjustment measured at the time of discharge from the acute hospitalization were prospectively related two months later with physical (SF-36 subscales: General Health, Bodily Pain) and psychosocial quality of life domains (SF-36 subscales: Mental Health, Vitality). These results remained robust when covarying TBSA, gender, age, and 1) preburn SF-36 physical function subscale was a covariant when dependent variable was two-month Physical Function, and 2) the preburn Mental Health subscale was covaried when the dependent variable was two-month Mental Health (Fauerbach et al., 2000).

Social Belonging as Core Survival Need

Belonging is understood as one of the core needs driving human social behavior. This experience of belonging is easily threatened when one has been or believes one has been excluded from important social groups. Exclusion is especially distressing when it is, or is perceived to be, on the basis of some aspect of one's appearance that cannot be readily changed (MacDonald & Leary, 2005). The pivotal sociometer theory posits that self-esteem is a marker for the degree of belonging one is experiencing (MacDonald & Leary, 2005). As belonging improves (e.g., invited to a party), self-esteem increases. When belonging decreases (e.g., excluded from an activity), self-esteem diminishes. A recent meta-analysis confirmed expectations that, following social exclusion, negative mood increases and both positive mood and self-esteem decline (Smart Richman, & Leary, 2009). Other researchers have obtained similar findings regarding the discomfort generated by being excluded and labeled it "social pain" and proposed that social pain and physical pain are processed through the same peripheral nerves and brain regions (Eisenberger & Lieberman, 2004). Although this proposition has inconsistent empirical support (Woo et al., 2014), this line of research has validated the viewpoint that social pain that results from feeling excluded is quite uncomfortable to one degree or another for almost everyone. Exclusion-related social pain stimulates neural structures that also effect mood and self-esteem and thus motivates adaptive coping to these threats to social belonging (Smart Richman & Leary, 2009).

An elegant series of experiments found that participants who were made to feel excluded, relative to those who were not made to feel excluded, afterward attended more to positive memories and interpreted ambiguous stimuli more positively (DeWall et al., 2011). This means of regulating the negative emotions that arose from being excluded raised the level of positive emotions and thus spurred new efforts at improving inclusion. Of note, this automatic emotion-regulation process was observed among individuals with high self-esteem and low depression but not among those with low self-esteem or high depression (DeWall et al., 2011). In addition, a study among participants whose self-esteem was strongly based on their appearance were subjected to social exclusion. Those with high self-esteem sought to reconnect to those who had excluded them, while those with low self-esteem avoided social contact (Park & Maner, 2009). Taken together, these findings suggest that high self-esteem along with low depression are good markers for resilience while low self-esteem in the presence of high depression are markers for increased vulnerability. These markers for vulnerability (low self-esteem, high depression) and resilience (high self-esteem, low depression) may serve as a means of identifying during the acute phase those burn survivors at high risk versus low risk for having difficulty with reintegrating into social roles and regaining comfort in public settings.

Appearance, Social Stigmatization, and Social Exclusion

Appearance norms are communicated to the individual both through the mass media and interpersonal behavior. Via the mass media and interpersonal reactions people are exposed to hundreds of images of "beautiful people" that, on the internet for example, may be enhanced through processes such as airbrushing, soft-focus camera shots, and manipulated digital images. The message, implicit or explicit, of cosmetic product advertisements is that one is an inadequate person unless one is very attractive, and this product will enhance one's appearance. There is also interpersonal pressure to conform to appearance norms. The most troubling challenge for many people re-entering society following major burns are their own appraisals of the scars and related changes in appearance and function—and their expectations of what others will think and do when they notice the scars.

Social stigmatization is a process in which people are socially rejected (put out) and ostracized (kept out) based on a negative stereotype. People with visible differences have long been stigmatized in various contexts, subcultures, and in Western communication and entertainment venues. In many movies and video games, the villain is a person who is visibly different (e.g., burn scars). Stigmatizing interpersonal behaviors experienced by burn survivors include an absence of friendliness and courtesy, staring, pointing, startled and disgusted reactions, ignoring, avoidance, confused behavior, teasing, bullying, and discrimination (Lawrence, Fauerbach, Heinberg, & Doctor, 2006).

This emphasis on an attractive appearance is an onerous barrier to inclusion and social participation for those with a visible difference. In addition, acquired disfigurement can be difficult to incorporate into preburn body image (Rybarczyk et al., 2004; Weaver et al., 2007). Body image, a facet of self-esteem, is formed at the nexus at which individual differences intersect with social group norms (Anthony et al., 2007). Consequently, injury-related disfigurement creates distress over both an altered body image and concern about its interference with being excluded from social groups and contexts on the basis of appearance. Burn injuries cause an immediate change in appearance, and, in addition, uncertainty about final appearance outcome persists as healing is followed by months or years of scar maturation during which appearance typically becomes worse before improving (Linares, 1996). To complicate matters, the scars may also serve as reminders of the traumatic injury event and/or the acute pain of the wound healing period (Weaver et al., 2007). This change in appearance thus represents an amalgam of threats—to safety, comfort, body image/self-esteem, and social belonging.

These effects may persist for years in some and, particularly among certain vulnerable individuals, may lead to social sensitivity and concern with exclusion or stigmatization. Today, the emphasis in many burn care and rehabilitations centers is on providing training and practice in effective social skills for managing awkward or hostile interactions as a means of self-management.

What are the psychosocial consequences for burn survivors living in a highly beauty-conscious society? Few studies have investigated the frequency of body-image dissatisfaction and perceived stigmatization and their correlates among burn survivors. Much more remains to be done in order to discern whether, with whom, and at what point in recovery burn survivors are most affected by altered appearance. Further, there remains much to do in order to firmly establish what person, injury, and social factors may protect against body-image dissatisfaction or promote recovery from it.

Factors Affecting Body-Image Dissatisfaction and Social Discomfort

Attractiveness in physical appearance optimized by augmenting body and hair features with culture-specific styles is an almost universal criterion for group membership (Oaten et al., 2011). Recently, a series of experiments found that social acceptance was more strongly contingent on physical appearance/attractiveness than on social attributes (Anthony et al., 2007). One perspective about where this emphasis on appearance may have originated suggests that through natural selection, evolution favored those who quickly learned to notice signs of ill health or threat by noticing individuals outside the range of appearance considered normal. For example, when individuals developed skin lesions associated with infectious diseases (e.g., smallpox) or physical signs on outsiders (e.g., certain types of tattoos, clothing, hair), the group excluded and ostracized them as possible threats of contagion or aggression, respectively (Neuberg et al., 2011). The degree to which one fits in with the group culture, including normative appearance, the greater likelihood one has of being included. The premise that threat is eliminated by excluding those with nonnormative appearance is problematic in that non-infectious, non-dangerous signs (e.g., burn scars) often change a person's appearance in a manner that unnecessarily leads to exclusion and reduces self-esteem of some burn survivors. This exclusion also then precludes the benefits that might accrue to the group by including these ostracized individuals (e.g., talents, intelligence, diversity in gene pool).

Perceived discrimination, similar in nature and impact to social exclusion, has also been linked to poor health outcomes (Parker, 2012). Proposed pathways suggest that discrimination activates physiological processes (e.g., blood pressure; inflammatory response; Townsend, 2011) that negatively impact health (Pascoe et al., 2009). A systematic review of 134 samples found strong evidence that discrimination increases the stress response and concluded that it is associated with increased engagement in health-risk behavior and decreased participation in protective health behaviors (Pascoe et al., 2009). Thus discrimination is a form of exclusion that is omnipresent culturally and globally, is distressing, and negatively impacts health and adjustment (Parker, 2012; Butler, Lee, & Grossm 2007).

Recent studies among burn survivors investigated the theory that social exclusion of individuals whose appearance is outside the range considered normal may be motivated by the fear of disease or injury (Oaten et al., 2011) or of intense emotions (Willebrand & Sveen, 2016). This view may, for example, help explain the initial reactions of some children or naïve adults on seeing someone with burn scars for the first time—it would seem to be based on automatic emotion regulation processes on the part of the observer. The initial reaction, likely to be genetically determined and distributed normally across the population, is the fear of external signs on the body or face that might connote disease, contagion, or tribal enemies and reactions are associated with intense emotion (e.g., disgust, horror; Oaten et al., 2011; Willebrand & Sveen, 2016). In fact, this reaction may, in some people, be so strong as to trigger avoidant behavior that is strongly, negatively reinforced, thus leading to "blood, injury, injection phobia" (American Psychiatric Association, 2013).

While this first reaction is automatic and largely beyond conscious choice, we propose that there is a second stage of reaction on viewing visible differences. This second stage is more likely to involve a higher order of cognitive emotion regulation (e.g., reappraisal) and socialization that is acquired through internalizing social norms, parental training, and peer conformity. This higher level of cognitive processing and emotion regulation involves conscious appraisal of appearance differences, takes into consideration their source and implications, and is most likely acquired through the same processes as are social norms for appropriate behavior, openness versus closed-mindedness, and altruism versus selfishness. Although this second level has not been empirically evaluated, it has been clinically reported by burn survivors to have been helpful when reintegrating and adjusting to community, work, school, and family.

Regarding risk factors for negative body image, severity of burn scarring has proven to have only a modest relationship with body image among both adult and child burn survivors. One study suggested that the relationship between perceived scar severity and body image is moderated by importance of appearance (Lawrence et al., 2006). For those burn survivors who placed little value on physical appearance, self-rated scar severity had no relationship with body image. For those burn survivors who highly valued physical appearance, scar severity was highly predictive of body-image dissatisfaction.

Visibility Hypothesis

Body image and self-perceived appearance is another domain of psychological functioning of salience for individuals with a history of burn injuries. Individuals with burn injuries experience skin changes, ranging from acutely altered appearance of redness in mild burns to hypopigmentation to hypertrophic scarring and skin grafts.

Within the literature, there has been a theoretical debate regarding the relationship between burn scar location and body image. The "visible hypothesis" posits that socially visible scars, such as scars on the face, will be highly related to body-image dissatisfaction because burn survivors with visible scars will experience more frequent stigmatizing reactions from others and self-stigmatization from themselves. The "hidden scar" hypothesis posits that because the person has fewer opportunities to learn how to deal with the reactions of others, he or she will live in fear of the scar being revealed and thus have a negative body image. There is little empirical evidence for either hypothesis. One notable exception found that burn-scar visibility was related to the degree to which one's body-esteem is based on appearance; however, this was only as the relationship was mediated by social stigmatization. (Lawrence et al., 2004) Further, when partialling the effect of stigmatization, the impact of scar visibility on body esteem-appearance was quite low (Lawrence et al., 2004).

Burn-Specific Interventions and Peer Support

Several programs designed to address one or more aspects of self-management are provided in burn centers, burn survivor camps, or school/community.

Programs Promoting Survivor Assistance to Other Survivors

The Survivor Outreach to Assist in Recovery of the Phoenix Society for Burn Survivors (United States) and the FaceIT (CBT online or in person) program of Changing Faces organization in cooperation with the Center for the Study of Appearance (United Kingdom) for example, train survivors in the knowledge and skills for conducting supportive therapy (1:1, group, family). The Phoenix Society's programs also include social skills, body language, image enhancement, and school re-entry. Some burn centers are developing resources for an umbrella of acute, rehabilitation, and reconstruction phase support funded by the National Institute on Disability and Independent Living Research (in the Agency for Community Living, Health and Human Services) directly and by engaging with outside agencies such as the Phoenix Society for Burn Survivors. Resources can be accessed on the websites for the Model System Knowledge Translation

Center (http://www.msktc.org/burn) and the Phoenix Society for Burn Survivors (https://www.phoenix-society.org/).

Qualitative phenomenological methods were used to construct themes from data collected by in-depth individual semistructured interviews of survivors' ($n = 21$) experiences with providing and receiving in-patient peer support (Kornhaber, Wilson, Abu-Qamar, McLean, & Vandervord, 2015). The emergent theme of "burn survivor peer support" identified five clusters of experiences giving/receiving support: (a) encouragement, inspiration, and hope; (b) reassurance; (c) the importance of timing (i.e., when inviting newly injured individuals to participate; (d) the same skin (i.e., concerns about source of cadaver skin or about appearance of scarred skin); and (e) appropriate matching (e.g., newly injured people sometimes benefit from survivor support from someone with similar injury characteristics, socioeconomic status, demographics, etc.). The authors conclude that peer support fosters reassurance, hope, and motivation among those still going through the changes of burn recovery.

Dutch adult burn survivors' views were surveyed with regard to peer support and group self-management activities that attract or repel them or the reasons that promote or prevent participation in activities (Papamikrouli et al., 2016). Descriptive analyses found that perceived benefits of participation are related to receiving and giving support rather than to "personal developmental reasons." The barriers that the survivors reported had inhibited them from participating in support group activities included the idea that since they were already feeling positive emotional states (e.g., confident, happy, connected), that this meant there was nothing for them to gain from attending the activities. Interestingly, the perceived benefits and barriers were the same among those who reported that they felt that they needed social support and those who did not report this need. Also of note, there were no differences noted among those who reported that they had attended peer-support activities and those who reported that they had not participated.

A synthesis of the peer-provider literature has recently been published by Tolley and Foroushami (2014). They conducted a literature review of several broad and relevant databases to assemble all acceptably rigorous and relevant studies. The two goals for the review were to (a) understand the state of knowledge regarding what is the reported benefit obtained by burn survivors who have obtained support from trained peer providers and (b) compile published information on those aspects of the peer-support program structure that were valued by the survivors who had utilized peer-support programs. Ten themes were derived regarding potential benefits. The most frequently endorsed "benefit obtained" items across the reviewed articles were reflected in the themes of positive impact, provide hope and inspiration, enhance motivation, create social connectedness/reduce isolation, and enhance self-esteem/self-image. Of note, the latter two benefits reflect the impact that belongingness has on enhancing self-esteem—as discussed previously. The authors also synthesized information across the reviewed articles regarding what aspects of the peer-support program structure that were considered to be highly valued by survivors. The most frequently endorsed "program structure" items across the reviewed articles were reflected in the themes of need for a screening/selecting method for peer providers and peer participants, adequate peer training, matching peer participants with trained peer providers, ensuring cooperating with hospital regulations, activities with a formal meeting structure, active facilitation of interactions, monitoring of group activities, and allowing for peers to choose to participate or not by respecting autonomy/choice/informed consent (Tolley & Foroushami, 2014).

Programs Promoting Professional Assistance to Survivor and Family

Specialized programs for survivors of burn injury targeting posttraumatic distress, body image, and social skills have been evaluated, validated, and published in Germany, the United Kingdom, and the United States.

ASD and PTSD, whether measured as symptom severity or using formal diagnostic criteria, are two of the most studied symptoms following burn injury. Somewhat surprisingly, only two investigators in the United States have developed and evaluated interventions targeting early symptoms of ASD/PTSD. Cukor, Wyka, Leahy, Yurt, and Difede (2015) published preliminary findings on an eight-session intervention suitable for the rehabilitation phase treating PTSD and also social anxiety related to discomfort from body image or social reactions. They conducted an uncontrolled pilot study evaluating the feasibility and preliminary efficacy of a manual-driven, 14-session protocol (imaginal and in vivo exposure for trauma reminders and for social situations), behavioral activation, and cognitive therapy for inaccurate or unhelpful thoughts about themselves) with adult burn survivors ($n = 9$ completers, 1 dropout). Significant improvements in pre- to posttreatment scores were obtained on the PTSD, depression, and community reintegration measures (Cukor et al., 2015). A great strength of the study was that it combined intervention components addressing ASD symptoms, social anxiety, and social skills.

Fauerbach and colleagues conducted a randomized, manual driven, proof of concept study of a 4-session, early intervention for adults from the in-patient setting that targeted symptoms of ASD and depression with the aim of preventing PTSD and mood disorder. The Safety, Meaning, Activation, and Reappraisal Therapy (SMART) study was conducted among acutely injured, hospitalized adults with burns and recently presented (Gehrke et al., 2017). The active components of SMART include stress management/mindfulness, behavioral activation, and cognitive therapy for inaccurate/unhelpful thoughts and seeking ways to improve safety and establish meaning from the event. The specific aims are to reduce symptoms of ASD and depression from pretest to posttest and to prevent PTSD and major depression at follow-up. The two groups included the active treatment, SMART ($n = 21$ treated) with completed assessments at pretreatment ($n = 16$), posttreatment completed ($n = 13$), and at one month ($n = 12$). The active treatment was contrasted with a viable control group, Supportive Counseling ($n = 19$ treated), with completed assessments at pretreatment ($n = 18$), 1 week posttreatment ($n = 15$) and at one month ($n = 13$). Importantly, the SMART group scores improved significantly from pretest (median 67.0) to posttest (median 16.0) and from pretest to one month (median 6.5). Interesting, the scores of the Supportive Counseling control group also improved significantly from pretest 60.5) to posttest (median= 30.0) and at one-month follow-up (median= 43.0). Of note, the participants in the SMART condition achieved clinically significant change (median scores below established cutoff for clinical severity - 40), while the control group participants initially dropped below clinical cutoff at the end of treatment, the control group median scores rose above cutoff by 1-month post-treatment. The trial successfully showed the clinical benefit and feasibility of CBT-based treatment of ASD in the acute burn center setting, all of which is perhaps more intriguing given the underpowered sample and without examining confounds (e.g., outliers, dropouts) that may have differentially effected group data.

Bessel and colleagues (2012) developed and evaluated a CBT-based intervention for burn survivors targeting body-image comfort and satisfaction, anxiety, depression, social anxiety, appearance-related distress (Derriford Appearance Scale-24), and body image (Body Image Quality of Life inventory). The randomized, controlled trial contrasted the CBT-based treatment presented either in person (Treatment as Usual, n = 15 completers) or via a new computerized version (PC-CBT, n = 19 completers) and a no-intervention control group (n = 14 completers). The components of the eight-session CBT treatment for both the in-person and PC versions were (a) introduction to model and appearance-related issues, (b) nonverbal communication, (c) verbal social skills, (d) goal-setting, (e) negative automatic thoughts, (f) social skills and goal-setting with practical examples and tips with a video, (g) exposure therapy rationale and methods with videotaped examples, and (h) summary of the material and process. The findings indicated that both the in-person and the PC versions resulted in reduced anxiety, depression, and concerns about appearance (DAS-24), while improving adjustment. These interventions have potential to make large contribution to the field and invite replication and extension.

Renneberg and colleagues (Seehausen et al., 2015) developed and evaluated an eight-session intervention for survivors in the postacute, rehabilitation phase. The aims were to promote social comfort, body-image satisfaction, and self-management and incorporated aspects of validated methods of reducing symptoms of distress, depression, and PTSD and of enhancing quality of life among individuals with differences in appearance. The intervention involved eight modules: introduction, discussion with expert on pain and scar formation/maturation, psychological distress, self-management with an altered body, coping with stress, dealing with social reactions, effect of avoidance on social distress and practicing social skills about scars and the event that caused them, and a review of the information. The participants were provided psychoeducation on psychological distress, scar formation, and the manner by which social withdrawal negatively impacts psychological and social adjustment. The process also involved role-plays by participants who were encouraged to discuss personal experiences. The intervention group showed significantly greater decrease in pre- to posttreatment scores and pre- to follow-up scores on general psychological distress and posttraumatic distress, as well as significant pre- to posttreatment improvement on the psychosocial (but not physical) quality of life and optimism.

CONCLUSION

Long-term impairments associated with burn injuries include physical consequences (e.g., hypertrophic scar contractures, pain, itch, range of motion, deconditioning), psychological function (e.g., depression with low energy and social withdrawal, body-image dissatisfaction due to scarring, posttraumatic distress with aversive memories, insomnia, hyperarousal), and social belonging (e.g., peer rejection/stigmatization due to altered appearance and reduced self-esteem due to perceived stigmatization by others and negative appraisals of oneself).

Self-management involves many domains of function following burn injury. These include cognition (problem-solving, self-monitoring, decision-making; Holroyd & Creer, 1986), behavior (attending appointments and completing tasks for scar management; Corbin & Strauss, 1988), emotion regulation (e.g., reappraisal of the emotions associated with wound care, sustaining motivation and effort in rehabilitation and then on one's own, persisting at difficult tasks such as pressure garments, range of motion), and social (e.g., assertive communication of needs and cooperating with caregivers and providers). Education is a key skill applicable to each of these domains in adapting means of self-management in light of specific needs related to the individual's chronic health conditions (Clark, Becker, Janz, Rakowski, & Anderson, 1991).

For individuals who survive a burn injury and for their families, emotion regulation involves learning to manage the logistic coordination, social experiences, and apprehensions and at the same time assimilating the meaning of the totality of this for oneself embedded in the psychological/emotional/interpersonal/community. Aspects of burns that challenge this meaning and require assimilating into existing schema or accommodating schema to incorporate these new experiences, include the circumstances of the traumatic event, the acute painful wound care, rehabilitation and deconditioning, and long-term implications of adjusting to disfigurement and social reactions. Maintaining a sense of psychological, social, and spiritual wholeness in the midst of all this can be emotionally overwhelming. Therefore, another cross-cutting skill for burn survivors is learning to regulate their emotions in order to restore a positive equilibrium when intensive negative emotions are generated whether through frustrating physical limitations (e.g., scar contractures), mood lability (e.g. after intrusive recollection of injury event), psychological strain (e.g., reduced self-efficacy), or social interactions (e.g., perceived or actual stigmatization/exclusion).

Great progress has been made in identifying, quantifying the prevalence, and tracking differences in trajectory of many burn-related conditions. Similarly, progress has been achieved in identifying individual characteristics that increase risk for adjustment difficulties (e.g., personality, suppressing emotion experience and expression, elevated acute symptoms), and some promising work has identified characteristics that reduce risk of initial and chronic conditions (e.g., optimism, resilience, self-efficacy). The emergence of interventions through the work of survivors and that of professional providers over the years has largely progressed by applying what has been learned elsewhere (e.g., support groups, trauma-focused CBT). New developments have recently emerged by adapting and integrating the clinical and experiential knowledge of dedicated survivors and clinicians (e.g., Social Skills Training interventions with the Phoenix Society for Burn Survivors and the FACEIT program collaboration between University of Bristol and Changing Faces peer support group in the United Kingdom). The framework provided by self-management and emotion regulation may direct refinements in these early efforts to enhance the focus on behaviors, skills, and knowledge that are most applicable to a given person's needs and are more operationally quantifiable in evaluating program results.

REFERENCES

American Burn Association. (2016). *Burn incidence and treatment in the United States: 2016*. Retrieved from http://www.ameriburn.org/resources_factsheet.php

American Psychiatric Association. (2013). *Diagnostic and statistical manual of mental disorders* (5th ed.). Washington, DC: Author.

Anthonissen, M., Daly, D., Janssens, T., & Van den Kerckhove, E. (2016). The effects of conservative treatments on burn scars: A systematic review. *Burns, 42*(3), 508–518. doi:10.1016/j.burns.2015.12.006.

Anthony, D. B., Holmes, J. G., & Wood, J. V. (2007). Social acceptance and self-esteem: Tuning the sociometer to interpersonal value. *Journal of Personality and Social Psychology, 92*(6), 1024–1039. doi:10.1037/0022-3514.92.6.1024

Austenfeld, J. L., & Stanton, A. L. (2004). Coping through emotional approach: A new look at emotion, coping, and health-related outcomes. *Journal of Personality, 72*(6), 1335–1363. doi:10.1111/j.1467-6494.2004.00299.x

Beck, J. S. (2010). Cognitive therapy. In I. B. Weiner & W. E. Craighead (Eds.), *The Corsini encyclopedia of psychology* (pp. 1–3). Hoboken, NJ: John Wiley. doi:10.1002/9780470479216.corpsy0198

Bessell, A., Brough, V., Clarke, A., Harcourt, D., Moss, T. P., & Rumsey, N. (2012). Evaluation of the effectiveness of Face IT, a computer-based psychosocial intervention for disfigurement-related distress. *Psychology, Health & Medicine, 17*(5), 565–577. doi:10.1080/13548506.2011.647701

Bosmans, M. G., Hofland, H. W., De Jong, A. E., & Van Loey, N. E. (2015). Coping with burns: The role of coping self-efficacy in the recovery from traumatic stress following burn injuries. *Journal of Behavioral Medicine, 38*(4), 642–651. doi:10.1007/s10865-015-9638-1

Bosmans, M. W., Van der Knaap, L. M., & Van der Velden, P. G. (2015). Personality traits as predictors of trauma-related coping self-efficacy: A three-wave prospective study. *Personality and Individual Differences, 76*, 44–48. doi:10.1016/j.paid.2014.11.052

Butler, E. A., Lee, T. L., & Gross, J. J. (2007). Emotion regulation and culture: Are the social consequences of emotion suppression culture-specific?. *Emotion, 7*(1), 30–48. doi:10.1037/1528-3542.7.1.30

Browne, A. L., Andrews, R., Schug, S. A., & Wood, F. (2011). Persistent pain outcomes and patient satisfaction with pain management after burn injury. *Clinical Journal of Pain*, 27(2), 136–145.

Campos, J. J., Campos, R. G., & Barrett, K. C. (1989). Emergent themes in the study of emotional development and emotion regulation. *Developmental Psychology*, 25(3), 394–402. doi:10.1037/0012-1649.25.3.394

Carr, T., Harris, D., & James, C. (2000). The Derriford Appearance Scale (DAS-59): A new scale to measure individual responses to living with problems of appearance. *British Journal of Health Psychology*, 5(Part2), 201–215. doi:10.1348/135910700168865

Carr, T., Moss, T., & Harris, D. (2005). The DAS24: A short form of the Derriford Appearance Scale DAS59 to measure individual responses to living with problems of appearance. *British Journal of Health Psychology*, 10(2), 285–298. doi:10.1348/135910705X27613

Chen, L., Wang, W., Tan, T., Han, H., & Dong, Z. (2016). GABA A receptors in the central nucleus of the amygdala are involved in pain-and itch-related responses. *The Journal of Pain*, 17(2), 181–189. doi:10.1016/j.jpain.2015.10.008

Cho, Y. S., Jeon, J. H., Hong, A., Yang, H. T., Yim, H., Cho, Y. S., . . . Seo, C. H. (2014). The effect of burn rehabilitation massage therapy on hypertrophic scar after burn: A randomized controlled trial. *Burns*, 40(8), 1513–1520. doi.org/10.1016/j.burns.2014.02.005

Clark, N. M., Becker, M. H., Janz, N. K., Lorig, K., Rakowski, W., & Anderson, L. (1991). Self-management of chronic disease by older adults: A review and questions for research. *Journal of Aging And Health*, 3(1), 3–27. doi:10.1177/089826439100300101

Corry, N. H., Klick, B., & Fauerbach, J. A. (2010). American Burn Association Clinical Research Award. Posttraumatic stress disorder and pain impact functioning and disability following major burn injury. *J Burn Care Research*, 31, 13–25.

Corbin, J. M., & Strauss, A. (1988). *Unending work and care: Managing chronic illness at home*. San Francisco, CA: Jossey-Bass.

Cukor, J., Wyka, K., Leahy, N., Yurt, R., & Difede, J. (2015). The treatment of posttraumatic stress disorder and related psychosocial consequences of burn injury: A pilot study. *Journal of Burn Care & Research*, 36(1), 184–192. doi:10.1097/BCR.0000000000000177

DeSouza, A. (2010). Psychological aspects of paediatric burns (a clinical review). *Annals of Burns and Fire Disasters*, 23(3), 155–159.

DeWall, C. N., Twenge, J. M., Koole, S. L., Baumeister, R. F., Marquez, A., & Reid, M. W. (2011). Automatic emotion regulation after social exclusion: Tuning to positivity. *Emotion*, 11(3), 623–636. doi:10.1037/a0023534

Edwards, R. R., Magyar-Russell, G., Thombs, B., Smith, M. T., Holavanahalli, R., Patterson, D. R., . . . Fauerbach, J. A. (2007). Acute pain at discharge from hospitalization for burn injury is a prospective predictor of long-term suicidal ideation. *Archives of Physical Medicine and Rehabilitation*, 88(12 Suppl. 2), S36–S42. doi:10.1016/j.apmr.2007.05.031

Edwards, R. R., Smith, M. T., Klick, B., Magyar-Russell, G., Haythornthwaite, J. A., Holavanahalli, R., . . . Fauerbach, J. A. (2007). Symptoms of depression and anxiety as unique predictors of pain-related outcomes following burn injury. *Annals of Behavioral Medicine*, 34(3), 313–322. doi:10.1007/BF02874556

Eisenberger, N. I., & Lieberman, M. D. (2004). Why rejection hurts: A common neural alarm system for physical and social pain. *Trends In Cognitive Sciences*, 8(7), 294–300. doi:10.1016/j.tics.2004.05.010

Fauerbach, J. A., Bresnick, M. G., & Smith, M. T. (2007). Coping with burn injury: Research summary and a new model of the influence of coping on psychological complications. In E. Martz & H. Livneh (Eds.), *Coping with chronic illness and disability* (pp. 173–190). New York: Springer.

Fauerbach, J. A., Heinberg, L. J., Lawrence, J. W., Bryant, A. G., Richter, L., & Spence, R. J. (2002). Coping with body image changes following a disfiguring burn injury. *Health Psychology, 21*(2), 115. doi:10.1037/0278-6133.21.2.115

Fauerbach, J. A., Lawrence, J., Haythornthwaite, J., Richter, D., McGuire, M., Schmidt, C., & Munster, A. (1997). Psychiatric history affects post trauma morbidity in a burn injured adult sample. *Psychosomatics, 38*, 374–385.

Fauerbach, J. A., Lawrence, J. W., Schmidt, C. W. Jr, Munster, A. M., & Costas, P. T. Jr. (2000). Personality predictors of injury-related posttraumatic stress disorder. *Journal of Nervous and Mental Disease, 188*(8), 510–517. doi:10.1097/00005053-200008000-00006

Gehrke, A., Mason, S. T., Sabo, A., McCann, U., Caffrey, J., & Milner, S., Fauerbach, J. A. (2017). Cognitive behavioral treatment for acute stress disorder: The Safety, Meaning, Activation, and Resilience Training trial. *Supplement to Journal of Burn Care and Research, Proceedings of the American Burn Association 49th Annual Meeting, 38*(2), S29.

Fauerbach, J. A., Rios, R., Immel, C., Mason, S. T., Price, L. A., & Milner, S. (2014, April). Perceived Stigmatization and Appearance Dissatisfaction Affect Psychological and Social Recovery from Disfiguring Burn Injury. Poster presented to the 32nd Annual Conference of the Anxiety Disorders Association of America, Washington D.C.

Forjuoh, S. N. (1998). The mechanisms, intensity of treatment, and outcomes of hospitalized burns: Issues for prevention. *Journal of Burn Care & Research, 19*(5), 455–460. doi:0273-8481/98/

Gross, J. J., & Thompson, R. A. (2007). Emotion regulation: Conceptual foundations. In J. J. Gross (Ed.), *Handbook of emotion regulation* (pp. 3–24). New York: Guilford Press.

Ho, F. Y. Y., Chan, C. S., & Tang, K. N. S. (2016). Cognitive-behavioral therapy for sleep disturbances in treating posttraumatic stress disorder symptoms: A meta-analysis of randomized controlled trials. *Clinical Psychology Review, 43*, 90–102. doi:10.1016/j.cpr.2015.09.005

Holroyd, K. A., & Creer, T. L. (Eds.). (1986). *Self-management of chronic disease: Handbook of clinical interventions and research.* New York: Academic Press.

James, A. C., James, G., Cowdrey, F. A., Soler, A., & Choke, A. (2015). Cognitive behavioural therapy for anxiety disorders in children and adolescents. *Cochrane Database of Systematic Reviews, 6*, CD004690. doi:10.1002/14651858.CD004690.pub4.

Jerant, A. F., von Friederichs-Fitzwater, M. M., & Moore, M. (2005). Patients' perceived barriers to active self-management of chronic conditions. *Patient Education and Counseling, 57*(3), 300–307. doi:10.1016/j.pec.2004.08.004

Kazak, A. E., Kassam-Adams, N., Schneider, S., Zelikovsky, N., Alderfer, M. A., & Rourke, M. (2006). An integrative model of pediatric medical traumatic stress. *Journal of Pediatric Psychology, 31*(4), 343–355. doi:10.1093/jpepsy/jsj054

Kornhaber, R., Wilson, A., Abu-Qamar, M., McLean, L., & Vandervord, J. (2015). Inpatient peer support for adult burn survivors—a valuable resource: A phenomenological analysis of the Australian experience. *Burns, 41*(1), 110–117. doi:10.1016/j.burns.2014.05.003

Lawrence, J. W., Fauerbach, J. A., Heinberg, L., & Doctor, M. (2004). The 2003 clinical research award: Visible vs hidden scars and their relation to body esteem. *Journal of Burn Care & Research, 25*(1), 25–32. doi:10.1097/01.BCR.0000105090.99736.48

Lawrence, J. W., Fauerbach, J. A., & Thombs, B. D. (2006). A test of the moderating role of importance of appearance in the relationship between perceived scar severity and body-esteem among adult burn survivors. *Body Image, 3*(2), 101–111. doi:10.1016/j.bodyim.2006.01.003

Lawrence, J. W., Heinberg, L. J., Roca, R., Munster, A., Spence, R., & Fauerbach, J. A. (1998). Development and validation of the Satisfaction with Appearance Scale: Assessing body image among burn-injured patients. *Psychological Assessment, 10*(1), 64–70. doi:10.1037/1040-3590.10.1.64

Lawrence, J. W, Fauerbach, J. A., Heinberg, L. J., & Doctor, M. (2006). The reliability and validity of the Perceived Stigmatization Questionnaire (PSQ) and the Social Comfort Questionnaire (SCQ) in an adult burn survivor sample. *Psychological Assessment, 18*(1), 106–111.

Linares, H. A. (1996). Pathophysiology of the burn scar. In D. N. Herndon (Ed.), *Total burn care* (pp. 383–397). Philadelphia, PA: Saunders Elsevier.

Livneh, H., & Antonak, R. F. (1997). *Psychosocial adaptation to chronic illness and disability*. Gaithersburg, MD: Aspen.

Logsetty, S., Shamlou, A., Gawaziuk, J. P., March, J., Doupe, M., Chateau, D., . . . Enns, M. W. (2016). Mental health outcomes of burn: A longitudinal population-based study of adults hospitalized for burns. *Burns, 42*(4), 738–744. doi:10.1016/j.burns.2016.03.006

Lorig, K. R., & Holman, H. R. (2003). Self-management education: History, definition, outcomes, and mechanisms. *Annals of Behavioral Medicine, 26*, 1–7. doi:10.1207/S15324796ABM2601_01

MacDonald, G., & Leary, M. R. (2005). Why does social exclusion hurt? The relationship between social and physical pain. *Psychological Bulletin, 131*(2), 202–223. doi:10.1037/0033-2909.131.2.202

Mason, S. T., Corry, N., Gould, N., Amoyal, N., Wiechman Askay, S., Holavanahalli, R., Banks, S., Arceneaux, L. L., & Fauerbach, J. A. (2010). Growth curve trajectories of distress in burn patients. *Journal of Burn Care Research, 31*, 64–72.

Mason, S. T., Lawrence, J. W., Plaff, J., Allen, L., Martinez, E. M., Jochai, D., . . . Fauerbach, J. A. (2011). Body image and social adjustment: Proceedings of the 43rd Annual Meeting of the American Burn Association, Chicago, March 29–April 1, 2011. *Journal of Burn Care Research, 36*(3 Suppl.).

McKibben, J. B., Bresnick, M. G., Askay, S. A. W., & Fauerbach, J. A. (2008). Acute stress disorder and posttraumatic stress disorder: A prospective study of prevalence, course, and predictors in a sample with major burn injuries. *Journal of Burn Care & Research, 29*(1), 22–35. doi:10.1097/BCR.0b013e31815f59c4

Modi, A. C., Pai, A. L., Hommel, K. A., Hood, K. K., Cortina, S., Hilliard, M. E., . . . Drotar, D. (2012). Pediatric self-management: A framework for research, practice, and policy. *Pediatrics, 129*(2), e473–e485. Retrieved from http://pediatrics.aappublications.org/content/129/2/e473.full

Neuberg, S. L., Kenrick, D. T., & Schaller, M. (2011). Human threat management systems: Self-protection and disease avoidance. *Neuroscience and Biobehavioral Reviews, 35*(4), 1042–1051. doi:10.1016/j.neubiorev.2010.08.011

Oaten, M. J., Stevenson, R. J., & Case, T. I. (2011). Disease avoidance as a functional basis for stigmatization. *Philosophical Transactions of the Royal Society, London, B, 366*, 3433–3452. doi:10.1098/rstb.2011.0095

Oster, C., Kildal, M., & Ekselius, L. (2010). Return to work after burn injury: Burn-injured individuals' perception of barriers and facilitators. *Journal of Burn Care and Research*, *31*(4), 540–550. doi:10.1097/BCR.0b013e3181e4d692

Papamikrouli, E., van Schie, C. M., Schoenmaker, J., Berge, A. B. V., & Gebhardt, W. A. (2016). Peer support needs among adults with burns. *Journal of Burn Care & Research*. Advance online publication. doi:10.1097/BCR.0000000000000424

Pascoe, E. A., & Smart Richman, L. (2009). Perceived discrimination and health: A meta-analytic review. *Psychological Bulletin*, *135*(4), 531–554. doi:10.1037/a0016059

Park, L. E., & Maner, J. K. (2009). Does self-threat promote social connection? The role of self-esteem and contingencies of self-worth. *Journal of Personality and Social Psychology*, *96*(1), 203–217. doi:10.1037/a0013933

Parker, R. (2012). Stigma, prejudice and discrimination in global public health. *Cadernos de Saúde Pública*, *28*(1), 164–169. doi: 10.1590/S0102-311X2012000100017

Peck, M. D. (2011). Epidemiology of burns throughout the world. Part I: Distribution and risk factors. *Burns*, *37*(7), 1087–1100. doi:10.1016/j.burns.2011.06.005

Perry, J. L., Sharp, S. A., Rosenberg, M. A., Rosenberg, L. E., & Meyer, W. J. (2012). Psychosocial aspects of pediatric burn care. In B. J. Phillips (Ed.), *Pediatric burns: From tragedy to hope* (pp. 374–392). Amherst, NY: Cambria Press.

Retrouvey, H., & Shahrokhi, S. (2015). Pain and the thermally injured patient-a review of current therapies. *Journal of Burn Care and Research*, *36*(2), 315–323. doi:10.1097/BCR.0000000000000073.

Rosenbach, C., & Renneberg, B. (2008). Positive change after severe burn injuries. *Journal of Burn Care and Research*, *29*(4), 638–643. doi:10.1097/BCR.0b013e31817de275.

Rybarczyk, B., Edwards, R., & Behel, J. (2004). Diversity in adjustment to a leg amputation: Case illustrations of common themes. *Disability and Rehabilitation: An International, Multidisciplinary Journal*, *26*(14–15), 944–953. doi:10.1080/09638280410001708986

Saffle, J. R., Davis, B., & Williams, P. (1995). Recent outcomes in the treatment of burn injury in the United States: A report from the American Burn Association Patient Registry. *Journal of Burn Care & Research*, *16*(3), 219–232. doi:0273-8481/95/

Schneider, K. A. (2006). Does attention alter appearance? *Perception & Psychophysics*, *68*(5), 800–814. doi:10.3758/BF03193703

Seehausen, A., Ripper, S., Germann, G., Hartmann, B., Wind, G., & Renneberg, B. (2015). Efficacy of a burn-specific cognitive-behavioral group training. *Burns*, *41*(2), 308–316. http://dx.doi.org/10.1016/j.burns.2014.07.006

Smart Richman, L., & Leary, M. R. (2009). Reactions to discrimination, stigmatization, ostracism, and other forms of interpersonal rejection: A multimotive model. *Psychological Review*, *116*(2), 365–383. doi:10.1037/a0015250

Smith, M. T., Klick, B., Kozachik, S., Edwards, R. R., Holavanahalli, R., Wiechman, S., ... Fauerbach, J. A. (2008). Sleep onset insomnia symptoms during hospitalization for major burn injury predict chronic pain. *Pain*, *138*(3), 497–506.

Suri, G., Whittaker, K., & Gross, J. J. (2015). Launching reappraisal: It's less common than you might think. *Emotion*, *15*(1), 73–77. doi:10.1037/emo0000011

Sveen, J., Ekselius, L., Gerdin, B., & Willebrand, M. (2011). A prospective longitudinal study of posttraumatic stress disorder symptom trajectories after burn injury. *Journal of Trauma and Acute Care Surgery*, *71*(6), 1808–1815. doi:10.1097/TA.0b013e31822a30b8

Szabo, M. M., Urich, M. A., Duncan, C. L., & Aballay, A. M. (2016). Patient adherence to burn care: A systematic review of the literature. *Burns*, *42*(3), 484–491. doi:10.1016/j.burns.2015.08.010

Thombs, B. D., Notes, L. D., Lawrence, J. W., Magyar-Russell, G., Bresnick, M. G., & Fauerbach, J. A. (2008). From survival to socialization: A longitudinal study of body image in survivors of severe burn injury. *Journal of Psychosomatic Research*, 64(2), 205–212. doi:10.1016/j.jpsychores.2007.09.003

Tolley, J. S., & Foroushani, P. S. (2014). What do we know about one-to-one peer support for adults with a burn injury? A scoping review. *Journal of Burn Care & Research*, 35(3), 233–242. doi:10.1097/BCR.0b013e3182957749

Townsend, S. S., Major, B., Gangi, C. E., & Mendes, W. B. (2011). From "in the air" to "under the skin": Cortisol responses to social identity threat. *Personality and Social Psychology Bulletin*, 37(2), 151–164. doi:10.1177/0146167210392384.

Van Loey, N. E., van Beeck, E. F., Faber, B. W., van de Schoot, R., & Bremer, M. (2012). Health-related quality of life after burns: A prospective multicenter cohort study with 18 months follow-up. *Journal of Trauma and Acute Care Surgery*, 72(2), 513–520. doi:10.1097/TA.0b013e3182199072.

Ware, J. E., Snow, K. K., Kosinski, M., & Gandek, B. (1993). *SF-36 Health Survey manual and interpretation guide*. Boston: Health Institute, New England Medical Center.

Watts, S. E., Turnell, A., Kladnitski, N., Newby, J. M., & Andrews, G. (2015). Treatment-as-usual (TAU) is anything but usual: A meta-analysis of CBT versus TAU for anxiety and depression. *Journal of Affective Disorders*, 175, 152–167. doi:10.1016/j.jad.2014.12.025

Weaver, T. L., Resnick, H. S., Kokoska, M. S., & Etzel, J. C. (2007). Appearance-related residual injury, posttraumatic stress, and body image: Associations within a sample of female victims of intimate partner violence. *Journal of Traumatic Stress*, 20(6), 999–1008. doi:10.1002/jts.2027

Willebrand, M., & Sveen, J. (2016). Injury-related fear-avoidance and symptoms of posttraumatic stress in parents of children with burns. *Burns*, 42(2), 414–420. doi:10.1016/j.burns.2015.08.004.

Williams, A. C. D. C., Eccleston, C., & Morley, S. (2012). Psychological therapies for the management of chronic pain (excluding headache) in adults. *Cochrane Database of Systematic Reviews*, 11, CD007407. doi:10.1002/14651858.CD007407.pub3

Woo, C. W., Koban, L., Kross, E., Lindquist, M. A., Banich, M. T., Ruzic, L., . . . Wager, T. D. (2014). Separate neural representations for physical pain and social rejection. *Nature Communications*, 5, 5380. doi:10.1038/ncomms6380

World Health Organization. (2008). *The global burden of disease: 2004 update*. Geneva: Author.

10

Self-Management of Cancer

AMY DECKERT AND GERALD M. DEVINS ∎

Behavioral self-management contributes importantly to the effective management of many medical conditions. The approach entails enlisting affected people in (a) understanding the processes that underlie their conditions and the treatments applied to them, (b) accepting responsibility for actively collaborating with healthcare providers to implement treatment and to alleviate symptoms and treatment side effects, and (c) acquiring the requisite skills to implement self-management effectively (Devins & Binik, 1996). The approach was initially applied in arthritis (Lorig & Fries, 2006), but its merits and relevance were quickly recognized by professionals working with other chronic conditions (witness the numerous chapters in the current volume that address the self-management of diverse health conditions). The chronic conditions to which self-management programs are traditionally applied usually progress slowly and, although often painful and disabling, are not typically fatal, although there are exceptions (e.g., cardiac conditions, untreated type 1 diabetes, and HIV, all of which are discussed in this book). The goal of medical treatment in these instances is not to *cure* the underlying biomedical condition but to minimize the deleterious effects of disease, retard its progression, and thereby help affected individuals to live as meaningfully and productively as possible. Over time, these conditions progress to stages of increasing severity and impact. Complications can develop, but most people can expect to live for many years.

In cancer, the situation is quite different: The biological processes that underlie the condition typically lead to death if untreated. The goal of treatment is to eliminate the underlying disease, although it is not possible to establish this definitively (the best possible outcome is to determine that there is "no evidence of disease"). Cancer is associated with a number of highly unpleasant symptoms (e.g., pain, dyspnea, fatigue) and treatment side effects (e.g., nausea, mouth sores, erectile dysfunction), but it does not usually produce the types of physical disability (e.g., impaired ambulation, paresthesia, tremor) that are evident in other chronic conditions for which self-management interventions exist (e.g., arthritis, multiple sclerosis). Self-management as applied to cancer, therefore, aims largely to minimize the suffering people experience due to the condition and its treatment. It also aims to reduce the burden on the healthcare system (e.g., reducing demands on nursing staff, transfer of healthcare responsibilities from treatment setting to home). Many programs focus on cancers associated with comparatively long periods of survival (e.g., the five-year relative survival rate for men affected by prostate cancer is 98.9%, and the rate for women affected by breast cancer is 89.7% [Howlader et al., 2016]), but self-management can play an important role in improving health outcomes across the cancer spectrum, regardless of diagnosis, treatment type, or prognosis. The collaborative relationship between healthcare provider and the person with cancer that is inherent in a self-management approach has the potential to benefit many important outcomes, including facilitating decision-making, enhancing treatment effectiveness, minimizing treatment side effects, and maximizing health outcomes. The self-management of cancer is particularly important in light of changes to the cancer-care system that rely on the affected person to administer and follow treatments (e.g., chemotherapy) and to initiate changes to lifestyle (e.g., fitness and activity levels) or health behavior (e.g., smoking cessation, weight loss) to maximize treatment benefits and prevent complications or recurrence. In this chapter, we highlight distinctions between chronic medical conditions and cancer and describe the essential elements of self-management programs and the application of self-management skills to the problems introduced by cancer. We review and critique the cancer self-management literature as a function of four categories of self-management targets and offer suggestions for future research.

DISTINCTIONS BETWEEN CHRONIC CONDITIONS AND CANCER

As indicated, cancer and its treatment differ from most other medical conditions for which self-management programs have been developed. Most cancers are fatal if left untreated. Many advance rapidly. Advances in technology, detection, and treatment innovations have resulted in increasing numbers of people surviving long after diagnosis and treatment (Howlader et al., 2016). In oncology care, the goal of treatment is to eliminate cancer, using means that require highly specialized expertise and advanced biomedical technology and are thus largely beyond the control of the affected person (e.g., surgery, chemotherapy, radiation). By contrast, in chronic medical conditions, such as multiple sclerosis, the disease cannot be eliminated or cured. As a result, people with such conditions must endure an ongoing threat that necessitates management of symptoms and the underlying disease process itself. To illustrate, for a person with arthritis, the primary focus of treatment is to retard progression and to prevent and manage symptoms and impairments. One of the primary concerns of people with arthritis is pain, and so self-management is informed within the context of pain management. Pain is exacerbated by tense or weakened muscles. Individuals with arthritis may, thus, be encouraged to engage in physical exercises to strengthen and relax the muscles, which can be expected, in turn, to reduce arthritis pain and related impairments.

Similarly, certain cancers cannot be eliminated, such as those that are advanced or metastatic (i.e., spread to other bodily locations or systems). Consequently, affected individuals may experience a variety of cancer-related impairments that require management. In many types of cancer, it is common, too, for impairments to arise long after treatment has been completed, despite no detectable cancer in the body. Among individuals treated for cancer, "no evidence of disease" means that the disease cannot be *detected*—it does not mean that no cancer is *present*, and so this desirable outcome does not necessarily mean that a person has been cured. Thus chronicity has a unique meaning in oncology, whereby "no evidence of disease" must be accompanied by residual management, surveillance, and monitoring for treatment late effects or recurrence. The ongoing threat of physical symptoms associated with treatment and the psychological threat of cancer recurrence require management that is distinct from that which is intended to eliminate the cancer. "Chronic cancer" is a term that has been used to describe cancers that are incurable with currently available treatments. Treatment in such instances, thus, aims to attenuate physical-symptom burden, retard progression, or extend life (Harley, Pini, Bartlett, & Velikova, 2015). Cancers that are considered chronic in nature are well-suited for self-management interventions as the targets are aligned with those of conventional programs (e.g., symptom control, preventing complications, maintaining abilities, and preserving quality of life).

SELF-MANAGEMENT PROGRAMS

Successful self-management has been described as a set of interventions that bolster individual capacity for self-monitoring of symptoms and illness while mobilizing the cognitive, affective, and behavioral responses necessary to preserve quality of life (Barlow, Wright, Sheasby, Turner, & Hainsworth, 2002). Self-management programs for individuals with chronic health conditions (e.g., chronic disease self-management [CDSM]) have been developed and evaluated extensively at the Stanford Patient Education Research Center (Lorig & Holman, 2003) and elsewhere. CDSM programs may target specific chronic health conditions, such as arthritis, or diagnostically mixed groups that include people with diverse chronic conditions. CDSM intervention components are grounded in principles of cognitive-behavior therapy and include self-monitoring of symptoms and side effects, goal-setting, and problem-solving techniques (Lorig & Holman, 2003). Findings from prospective cohort studies demonstrate adaptive behavior change postintervention, which includes increased engagement in prescribed self-management techniques and self-reported improvements in communicating with physicians. In a large, randomized controlled trial of individuals with mixed chronic conditions excluding cancer ($N = 952$), participants randomized to CDSM increased their participation in relevant health behaviors (e.g., aerobic and resistance exercise), increased their use of symptom-management strategies (e.g., to attenuate pain or other symptoms), communicated more frequently with healthcare providers, and used fewer health services (e.g., hospitalization; Lorig et al., 1998).

Effective uptake and completion of self-management programs have been studied extensively and necessitate a comprehensive set of tasks and core skills. Lorig and Holman (2003) delineate a problem-based framework derived from the ways in which people perceive their health conditions (Corbin & Strauss, 1988). Within this framework, three tasks are essential to the effective self-management of chronic conditions: (a) medical management (e.g., following medication or treatment protocols); (b) role management (e.g., adoption or maintenance of new meaningful behaviors or life roles); and (c) emotional management (e.g., management of emotional consequence of illness). Lorig and Holman posited that these tasks are accomplished through the practice of the following core skills: (a) problem-solving, (b) decision-making, (c) resource identification and utilization, (d) partnership between the recipient of healthcare and the provider, (e) action planning for behavioral change, and (f) individual capacity for self-tailoring, or personalizing the application of the intervention to meet the individual's situation and needs (Lorig & Holman, 2003).

APPLYING SELF-MANAGEMENT SKILLS TO CANCER

Self-management tasks and core skills may require modification before they can be implemented for cancer self-management, particularly due to practical concerns. Individuals have limited resources, including financial and time constraints. In addition, the comprehensive and complex processes delineated for the application of self-management to one's chronic health condition requires considerable attentional reserve, effort, and psychological sophistication. Self-efficacy has been identified as the mechanism responsible for change attributable to self-management enactment. In this context, self-efficacy is defined as expectations of personal competence to organize and execute the actions required to manage the medical, behavioral, and emotional consequences of a given condition (Bandura, 1997). It is measured as the confidence that one can perform certain behaviors or achieve given physiological states under specific conditions (Bandura, 1997). In CDSM research, baseline and changes in self-efficacy induced by self-management have been associated with improvements in future health status (Lorig et al., 1998). By contrast, improving self-efficacy to manage cancer-related medical consequences or treatment side effects may not reflect a credible goal inasmuch as the healthcare recipient's role does not typically extend beyond attending and completing curative treatments (e.g., chemotherapy or radiotherapy). People with cancer cannot exert control over medical consequences to the extent that may be possible in other chronic health conditions, such as diabetes or arthritis. There are elements of self-management that cannot be implemented or achieved in cancer. For example, blood-glucose monitoring and physical activity are effective in slowing diabetes progression and delaying the inevitable occurrence of associated complications (Fisher et al., 2005; Norris & Narayan, 2001), but the notion that similar self-monitoring and lifestyle changes can slow the progression of an aggressive cancer or prevent metastasis has not been substantiated (Ligibel, 2012; Smith-Turchyn, Morgan, & Richardson, 2016).

When considering the application of self-management programs to cancer, it is important to remember the distinction between cancer and chronic medical conditions with respect to their anticipated illness trajectories. The diagnosis of many forms of arthritis, multiple sclerosis, or type 2 diabetes do not typically invoke the same sense of intense threat and urgency as does the diagnosis of cancer, although type 1 diabetes, HIV, and cardiac conditions can be urgent and life-threatening at the time of diagnosis when not yet treated (see chapters 11, 12, and 15 in this volume). The necessarily prompt response to a cancer diagnosis often triggers additional medical developments in rapid succession, such as further diagnostic testing and decision-making regarding treatment plans and goals that are unique to cancer (e.g., pretreatment staging including imaging, bloodwork, and biopsies). In many cases, the urgency of a cancer diagnosis invokes the need for immediate action. With the evolution of personalized and precision medicine, it is often necessary to conduct multiple diagnostic tests in close succession once cancer has been detected. In modern-day healthcare, people must be informed of their diagnoses, told about treatment alternatives, and provided with opportunities to exercise autonomy in decision-making. A cancer diagnosis often involves urgent demands for action. Unlike many conditions, most treatment-related decisions in cancer must be taken very shortly after diagnosis, and this often precludes participation in self-management interventions to acquire or bolster decision-making skills. For example, the general curative therapeutic regimen for acute myeloid leukemia includes an immediate course of intensive, induction chemotherapy (Döhner, Weisdorf, & Bloomfield, 2015). Following pathologic confirmation of cytogenetic and chromosomal abnormalities, treatment plans must be tailored accordingly. The context in which this unfolds presents constraints and challenges that are quite different from the contexts characteristic of many progressive, chronic medical conditions, such as rheumatoid or osteoarthritis, and therefore requires unique consideration. A diagnosis of arthritis is not accompanied by the urgency to establish diagnostic characteristics and introduce life-saving treatment without delay. The consequences of watching and waiting are much less severe in a more slowly evolving, chronic condition than in the case of people diagnosed with acute myeloid leukemia or other malignancies. During the time of diagnosis and initiation of treatment, people affected by cancer may not have the time, mindset, or cognitive reserves necessary to participate in weekly sessions to develop and practice the tasks and skills delineated for the self-management of chronic conditions. Self-management becomes much more relevant and useful at later stages in the disease trajectory (e.g., learning how to take medication as prescribed, managing disruptive treatment side effects).

The principles of self-management as articulated in the self-management literature are certainly applicable to cancer, but some elements require modification before they can be applied effectively. Helping people to acquire decision-making skills can contribute adaptively to the self-management of many chronic conditions, for example, but the urgency associated with diagnosing and initiating treatment in cancer renders this impractical in many instances. Similarly, there simply may not be sufficient time to introduce interventions to help people develop strategies to identify and take advantage of relevant resources. In some cancers, action planning to facilitate health-behavior change is important (e.g., dietary and activity uptake in colorectal cancer), but there may not be sufficient time to provide instruction or intervene to help people develop the requisite skills and strategies to facilitate such change until they reach the posttreatment recovery phase.

The literature over the past decade has focused increasingly on the development and evaluation of self-management interventions tailored for cancer. Three reviews address self-management interventions across the cancer continuum (Gao et al., 2011; Hammer et al., 2015; McCorkle et al., 2011). Other reviews consider self-management interventions specific to cancer subgroups, such as adults with advanced cancer at the end of life (Johnston et al., 2009), posttreatment prostate cancer survivors (Paterson, Jones, Rattray, & Lauder, 2015), and hormone receptor-positive breast cancer survivors (Van Liew, Christensen, & de Moor, 2014). Some reviews attempt to synthesize and critique the evidence base for symptom-specific interventions, such as the self-management of cancer pain (Koller, Miaskowski, De Geest, Opitz, & Spichiger, 2012; Lovell et al., 2014) and chemotherapy-induced nausea and vomiting (Richardson, 1992). The characteristics of the facilitators employed to deliver these programs vary considerably, including professional discipline (e.g., psychology, nursing) and levels of experience and expertise (e.g., clinicians, researchers, trained laypeople, and peer volunteers). Self-management interventions that focus on cancer can be delivered by diverse modalities, including face-to-face meetings, telephone exchanges, and web-based programs. In general, the therapeutic elements of self-management have not been described in sufficient detail in the cancer literature. Critical gaps remain. This, of course, renders it difficult to draw firm conclusions or offer recommendations with authority. Despite these gaps and the infancy of the literature, patient education (Hammer et al., 2015) and the partnership between healthcare recipients and providers (McCorkle et al., 2011) have been highlighted as integral to the management of pain and other cancer-related symptoms or impairments (Lovell et al., 2014).

In the following sections, we critique the extant literature concerning the self-management of cancer and offer suggestions for future research. Published reviews have limited their focus to studies involving cancer only but have not considered how the approach may require tailoring to address the unique needs or constraints people experience when they are affected by these conditions. Published literature reviews have not distinguished among diverse targets for cancer self-management interventions. This raises important implications for effectiveness (e.g., do self-management interventions target outcomes that they might reasonably be expected to influence?). The literature provides insufficient information about the types of self-management interventions that have been applied to people affected by cancer or about the specific, therapeutic components they comprise, limiting possibilities for replication and precluding the extension of this work to cancer sites other than those investigated. Reviews, to date, have been highly selective and are, thus, likely biased: In one review, for example, the search was limited to studies in which a nurse was principal investigator (Hammer et al., 2015), although this was not justified. The field is more likely to advance meaningfully when investigators and scholars adopt a wide-ranging perspective that seeks to learn from relevant research that originates across a broad range of disciplines and clinical populations and that is careful to document important and relevant details (e.g., providing descriptions of self-management intervention components in sufficient detail to permit others to adopt them effectively).

READING THE LITERATURE ON SELF-MANAGEMENT IN CANCER

In order to improve clinical outcomes and to attenuate the burden of physical and psychological symptoms, we propose that people affected by cancer require the following skills for effective self-management: (a) knowledge about their specific cancer, treatment, and symptoms; (b) collaboration with their healthcare provider(s); and (c) a repertoire of effective self-management skills (i.e., behavioral repertoire). The effectiveness of self-management in improving clinical outcomes has been demonstrated in relation to specific cancer-related symptoms (e.g., pain, fatigue).

We propose that the effective self-management of cancer is predicated on three principal elements: (a) people must acquire knowledge about their cancer and its treatment, (b) they must accept responsibility for collaborating and communicating with their healthcare providers, and (c) they must master the skills needed to implement self-management effectively. Although published studies of cancer self-management have been variously labeled "self-care," "patient education," and "cognitive-behavioral interventions" (among others), this chapter applies these principles to identify the self-management interventions to be reviewed regardless of the descriptive label assigned to them. Overall, few randomized controlled trials meet these criteria. Many studies are exploratory or descriptive in nature. The majority of published studies about cancer self-management comprise quantitative or qualitative assessments of needs, preferences, cancer-related self-management barriers, and facilitators. They report the perspectives of people directly affected by the condition, their family members, and their healthcare providers.

SELF-MANAGEMENT TARGETS

Four levels of self-management targets are relevant to cancer. *Primary targets* entail elements of the disease process that can be influenced by self-management efforts (e.g., weight loss to enhance the effectiveness of radiation treatment for breast cancer). *Secondary targets* involve symptoms (e.g., fatigue, pain) and treatment side effects (e.g., nausea, difficulty swallowing). *Tertiary targets* involve psychosocial consequences (e.g., illness intrusiveness, quality of life, or empowerment). *Quaternary targets* involve the prevention of developments that have not yet occurred but can be avoided through appropriate action. Quaternary targets include anticipated treatment side effects (e.g., mucositis, fatigue, nausea, and vomiting), cancer recurrence, or the untoward consequences that follow from them.

In many instances, effective self-management of secondary targets can also result in benefits at the tertiary level. For example, self-management steps relevant to a person experiencing cancer-related pain include acquiring knowledge and understanding of the disease and treatment(s) and a behavioral repertoire that includes communicating with healthcare providers about pain intensity when indicated. This informed and collaborative approach is necessary to attenuate pain as a secondary target of self-management. Effective pain management, of course, can be expected also to preserve or enhance quality of life. Knowledge about one's condition and its treatment can help to mitigate medical treatment errors and improve completion of treatment protocols and engagement in health behaviors. Collectively, these direct and indirect effects may produce additional psychosocial benefits, including reducing stigma, minimizing destructive intrusions into valued roles and relationships (i.e., illness intrusiveness), and thereby reducing emotional distress.

Effective interventions require that self-management targets be clearly defined and measurable. For example, an intervention designed to impact fatigue, a secondary self-management target, is likely to be most effective when it directly addresses factors known to cause fatigue, such as physical deconditioning, which can be reversed by exercise and activity. Establishing the benefit of interventions that increase exercise and activity can best be accomplished by identifying and measuring fatigue as the outcome of primary interest.

Primary Targets

Primary self-management targets involve aspects of cancer itself (e.g., tumor reduction). Self-management tactics to achieve improvement in primary targets include strategies to facilitate and improve treatment completion (e.g., oral chemotherapy agents), facilitating uptake of ancillary health behaviors to enhance treatment or diagnostic effectiveness (e.g., weight loss for women with breast cancer), preventing treatment errors, or bringing relevant, new symptoms or other changes to the attention of healthcare providers. Primary targets represent an increasingly important focus for future self-management interventions in cancer. The self-administration of cytotoxic and targeted oral chemotherapeutic agents is likely to be especially important because the medications are self-administered at home and present unique challenges in terms of monitoring, dose variability, and complications (Greer et al., 2016; Partridge, Avorn, Wang, & Winer, 2002). Self-assessment and symptom management can contribute usefully to improvements in primary self-management targets. It has been estimated that only 50% of medications are taken as prescribed across the entire spectrum of medical practice (Haynes et al., 1976). Unfortunately, despite considerable efforts, this statistic remains unchanged (Brown & Bussell, 2011). Additional complications relevant to oral cancer therapies include side effects attributable to other (i.e., non-cancer) medications that can impact treatment outcomes (e.g., cognitive impairments, fatigue) and interactions with nonprescription pharmaceuticals or complementary and alternative medicines (e.g., ginseng, cat's claw) that can result in subtherapeutic dosages or increases in the toxicity of chemotherapy agents. Interventions that target primary self-management targets are likely to become even more important as oral anticancer agents become increasingly common adjuvant treatments (e.g., capecitabine for stage III colon cancer; Twelves et al., 2005). Oral agents are becoming increasingly common as first-line anticancer therapies for breast (Murphy, Bartholomew, Carpentier, Bluethmann, & Vernon, 2012) and prostate (Greer et al., 2016) cancers. They are equivalent or even more effective in achieving disease-free survival as compared to their intravenous counterparts (O'Neill & Twelves, 2002; Twelves et al., 2005). Of course, people must follow the treatment protocol accurately to maximize the effectiveness of prescribed oral agents. This objective will likely be more attainable when those for whom oral cancer therapies are prescribed possess the knowledge and behavioral repertoires necessary to recognize adverse events when they occur, know when to discontinue treatment when indicated, and communicate clearly with oncologists in a timely manner, as has been demonstrated in other medical conditions (Edworthy, Devins, & the Patient Education Study Group, 1999). Clearly, this is a highly promising direction for future cancer self-management efforts.

Secondary Targets

Cancer-related impairments often impact people during the acute phase of treatment and may persist or present as long-term or "late effects." Information and resources to anticipate and manage common treatment side effects are widely available through national and international medical research consortia and community organizations (e.g., National Cancer Institute, Canadian Cancer Society). The American Cancer Society (http://www.cancer.org) has consolidated a comprehensive list of the potential acute, long-term, and late side effects of chemotherapy; including fatigue, alopecia, anemia, cognitive impairment, constipation, and diarrhea (American Cancer Society, 2016). Chemotherapy can cause changes in mood, taste, appetite, body weight, skin, nails, libido, sexual function, and urinary and bladder function, in addition to problems with the kidneys, fertility, mouth and tongue (e.g., mucositis), swallowing, and nerve and muscle problems (e.g., numbness and pain). Medical treatments are available to prevent or alleviate the suffering associated with many of these. For example, mucositis can be prevented or treated with medicinal mouthwash; pain can be managed with analgesics and opioids. Some symptoms, such as alopecia (i.e., hair loss), may not be as amenable to self-management but can be resolved using nonmedical prostheses (e.g., wigs) or with no intervention at all (e.g., some people prefer not to disguise cancer-related hair loss). Chemotherapy side effects generally resolve within months after completing treatment, but some, such as complications to solid organs (e.g., the heart), may persist until the end of life; others (e.g., secondary cancers) may not present until years later.

Common, acute side effects of radiation therapy reported by the American Cancer Society (http://www.cancer.org) include fatigue, skin problems, alopecia, decreased platelets and white blood cells (this can compromise immune function), and difficulties with eating and digestion. People undergoing radiation therapy for cancer may be informed of these potential side effects prior to treatment and can be provided with strategies to mitigate their occurrence and associated discomfort. For example, people may receive information about the possibility of radiation dermatitis (i.e., damaged skin following radiotherapy) and can be offered recommendations to minimize the associated discomfort, such as wearing loose-fitting apparel made of gentle textiles (e.g., cotton). Self-management may be particularly relevant for side effects such as problems with the skin or eating and digestion, because preventive measures can be taken in collaboration with the radiation oncology healthcare team. Long-term side effects of radiation therapy include cell and tissue damage specific to the treatment area. The lungs and heart can be damaged by radiation to the chest; problems with the bladder, bowels, fertility, and sexual function are often consequences of radiation to the abdomen or pelvis. Although the long-term and late effects of radiation, such as organ damage, may not be amenable to self-management, it is essential for affected individuals to be informed about them and to identify symptoms or other changes that must be reported to the treating oncologist, who can intervene to treat them. The potential for harm to a person is great when these go unrecognized or unreported, underscoring the importance of a collaborative relationship between people who undergo treatment for cancer and their service providers.

The management of symptoms and side effects (e.g., fatigue, pain, dyspnea) is fundamental in preserving quality of life for people living with cancer. Secondary targets, such as physical symptoms and treatment side effects, can be overwhelming for people and can compromise quality of life increasingly over time. Cancer-related fatigue is the most commonly reported symptom across the cancer trajectory, even when the disease can no longer be detected (Minton, 2008). Fatigue is especially distressing because it can be highly debilitating and interferes significantly with lifestyles, activities, and interests. Fatigue often persists for months or years after treatment completion (Pachman, 2012), rendering it puzzling and especially pernicious. Although somewhat counterintuitive, aerobic exercise has been shown to be effective in reducing cancer-related fatigue in people with solid tumor cancers (Cramp & Byron-Daniel, 2012). Self-management efforts to reduce this distressing symptom should enhance understanding about fatigue and its relation to cancer and should introduce strategies and tactics to minimize it. This can be especially challenging because many people are not especially physically active (Kohl et al., 2012) and, in fact, appear to be averse to engaging in exercise even when they are physically healthy (Bauman et al., 2012). People diagnosed with a life-threatening condition like cancer, and especially those experiencing significant fatigue, may be especially difficult to reach (Oldervoll, Kaasa, Hjermstad, Lund, & Loge, 2004). It is crucial, therefore, to address the individual's acceptance of exercise-based self-management interventions for fatigue and to enhance this to facilitate uptake and maintenance. This can be achieved by providing psychoeducation about the fatigue-reducing benefits of exercise, by introducing exercise regimens that are relevant to cancer-related fatigue and are congruent with the constraints associated with the individual's particular type of cancer, and by helping people to acquire and master relevant cognitive-behavioral techniques, including self-monitoring and goal-setting, to enhance maintenance of exercise behavior. Additional benefit will likely accrue by including intervention components that attenuate the disruptive impact of fatigue on daily life (e.g., social support for the uptake and safe participation in physical exercise). Relevant practice guidelines to ensure that healthcare team members communicate appropriately about fatigue and other secondary targets (e.g., dyspnea, pain) can also contribute valuably (e.g., BC Cancer Agency, 2016); Cancer Care Ontario, 2016); National Comprehensive Cancer Network, 2016).

The management of secondary targets (i.e., symptoms and side effects) has important implications for quality of life across the cancer continuum. In people with advanced cancer, pain caused by bone metastases is a common and particularly debilitating symptom (Falk & Dickenson, 2014). Reductions to pain intensity have been observed in people with radiographic confirmation of metastasis to the bone after they participated in a self-management program that specifically addressed pain control (PRO-SELF Pain Control Program; Miaskowski et al., 2004). This nurse-delivered pain-control intervention includes self-management techniques acquired and mastered through psychoeducation and coaching (West et al., 2003). In telephone and face-to-face exchanges, participants learn the information necessary to optimize pain self-control. Psychoeducation sessions focus on monitoring pain intensity, tools for recording and managing prescriptions (e.g., pain diary and pillbox), and information and guidance to modify analgesic intake appropriately. Skills acquired through coaching sessions include communication with the medical team about pain relief, managing side effects of analgesics, planning the medication regimen, and adjusting dosage when required. Appropriate self-management behaviors are reinforced by the interventionist, and support is provided by the nurse-coach and family caregivers (where available). Evidence from randomized controlled trials indicates that this intervention is effective in increasing knowledge about cancer pain management and in reducing reported pain intensity (Miaskowski et al., 2004; Rustøen et al., 2012).

Tertiary Targets

People living with cancer-related impairments may experience psychosocial and emotional sequelae, which can have deleterious impacts on quality of life.

A diagnosis and treatment for cancer can contribute to changes in one's sense of self and relationships with others. These issues are addressed in Chapter 5, "Illness Intrusiveness and Self-Management of Medical Conditions." It is important to note that self-management programs that address tertiary targets, such as quality of life, require specificity in the intervention design and evaluation. When evaluating tertiary targets, one must always consider the impact of variables unrelated to cancer that may also influence these outcomes importantly (e.g., independent, stressful life events). Some of these factors may be unique to cancer. For example, as noted, people can be declared to present "no evidence of disease," but this does not mean that they are cancer-free. They must contend with uncertainty about the possibility of remission and potential recurrence. Tertiary targets are important to consider in the self-management of cancer and are frequently used to assess the impact of cancer treatments, although it remains a challenge to discern the unique impact of self-management on quality of life and other tertiary targets. One important confounding factor that cannot be ignored is the recovery process that may occur over time independent of self-management intervention. Unlike a stable or slowly evolving chronic medical condition, cancer is often situated in the context of a life-or-death crisis, with the potential for dramatic shifts in physical-symptom burden. Alleviation of physical symptoms can occur with or without medical treatment or symptom control. Efforts to evaluate the benefits of cancer self-management must take such factors into consideration and must rule out their effects before drawing conclusions about the effectiveness of the intervention.

The physical-symptom burden experienced by people with cancer contributes to important tertiary targets of self-management because of their potential to compromise physical and psychological well-being. Cognitive-behavioral intervention elements, such as problem-solving strategies, can attenuate the interference caused by physical symptoms in people undergoing chemotherapy for newly diagnosed solid-tumor cancers (Doorenbos, Given, Given, Verbitsky, Cimprich, & McCorkle, 2005). In this intervention (Doorenbos et al., 2005), a nurse collaborates with a person undergoing cancer treatment to select and address up to four physical symptoms (e.g., pain, fatigue, insomnia) as targets for self-management using a problem-solving cognitive-behavioral intervention. The participant and interventionist meet face-to-face and by telephone for a total of 10 visits to apply problem-solving techniques to the targeted symptoms. Intervention components include education about the symptoms and other information relevant to decision-making, supportive counseling, and problem-solving strategies to improve communication with the medical team and for self-care. Interventionists review session recordings and participant feedback to evaluate the application of problem-solving strategies and to suggest refinements where necessary to monitor the fidelity and quality of the intervention. Research evaluating this approach demonstrates that people who receive the intervention report significantly reduced "symptom limitations," which was maintained over a 10-week follow-up period (Doorenbos et al., 2005).

Empowerment (i.e., the generalized sense that one can exercise control over important life outcomes; Kaur, 2014; Maunsell et al., 2014) and *patient activation* (defined as managing one's health through the acquisition of knowledge, skills, and the confidence required to apply them effectively and as needed; Hibbard, Stockard, Mahoney, & Tusler, 2004) are frequently mentioned constructs in the cancer self-management literature. Although not related specifically to cancer, "empowerment" and "patient activation" may be considered tertiary targets because they are expected to have an impact on self-management in cancer care. Acquiring and executing such self-management skills as problem-solving, planning, and communication with healthcare providers will inevitably influence the sense of control over one's cancer experience and influence perceived knowledge, skill, and confidence in managing health. Empowerment and patient activation have been described both as outcomes and as mechanisms of action in the cancer self-management literature. It is suggested that people with cancer become empowered by their actions and interactions with others when they engage in self-management because this provides evidence that they can influence the outcomes that they consider important and worthwhile (e.g., empowerment as outcome; van den Berg, Gielissen, Ottevanger, & Prins, 2012). Self-management programs that aim to inculcate empowerment comprise intervention components, such as psychoeducation, cognitive reframing, and goal-setting (van den Berg et al., 2012). Traditional self-management programs (e.g., CDSM) for chronic health conditions enhance patient activation through increased engagement in self-management behaviors (Hibbard, Mahoney, Stock, & Tusler, 2007).

Patient activation is described as a prerequisite to engaging in cancer self-management, but it is often treated as an outcome of self-management interventions (i.e., as a treatment target). Patient activation is an intervening variable that enables people who want to engage in cancer self-management to enact and implement it. Patient activation is certainly relevant to cancer self-management, but it can be misleading when authors and researchers do not articulate specifically whether it is being considered as an intervening (i.e., a so-called process) variable or as a treatment target. Patient activation is a process variable that influences whether and to what extent a person engages in self-management, but it does not influence health states or outcomes (e.g., quality of life) by itself. Future research concerning patient activation must recognize this conceptual inconsistency and articulate clearly whether patient activation is being examined as an outcome or a process variable. Failure to recognize and address this problem will continue to undermine the contribution of self-management research in cancer.

The measurement of patient activation bears special consideration. Activation requires action, yet the items employed to assess patient activation in psychometric instruments developed for this purpose actually tap related concepts that extend beyond self-management behavior. For example, items intended to tap patient activation address respondents' *confidence* that they can engage in self-management behavior or their *intentions* to do so, but they do not actually address the *initiation of self-management behavior*. Patient activation has been defined as comprising the knowledge, skills, and confidence required to manage one's health (Greene & Hibbard, 2012), which goes far beyond the non-technical meaning of the term as it might apply to cancer self-management, that is, that it entails the *implementation of ideas into action*. The concept of patient activation has been defined as knowledge, skills, and confidence to manage health. This definition is complex and overlaps significantly with self-management itself (e.g., incorporating and combining two of the three essential elements of self-management—knowledge and skills). It is no surprise, therefore, that "patient activation" so defined is associated with improved health outcomes, such as cancer screening and adaptive health behavior. Tailored CDSM programs for chronic conditions have been observed to increase activation (Hibbard, Greene, & Tusler, 2009). Conceptual problems, such as the misspecification of a process variable (i.e., activation) as a self-management target, and methodologic problems, such as measurement redundancy (i.e., item-content overlap) in the instruments employed to measure central concepts (i.e., activation) must be overcome before research can effectively delineate its role in effective cancer self-management.

Quaternary Targets

Cancer self-management should include interventions to address anticipated treatment demands (e.g., coordination of care), predictable stressors (e.g., financial concerns, strain on family and relationships), and minimize anticipated symptoms and side effects (e.g., nausea, vomiting, and mucositis). Active collaboration that includes the affected person and healthcare professionals across the entire cancer trajectory offers the potential to prevent or reduce the severity of symptoms and minimize treatment side-effects. By applying principles of *prehabilitation* (Carli & Zavorsky, 2005; Ditmeyer, Topp, & Pifer, 2002), people may be able to achieve this if cancer self-management interventions can be introduced early in the process of diagnosis and treatment. Prehabilitation entails early intervention to prepare the recipient of healthcare for an anticipated external stressor to minimize its destructive effects (e.g., resistance training to strengthen leg muscles prior to total knee arthroplasty). It can include physical conditioning (e.g., aerobic exercise), psychological support for anxiety reduction (e.g., training in progressive relaxation or meditation for stress management or cognitive reframing), and dietary intervention (e.g., nutritional counseling; Gillis et al., 2014). In cancer, interventions adopting a prehabilitation framework are gaining attention to prepare people for surgery, for intensive chemotherapeutic regimens, and for stem-cell transplantation. The application of prehabilitation as a model of early self-management interventions across the cancer trajectory may facilitate recovery or ameliorate deterioration in physical functioning and quality of life. Prehabilitation efforts may also enhance the effectiveness of self-management efforts that address secondary or tertiary outcomes. For example, collaboration with the oncology care team to understand the appropriate timing and administration of prophylactic medicines to prevent nausea, vomiting, or mucositis during chemotherapy can directly impact side effects of treatment (i.e., secondary targets). In addition, accepting responsibility to work with a mental health professional (e.g., psychologist) to acquire stress-management skills prior to cancer treatment can improve tertiary targets (e.g., distress).

Notwithstanding its promise in helping to maximize healthcare outcomes and minimize suffering and distress, self-management efforts to achieve prehabilitation must be tempered by the recognition that the early stages of cancer diagnosis and treatment are tumultuous and introduce significant stressors and adaptive challenges. It will be crucial to titrate the intensity of self-management efforts to achieve prehabilitation against the added psychosocial burden and stress (e.g., attributable to fear, threat, and limited cognitive capabilities) that operate on people at this stage of the cancer trajectory.

SELF-MANAGEMENT INTERVENTIONS IN CANCER

Table 10.1 presents a summary of the evidence from experimental studies of self-management interventions according to their primary, secondary, tertiary, or quaternary targets. Although many studies have focused on "self-management" interventions in various cancer populations, many of these do not incorporate all of the essential elements we identified at the beginning of this chapter. Essential elements of self-management interventions in cancer include education about cancer, its treatment, and common side effects; cultivating a collaborative partnership with healthcare providers; and helping people to acquire a behavioral repertoire to accomplish self-management tasks. Table 10.1 is limited to interventions that include all of these elements. It is challenging to identify and include all of the published literature bearing on cancer self-management because authors have employed different terms to describe it. Table 10.1 includes published studies on the basis of the component interventions delivered to participants rather than the labels by which authors referred to them. Unfortunately, nomenclature differences may have resulted in some relevant, published work being overlooked and omitted from the current review. Self-management researchers should adopt a common nomenclature and standard keywords to facilitate the identification of relevant research.

Published studies investigating cancer self-management, to date, primarily address tertiary targets in people who have completed cancer treatment with curative intent. Unfortunately, the studies that identify a tertiary target as their primary outcomes (e.g., quality of life) have not always included interventions that directly address the intended target. For example, physical exercise has demonstrated positive effects on psychological and physical outcomes in people with cancer, but the mechanisms by which exercise impacts these outcomes are not well understood (Fong, 2012). Therefore, it is not surprising that the application of cognitive-behavioral strategies to improve uptake of physical exercise does not necessarily achieve additional effects on a tertiary target such as quality of life (Korstjens et al., 2008). Interventions that directly address knowledge, skills, and behaviors relevant to the self-management target have been most successful in achieving meaningful results. In general, interventions that have been effective

Table 10.1. Overview of Self-Management Interventions in the Field of Cancer

Study	Patient Population	Self-Management Target	Target Category	Study Design and Intervention	Major Findings
Ahlberg et al.[a] (2011)	Adults with head and neck cancer scheduled to receive external beam radiotherapy with curative intent ($N = 374$)	Weight loss and two-year survival (primary outcomes)	Secondary	Prospective parallel group non-randomized trial • early preventive rehabilitation conducted by speech/language pathologist and physiotherapist vs. standard care	No significant between-groups difference in weight loss or overall survival

Comment: This paper reports on a preventive self-management intervention targeting weight loss and survival in people undergoing treatment for head and neck cancer.
- Participants in the experimental and control groups were treated in different settings. Limited information is presented about standard care.
- Although the intervention focused primarily on relevant exercises and nutrition, these behavioral outcomes were not assessed (i.e., exercise behavior, caloric intake). Therefore, it is difficult to attribute changes in body weight to the intervention without knowing the caloric intake of the study participants.

Study	Patient Population	Self-Management Target	Target Category	Study Design and Intervention	Major Findings
Chambers et al. (2014)	Adults with cancer (mixed cancer sites; $n = 354$) and unmatched caregivers ($n = 336$) who had contacted an Australian cancer support helpline	Psychological distress (primary outcome); cancer-specific distress (secondary outcome)	Tertiary	RCT • single telephone self-management support and brief psychoeducation session with oncology nurse ($n = 345$) vs. five psychologist-led telephone sessions of CBT and self-management support ($n = 345$)	Participants in both treatment groups demonstrated significant decreases in psychological and cancer-specific distress

Comment: This paper reports on two self-management interventions targeting psychological distress through psychoeducation and self-management support. One group received support from a specialized oncology nurse; the other engaged with a clinical psychologist who provided telephone support.
- The mechanism hypothesized to cause distress is not clearly articulated. Therefore, it is difficult to discern how psychoeducation and CBT were hypothesized to alleviate the target problem.
- The support provided in these treatment groups is likely to reduce distress in addition to the information and skills delivered in the experimental intervention, but it is not possible to delineate the extent to which observed benefits were attributable to the self-management component interventions as compared to the effects of support alone.

Doorenbos et al. (2005)	Adults with newly diagnosed solid-tumor cancer undergoing chemotherapy ($N = 237$)	Decreased symptom limitations (primary outcome)	Tertiary	Multicenter RCT • tailored problem-solving cognitive-behavioral nursing intervention • 18-week intervention (10 sessions) • 32-week follow-up period	Significant reduction of symptom limitations over time in intervention group

Comment: This paper reports on a self-management intervention to reduce interference caused by physical-symptom burden during chemotherapy.
- This was a carefully planned and well-executed trial. The theoretical underpinnings were well articulated, which resulted in meaningful findings.

Gaston-Johansson et al. (2013)	Women with breast cancer undergoing high-dose chemotherapy and scheduled for autologous hematopoietic stem-cell transplant ($N = 110$)	QOL (primary outcome)	Tertiary	RCT • comprehensive coping strategy program: preparatory education + cognitive-behavioral skills + guided imagery vs. standard care	Experimental group demonstrated significantly higher overall QOL in treatment group as compared to controls at one-year follow-up

Comment: This paper reports on a self-management cognitive-behavioral intervention that was effective in improving QOL, which was sustained at one-year follow-up.
- This study illustrates that useful findings are more likely to be observed when the intervention is aligned with the self-management target.

Jahn et al. (2014)	Adults diagnosed with cancer who report persistent pain of moderate intensity ($N = 263$)	Cognitive pain-related barriers (primary outcome)	Tertiary	Cluster-randomized RCT • nurse-administered psychoeducational intervention vs. standard care (pharmacologic pain treatment)	Experimental group demonstrated a significant reduction in pain-related barriers compared to controls

Comment: This paper reports on an intervention to improve self-management of cancer pain.
- Repeated visits with the interventionist that included supportive counselling introduce the possibility that demand characteristics (Orne, 1962) may have threated the validity of study findings.

(*continued*)

Table 10.1. CONTINUED

Study	Patient Population	Self-Management Target	Target Category	Study Design and Intervention	Major Findings
Korstjens et al. (2008)[a]	Adults ≥3 months posttreatment for cancer; referred by medical provider when ≥3 psychological and/or physical impairments were evident ($N = 147$)	QOL (primary outcome)	Tertiary	Multicenter RCT • Exercise + CBT vs. Exercise vs. Wait-list control • CBT comprised psychoeducation + structured self-management skills	Intervention groups did not differ in QOL at three-month follow-up (no added benefit of CBT); significant improvement to QOL in both treatment groups as compared to control

Comment: This paper describes an exercise intervention with two treatment groups exposed to physical training compared to a wait-list control. One treatment group received physical training alone and one received this plus CBT for additional support and to enhance exercise self-regulation, but no incremental benefit was associated with the inclusion of CBT.

- The group component of the physical training was designed to foster self-efficacy and enjoyment of exercise. It is not surprising, therefore, that both experimental groups demonstrated similar QOL benefits.
- The mechanism by which exercise was expected to influence QOL was not articulated. A component analysis would have been useful to verify the effects of exercise on QOL and rule out the confounded, potential benefits of group support.

| Lee, Lee, Oh, and Kim (2013) | Women newly diagnosed with Stage I–III breast cancer; score ≥8 on HADS ($N = 129$) | Self-efficacy for self-management of breast cancer (primary outcome); anxiety and depression (secondary outcome); mental adjustment (tertiary outcome) | Tertiary | RCT
• Six-week dyadic peer-support intervention vs. usual care: dyadic support partner selected based on completion of primary cancer treatment ≥1 year prior to the intervention | Experimental group demonstrated improvement in self-efficacy for self-management; no group differences in secondary or tertiary outcomes |

Comment: This paper reports on an intervention to promote self-efficacy for the self-management of breast cancer through dyadic peer-support.

- The study did not articulate the link between theoretical underpinnings (i.e., self-efficacy and social support) and the self-management intervention. No hypotheses specify the mechanisms believed responsible for the anticipated outcomes.
- Although coping with cancer and promoting self-efficacy and confidence were involved in the intervention, participants were not involved in direct management of cancer. The experimental design did not rule out the possibility that observed benefits may reflect the effects of demand characteristics rather than the intervention.

Study	Sample	Outcomes	Level	Design/Description	Results
Loh, Packer, Chinna, and Quek (2013)[b]	Multiethnic women within one year of non-metastatic breast cancer diagnosis (Stages I–III; $N = 147$)	QOL physical composite score (primary outcome); psychological distress (secondary outcome)	Tertiary	Non-randomized controlled trial • four-week therapist-led support and educational sessions • experimental vs. usual care with lagged recruitment to avoid contamination	Experimental group demonstrated significant improvements in QOL (physical composite score) at four-week follow-up; stress and depression postintervention and at four-week follow-up

Comment: This paper reports on a self-management intervention to improve QOL and attenuate levels of distress among multiethnic women with early stage breast cancer. Self-efficacy was identified a priori as the theoretical link between self-management and QOL.

- The aspects of QOL that differed significantly between groups were specific to physical symptoms that are amenable to improvement due to medical intervention. Therefore, observed improvements in physical symptoms may be due to medical treatment rather than self-management training.
- Statistical analyses involved comparing change scores, which are unreliable and may result in spurious results.

Study	Sample	Outcomes	Level	Design/Description	Results
May et al. (2009)	Adults ≥3 months after curative treatment for cancer with ≥1 year life expectancy and medical referral for rehabilitation ($N = 147$)	QOL (primary outcome) PA behavior (secondary outcome)	Tertiary	Multicenter RCT • group-based self-management program including exercise + CBT problem-solving vs. exercise alone	Significant improvement to QOL and increased PA behavior in both treatment groups

Comment: This paper describes a group-exercise intervention with an additional experimental condition in which group exercise was supplemented by CBT-based problem-solving to facilitate self-management of exercise for improved QOL.

- No theoretical mechanism links the intervention and outcome. It would have been more informative if the mechanism by which problem-solving potentiates the benefits of exercise had been articulated. Maximum potential benefit may be limited and may be achievable either by exercise or problem-solving, but incremental improvement due to the combination of these two components may not be possible.
- This paper is presented as a study of self-management but is actually a study of self-regulation in applying self-management tactics to achieve personal goals (e.g., physical activity, vocational, relational, etc.). The primary outcome is QOL, but the self-management target is not specified and is based on individual goals. Therefore, participants' goals could align with multiple domains of QOL (e.g., physical, social), making it difficult to attribute the impact of the intervention to improvements in QOL.
- It is important to specify the self-management target and to articulate explicitly the mechanism by which the two hypothesized intervention components influence the target (e.g., an interaction that potentiates individual effects vs. compensatory, independent benefits).

(continued)

Table 10.1. CONTINUED

Study	Patient Population	Self-Management Target	Target Category	Study Design and Intervention	Major Findings
Miaskowski et al. (2004)	English-speaking adults with cancer under care of oncology ambulatory unit and reporting pain from bone metastases (N = 174)	Pain intensity (primary outcome); opioid analgesic intake (secondary outcome); appropriate analgesic prescriptions (tertiary outcome)	Secondary	Multicenter RCT • PRO-SELF®-Pain Control Program: nurse-led psychoeducation vs. standard care, pain monitoring, and provision of cancer pain guidelines	Significant decrease in pain intensity for experimental group; no significant between-group differences in opioid intake or appropriate type of analgesic prescriptions

Comment: This intervention included psychoeducation and coaching about pain control for people experiencing pain caused by bone metastases. In addition to standard care, the control group received written guidelines for pain management and monitored their pain intensity daily using the same diary as participants in the experimental group.

- The information and attention provided to the control group may have influenced their pain management behavior.
- The lack of an effect on behavioral outcomes (i.e., secondary and tertiary outcomes that did not involve pain but might be expected to improve with increased pain control) suggests that demand characteristics cannot be ruled out when explaining the effect on pain intensity.

Miaskowski et al. (2007)[c] *data from PRO-SELF® Pain Control Program RCT analyzed using responder analysis*	English-speaking adults with cancer under care of oncology ambulatory unit and reporting pain from bone metastases; pain intensity scores required for responder analysis (N = 167)	Mood states (primary outcome); QOL (secondary outcome); pain interference (tertiary outcome)	Tertiary	Multicenter RCT • PROSELF® Pain Control Program: nurse-led psychoeducation vs. standard care and provision of cancer pain guidelines	No significant changes in mood; improved depression scores in experimental group ("partial responders" only); significant improvement to QOL in all responder categories; significant improvements to pain interference in all responder groups exposed to the intervention

Comment: This paper presents ad hoc statistical analyses that do not provide a comprehensive test of the hypothesis (e.g., in some cases, responder analysis was limited to the experimental group despite the relevance of some control-group participants).

- Few statistically significant results were evident and the importance of these is emphasized without acknowledging the context of numerous non-significant findings (i.e., interpretation focused on significant findings).
- Despite these limitations, the idea that people can be taught how to use pain medications effectively is promising and merits further investigation.

Oliver, Kravitz, Kaplan, and Meyers (2001)	Adults with cancer reporting "moderate" or more severe pain ($N = 67$)	Average pain (primary outcome); pain-related impairment (secondary outcome); pain frequency (tertiary outcome)	Secondary Tertiary	RCT	• single session of individualized education and coaching (experimental) vs. standard educational session (control)	Experimental group demonstrated statistically significant improvements in all outcomes at follow-up assessment

Comment: This paper reports on an educational and coaching intervention to improve pain outcomes in people experiencing cancer-related pain. Participants and physicians were blinded to group assignment by providing general pain-control education to control group members as part of standard care.
- Information about medications prescribed at baseline was not available for all study participants.
- All intervention outcomes were collected by self-report and were not cross-validated by independent evidence. This limitation threatens the validity of the findings.

Ruland et al. (2013)	Adults diagnosed with and undergoing treatment for breast or prostate cancer ($N = 162$)	Physical symptom distress (primary outcome); depression (secondary outcome); self-efficacy (tertiary outcome); HRQOL (quaternary outcome); Social support (quinary outcome)	Tertiary	RCT	• web-based self-management support vs. access to publicly available cancer-related websites	Experimental group demonstrated a significant reduction in global symptom distress; no significant differences between groups on other study outcomes

Comment: This paper reports on the outcomes of web-based self-management support for people undergoing treatment for breast or prostate cancer.
- The results of this study indicate equivocal improvement in symptom distress.
- The effect demonstrated on the global distress index (GDI) should be interpreted with caution. The GDI is calculated as a weighted composite score (the summed products of symptom frequency × distress ratings). Therefore, it is not clear whether the intervention reduced the occurrence of symptoms, changed the reported appraisal of distress associated with symptoms, or both.

(continued)

Table 10.1. CONTINUED

Study	Patient Population	Self-Management Target	Target Category	Study Design and Intervention	Major Findings
Sherwood et al. (2005)	Adults undergoing chemotherapy for newly diagnosed or recurrent advanced cancer ($N = 124$)	Symptom severity (primary outcome)	Secondary	RCT • problem-solving cognitive-behavioral intervention vs. control • eight-week nurse-led face-to-face and telephone sessions (five contacts in total)	Experimental group demonstrated significantly lower symptom severity at the 10- and 20-week follow-up assessments compared to the control group

Comment: This paper describes a self-management intervention to mitigate the severity of physical symptoms among people undergoing chemotherapy for advanced cancer.
- The experimental group clearly received useful information and behavioral support to enhance symptom self-management.
- The underlying mechanisms are clearly articulated.
- The treatments received by the control group are not described. Therefore, it is difficult to discern the added benefit of the problem-solving element.

| van den Berg et al. (2015) | Women two to four months following curative treatment for breast cancer ($N = 151$) | Psychological distress and psychological empowerment (primary outcomes); 14 additional outcomes related to psychological adjustment | Tertiary | Multicenter RCT
• 16-week self-administered web-based cognitive behavioral self-management intervention vs. usual care | Experimental group demonstrated significant reduction in distress; no effects on empowerment. Reductions in distress at follow-up were evident regardless of group assignment |

Comment: This paper reports on a web-based self-management intervention to attenuate distress and foster empowerment among women who recently completed curative treatment for breast cancer.
- The self-management targets addressed by this web-based intervention were not defined.
- The mechanism by which the intervention was expected to enhance control and empowerment was not specified explicitly, and it was not clear that the therapeutic elements of the self-management components actually influenced the outcomes of interest.
- The more rapid reduction in psychological distress demonstrated by the experimental—as compared to the control—group is encouraging, but the lack of between-group differences at follow-up suggests that the intervention may not produce sustainable change and leaves plausible the alternative interpretation that other factors may account for the results (e.g., regression to the mean).

Study	Sample	Outcomes	Prevention Level	Design and Intervention	Findings
Yates et al. (2005)	Women with early-stage breast cancer scheduled for adjuvant chemotherapy ($N = 109$)	Fatigue, fatigue-management behaviors, confidence in managing fatigue (primary outcomes); cancer self-efficacy, QOL, psychological well-being (secondary outcomes)	Secondary	Multicenter RCT • nurse-delivered psychoeducation intervention vs. general cancer-education sessions (control)	Significant reduction in fatigue at T2 (one to two weeks postintervention); no group differences in fatigue management behaviors or secondary outcomes

Comment: This paper describes a psychoeducation intervention targeting fatigue in women with early-stage breast cancer who are scheduled for adjuvant chemotherapy. The intervention included strategies for fatigue self-management and the experimental group demonstrated increases in self-management behaviors.
- More than half of the fatigue self-management behaviors involved rest or relaxation, which can further weaken the body if not balanced with physical activity.
- Key elements of self-management, including partnership with the healthcare team and accepting responsibility for engagement, were not addressed.
- Participants were enrolled in the intervention at the start of cancer treatment, prior to the onset of treatment-related fatigue. Therefore, the timing of the intervention may have undermined the potential to demonstrate effectiveness in mitigating fatigue.

Study	Sample	Outcomes	Prevention Level	Design and Intervention	Findings
Zhang et al. (2014)	Chinese-speaking adults diagnosed with nonmetastatic colorectal cancer within past six months; scheduled to receive postsurgical adjuvant chemotherapy ($N = 128$)	Self-efficacy (primary outcome); symptom distress (secondary outcome); anxiety and depression (tertiary outcome); QOL (quaternary outcome)	Tertiary	Multicenter RCT • six-month nurse-led self-efficacy intervention vs usual care	Experimental group demonstrated significant improvements to self-efficacy at baseline, three-, and six-month assessments; reductions to symptom distress, anxiety and depression; no change to QOL

Comment: This paper describes an intervention that incorporates elements (i.e., self-efficacy theory) that correspond closely with the self-management targets it intended to change (i.e., self-efficacy). The intervention was tested in Chinese-speaking adults with colorectal cancer, who were scheduled to receive postsurgical adjuvant chemotherapy.
- The positive impact of the intervention on self-efficacy substantiates the importance of clearly delineating the underlying mechanisms for effective self-management interventions. It is not surprising that there were no effects on QOL because it was not directly addressed in the intervention.

NOTE: RCT = randomized controlled trial; CBT = cognitive behavioral therapy; QOL = quality of life; HADS = Hospital Anxiety and Depression Scale; PA = physical activity; HRQOL = health-related quality of life; CEQ = Cancer Empowerment Questionnaire

[a] See also Korstjens et al. (2011): same study group, different outcomes. [b] See also Loh et al. (2012) for findings from same RCT with distress as primary outcome. [c] See also Rustoen et al. (2014) for evaluation of PRO-SELF® Pain Control Program, modified for Norwegian cancer population and healthcare system.

in cancer were carefully designed and implemented; they adapted cognitive-behavioral skills that were developed to manage (non-cancer) chronic medical conditions in a manner that is appropriate for people with cancer.

WORKS IN PROGRESS

Numerous studies of self-management are currently in progress. A search of the international clinical trials registry identified protocols for completed clinical trials and those in progress. Although they do not report results that bear on the efficacy or effectiveness of an intervention, published trial protocols can be a valuable asset for scientists who wish to develop self-management interventions for people affected by cancer. These trials have passed peer review and provide detailed descriptions of intervention elements and trial procedures. Table 10.2 summarizes published protocols for studies that aim to test hypotheses relevant to cancer self-management. The study protocols focus predominantly on the post-treatment period and on self-management interventions for identified secondary targets, such as pain or fatigue. Increased attention to self-management interventions facilitated by technology or web-based content and delivery is evident.

A search identified 61 registered clinical-trials in the World Health Organization International Clinical Trials Registry (June 2016; http://www.who.int/ictrp/search/en/), highlighting the direction of research in this field. Overall, primary trial objectives related to the feasibility of self-management interventions in attenuating physical symptoms and psychological distress in individuals living with a variety of cancers at diverse stages and loci along the care trajectory. One-third of the identified trials involved interventions delivered or facilitated by technology (e.g., mobile-phone applications, web-based platforms) to provide education, care coordination, cognitive-behavioral skills, peer support, communication skills, or decisional aids. Primary self-management targets were identified as the treatment objective in four trials that aimed to improve implementation of adjuvant therapies as prescribed. Secondary and tertiary self-management targets were the most commonly identified aims of the registered trials. Secondary targets included reducing symptom burden and distress, particularly related to fatigue, pain, and lymphedema. Lifestyle and behavior change was a common intervention, including smoking cessation, nutrition enhancement, and a variety of physical-rehabilitation interventions to attenuate physical symptoms and psychological distress associated with cancer and/or treatment effects. Tertiary targets were generally related to coping and distress. Self-management support in these ongoing trials was described as facilitated or led by nurses, clinical psychologists, unspecified healthcare professionals, counselors, or coaches. Interventions were offered for both individuals and groups and delivered using diverse technologies or face-to-face and in a variety of settings, including cancer hospitals, participants' homes, or community-based settings. Generally, interventions were coordinated with a phase in the disease trajectory when care needs were aligned with the principles of self-management, including transitions to ambulatory care, undergoing

Table 10.2. Overview of Published Study Protocols

Reference	Country of Origin	Cancer Type(s)	Treatment Target	Self-Management Intervention Component(s)
Corbett, Walsh, Groarke, Moss-Morris, and McGuire (2016)	Ireland	Adults who have completed primary treatment for nonmetastatic cancer (mixed types) and are experiencing fatigue	Fatigue (primary outcome) QOL (secondary outcome)	Cognitive-behavioral intervention techniques, including • education • self-monitoring • cognitive reappraisal • problem-solving • attentional control • assertiveness skills training
Cormie et al. (2014)	Australia	Adult men who are undergoing or have completed treatment for prostate cancer and are experiencing concerns about sexual health	Sexual health (primary outcome)	Aerobic and resistance exercise + cognitive behavioral strategies to support psychosexual self-management, including • education • stress management • problem-solving • goal-setting
Foster et al. (2015)[a]	United Kingdom	Adults who have completed primary cancer treatment (no cancer site specified) and are experiencing cancer-related fatigue	Self-efficacy for the management of cancer-related fatigue	Web-based cognitive-behavioral techniques, including • education • self-monitoring • goal-setting and planning • stress management • communication in relationships

(continued)

Table 10.2. CONTINUED

Reference	Country of Origin	Cancer Type(s)	Treatment Target	Self-Management Intervention Component(s)
James et al. (2011)	Australia	Ambulatory adults who have completed active treatment for cancer (any type or stage) and their caregivers	QOL (secondary outcome). The primary outcome and other secondary outcomes include the targeted lifestyle behaviors and related outcomes	Supervised exercise sessions and techniques adopted from chronic disease self-management, including · education · self-monitoring · goal-setting
McCaughan et al. (2013)	Northern Ireland	Adult men who have completed treatment with curative intent for prostate cancer and their spouse/partner	QOL (secondary outcome). Primary outcome and other secondary outcomes include self-efficacy and health behaviors intended to improve QOL	Group sessions over nine weeks, including · education · social support · emotional regulation · self-efficacy enhancement · planning and goal-setting
te Boveldt et al. (2011)	The Netherlands	Adults with cancer experiencing pain who are familiar with mobile phone technology	Pain intensity (second primary outcome). The first primary outcome is related to feasibility of implementation.	Multifaceted intervention delivered by telephone and SMS-IVR, including · self-monitoring · education · feedback

Turner et al. (2014)	Australia	Adults who have completed treatment for head and neck cancer	QOL (primary outcome)	Self-Management Care Plan, focused on techniques to promote self-efficacy, including · mastery · modeling · verbal persuasion · attention to physiological states
van den Berg, Gielissen, Ottevanger, and Prins (2012)	The Netherlands	Dutch-speaking women who have completed treatment with curative intent for breast cancer and have basic Internet skills	Psychological distress and psychological empowerment (co-primary outcomes).	Web-based cognitive behavioral techniques, including · psychoeducation · cognitive reframing · goal planning · process evaluation

NOTE: QOL = quality of life; Short Message Service with Interactive Voice Response = SMS-IVR.
aSee also Grimmett et al. (2013).

treatments, or the emergence of side effects that require skillful communication with healthcare providers and the knowledge and behavioral repertoire required for symptom monitoring and management.

SELF-MANAGEMENT OR SELF-REGULATION?

A number of interventions do not focus specifically on the self-management of cancer. The term "self-management" has often been used to describe behavioral change or lifestyle programs that do not necessarily involve self-management (Risendal et al., 2014). Health behaviors such as physical activity may be essential to the effective management of fatigue (a secondary self-management target), but many interventions involving physical activity that are presented as cancer self-management do not actually focus on the management of a cancer-related target. Rather they focus on the regulation of a health behavior, such as exercise, that is linked to a secondary target, such as fatigue. This distinction is important when considering the goals of the intervention, because the health behavior in question may, in fact, influence secondary self-management targets, but this is not actually addressed in the studies (i.e., the research concerns how to engage people in physical activity rather than addressing whether or how physical activity may ameliorate cancer-related fatigue). It may be reasonable to assume that the self-regulated behavior that is the focus of the research (e.g., physical activity) will alleviate a given symptom (e.g., fatigue), but it is premature to draw this conclusion unless the premise has been tested and supported empirically. Even after this has been achieved, interventions that increase participation in self-management behavior are not self-management interventions in themselves.

CANCER SELF-MANAGEMENT: JUST DO IT!

A number of investigators provide evaluations or recommendations in the absence of scientific evidence. We encountered such statements in many published works, including study protocols that described works in progress with no reported results, descriptive studies of self-reported needs and barriers relevant to cancer self-management, and qualitative studies of perceptions and experiences of self-management in cancer. We encountered a number of published pilot and feasibility studies in which the investigators recommended the implementation of their interventions (i.e., adoption into clinical practice) without presenting empirical evidence to support their effectiveness. Similarly, many published papers that report the results of cross-sectional, qualitative, and pilot or feasibility studies highlight important self-management goals for cancer care that have not been substantiated by research findings. Further research must confirm the benefits of such interventions before one can responsibly recommend implementation.

Many studies engaged in "HARKing"—that is, Hypothesizing After the Results are Known (Kerr, 1998)—which raises serious questions about the validity of evidence on which their clinical recommendations have been based. Conclusions and recommendations that lack credible scientific support must be interpreted with caution and, unfortunately, often with skepticism.

BARRIERS TO SELF-MANAGEMENT OF CANCER

Barriers to the implementation of self-management models of care include the need for trained personnel to deliver self-management programs, financial costs that may not be covered by government programs or health insurance, and the large number of self-management component interventions that comprise the self-management framework, which may prove difficult to implement in cancer given the challenges identified earlier (e.g., time pressures, intense threats to life and well-being). Additional barriers may include cultural biases (e.g., deference to the authority of the doctor; Bedi & Devins, 2016), stigma (Allen, Wright, Harding, & Broffman, 2014), health literacy (Berkman, Sheridan, Donahue, Halpern, & Crotty, 2011), or healthcare inequalities attributable to sex ("Unfinished Business," 2016) or race (National Center for Health Statistics, 2016), and socioeconomic status (Adler et al., 1994). Even in countries where government funding purports to make healthcare universally accessible, these barriers continue to persist (Hajizadeh, Mitnitski, & Rockwood, 2016). The importance of cancer-related knowledge and collaboration with healthcare providers for effective self-management require that these factors receive attention in designing interventions.

CONSIDERATIONS AND FUTURE DIRECTIONS

There is clearly enthusiasm for research and implementation of self-management to ease the growing burden on the people and systems that cancer affects. This is a particularly compelling area of research given the financial and practical demands imposed on the healthcare system by an aging population that now includes people who live for many years after cancer has been diagnosed. The implementation of survivorship care-plans to coordinate care for long-term and late effects of cancer and its treatment outside of the cancer center may provide a promising solution, because such plans provide a summary of the cancer diagnosis and treatment received to date, in addition to providing a comprehensive blueprint for follow-up care coordination that includes strategies for the self-management of long-term and "late" treatment effects (Brennan, Gormally, Butow, Boyle, & Spillane, 2014). The extensive and generally successful application of self-management in chronic health conditions provides an enticing template for intervention development for people affected by cancer. It will be crucial, however, to consider the conceptual distinctions between cancer and chronic conditions, particularly in relation to their trajectories and the associated expectations of those who are diagnosed and undergo treatment for cancer as compared to those who are required to monitor and manage life-long symptoms of chronic health conditions.

A number of published, descriptive studies address cancer self-management (e.g., cross-sectional surveys, qualitative inquiries), particularly in relation to the needs and preferences for tailoring interventions. Many have advanced recommendations for implementation, but, as noted, few have contributed formal evaluations. We encourage future researchers to formulate testable a priori hypotheses that are aligned with a relevant and appropriate self-management target and to employ scientifically sound methods to design and evaluate the intervention. As research evolves in the self-management of cancer, studies will be needed to elucidate the mechanisms of action by which self-management interventions achieve uptake and effectiveness. The continued evolution of biomedical cancer treatments, including oral cancer therapies, underscores the need for concrete self-management tactics (e.g., partnerships with the medical team and communication of all relevant information) to protect the affected individual and facilitate treatment completion and efficacy.

The implementation of self-management programs in cancer care requires adaptation from the types of self-management approaches that have been implemented traditionally for chronic health conditions. Future research efforts should not only take into consideration the appropriate targets for self-management in cancer but also be mindful to avoid inappropriate targets. We must consider not only the demands on the healthcare system but also the demands on the people affected by cancer and the extent to which they have the time and capacity to engage in comprehensive programs to facilitate the management of the psychological and physical sequelae of their conditions. There may be instances in which self-management can be detrimental for people with cancer, and therefore we must consider when self-management is indicated and when it is not. For example, people may misunderstand the limits of the benefits of self-management. It is important to provide self-management support with the understanding that it may not always be sufficient to manage the effects of cancer and its treatment. It is important to consider the limits to self-management interventions in cancer, including identifying those for whom self-management is appropriate, and to establish realistic expectations about what it can accomplish. Future challenges will include seamless integration of self-management programs into routine cancer care, delineation of the optimal setting and professional or system responsible for providing this support, and design of a sustainable model despite the multiple healthcare providers involved in each person's care across the cancer continuum. A critical lens will be required to provide meaningful advances to the self-management of cancer. We must question the boundaries of self-management as it applies to the specific needs of people affected by cancer and the direct and indirect benefits that may result from its effective application.

REFERENCES

Adler, N. E., Boyce, T., Chesney, M. A., Cohen, S., Folkman, S., Kahn, R. L., & Syme, S. L. (1994). Socioeconomic status and health: The challenge of the gradient. *American Psychologist, 49*(1), 15–24.

Ahlberg, A., Engstrom, T., Nikolaidis, P., Gunnarsson, K., Johansson, H., Sharp, L., & Laurell, G. (2011). Early self-care rehabilitation of head and neck cancer patients. *Acta Oto-Laryngologica, 131*(5), 552–561.

Allen, H., Wright, B. J., Harding, K., & Broffman, L. (2014). The role of stigma in access to health care for the poor. *Milbank Quarterly, 92*(2), 289–318.

American Cancer Society. (2016). *Treatments and side effects* Atlanta: Author.

Bandura, A. (1997). *Self-efficacy: The Exercise of Control*. New York: W. H. Freeman.

Barlow, J., Wright, C., Sheasby, J., Turner, A., & Hainsworth, J. (2002). Self-management approaches for people with chronic conditions: A review. *Patient Education and Counseling, 48*(2), 177–187.

Bauman, A. E., Reis, R. S., Sallis, J. F., Wells, J. C., Loos, R. J. F., & Martin, B. W. (2012). Correlates of physical activity: Why are some people physically active and others not? *The Lancet, 380*(9838), 258–271. http://dx.doi.org/10.1016/S0140-6736(12)60735-1

BC Cancer Agency. (2016). *Symptom management*. Vancouver: Author.

Bedi, M., & Devins, G. M. (2016). Cultural considerations for South Asian women with breast cancer. *Journal of Cancer Survivorship, 10*(1), 31–50.

Berkman, N. D., Sheridan, S. L., Donahue, K. E., Halpern, D. J., & Crotty, K. (2011). Low health literacy and health outcomes: An updated systematic review. *Annals of Internal Medicine, 155*(2), 97–107.

Brennan, M. E., Gormally, J. F., Butow, P., Boyle, F. M., & Spillane, A. J. (2014). Survivorship care plans in cancer: A systematic review of care plan outcomes. *British Journal of Cancer, 111*(10), 1899–1908. doi:10.1038/bjc.2014.505

Brown, M. T., & Bussell, J. K. (2011). Medication adherence: WHO Cares? *Mayo Clinic Proceedings, 86*(4), 304–314. doi:10.4065/mcp.2010.0575

Cancer Care Ontario. (2016). *Symptom management guides*. Retrieved from https://smg.cancercare.on.ca/

Carli, F., & Zavorsky, G. S. (2005). Optimizing functional exercise capacity in the elderly surgical population. *Current Opinion in Clinical Nutrition & Metabolic Care, 8*(1), 23–32.

Chambers, S. K., Girgis, A., Occhipinti, S., Hutchison, S., Turner, J., McDowell, M., . . . Dunn, J. C. (2014). A randomized trial comparing two low-intensity psychological interventions for distressed patients with cancer and their caregivers. *Oncology Nursing Forum, 41*(4), E256–E266.

Corbett, T., Walsh, J. C., Groarke, A., Moss-Morris, R., & McGuire, B. E. (2016). Protocol for a pilot randomised controlled trial of an online intervention for post-treatment cancer survivors with persistent fatigue. *BMJ Open, 6*(6), e011485. doi:10.1136/bmjopen-2016-011485

Corbin, J., & Strauss, A. (1988). *Unending work and care: Managing chronic illness at home*. San Francisco, CA: Jossey-Bass.

Cormie, P., Chambers, S. K., Newton, R. U., Gardiner, R. A., Spry, N., Taaffe, D. R., . . . Galvao, D. A. (2014). Improving sexual health in men with prostate cancer: Randomised controlled trial of exercise and psychosexual therapies. *BMC Cancer, 14*, 199.

Cramp, F., & Byron-Daniel, J. (2012). Exercise for the management of cancer-related fatigue in adults. *Cochrane Database of Systematic Reviews, 11*, CD006145.

Devins, G. M., & Binik, Y. M. (1996). Predialysis psychoeducational interventions: Establishing collaborative relationships between health service providers and recipients. *Seminars in Dialysis, 9*(1), 51–55.

Ditmeyer, M., Topp, R., & Pifer, M. (2002). Prehabilitation in preparation for orthopaedic surgery. *Orthopaedic Nursing, 21*(5), 43–54.

Döhner, H., Weisdorf, D. J., & Bloomfield, C. D. (2015). Acute myeloid leukemia. *The New England Journal of Medicine, 373*(12), 1136–1152. doi:doi:10.1056/NEJMra1406184

Doorenbos, A., Given, B., Given, C., Verbitsky, N., Cimprich, B., & McCorkle, R. (2005). Reducing symptom limitations: A cognitive behavioral intervention randomized trial. *Psycho-Oncology, 14*(7), 574–584. doi:10.1002/pon.874

Edworthy, S.M., Devins, G.M., & Patient Education Study Group (1999). Improving medication adherence through patient education distinguishing between appropriate and inappropriate utilization. *Journal of Rheumatology, 26*, 1793–1801).

Falk, S., & Dickenson, A. H. (2014). Pain and nociception: Mechanisms of cancer-induced bone pain. *Journal of Clinical Oncology, 32*(16), 1647–1654.

Fisher, E. B., Brownson, C. A., O'Toole, M. L., Shetty, G., Anwuri, V. V., & Glasgow, R. E. (2005). Ecological approaches to self-management: The case of diabetes. *American Journal of Public Health, 95*(9), 1523–1535. doi:10.2105/AJPH.2005.066084

Fong, D. Ho, J., Hui, B., Lee, A. M., Macfarlane, D. J., Leung, S. S. K., . . . Cheng, K. (2012). Physical activity for cancer survivors: Meta-analysis of randomised controlled trials. *BMJ, 34*, e70.

Foster, C., Calman, L., Grimmett, C., Breckons, M., Cotterell, P., Yardley, L., . . . Richardson, A. (2015). Managing fatigue after cancer treatment: Development of RESTORE, a web-based resource to support self-management. *Psycho-Oncology, 24*(8), 940–949.

Gao, W. J., & Yuan, C. R. (2011). Self-management programme for cancer patients: A literature review. *International Nursing Review, 58*(3), 288–295.

Gaston-Johansson, F., Fall-Dickson, J. M., Nanda, J. P., Sarenmalm, E. K., Browall, M., & Goldstein, N. (2013). Long-term effect of the self-management comprehensive coping strategy program on quality of life in patients with breast cancer treated with high-dose chemotherapy. *Psycho-Oncology, 22*(3), 530–539.

Gillis, C., Li, C., Lee, L., Awasthi, R., Gamsa, A., Liberman, A. S., . . . Carli, F. (2014). Prehabilitation versus rehabilitation: A randomized control trial in patients undergoing colorectal resection for cancer. *Anesthesiology, 121*(5), 937–947.

Greene, J., & Hibbard, J. H. (2012). Why does patient activation matter? An examination of the relationships between patient activation and health-related outcomes. *Journal of General Internal Medicine, 27*(5), 520–526. doi:10.1007/s11606-011-1931-2

Greer, J. A., Amoyal, N., Nisotel, L., Fishbein, J. N., MacDonald, J., Stagl, J., . . . Pirl, W. F. (2016). A systematic review of adherence to oral antineoplastic therapies. *The Oncologist, 21*(3), 354–376. doi:10.1634/theoncologist.2015-0405

Grimmett, C., Armes, J., Breckons, M., Calman, L., Corner, J., Fenlon, D., ... Foster, C. (2013). RESTORE: An exploratory trial of an online intervention to enhance self-efficacy to manage problems associated with cancer-related fatigue following primary cancer treatment: Study protocol for a randomized controlled trial. *Trials, 14*, 184.

Hajizadeh, M., Mitnitski, A., & Rockwood, K. (2016). Socioeconomic gradient in health in Canada: Is the gap widening or narrowing? *Health Policy, 120*(9), 1040-1050.

Hammer, M. J., Ercolano, E. A., Wright, F., Dickson, V. V., Chyun, D., & Melkus, G. D. E. (2015). Self-management for adult patients with cancer: An integrative review. *Cancer Nursing, 38*(2), E10–E26.

Harley, C., Pini, S., Bartlett, Y. K., & Velikova, G. (2015). Defining chronic cancer: Patient experiences and self-management needs. *BMJ Supportive & Palliative Care, 5*(4), 343–350.

Haynes, R. B., Gibson, E., Hackett, B., Sackett, D., Taylor, D. W., Roberts, R., & Johnson, A. (1976). Improvement of medication compliance in uncontrolled hypertension. *The Lancet, 307*(7972), 1265–1268.

Hibbard, J. H., Greene, J., & Tusler, M. (2009). Improving the outcomes of disease management by tailoring care to the patient's level of activation. *American Journal of Managed Care, 15*(6), 353–360.

Hibbard, J. H., Mahoney, E. R., Stock, R., & Tusler, M. (2007). Do increases in patient activation result in improved self-management behaviors? *Health Services Research, 42*(4), 1443–1463. doi:10.1111/j.1475-6773.2006.00669.x

Hibbard, J. H., Stockard, J., Mahoney, E. R., & Tusler, M. (2004). Development of the Patient Activation Measure (PAM): Conceptualizing and measuring activation in patients and consumers. *Health Services Research, 39*(4 Pt. 1), 1005–1026. doi:10.1111/j.1475-6773.2004.00269.x

Howlader, N., Noone, A., Krapcho, M., Miller, D., Bishop, K., Altekruse, S., ... Cronin, K. (Eds.). (2016). SEER cancer statistics review, 1975–2013. Bethesda, MD: National Cancer Institute. http://seer.cancer.gov/csr/1975_2013/

Jahn, P., Kuss, O., Schmidt, H., Bauer, A., Kitzmantel, M., Jordan, K., ... Landenberger, M. (2014). Improvement of pain-related self-management for cancer patients through a modular transitional nursing intervention: A cluster-randomized multicenter trial. *Pain, 155*(4), 746–754.

James, E. L., Stacey, F., Chapman, K., Lubans, D. R., Asprey, G., Sundquist, K., ... Girgis, A. (2011). Exercise and nutrition routine improving cancer health (ENRICH): The protocol for a randomized efficacy trial of a nutrition and physical activity program for adult cancer survivors and carers. *BMC Public Health, 11*, 236.

Johnston, B., McGill, M., Milligan, S., McElroy, D., Foster, C., & Kearney, N. (2009). Self care and end of life care in advanced cancer: Literature review. *European Journal of Oncology Nursing, 13*(5), 386–398.

Kaur, J. S. (2014). How should we "empower" cancer patients? *Cancer, 120*(20), 3108–3110. doi:10.1002/cncr.28852

Kerr, N. L. (1998). HARKing: Hypothesizing after the results are known. *Personality and Social Psychology Review, 2*(3), 196–217.

Kohl, H. W., Craig, C. L., Lambert, E. V., Inoue, S., Alkandari, J. R., Leetongin, G., & Kahlmeier, S. (2012). The pandemic of physical inactivity: Global action for public health. *The Lancet, 380*(9838), 294–305. doi:http://dx.doi.org/10.1016/S0140-6736(12)60898-8

Koller, A., Miaskowski, C., De Geest, S., Opitz, O., & Spichiger, E. (2012). A systematic evaluation of content, structure, and efficacy of interventions to improve patients' self-management of cancer pain. *Journal of Pain and Symptom Management, 44*(2), 264–284.

Korstjens, I., May, A. M., van Weert, E., Mesters, I., Tan, F., Ros, W. J. G., . . . van den Borne, B. (2008). Quality of life after self-management cancer rehabilitation: A randomized controlled trial comparing physical and cognitive-behavioral training versus physical training. *Psychosomatic Medicine, 70*(4), 422–429.

Korstjens, I., Mesters, I., May, A. M., van Weert, E., van den Hout, J. H. C., Ros, W., . . . van den Borne, B. (2011). Effects of cancer rehabilitation on problem-solving, anxiety and depression: A RCT comparing physical and cognitive-behavioural training versus physical training. *Psychology & Health, 26*(Suppl. 1), 63–82.

Lee, R., Lee, K. S., Oh, E.-G., & Kim, S. H. (2013). A randomized trial of dyadic peer support intervention for newly diagnosed breast cancer patients in Korea. *Cancer Nursing, 36*(3), E15–E22.

Ligibel, J. (2012). Lifestyle factors in cancer survivorship. *Journal of Clinical Oncology, 30*(30), 3697–3704. doi:10.1200/JCO.2012.42.0638

Loh, S. Y., Packer, T., Chinna, K., & Quek, K. F. (2013). Effectiveness of a patient self-management programme for breast cancer as a chronic illness: A non-randomised controlled clinical trial. *Journal of Cancer Survivorship: Research and Practice, 7*(3), 331–342.

Loh, S. Y., Packer, T., Tan, F. L., Xavier, M., Quek, K. F., & Yip, C. H. (2012). Does a self management intervention lower distress in woman diagnosed with breast cancer? *Japanese Psychological Research, 54*(2), 159–169.

Lorig, K., & Fries, J. (2006). *The arthritis helpbook* (6th ed.). Cambridge MA: Da Capo Press.

Lorig, K., & Holman, H. (2003). Self-management education: History, definition, outcomes, and mechanisms. *Annals of Behavioral Medicine, 26*(1), 1–7. doi:10.1207/S15324796ABM2601_01

Lorig, K., Sobel, D., Stewart, A., Brown, B., Bandura, A., Ritter, P., . . . Holman, H. (1998). Evidence suggesting that a Chronic Disease Self-Management Program can improve health status while reducing hospitalization: A randomized trial. *Medical Care, 37*(1), 5–14.

Lovell, M. R., Luckett, T., Boyle, F. M., Phillips, J., Agar, M., & Davidson, P. M. (2014). Patient education, coaching, and self-management for cancer pain. *Journal of Clinical Oncology, 32*(16), 1712–1720.

Maunsell, E., Lauzier, S., Brunet, J., Pelletier, S., Osborne, R., & Campbell, S. (2014). Health-related empowerment in cancer: Validity of scales from the Health Education Impact Questionnaire. *Cancer, 120*, 3228–3236.

May, A. M., Korstjens, I., van Weert, E., van den Borne, B., Hoekstra-Weebers, J. E. H. M., van der Schans, C. P., . . . Ros, W. J. G. (2009). Long-term effects on cancer survivors' quality of life of physical training versus physical training combined with cognitive-behavioral therapy: Results from a randomized trial. *Supportive Care in Cancer, 17*(6), 653–663.

McCaughan, E., Prue, G., McSorley, O., Northouse, L., Schafenacker, A., & Parahoo, K. (2013). A randomized controlled trial of a self-management psychosocial intervention for men with prostate cancer and their partners: A study protocol. *Journal of Advanced Nursing, 69*(11), 2572–2583.

McCorkle, R., Ercolano, E., Lazenby, M., Schulman-Green, D., Schilling, L. S., Lorig, K., & Wagner, E. H. (2011). Self-management: Enabling and empowering patients living with cancer as a chronic illness. *CA: A Cancer Journal for Clinicians, 61*(1), 50–62.

Miaskowski, C., Dodd, M., West, C., Paul, S. M., Schumacher, K., Tripathy, D., & Koo, P. (2007). The use of a responder analysis to identify differences in patient outcomes following a self-care intervention to improve cancer pain management. *Pain, 129*(1–2), 55–63.

Miaskowski, C., Dodd, M., West, C., Schumacher, K., Paul, S. M., Tripathy, D., & Koo, P. (2004). Randomized clinical trial of the effectiveness of a self-care intervention to improve cancer pain management. *Journal of Clinical Oncology, 22*(9), 1713–1720.

Minton, O. (2008). A systematic review and meta-analysis of the pharmacological treatment of cancer-related fatigue. *Journal of the National Cancer Institute, 100*, 1155–1166.

Mitnitski, A., Rockwood, K., & Hajizadeh, M. (2016). Socioeconomic gradient in health in Canada: Is the gap widening or narrowing? *Health Policy, 120*(9), 1040–1050.

Murphy, C. C., Bartholomew, L. K., Carpentier, M. Y., Bluethmann, S. M., & Vernon, S. W. (2012). Adherence to adjuvant hormonal therapy among breast cancer survivors in clinical practice: A systematic review. *Breast Cancer Research and Treatment, 134*(2), 459–478.

National Center for Health Statistics. (2016, May). *Health, United States, 2015: With special feature on racial and ethnic health disparities.* Report No. 2016-1232. Hyattsville, MD: Author.

National Comprehensive Cancer Network. (2016). *Clinical practice guidelines in oncology.* Retrieved from https://www.nccn.org/professionals/physician_gls/f_guidelines.asp#supportive

Norris, S. L., M., E. M., & Narayan, K. M. (2001). Effectiveness of self-management training in type 2 diabetes: A systematic review of randomized controlled trials. *Diabetes Care, 24*(3), 561–587.

Oliver, J. W., Kravitz, R. L., Kaplan, S. H., & Meyers, F. J. (2001). Individualized patient education and coaching to improve pain control among cancer outpatients. *Journal of Clinical Oncology, 19*(8), 2206–2212.

O'Neill, V. J., & Twelves, C. J. (2002). Oral cancer treatment: Developments in chemotherapy and beyond. *British Journal of Cancer, 87*(9), 933–937. doi:10.1038/sj.bjc.6600591

Oldervoll, L. M., Kaasa, S., Hjermstad, M. J., Lund, J. A., & Loge, J. H. (2004). Physical exercise results in the improved subjective well-being of a few or is effective rehabilitation for all cancer patients? *European Journal of Cancer, 40*(7), 951–962. doi:10.1016/j.ejca.2003.12.005

Orne, M. T. (1962). On the social psychology of the psychological experiment: With particular reference to demand characteristics and their implications. *American Psychologist, 17*(11), 776–783.

Pachman, D. R. (2012). Troublesome symptoms in cancer survivors: Fatigue, insomnia, neuropathy, and pain. *Journal of Clinical Oncology, 30*, 3687–3696.

Partridge, A. H., Avorn, J., Wang, P. S., & Winer, E. P. (2002). Adherence to therapy with oral antineoplastic agents. *Journal of the National Cancer Institute, 94*(9), 652–661. doi:10.1093/jnci/94.9.652

Paterson, C., Jones, M., Rattray, J., & Lauder, W. (2015). Identifying the self-management behaviours performed by prostate cancer survivors: A systematic review of the evidence. *Journal of Research in Nursing, 20*(2), 96–111.

Richardson, A. (1992). Studies exploring self-care for the person coping with cancer treatment: A review. *International Journal of Nursing Studies, 29*(2), 191–204.

Ruland, C. M., Maffei, R. M., Borosund, E., Krahn, A., Andersen, T., & Grimsbo, G. H. (2013). Evaluation of different features of an eHealth application for personalized illness management support: Cancer patients' use and appraisal of usefulness. *International Journal of Medical Informatics, 82*(7), 593–603.

Rustøen, T., Valeberg, B. T., Kolstad, E., Wist, E., Paul, S., & Miaskowski, C. (2012). The Pro-Self(©) Pain Control program improves patients' knowledge of cancer pain management tone. *Journal of Pain and Symptom Management, 44*(3), 321–330.

Rustøen, T., Valeberg, B. T., Kolstad, E., Wist, E., Paul, S., & Miaskowski, C. (2014). A randomized clinical trial of the efficacy of a self-care intervention to improve cancer pain management. *Cancer Nursing, 37*(1), 34–43.

Sherwood, P., Given, B. A., Given, C. W., Champion, V. L., Doorenbos, A. Z., Azzouz, F., . . . Monahan, P. O. (2005). A cognitive behavioral intervention for symptom management in patients with advanced cancer. *Oncology Nursing Forum, 32*(6), 1190–1198.

Smith-Turchyn, J., Morgan, A., & Richardson, J. (2016). The effectiveness of group-based self-management programmes to improve physical and psychological outcomes in patients with cancer: A systematic review and meta-analysis of randomised controlled trials. *Clinical Oncology, 28*, 292–305.

te Boveldt, N., Engels, Y., Besse, K., Vissers, K., & Vernooij-Dassen, M. (2011). Rationale, design, and implementation protocol of the Dutch clinical practice guideline pain in patients with cancer: A cluster randomised controlled trial with short message service (SMS) and interactive voice response (IVR). *Implementation Science, 6*, 126.

Turner, J., Yates, P., Kenny, L., Gordon, L. G., Burmeister, B., Thomson, D., . . . Carswell, K. (2014). The ENHANCES study—Enhancing Head and Neck Cancer patients' Experiences of Survivorship: Study protocol for a randomized controlled trial. *Trials, 15*, 191.

Twelves, C., Wong, A., Nowacki, M. P., Abt, M., Burris, H. I., Carrato, A., . . . Scheithauer, W. (2005). Capecitabine as adjuvant treatment for stage III colon cancer. *The New England Journal of Medicine, 352*(26), 2696–2704. doi:doi:10.1056/NEJMoa043116

Unfinished business: Women's health inequality in the USA. (2016). *The Lancet, 388*(10047), 842–842.

van den Berg, S. W., Gielissen, M. F. M., Custers, J. A. E., van der Graaf, W. T. A., Ottevanger, P. B., & Prins, J. B. (2015). BREATH: Web-based self-management for psychological adjustment after primary breast cancer: Results of a multicenter randomized controlled trial. *Journal of Clinical Oncology, 33*(25), 2763–2771. doi:10.1200/jco.2013.54.9386

van den Berg, S. W., Gielissen, M. F. M., Ottevanger, P. B., & Prins, J. B. (2012). Rationale of the BREAst cancer e-healTH [BREATH] multicentre randomised controlled trial: An Internet-based self-management intervention to foster adjustment after curative breast cancer by decreasing distress and increasing empowerment. *BMC Cancer, 12*, 394.

Van Liew, J. R., Christensen, A. J., & de Moor, J. S. (2014). Psychosocial factors in adjuvant hormone therapy for breast cancer: An emerging context for adherence research. *Journal of Cancer Survivorship: Research and Practice, 8*(3), 521–531.

West, C. M., Dodd, M. J., Paul, S. M., Schumacher, K., Tripathy, D., Koo, P., & Miaskowski, C. (2003). The PRO-SELF: Pain Control Program: An effective approach for cancer pain management. *Oncology Nursing Forum, 30,* 65–73.

Yates, P., Aranda, S., Hargraves, M., Mirolo, B., Clavarino, A., McLachlan, S., & Skerman, H. (2005). Randomized controlled trial of an educational intervention for managing fatigue in women receiving adjuvant chemotherapy for early-stage breast cancer. *Journal of Clinical Oncology, 23*(25), 6027–6036. doi:10.1200/JCO.2005.01.271

Zhang, M., Chan, S. W., You, L., Wen, Y., Peng, L., Liu, W., & Zheng, M. (2014). The effectiveness of a self-efficacy-enhancing intervention for Chinese patients with colorectal cancer: A randomized controlled trial with 6-month follow up. *International Journal of Nursing Studies, 51*(8), 1083–1092.

11

Self-Management of Cardiac-Related Health Issues

NOA VILCHINSKY ■

"How can I stop eating fatty foods? I'm a Frenchman! I eat foie gras . . . I eat buttered croissants. . . . This is who I am."

"I'm furious about the need to exercise and change my diet. I'm a prominent professor in my field, I can't stand the idea that I'm being told what to do!"

"I can't fast-walk or do any kind of outdoor exercise in my village. . . . Everyone will know I'm ill. . . . I will lose everyone's respect."

(Excerpts from oral statements made by individuals with cardiac-related health issues at the Meir Medical Center, Israel)

Each of these examples portrays the difficulty of changing one's lifelong and ingrained habits, even in the face of a life-threatening condition, such as impaired cardiac functioning. The mere taking on of positive behaviors—that is, those known to be health-promoting—can be conceived as a threat to one's identity and social role, simply because it constitutes a change to who one is/was.

The goals of this chapter are to provide an overview of the self-management behaviors most recommended in the context of impaired cardiac function and the sociocultural, gender-related, and psychological barriers that prevent individuals from optimally applying them. Ways of overcoming these barriers are also introduced and reviewed.

IMPAIRMENT TO CARDIAC FUNCTION: NATURE AND PREVALENCE

Cardiovascular disease (CVD) is one of the major causes of death, disability, and activity limitations in developed countries (Centers for Disease Control and Prevention, 2016). The most frequently seen type of CVD is ischemic heart disease, which is precipitated by coronary atherosclerosis. In this condition, blockages in the coronary arteries cause diminished blood flow to the heart muscle, or myocardium (Falvo, 2014). When the myocardium receives insufficient blood supply, the result is myocardial ischemia, which may cause acute coronary syndromes (i.e., myocardial infarction [MI] or unstable angina); this, in turn, can lead to disability and death (Falvo, 2014). Another type of acute cardiac event is cardiac arrest: an emergency situation in which unexpected circulatory arrest occurs within one hour of symptom onset. Cardiac arrest usually leads within minutes to sudden cardiac death and therefore requires immediate resuscitation efforts (Allan, 2012). Another common cardiac impairment is congestive heart disease or heart failure. Heart failure occurs when the heart's ability to pump blood is chronically impaired (Falvo, 2014).

The number of non-institutionalized adults with diagnosed cardiac-related health issues in the United States alone is 26.6 million (Blackwell, Lucas, & Clarke, 2014), of whom more than 17 million survived an acute coronary event (Edmondson, 2014). Cardiac-related health issues led to 13% of all deaths that took place in 2010 in EU member states, according to the Organisation for Economic Co-operation and Development (Bansilal, Castellano, & Fuster, 2016).

Beyond the concrete danger of death and possible limitations in physical activity, impaired cardiac function may also have substantive psychological ramifications, such as depression, anxiety, and posttraumatic stress disorder, which reduce individuals' quality of life and may even lead to a recurrence of cardiac impairments and higher mortality rates (Ginzburg & Ein-Dor, 2011; Lett, Sherwood, Watkins, & Blumenthal, 2007).

The treatment for impaired cardiac function is mostly interventional, that is, catheterization, heart surgery, and, in the case of irregular heartbeat, implantation of a pacemaker (Falvo, 2014). Cases in which heart failure is so severe that neither medication nor other interventions have been effective may call for heart transplantation (Lund, 2013).

Although the aforementioned medical procedures may save individuals' lives, they do not prevent the chronic processes of cardiac conditions (e.g. inflammation, atherosclerosis) from continuing to progress (Allan, 2012). Many of the risk factors for recurrent cardiac-related health issues, such as older age, male gender, family history, and genetic vulnerability, are, unfortunately, unmodifiable (Allan, 2012). However, other risk factors, such as hypertension, high blood cholesterol levels, smoking, obesity, sedentary lifestyle, and emotional stress, *are* modifiable (Allan, 2012), and altering them is known to greatly improve individuals' health (American Association of Cardiovascular and Pulmonary Rehabilitation, 2004; Baigent et al., 2009; Eyre et al., 2004; Mills et al., 2011; Smith et al., 2001; Zafari & Wenger, 1998). Therefore, one of the best means by which to reduce the risk of cardiovascular event recurrence and mortality is via self-managing one's lifestyle (Chow et al., 2010). Yet reducing the risk is easier said than done. The many putative barriers to self-management that have been discussed in the literature are portrayed in the next section of this chapter.

Lifestyle Areas for Intervention

It is well-documented that difficulties in managing lifestyle changes exist among many individuals with cardiac-related health issues, regardless of their particular condition (Crowley, Grubber, Olsen, & Bosworth, 2013; Fix & Bokhour, 2012) and that these difficulties are experienced in regard to all of the following recommended health-promoting behaviors.

Smoking Cessation

Cigarette smoke is known to damage the endothelium, the thin narrow layer of cells that lines the interior surface of blood vessels. This kind of damage increases the odds for inflammation, leads to the development of atherosclerosis, increases the risk for plaque rupture, and thus contributes to the occurrence of acute coronary syndromes (Allan, 2012). Panagiotakos, Rallidis, Pitsavos, Stefanadis, and Kremastinos (2007) suggest that cigarette smoking is the risk factor that plays the largest role in MIs occurring among individuals under the age of 36. Smoking *cessation,* by contrast, is strongly correlated with a decrease in cardiac-related impairment and mortality (Edwards, 2004; Perez, Nicolau, Romano, & Laranjeira, 2007) and is therefore considered a high priority in the management of individuals with impaired cardiac function (Pipe, Papadakis, & Reid, 2010).

Unfortunately, the vast majority of smokers are unable to quit smoking, and relapse is very common among individuals with cardiac-related health issues who even try to quit (Dornelas, Sampson, Gray, Waters, & Thompson, 2000). In a Cochrane Collaboration review of smoking-cessation interventions, the rates of cessation ranged between 39% and 70% in intervention groups but were as low as 25% among individuals in control groups one year after they experienced an acute cardiac event (Barth, Critchley, & Bengel, 2008).

Exercise

A lack of physical activity is one of the greatest contributors to the progression of cardiac-related health issues (Franklin & Cushman, 2011; Mozaffarian, Wilson, & Kannel, 2008). Evidence suggests that increased physical activity and cardiorespiratory fitness can significantly reduce impairment and mortality in individuals with cardiac health issues (Franklin & Cushman, 2011; Mozaffarian et al., 2008). For example, Davies et al. (2010), in a Cochrane systematic review and meta-analysis of the role played by physical exercise in the recovery of individuals coping with heart failure, concluded that physical exercise reduces heart failure–related hospitalizations and results in clinical improvements in quality of life when compared to care as usual. Individuals with impaired cardiac function are therefore advised to exercise on a regular basis, either on their own or via formal cardiac prevention and rehabilitation programs (Eyre et al., 2004; Smith et al., 2001).

Despite these consistent recommendations, a large number of individuals with cardiac-related health issues do not exercise voluntarily, nor do they avail themselves of organized rehabilitation services (Chow et al., 2010; Reges et al., 2013a; Reges et al., 2015; Suaya et al., 2007), for a variety of reasons, which will be elaborated upon later in this chapter.

Changing Eating Habits

Harmful dietary factors include the intake of trans-fatty acids and foods with a high glycemic index or load, as well as the consumption of monounsaturated fatty acids and keeping a "Western-style" diet. Protective dietary factors, by contrast, include the intake of vegetables, nuts, and the adoption of a "Mediterranean-style" diet. In their systematic review of over 600 randomized controlled trials and prospective studies, Mente, de Koning, Shannon, and Anand (2009) found strong evidence supporting a causal link between dietary factors and cardiac illness. In the years since this review, much additional evidence has attested to the important role played by a healthy diet in reducing the risk of coronary death or non-fatal myocardial events (de Oliveira Otto et al., 2012; Estruch et al., 2013; Luszczynska & Cieslak, 2009). Thus individuals with cardiac-related health issues are advised to eat a variety of nutritious foods (e.g., fruits and vegetables, whole grains, low-fat dairy products) while avoiding, or at least limiting, the consumption of saturated fat, trans fat, sodium, red meat, sweets, and sugar-sweetened beverages and to take in only as many calories as they will use up (Anderson et al., 2013; Mozaffarian et al., 2012).

Maintaining a healthy diet also presents a challenge to individuals with cardiovascular conditions (Leslie, Hankey, Matthews, Currall & Lean, 2004), although it is true that once they have experienced a cardiac event individuals very often increase their fruit and vegetable intake. Yet, they generally do not achieve the recommended daily intake, and the increases they do achieve tend to be reduced by the time of follow-up assessment (Luszczynska & Cieslak, 2009).

Medication-Taking

Faithfully observing one's prescribed medication regimen is considered the major ongoing treatment for individuals with cardiovascular conditions (Ens, Seneviratne, Jones, & King-Shier, 2014). Optimal medication management is generally defined as individuals taking their medications as prescribed (e.g., twice daily) and on a continuing and regular basis (Ho, Bryson, & Rumsfeld, 2009).

Less-than-optimal medication management has been associated with a substantial worsening of cardiovascular conditions, increased healthcare costs, greater chance of hospitalization, and even increased risk of mortality (Granger et al., 2005; Ho et al., 2009). These findings highlight the importance of informing individuals about the contribution of properly managing their medication-taking to successful health outcomes.

Despite the fact that individuals with cardiac-related health issues acknowledge the effectiveness of their medications (Sud et al., 2005) and that side effects are reportedly few and well-tolerated (Bagnall et al., 2010), a high percentage of these individuals do not manage their medication regime adequately (Ho et al., 2009; Naderi, Bestwick, & Wald, 2012). In a systematic review and meta-analysis of 44 unique prospective studies, looking at a total of 1,978,919 non-overlapping participants with cardiac-related health issues, findings revealed that only 60% of participants demonstrated satisfactory medication self-management (Chowdhury et al., 2013).

In conclusion, the effectiveness of lifestyle changes in the prevention of cardiac event recurrence is well-established in the literature. Individuals with cardiovascular conditions who increase their physical activity, maintain a low-fat diet, and reliably take their medications have substantially lower rates of recurrent cardiac-related events and mortality (Chow et al., 2010; Sher et al., 2014).

Nevertheless, these recommended health-promoting behaviors are extremely difficult to follow.

BARRIERS TO SELF-MANAGEMENT

An examination of barriers to self-management is therefore essential in the promotion of healthy behaviors among individuals with cardiac-related health issues. In the following lines, we discuss these putative barriers—including systemic and sociocultural, gender-related, and psychological barriers.

Systemic and Sociocultural Barriers

As has been illustrated, less-than-optimal self-management typifies the vast majority of individuals with cardiovascular conditions. Yet, this problem is even more pervasive among individuals from minority and socioeconomically disadvantaged groups. Minority groups are known to be more vulnerable to cardiac impairment and mortality than majority groups and to engage in cardiac rehabilitative and preventive activities to a lesser degree (Kark, Fink, Adler, Goldberger, & Goldman, 2006; Kark, Gordon, & Haklai, 2000; Valencia, Savage, & Ades, 2011). Further, Mead (2010) claims that minority groups, as well as low-income groups, are less likely than majority/high-income groups to have the resources necessary to manage their medical conditions. Indeed, socioeconomic status has been found to be highly predictive of survival rates among individuals with cardiovascular conditions (Gerber et al., 2010).

With regard to specific health-promoting behaviors, Reges et al. (2015), in a series of studies conducted in Israel, showed a significant gap in smoking prevalence between Arab and Jewish men six months after they underwent a cardiac event (47% among Arabs vs. 15.5% among Jews). In addition, physical inactivity was substantially higher among Arab men with cardiac-related health issues than among Jewish men at hospital admission, and this difference was even larger at the six-month follow-up (Reges et al., 2015).

A consistent gap between majority and minority groups exists with regard to cardiac prevention and rehabilitation program (CPRP) participation (Allen, Scott, Stewart, & Young, 2004; Mochari, Lee, Kligfield, & Mosca, 2006; Reges et al., 2013a; Suaya et al., 2007). Beauchamp, Peeters, Tonkin, & Turrell (2010) suggest that multiple factors associated with the lives of disadvantaged populations—that is, material, social, and environmental—may create significant barriers to CPRP attendance.

These findings also raise the possibility of referral bias. Indeed, Gregory, LaVeist, and Simpson, (2006) found that African Americans were referred less often to CPRP than Caucasian Americans. The same bias was discovered by Allen and colleagues (2004), who found that the rate of referral to CPRP was significantly lower for African American women than it was for White women.

Gender-Related Barriers

Despite the fact that cardiovascular conditions are known to be the leading cause of death among women and men (Mehta et al., 2016), women themselves are not aware of the dangers these conditions pose for them (Hart, 2005). There are a few critical differences between men with cardiovascular conditions and women with those conditions. First, on average, women with cardiac-related health issues are older than their male counterparts (Mehta et al., 2016). Thus, they are more prone to having co-occurring impairments (Stramba- Badiale et al., 2006), as well as to lacking social support because of a loss of their spouse (Kristofferzon, Löfmark, & Carlsson, 2005; Lemos, Suls, Jenson, Lounsbury & Gordon, 2003).

Overall, it is possible that these gender differences in baseline cardiac profiles may cumulatively explain, at least in part, why women with cardiac-related health issues are less likely than their male counterparts to maintain an active lifestyle (Jason, McGannon, Blanchard, Rainham, & Dechman, 2015). In addition, several researchers have suggested that low self-management tendencies among women might be attributed to the difficulty they have in balancing their own needs with the needs of others, as they tend to assume the "caregiver" role in the family and may therefore lack the time and energy necessary to care for themselves in accordance with recommended heart-healthy behaviors (Jensen & King, 1997; Revenson et al., 2015). Other possible barriers for women include financial difficulties, environmental factors (e.g., neighborhoods with safety issues), and experiencing exercise as tiring or painful (Grace et al., 2009).

Another, rather disturbing, explanation may be that women are universally referred less often to CPRP by their physicians than are men (Allen et al., 2004; Menezes et al., 2014; Scott, 2010; Yohannes, Yalfani, Doherty, & Bundy, 2007). Indeed, despite the finding that women benefit just as much as men do from cardiac rehabilitation programs (Bjarnason-Wehrens, Grande, Loewel, Völler, & Mittag, 2007), and the fact that CPRP is integrated in effectiveness-based guidelines for women (Mosca et al., 2011), women have a lower participation rate in CPRPs than do men (Mehta et al., 2016).

Psychological Barriers

In the following section, we focused on both emotional as well as cognitive barriers for self management among cardiac patients.

Mental Health

Major depressive disorder is considerably more prevalent among individuals with cardiac health conditions (15% to 40%) than it is among the general population (2.3% to 9.3%; Kop & Plumhoff, 2012). The presence of depression has been found to increase the risk of cardiac impairment and mortality, as well as other severe clinical outcomes (Lett et al., 2007). In addition, posttraumatic stress disorder as a consequence of a cardiac event has been associated with subsequent major adverse cardiac events and all-cause mortality (Edmondson et al., 2011).

These associations between compromised mental health and negative cardiac outcomes may be explained via the mediating role of low self-management. Indeed, depression and anxiety are consistently associated with low motivation and reduced tendency to practice health-promoting behaviors, such as smoking cessation (Perez, Nicolau, Romano, & Laranjeira, 2008); exercising (Bennett, Mayfield, Norman, Lowe, & Morgan, 1999); maintaining a healthy diet (Ziegelstein et al., 2000); taking medications as prescribed (Bauer et al., 2012); and regularly attending CPRP (Glazer, Emery, Frid, & Banyasz, 2002; Kronish et al., 2006; McGrady, McGinnis, Badenhop, Bentle, & Rajput, 2009; Reges et al., 2014). In addition, posttraumatic stress symptoms among individuals with cardiovascular conditions were associated with non-optimal medication management (Shemesh et al., 2004).

Cognitive Attributions

According to Bennet et al. (1999), any relationship between negative emotionality and the practice of health behaviors is likely to be mediated through cognitive processes. For example, depression and anxiety can lead to cognitive perspectives that prevent people from trying to change their behavior. Indeed, theories of health behavior emphasize that the way people perceive their health situation is a crucial determinant of whether and how they will engage in health-promoting behaviors (Naidoo & Wills, 2000). Huffman et al. (2015) found that those individuals, who felt that the barriers to change were insurmountable, were less likely to maintain health-promoting behaviors than those who were more optimistic. One study found that perceptions about cardiac risk were significantly and negatively associated with smoking (Perez et al., 2007). Another study showed that people who held onto irrational ideas about health—that is, those not based on medical facts—had a tendency to stop attending cardiac rehabilitation before their recovery was complete (Anderson & Emery, 2014).

Another putative cognitive barrier preventing the adoption and maintenance of heart-healthy behaviors may be the notion that once one has been catheterized or undergone a coronary artery bypass grafting (CABG), one is essentially cured. For example, Fix and Bokhour (2012) found that some individuals who experienced CABG felt that the surgery had ameliorated both their health problems and their need for any concomitant behavioral changes. This finding, which highlights the dangers of misinformation and/or misunderstanding, is crucial because it emphasizes how important it is for individuals to be educated about their medical condition as early as possible upon hospitalization. Being properly informed can greatly influence the way individuals perceive their situation and, further on down the road, their motivation to maintain their new health regimen.

Finally, low levels of self-efficacy—that is, an individual's belief in his or her capacity to do what he or she needs to do in order to achieve a certain goal—have been found to predict low levels of self-management (physical activity in this case) among individuals with cardiovascular conditions (Jason, McGannon, Blanchard, Rainham, & Dechman, 2015). High levels of self-efficacy, by contrast, may do just the opposite and have been found to predict all-around better maintenance of a number of health-promoting behaviors (see Steca et al., 2015 for a review).

In light of the multifaceted barriers one is faced with when coping with cardiac-related health issues, innovative ideas for optimizing self-management are very much needed.

PRACTICES AND INTERVENTIONS TO IMPROVE CARDIAC SELF-MANAGEMENT

In the following section, possible pathways to facilitate self-management among individuals with cardiovascular conditions are reviewed.

Provision of Knowledge

Fix and Bokhour (2012) found that oftentimes individuals who underwent CABG did not understand why they had to go through it, what its purpose was, or how they were supposed to take care of themselves afterward. Not receiving comprehensive instructions regarding their postoperative healthcare is particularly problematic for individuals with cardiovascular conditions, as this kind of care can be complex and multifaceted, involving matters of physical exercise, diet, medication-taking, and smoking cessation to name a few examples. It has been shown that properly educating people motivates them to manage their own healthcare and change their behaviors, whereas not providing this education may have just the opposite effect, causing them to disregard medical recommendations altogether (Alm-Roijera, Stagmoa, Udénc, & Erhardt, 2004; de Melo et al., 2014).

In order to effectively educate individuals with cardiac-related health issues about their condition, the course it might take, and its management, a number of points must be addressed. Individuals must be taught (a) how to recognize and manage symptoms; (b) to change behaviors with the goal of ameliorating risk factors; (c) to familiarize themselves with all aspects of their medications (names, dosages, side effects, etc.); and (d) to understand what to do in case of emergency (de Melo Ghisi et al., 2014). Nevertheless, to date, studies assessing the effectiveness of education programs for individuals with cardiovascular conditions have shown inconsistent results (e.g., Meng et al., 2014; Song, Lindquist, Windenburg, Cairns, & Thakur, 2011). This inconsistency may imply that individuals' other needs—besides becoming knowledgeable about their health issues—should also be incorporated into these interventions.

Formal Interventions and Techniques for Improving Self-Management

Meade and Cronin (2012) suggest that an effective self-management program will teach individuals who are coping with a medical crisis how to monitor themselves, communicate with others, solve problems, and cope with their stress. They also point out that treatment recommendations are most successful when they are tailored to the needs and expectations of the specific individual.

Despite findings from randomized controlled trials that have shown self-management interventions to yield beneficial health effects for individuals with cardiovascular conditions (Clark et al., 2000; Clark et al., 1997), it is important to note that improvement has not been detected for all interventions. For example, Ho et al. (2009) claimed that interventions targeting maintenance of medication regimen produced only modest success. Radhakrishnan (2012), in her review of 10 reports of tailored interventions to improve self-management among individuals with type 2 diabetes, hypertension, and cardiac-related health issues, found no intervention impact on self-management activities, such as medication-taking, physical activity, smoking, or dietary regimen. In their review, Song et al. (2011) also detected that while most cardiac support groups had a positive effect on individuals self-management, results did not differ in a statistically significant way from those of individuals who had been in control groups. Finally, Rozansky (2014), in his review of the field of behavioral cardiology, also stated that conflicting results seem to be the norm in large studies looking at the effectiveness of behavioral interventions. The authors provided several explanations for these modest findings. For example, it was suggested that individuals merely talked about their feelings with each other, but without a structured program to manage the stress they experienced or deal directly with the feelings that surfaced no positive effect on psychological outcomes was detected (Song et al., 2011). With regard to the relatively low success rate of formal interventions, Rozansky claims that they may not have been comprehensive and flexible enough to meet the specific and all-encompassing needs of the individual. Despite these shortcomings, however, Rozansky acknowledged that as these interventions become more individually tailored and sophisticated, there is also more evidence pointing to the effectiveness of their use with individuals who have cardiac-related health issues.

CARDIAC PREVENTION AND REHABILITATION PROGRAMS

Of all the interventions designed to improve cardiac self-management, CPRP has probably received the most scientific corroboration. CPRP refers to a comprehensive program tailored to the individual; it applies a multidisciplinary approach and provides appropriate individualized exercise programs, dietary consultations, assistance in smoking cessation, and relevant education and psychosocial counseling (Beswick et al., 2005; Falvo, 2014) for people with cardiac-related health issues. The main goals of most CPRPs are to promote healthy habits and to facilitate the individual's emotional and physical adjustment to his or her cardiovascular condition (Bennet, 2012). Indeed, in the aftermath of an acute coronary event, all major international guidelines call for participation in a CPRP (Anderson et al., 2013; Antman et al., 2004; Perk et al., 2012).

Two very well-established meta-analyses have concluded that CPRPs are beneficial in reducing cardiac mortality and recurrence of MI and in creating positive effects on blood pressure, cholesterol, body weight, smoking behavior, physical exercise, and eating habits (Dusseldorp, Elderen, Maes, Meulman, & Kraaij, 1999; Miller, Balady, & Fletcher, 1997). More recent studies (Goel, Lennon, Tilbury, Squires, & Thomas, 2011; Hammill, Curtis, Schulman, & Whellan, 2010; Martin et al., 2012), including a recent Cochrane systematic review (Heran et al., 2011), also point to the positive role played by CPRPs. In addition, CPRPs have been found to reduce psychological symptoms associated with cardiac-related health issues, including depression and hostility (Lavie & Milani, 2005). Unfortunately, despite the numerous benefits to be gained by participating in CPRPs, they remain significantly underutilized worldwide (Cooper, Lloyd, Weinman, & Jackson, 1999; Reges et al., 2013a). Accordingly, there is a call for more efficient and easy-to- follow interventions.

WEB-BASED INTERVENTIONS

One particularly novel and promising venue for conducting successful interventions involves the use of Internet and mobile phone applications (Mehta 2016; Rozanski, 2014). With the rapid expansion of cellular networks and substantial advances in smartphone technologies, it is now both possible and affordable to digitally transmit medical data from wherever individuals are located to specialists in urban areas; in addition, individuals can receive real-time feedback and consultations. These mobile health tools have the potential to greatly improve individual–provider communication and self-management of chronic conditions. Indeed, the use of mobile phones, the Internet, and other cutting-edge communication technologies to deliver cardiac rehabilitation services to individuals in their homes may very well revolutionize the field and has already shown promising results (see Inglis et al., 2011 for a Cochrane review; Piette et al., 2015). More detailed observations of the use of these technologies to enhance individuals' health-promoting behaviors can be found in Section III of this book.

Partners' Support: *Self*–Management Does Not Mean One Needs to Do It All by *Oneself*

Social isolation and lack of social support are well-known risk factors for the likelihood of adverse cardiac events (Lett et al., 2005). Social integration, on the other hand, has been associated with many positive outcomes such as better adaptation to and recovery from cardiovascular conditions (King & Reis, 2012; Rozansky, 2014). Another consistent finding is the positive association between social support and better self-management among individuals with cardiac-related health issues (DiMatteo, 2004; Gallant, 2003). This finding may be linked to the fact that those who are isolated are less likely to push themselves to exercise and eat right, keep up with their medication-taking, and schedule doctor appointments (Pryor, Page, Patsamanis, & Jolly, 2014). One example of the effects of living alone versus living with others was provided by Bucholz et al. (2011), whose study revealed that people who lived alone after a heart attack were twice as likely to smoke as people who lived with others.

A close intimate relationship (marriage, cohabitation) can be a particularly good source of support and a strong link to other social outlets; indeed, being married—as opposed to widowed, divorced, or never married—has been associated with reduced cardiac risk (Bucholz et al., 2011; Smith, Baron, & Grove, 2014). Many researchers suggest that the response to medical situations in general, and to cardiac-related health conditions in particular, must be conceptualized as a dyadic rather than an individual process (Bennett, & Connell, 1999; Coyne & Smith, 1991; Dekel et al., 2013; Revenson, Kayser, & Bodenmann, 2005; Vilchinsky et al., 2010).

A study conducted on men with cardiovascular conditions and their female partners showed that women's support (i.e., active engagement, protective buffering, and overprotection) was associated with men's greater health-promoting behavior, such as smoking cessation (Vilchinsky et al., 2011). Another recent study detected that providers' support style predicted individuals' higher tendencies toward cardiac medication-taking (George-Levi et al., 2016). In addition, Bertoni, Donato, Graffigna, Barello, and Parise (2015) found that individuals with cardiac-related health issues who were part of a couple were more involved in their own healthcare than individuals who were single.

Sher et al. (2014) summarized the putative pathways through which a partner can influence behavior change in the other partner, including the provision of social support, offering the opportunity to make decisions and manage lifestyle choices together, providing emotional support and intimacy, as well as offering constructive criticism when needed and being solicitous, open, and communicative. All of these pathways should be targeted in psychological interventions designed for couples coping with one member's cardiac-related health issues.

RECOMMENDATIONS

Beginning at the healthcare-system level, there should be a push for more advanced and sophisticated ways of enrolling and keeping individuals in facilities that enhance self-management, such as CPRPs. For example, an automatic referral system with a built-in mechanism to provide feedback to the referring doctor should be considered in order to increase utilization and reduce disparities (Allen et al., 2004). According to Beswick et al. (2005), two additional venues for improving the CPRP referral process were linked with a notable increase in individuals' utilization of cardiac rehabilitation. One process was putting in place an educational intervention for healthcare providers themselves, so that they could better understand the comprehensive nature of cardiac rehabilitation and its benefits. The other, carried out by cardiac nurses serving as liaisons, was the co-ordination of postdischarge care between hospital practitioners and outside practitioners. Overall, having supervising medical staff refer all eligible individuals to CPRP—while giving special attention to vulnerable populations and tailoring recommendations in accordance with an individual's culture and gender—can improve participation in CPRP and is therefore warranted (Reges et al., 2013b).

Healthcare professionals who wish to facilitate their clients' self-management must do more than merely provide information; they must also help individuals believe in themselves and make choices that will foster healthier lives. There is much that healthcare professionals inside the hospital can do, including helping individuals locate primary-care physicians or cardiologists for follow-up care after their release; helping them obtain necessary medications; asking the in-hospital physician for a written referral to CPRP; helping individuals master their fears and anxieties about their recovery and future; and encouraging them to start exercising, stop smoking, and observe a healthy diet.

Once the individual is out of the hospital and back home, family physicians can support self-management by, for example, encouraging individuals to talk openly with them about particular areas of difficulty and directly and individually educating the individual or steering him or her toward appropriate resources in the greater community (Coleman & Newton, 2005).

Family members and spouses in particular are great sources of social support and should therefore be recruited to the "team." In addition, couples having difficulty coping with their partners' health situation should be offered assistance, as improved dyadic coping may eventually contribute to enhanced levels of self-management among the partners who have the health issues (Goldsmith, Lindholm, & Bute, 2006; Piette et al., 2008; Sher et al., 2002), which in turn might lead to improved health and saved lives. Finally, as it is the individuals themselves who must carry the burden of overhauling long-standing lifestyle habits, interventions should be designed and subsidized in order to help people achieve this goal.

CONCLUSIONS AND LIMITATIONS

It is important to emphasize that the fate of individuals with cardiovascular conditions is not predetermined; to the contrary, people can choose to manage their healthcare in ways that will make a significant difference in their quality of life and longevity. Therefore, much can and should be done to facilitate their health-promoting behaviors (Crowley, Grubber, Olsen, & Bosworth, 2013). Becoming knowledgeable about the barriers to and facilitators of self-management may lead to the development of more beneficial interventions that will help individuals make healthy and long-lasting changes in their lifestyles. Most importantly, assisting individuals to improve their self-management should be conceived of as a joint and comprehensive enterprise that involves the efforts of individuals and their family members, as well as their healthcare providers (i.e., physicians, psychologists) and the healthcare systems to which they belong.

Two limitations of this chapter should be noted: first, as its primary focus was on self-management in the context of acute cardiovascular conditions and heart failure, other cardiovascular conditions, such as congenital heart problems, valvular diseases, or cardiomyopathies, were not covered. Second, while this chapter focused specifically on three global barriers commonly found among individuals with cardiac-related health issues—systemic and cultural, gender-related, and psychological—many others barriers (see for example, Mead, Andres, Ramos, Siegel, & Regenstein, 2010) were not covered. For example, it was found that the regular maintenance of a medication regimen was especially low among individuals whose treatment required multiple medications to be taken on a chronic basis (Bansilal et al., 2016). Thus, in order to maximize self-management, the specific context of each modifiable behavior must be taken into consideration.

REFERENCES

Allan, R. (2012). The evolution of cardiac psychology. In R. Allan & J. Fisher (Eds.), *Heart and mind: The practice of cardiac psychology* (2nd ed., pp. 143–168). Washington, DC: American Psychological Association.

Allen, J. K., Scott, L. B., Stewart, K. J., & Young, D. R. (2004). Disparities in women's referral to and enrollment in outpatient cardiac rehabilitation. *Journal of General Internal Medicine, 19*(7), 747–753.

Alm-Roijer, C., Stagmo, M., Udén, G., & Erhardt, L. (2004). Better knowledge improves adherence to lifestyle changes and medication in patients with coronary heart disease. *European Journal of Cardiovascular Nursing, 3*(4), 321–330.

American Association of Cardiovascular and Pulmonary Rehabilitation. (2004). *Guidelines for cardiac rehabilitation and secondary prevention programs* (4th ed.). Champaign, IL: Human Kinetics.

Anderson, D. R., & Emery, C. F. (2014). Irrational health beliefs predict adherence to cardiac rehabilitation: A pilot study. *Health Psychology, 33*(12), 1614–1617.

Anderson, J. L., Adams, C. D., Antman, E. M., Bridges, C. R., Califf, R. M., Casey, D. E., . . . Lincoff, A. M. (2013). 2012 ACCF/AHA focused update incorporated into the ACCF/AHA 2007 guidelines for the management of patients with unstable angina/non-ST-elevation myocardial infarction: A report of the American College of Cardiology Foundation/American Heart Association Task Force on Practice Guidelines. *Journal of the American College of Cardiology, 61*(23), e179–e347.

Antman, E. M., Anbe, D. T., Armstrong, P. W., Bates, E. R., Green, L. A., Hand, M., . . . Mullany, C. J. (2004). ACC/AHA guidelines for the management of patients with ST-elevation myocardial infarction: A report of the American College of Cardiology/American Heart Association Task Force on Practice Guidelines (Committee to Revise the 1999 Guidelines for the Management of Patients with Acute Myocardial Infarction). *Journal of the American College of Cardiology, 44*(3), E1–E211.

Bagnall, A. J., Yan, A. T., Yan, R. T., Lee, C. H., Tan, M., Baer, C., . . . Canadian Acute Coronary Syndromes Registry II Investigators. (2010). Optimal medical therapy for non-ST-segment-elevation acute coronary syndromes: Exploring why physicians do not prescribe evidence-based treatment and why patients discontinue medications after discharge. *Circulation. Cardiovascular Quality and Outcomes, 3*(5), 530–537.

Baigent, C., Blackwell, L., Collins, R., Emberson, J., Godwin, J., Peto, R., . . . Meade, T. (2009). Aspirin in the primary and secondary prevention of vascular disease: Collaborative meta-analysis of individual participant data from randomized trials. *Lancet, 373*(9678), 1849–1860.

Bansilal, S., Castellano, J. M., & Fuster, V. (2016). Global burden of CVD: Focus on secondary prevention of cardiovascular disease. *International Journal of Cardiology, 201*(Suppl. 1), S1–S7.

Barth, J., Critchley, J., & Bengel, J. (2008). Psychosocial interventions for smoking cessation in patients with coronary heart disease. *Cochrane Database of Systematic Reviews, 1*, CD006886.

Bauer, L. K., Caro, M. A., Beach, S. R., Mastromauro, C. A., Lenihan, E., Januzzi, J. L., & Huffman, J. C. (2012). Effects of depression and anxiety improvement on adherence to medication and health behaviors in recently hospitalized cardiac patients. *The American Journal of Cardiology, 109*(9), 1266–1271.

Beauchamp, A., Peeters, A., Tonkin, A., & Turrell, G. (2010). Best practice for prevention and treatment of cardiovascular disease through an equity lens: A review. *European Journal of Cardiovascular Prevention & Rehabilitation, 17*(5), 599–606.

Bennett, P. (2012). Cardiovascular rehabilitation. In *The Oxford Handbook of Rehabilitation Psychology*. Edited by Paul Kennedy (pp. 337–350). Oxford: Oxford University Press.

Bennett, P., & Connell, H. (1999). Dyadic processes in response to myocardial infarction. *Psychology, Health & Medicine, 4*, 45–55.

Bennett, P., Mayfield, T., Norman, P., Lowe, R., & Morgan, M. (1999). Affective and social--cognitive predictors of behavioural change following first myocardial infarction. *British Journal of Health Psychology, 4*, 247–256.

Bertoni, A., Donato, S., Graffigna, G., Barello, S., & Parise, M. (2015). Engaged patients, engaged partnerships: Singles and partners dealing with an acute cardiac event. *Psychology, Health & Medicine, 20*(5), 505–517.

Beswick, A. D., Rees, K., West, R. R., Taylor, F. C., Burke, M., Griebsch, I., . . . Ebrahim, S. (2005). Improving uptake and adherence in cardiac rehabilitation: Literature review. *Journal of Advanced Nursing, 49*(5), 538–555.

Bjarnason-Wehrens, B., Grande, G., Loewel, H., Völler, H., & Mittag, O. (2007). Gender-specific issues in cardiac rehabilitation: Do women with ischaemic heart disease need specially tailored programmes? *European Journal of Cardiovascular Prevention & Rehabilitation, 14*(2), 163–171.

Blackwell, D. L., Lucas, J. W., & Clarke, T. C. (2014). Summary health statistics for U.S. adults: National Health Interview Survey, 2012. *Vital and Health Statistics, 10*(260), 1–171.

Bucholz, E. M., Rathore, S. S., Gosch, K., Schoenfeld, A., Jones, P.G., Buchanan, D. M., ... Krumholz, H. M. (2011) Effect of living alone on patient outcomes after hospitalization for acute myocardial infarction. *American Journal of Cardiology 108*, 943–948.

Centers for Disease Control and Prevention. (2016, March 10). *Heart disease facts.* Retrieved from http://www.cdc.gov/HeartDisease/facts.htm

Chow, C. K., Jolly, S., Rao-Melacini, P., Fox, K. A., Anand, S. S., & Yusuf, S. (2010). Association of diet, exercise, and smoking modification with risk of early cardiovascular events after acute coronary syndromes. *Circulation, 121,* 750–758.

Chowdhury, R., Khan, H., Heydon, E., Shroufi, A., Fahimi, S., Moore, C., ... Franco, O. H. (2013). Adherence to cardiovascular therapy: A meta-analysis of prevalence and clinical consequences. *European Heart Journal, 34*(38), 2940–2948.

Clark, N. M., Janz, N. K., Dodge, J. A., Schork, M. A., Fingerlin, T. E., Wheeler, J. R., ... Santinga, J. T. (2000). Changes in functional health status of older women with heart disease evaluation of a program based on self-regulation. *Journals of Gerontology Series B: Psychological Sciences and Social Sciences, 55*(2), S117–S126.

Clark, N. M., Janz, N. K., Dodge, J. A., Schork, M. A., Wheeler, J. R., Liang, J., ... Santinga, J. T. (1997). Self-management of heart disease by older adults: Assessment of an intervention based on social cognitive theory. *Research on Aging, 19*(3), 362–382.

Coleman, M. T., & Newton, K. S. (2005). Supporting self-management in patients with chronic illness. *American Journal of Family Physician, 72*(8), 1503–1510.

Cooper, A., Lloyd, G., Weinman, J., & Jackson, G. (1999). Why patients do not attend cardiac rehabilitation: Role of intentions and illness beliefs. *Heart, 82,* 234–236.

Coyne, J. C., & Smith, D. A. (1991). Couples coping with a myocardial infarction: A contextual perspective on wives' distress. *Journal of Personality and Social Psychology, 61,* 404–412.

Crowley, M. J., Grubber, J. M., Olsen, M. K., & Bosworth, H. B. (2013). Factors associated with non-adherence to three hypertension self-management behaviors: Preliminary data for a new instrument. *Journal of General Internal Medicine, 28*(1), 99–106.

Davies, E. J., Moxham, T., Rees, K., Singh, S., Coats, A. J., Ebrahim, S., ... Taylor, R. S. (2010). Exercise training for systolic heart failure: Cochrane systematic review and meta-analysis. *European Journal of Heart Failure, 12*(7), 706–715.

Dekel, R., Vilchinsky, N., Liberman, G., Leibowitz, Khaskia, A., & Mosseri, M. (2013). Marital satisfaction and depression among couples following men's acute coronary syndrome: Testing dyadic dynamics in a longitudinal design. *British Journal of Health Psychology, 19,* 347–362.

de Melo Ghisi, G. L., Grace, S. L., Thomas, S., Evans, M. F., Sawula, H., & Oh, P. (2014). Healthcare providers' awareness of the information needs of their cardiac rehabilitation patients throughout the program continuum. *Patient Education and Counseling, 95*(1), 143–150.

de Oliveira Otto, M. C., Mozaffarian, D., Kromhout, D., Bertoni, A. G., Sibley, C. T., Jacobs, D. R., & Nettleton, J. A. (2012). Dietary intake of saturated fat by food source and incident cardiovascular disease: The Multi-Ethnic Study of Atherosclerosis. *The American Journal of Clinical Nutrition, 96*(2), 397–404.

DiMatteo, M.R. (2004). Social support and patient adherence to medical treatment: A meta-analysis. *Health Psychology, 23,* 207–218.

Dornelas, E. A., Sampson, R. A., Gray, J. F., Waters, D., & Thompson, P. D. (2000). A randomized controlled trial of smoking cessation counseling after myocardial infarction. *Preventive Medicine, 30*(4), 261–268.

Dusseldorp, E., Elderen, T., Maes, S., Meulman, J., & Kraaij, V. (1999). A meta-analysis of psychoeducational programs for coronary heart disease patients. *Health Psychology, 18,* 506–519.

Edmondson, D. (2014). An enduring somatic threat model of posttraumatic stress disorder due to acute life threatening medical events. *Social and Personality Psychology Compass, 8,* 118–134.

Edmondson, D., Rieckmann, N., Shaffer, J. A., Schwartz, J. E., Burg, M. M., Davidson, K. W., ... Kronish, I. M. (2011). Posttraumatic stress due to an acute coronary syndrome increases risk of 42 month major adverse cardiac events and all-cause mortality. *Journal of Psychiatric Research, 45,* 1621–1626.

Edwards, R. (2004) ABC of smoking cessation: The problem of tobacco smoking. *British Medical Journal 328,* 217–219.

Ens, T. A., Seneviratne, C. C., Jones, C., & King-Shier, K. M. (2014). Factors influencing medication adherence in South Asian people with cardiac disorders: An ethnographic study. *International Journal of Nursing Studies, 51*(11), 1472–1481.

Estruch, R., Ros, E., Salas-Salvadó, J., Covas, M. I., Corella, D., Arós, F., ... Lamuela-Raventos, R. M. (2013). Primary prevention of cardiovascular disease with a Mediterranean diet. *The New England Journal of Medicine, 368*(14), 1279–1290.

Eyre, H., Kahn, R., Robertson, R. M., Clark, N. G., Doyle, C., Gansler, T., ... Thun, M. J. (2004). Preventing cancer, cardiovascular disease, and diabetes: A common agenda for the American Cancer Society, the American Diabetes Association, and the American Heart Association. *CA: A Cancer Journal for Clinicians, 54*(4), 190–207.

Falvo, D. R. (2014). *Medical and psychosocial aspects of chronic illness and disability.* Sudbury, MA: Jones and Bartlett.

Fix, G. M., & Bokhour, B. G. (2012). Understanding the context of patient experiences in order to explore adherence to secondary prevention guidelines after heart surgery. *Chronic Illness, 8*(4), 265–277.

Franklin, B. A., & Cushman, M. (2011). Recent advances in preventive cardiology and lifestyle medicine: A themed series. *Circulation, 123*(20), 2274–2283.

Gallant, M. P. (2003). The influence of social support on chronic illness self-management: A review and directions for research. *Health Education & Behavior, 30*(2), 170–195.

George-Levi, S., Vilchinsky, N., Tolmatcz, R., Khaskia, A., Mosseri, & Hod, H. (2016). "It takes two to take": Relational entitlement, caregiving styles, and cardiac patients' medication taking. *Journal of Family Psychology, 30*(6), 743–751.

Gerber, Y., Benyamini, Y., Goldbourt, U., Drory, Y., & Israel Study Group on First Acute Myocardial Infarction. (2010). Neighborhood socioeconomic context and long-term survival after myocardial infarction. *Circulation, 121*(3), 375–383.

Ginzburg, K., & Ein-Dor, T. (2011). Posttraumatic stress syndromes and health-related quality of life following myocardial infarction: 8-year follow-up. *General Hospital Psychiatry, 33*(6), 565–571.

Grace, S. L., Gravely-Witte, S., Kayaniyil, S., Brual, J., Suskin, N., & Stewart, D. E. (2009). A multisite examination of sex differences in cardiac rehabilitation barriers by participation status. *Journal of Women's Health, 18*(2), 209–216.

Gregory, P. C., LaVeist, T. A., & Simpson, C. (2006). Racial disparities in access to cardiac rehabilitation. *American Journal of Physical Medicine & Rehabilitation, 85*(9), 705–710.

Glazer, K. M., Emery, C. F., Frid, D. J., & Banyasz, R. E. (2002). Psychological predictors of adherence and outcomes among patients in cardiac rehabilitation. *Journal of Cardiopulmonary Rehabilitation, 22*, 40–46.

Goel, K., Lennon, R. J., Tilbury, R. T., Squires, R. W., & Thomas, R. J. (2011). Impact of cardiac rehabilitation on mortality and cardiovascular events after percutaneous coronary intervention in the community. *Circulation, 123*, 2344–2352.

Goldsmith, D. J., Lindholm, K. A., & Bute, J. J. (2006). Dilemmas of talking about lifestyle changes among couples coping with a cardiac event. *Social Science & Medicine, 63*(8), 2079–2090.

Granger, B. B., Swedberg, K., Ekman, I., Granger, C. B., Olofsson, B., McMurray, J. J., . . . Pfeffer, M. A. (2005). Adherence to candesartan and placebo and outcomes in chronic heart failure in the CHARM program: Double-blind, randomized, controlled clinical trial. *The Lancet, 366*(9502), 2005–2011.

Hammill, B. G., Curtis, L. H., Schulman, K. A., & Whellan, D. J. (2010). Relationship between cardiac rehabilitation and long-term risks of death and myocardial infarction among elderly Medicare beneficiaries. *Circulation, 121*, 63–70.

Hart, P. L. (2005). Women's perceptions of coronary heart disease: An integrative review. *Journal of Cardiovascular Nursing, 20*(3), 170–176.

Heran, B. S., Chen, J. M., Ebrahim, S., Moxham, T., Oldridge, N., Rees, K., . . . Taylor, R. S. (2011). Exercise-based cardiac rehabilitation for coronary heart disease. *Cochrane Database Systemic Review, 6*(7), CD001800.

Ho, P. M., Bryson, C. L., & Rumsfeld, J. S. (2009). Medication adherence: Its importance in cardiovascular outcomes. *Circulation, 119*(23), 3028–3035.

Huffman, J. C., Moore, S. V., DuBois, C. M., Mastromauro, C. A., Suarez, L., & Park, E. R. (2015). An exploratory mixed methods analysis of adherence predictors following acute coronary syndrome. *Psychology, Health & Medicine, 20*(5), 541–550.

Inglis, S. C., Clark, R. A., & Cleland, J. G. (2011). Cochrane Systematic Review Team: Telemonitoring in patients with heart failure. *The New England Journal of Medicine, 364*(11), 1078–1080.

Jason, T., McGannon, K. R., Blanchard, C. M., Rainham, D., & Dechman, G. (2015). A systematic gender-based review of physical activity correlates in coronary heart disease patients. *International Review of Sport and Exercise Psychology, 8*(1), 1–23.

Jensen, L., & King, K. M. (1997). Women and heart disease: The issues. *Critical Care Nurse, 17*(2), 45–53.

Kark, J. D., Fink, R., Adler, B., Goldberger, N., & Goldman, S. (2006). The incidence of coronary heart disease among Palestinians and Israelis in Jerusalem. *International Journal of Epidemiology, 35*(2), 448–457.

Kark, J. D., Gordon, E. S., & Haklai, Z. (2000). Coronary heart disease mortality among Arab and Jewish residents of Jerusalem. *The Lancet, 356*(9239), 1410–1411.

King, K. B., & Reis, H. T. (2012). Marriage and long-term survival after coronary artery bypass grafting. *Health Psychology, 31*(1), 55–62.

Kop, W. J., & Plumhoff, J. E. (2012). Depression and coronary heart disease: Diagnosis, predictive value, biobehavioral mechanisms, and intervention. In R. Allan & J. Fisher (Eds.), *Heart and mind: The practice of cardiac psychology* (2nd ed., pp. 143–168). Washington, DC: American Psychological Association.

Kristofferzon, M. L., Löfmark, R., & Carlsson, M. (2005). Perceived coping, social support, and quality of life 1 month after myocardial infarction: A comparison between Swedish women and men. *Heart & Lung: The Journal of Acute and Critical Care, 34*(1), 39–50.

Kronish, I. M., Rieckmann, N., Halm, E. A., Shimbo, D., Vorchheimer, D., Haas, D. C., & Davidson, K. W. (2006). Persistent depression affects adherence to secondary prevention behaviors after acute coronary syndromes. *Journal of General Internal Medicine, 21*, 1178–1183.

Lavie, C. J., & Milani, R. V. (2005). Cardiac rehabilitation and exercise training programs in metabolic syndrome and diabetes. *Journal of Cardiopulmonary Rehabilitation and Prevention, 25*(2), 59–66.

Lemos, K., Suls, J., Jenson, M., Lounsbury, P., & Gordon, E. E. I. (2003). How do female and male cardiac patients and their spouses share responsibilities after discharge from the hospital? *Annals of Behavioral Medicine, 25*, 8–15.

Leslie, W. S., Hankey, C. R., Matthews, D., Currall, J. E. P., & Lean, M. E. J. (2004). A transferable program of nutritional counselling for rehabilitation following myocardial infarction: A randomized controlled study. *European Journal of Clinical Nutrition, 58*(5), 778–786.

Lett, H. S., Blumenthal, J. A., Babyak, M. A., Strauman, T. J., Robins, C., & Sherwood, A. (2005). Social support and coronary heart disease: Epidemiologic evidence and implications for treatment. *Psychosomatic Medicine, 67*(6), 869–878.

Lett, H. S., Sherwood, A., Watkins, L., & Blumenthal, J. A. (2007). Depression and prognosis in cardiac patients. In A. Steptoe (Ed.), *Depression and physical illness* (pp. 87–108). Cambridge, UK: Cambridge University Press.

Lund, L. H., Edwards, L. B., Kucheryavaya, A. Y., Dipchand, A. I., Benden, C., Christie, J. D., . . . Stehlik, J. (2013). The Registry of the International Society for Heart and Lung Transplantation: Thirtieth official adult heart transplant report—2013; focus theme: Age. *Journal of Heart and Lung Transplant, 32*(10), 951–964.

Luszczynska, A., & Cieslak, R. (2009). Mediated effects of social support for healthy nutrition: Fruit and vegetable intake across 8 months after myocardial infarction. *Behavioral Medicine, 35*, 30–38.

Martin, B. J., Hauer, T., Arena, R., Austford, L. D., Galbraith, P. D., Lewin, A. M., . . . Aggarwal, S. (2012). Cardiac rehabilitation attendance and outcomes in coronary artery disease patients. *Circulation, 111*, 677–687.

McGrady, A., McGinnis, R., Badenhop, D., Bentle, M., & Rajput, M. (2009). Effects of depression and anxiety on adherence to cardiac rehabilitation. *Journal of Cardiopulmonary Rehabilitation and Prevention, 29*(6), 358–364.

Mead, H., Andres, E., Ramos, C., Siegel, B., & Regenstein, M. (2010). Barriers to effective self-management in cardiac patients: The patient's experience. *Patient Education and Counseling, 79*(1), 69–76.

Meade, M. A., & Cronin, L. (2012). The expert patient and the self-management of chronic conditions and disabilities. In P. Kennedy (Ed.), *The Oxford handbook of rehabilitation psychology* (pp. 492–510). Oxford: Oxford University Press.

Mehta, L. S., Beckie, T. M., DeVon, H. A., Grines, C. L., Krumholz, H. M., Johnson, M. N., . . . Wenger, N. K. (2016). Acute myocardial infarction in women: A scientific statement from the American Heart Association. *Circulation*. doi.org/10.1161/CIR.0000000000000351

Meng, K., Seekatz, B., Haug, G., Mosler, G., Schwaab, B., Worringen, U., & Faller, H. (2014). Evaluation of a standardized patient education program for inpatient cardiac rehabilitation: Impact on illness knowledge and self-management behaviors up to 1 year. *Health Education Research, 29*(2), 235–246.

Mente, A., de Koning, L., Shannon, H. S., & Anand, S. S. (2009). A systematic review of the evidence supporting a causal link between dietary factors and coronary heart disease. *Archives of Internal Medicine, 169*(7), 659–669.

Menezes, A. R., Lavie, C. J., Milani, R. V., Forman, D. E., King, M., & Williams, M. A. (2014). Cardiac rehabilitation in the United States. *Progress in Cardiovascular Diseases, 56*(5), 522–529.

Miller, T. D., Balady, G. J., & Fletcher, G. F. (1997). Exercise and its role in the prevention and rehabilitation of cardiovascular disease. *Annals of Behavioral Medicine, 19*(3), 220–229.

Mills, E. J., O'Regan, C., Eyawo, O., Wu, P., Mills, F., Berwanger, O., & Briel, M. (2011). Intensive statin therapy compared with moderate dosing for prevention of cardiovascular events: A meta-analysis of >40 000 patients. *European Heart Journal, 32*(11), 1409–1415.

Mochari, H., Lee, J. R., Kligfield, P., & Mosca, L. (2006). Ethnic differences in barriers and referral to cardiac rehabilitation among women hospitalized with coronary heart disease. *Preventive Cardiology, 9*(1), 8–13.

Mosca, L., Benjamin, E. J., Berra, K., Bezanson, J. L., Dolor, R. J., Lloyd-Jones, D. M., . . . Zhao, D. (2011). Effectiveness-based guidelines for the prevention of cardiovascular disease in women—2011 update: A guideline from the American Heart Association. *Journal of the American College of Cardiology, 57*(12), 1404–1423.

Mozaffarian, D., Afshin, A., Benowitz, N. L., Bittner, V., Daniels, S. R., Franch, H. A., . . . Popkin, B. M. (2012). On behalf of the American Heart Association Council on Epidemiology and Prevention, Council on Nutrition, Physical Activity and Metabolism, Council on Clinical Cardiology, Council on Cardiovascular Disease in the Young, Council on the Kidney in Cardiovascular Disease, Council on Peripheral Vascular Disease, and the Advocacy Coordinating Committee. Population approaches to improve diet, physical activity, and smoking habits: A scientific statement from the American Heart Association. *Circulation, 126*, 1514–1563.

Mozaffarian, D., Wilson, P. W., & Kannel, W. B. (2008). Beyond established and novel risk factors: Lifestyle risk factors for cardiovascular disease. *Circulation, 117*(23), 3031–3038.

Naderi, S. H., Bestwick, J. P., & Wald, D. S. (2012). Adherence to drugs that prevent cardiovascular disease: Meta-analysis on 376,162 patients. *The American Journal of Medicine, 125*(9), 882–887.

Naidoo, J., & Wills, J. (2000). *Health promotion: Foundations for practice*. London: Elsevier Health Sciences.

Panagiotakos, D. B., Rallidis, L. S., Pitsavos, C., Stefanadis, C., & Kremastinos, D. (2007). Cigarette smoking and myocardial infarction in young men and women: A case-control study. *International Journal of Cardiology, 116*(3), 371–375.

Perk, J., De Backer, G., Gohlke, H., Graham, I., Reiner, Ž., Verschuren, M., . . . Deaton, C. (2012). European guidelines on cardiovascular disease prevention in clinical practice (version 2012). *European Heart Journal, 33*(13), 1635–1701.

Perez, G. H., Nicolau, J. C., Romano, B. W., & Laranjeira, R. (2007). Smoking-associated factors in myocardial infarction and unstable angina: Do gender differences exist? *Addictive Behaviors, 32*(6), 1295–1301.

Perez, G. H., Nicolau, J. C., Romano, B. W., & Laranjeira, R. (2008). Depression: A predictor of smoking relapse in a 6-month follow-up after hospitalization for acute coronary syndrome. *European Journal of Cardiovascular Prevention & Rehabilitation, 15*(1), 89–94.

Piette, J. D., Gregor, M. A., Share, D., Heisler, M., Bernstein, S. J., Koelling, T., & Chan, P. (2008). Improving heart failure self-management support by actively engaging out-of-home caregivers: Results of a feasibility study. *Congestive Heart Failure, 14*(1), 12–18.

Piette, J. D., Striplin, D., Marinec, N., Chen, J., Trivedi, R. B., Aron, D. C., . . . Aikens, J. E. (2015). A mobile health intervention supporting heart failure patients and their informal caregivers: A randomized comparative effectiveness trial. *Journal of Medical Internet Research, 17*(6), e142.

Pipe, A. L., Papadakis, S., & Reid, R. D. (2010). The role of smoking cessation in the prevention of coronary artery disease. *Current Atherosclerosis Reports, 12*(2), 145–150.

Pryor, T., Page, K., Patsamanis, H., & Jolly, K. A. (2014). Investigating support needs for people living with heart disease. *Journal of Clinical Nursing, 23*(1-2), 166–172.

Radhakrishnan, K. (2012). The efficacy of tailored interventions for self-management outcomes of type 2 diabetes, hypertension or heart disease: A systematic review. *Journal of Advanced Nursing, 68*(3), 496–510.

Reges, O., Vilchinsky, N., Leibowitz, M., Khaskia, A., Mosseri, M., & Kark, J. D. (2013a). Arab–Jewish differences in attending cardiac rehabilitation programs following acute coronary syndrome. *International Journal of Cardiology, 163*, 218–219.

Reges, O., Vilchinsky, N., Leibowitz, M., Khaskia, A., Mosseri, M., & Kark, J. D. (2013b). Systemic determinants as barriers to participation in cardiac prevention and rehabilitation services after acute coronary syndrome. *International Journal of Cardiology, 168*(5), 4865.

Reges, O., Vilchinsky, N., Leibowitz, M., Khaskia, A., Mosseri, M., & Kark, J. D. (2014). Identifying barriers to participation in cardiac prevention and rehabilitation programs via decision tree analysis: Establishing targets for remedial interventions. *Open Heart, 1*(1), e000097.

Reges, O., Vilchinsky, N., Leibowitz, M., Khaskia, A., Mosseri, M., & Kark, J. D. (2015). Change in health behaviors following acute coronary syndrome: Arab–Jewish differences. *European Journal of Preventive Cardiology, 22*(4), 458–467.

Revenson, T. A., Griva, K., Luszczynska, A., Morrison, V. Panagopoulu, E., Vilchinsky, N., & Hagedoorn, M. (2015). *Caregiving in the illness context*. Hampshire, UK: Palgrave Macmillan.

Revenson, T., Kayser, K., & Bodenmann, G. (Eds.).(2005). *Emerging perspectives on couples' coping with stress*. Washington, DC: American Psychological Association.

Rozanski, A. (2014). Behavioral cardiology: Current advances and future directions. *Journal of the American College of Cardiology, 64*(1), 100–110.

Shemesh, E., Yehuda, R., Milo, O., Dinur, I., Rudnick, A., Vered, Z., & Cotter, G. (2004). Posttraumatic stress, non-adherence, and adverse outcomes on survivors of a myocardial Infarction. *Psychosomatic Medicine, 66*, 521–526.

Sher, T., Braun, L., Domas, A., Bellg, A., Baucom, D. H., & Houle, T. T. (2014). The Partners for Life program: A couples approach to cardiac risk reduction. *Family Process, 53*(1), 131–149.

Sher, T. G., Bellg, A. J., Braun, L., Domas, A., Rosenson, R., & Canar, W. J. (2002). Partners for Life: A theoretical approach to developing an intervention for cardiac risk reduction. *Health Education Research, 17*(5), 597–605.

Smith, S. D., Blair, S. N., Bonow, R. O., Brass, L. M., Cerqueira, M. D., Dracup, K., . . . Taubert, K. A. (2001). AHA/ACC guidelines for preventing heart attack and death in patients with atherosclerotic cardiovascular disease: 2001 update. *Circulation, 104*, 1577–1579.

Smith, T. W., Baron, C. E., & Grove, J. L. (2014). Personality, emotional adjustment, and cardiovascular risk: Marriage as a mechanism. *Journal of Personality, 82*(6), 502–514.

Scott, L. B. (2010). A call for intervention research to overcome barriers to women's enrollment in outpatient cardiac rehabilitation programs. *Journal of Women's Health, 19*(11), 1951–1953.

Song, Y., Lindquist, R., Windenburg, D., Cairns, B., & Thakur, A. (2011). Review of outcomes of cardiac support groups after cardiac events. *Western Journal of Nursing Research, 33*(2), 224–246.

Steca, P., Greco, A., Cappelletti, E., D'Addario, M., Monzani, D., Pancani, L., . . . Parati, G. (2015). Cardiovascular management self-efficacy: Psychometric properties of a new scale and its usefulness in a rehabilitation context. *Annals of Behavioral Medicine, 49*(5), 660–674.

Stramba-Badiale, M., Fox, K. M., Priori, S. G., Collins, P., Daly, C., Graham, I., . . . Tendera, M. (2006). Cardiovascular disease in women: A statement from the policy conference of the European Society of Cardiology. *European Heart Journal, 27*, 994–1005.

Suaya, J. A., Shepard, D. S., Normand, S. L. T., Ades, P. A., Prottas, J., & Stason, W. B. (2007). Use of cardiac rehabilitation by Medicare beneficiaries after myocardial infarction or coronary bypass surgery. *Circulation, 116*(15), 1653–1662.

Sud, A., Kline-Rogers, E. M., Eagle, K. A., Fang, J., Armstrong, D. F., Rangarajan, K., . . . Erickson, S. R. (2005). Adherence to medications by patients after acute coronary syndromes. *The Annals of Pharmacotherapy, 39*(11), 1792–1797.

Valencia, H. E., Savage, P. D., & Ades, P. A. (2011). Cardiac rehabilitation participation in underserved populations. *Journal of Cardiopulmonary Rehabilitation and Prevention, 31*(4), 203–210.

Vilchinsky, N., Dekel, R., Leibowitz, M., Reges, O., Khaskia, A., & Mosseri, M. (2011). Dynamics of support perceptions among couples coping with cardiac illness: The effect on recovery outcomes. *Health Psychology, 30*, 411–419.

Vilchinsky, N., Haze-Filderman, L., Leibowitz, M., Reges, O., Khaskia, A., & Mosseri, M. (2010). Spousal support and cardiac patients' distress: The moderating role of attachment orientation. *Journal of Family Psychology, 24*(4), 508–512.

Yohannes, A. M., Yalfani, A., Doherty, P., & Bundy, C. (2007). Predictors of drop-out from an outpatient cardiac rehabilitation programme. *Clinical Rehabilitation, 21*(3), 222–229.

Zafari, A. M., & Wenger, N. K. (1998). Secondary prevention of coronary heart disease. *Archives of Physical Medicine and Rehabilitation, 79*, 1006–1017.

Ziegelstein, R. C., Fauerbach, J. A., Stevens, S. S., Romanelli, J., Richter, D. P., & Bush, D. E. (2000). Patients with depression are less likely to follow recommendations to reduce cardiac risk during recovery from a myocardial infarction. *Archives of Internal Medicine, 160*(12), 1818–1823.

12

Self-Management of Diabetes

JONATHAN F. DEICHES, EMRE UMUCU, AND FONG CHAN ■

Diabetes mellitus is a group of metabolic conditions characterized by impaired blood glucose regulation and hyperglycemia (American Diabetes Association [ADA], 2016a). Most cases of diabetes fall into two broad categories: (a) type 1 diabetes mellitus (T1DM) and (b) type 2 diabetes mellitus (T2DM). These two types are distinguished by pathogenesis (Cnop et al., 2005). T1DM is generally caused by an autoimmune response that destroys the pancreatic β-cells that produce insulin. In contrast, T2DM is caused by a combination of resistance to insulin action and inadequate compensatory insulin secretion due to β-cell dysfunction.

Diabetes is one of the most substantial public health problems currently facing the United States (Bonow & Gheorghiade, 2004; Steinbrook, 2006) and many other countries across the globe (Kolb & Mandrup-Poulsen, 2010). Approximately 415 million adults are affected worldwide, with an international prevalence rate of 8.8% (International Diabetes Federation, 2015). In the United States, an estimated 29.1 million people ages 12 and older have diabetes, corresponding to a prevalence rate of 9.3% (Centers for Disease Control and Prevention [CDC], 2014). The vast majority of diabetes cases in the United States are T2DM, accounting for 90% to 95% of all cases. Approximately 5% are T1DM, and the remaining 1% to 5% of diabetes cases are other types of diabetes, such as gestational diabetes and diabetes caused by specific genetic conditions or from surgery, medications, or other health conditions (CDC, 2014). Over the past few decades, T2DM has become a global public health crisis, and incidence rates have risen dramatically (Fox et al., 2006; Geiss et al., 2014).

This chapter provides essential knowledge for healthcare providers and individuals with diabetes and describes the current state of management practices and research. We begin with an overview of the biopsychosocial aspects of diabetes, followed by a review of diabetes self-management practices and interventions.

BIOLOGICAL, PSYCHOLOGICAL, AND SOCIAL ASPECTS OF DIABETES

Diabetes not only affects a person's biology and physical health, it also influences one's psychological health and social functioning. Changes in any one of these areas may have significant implications for the other domains of functioning, as well as a person's overall quality of life. Thus, to fully appreciate the experience of living with diabetes, each area of functioning must be considered.

Biological Aspects of Diabetes

T1DM is a metabolic disorder typically caused by an autoimmune response that leads to the destruction of insulin-producing pancreatic β-cells (Atkinson, Eisenbarth, & Michels, 2014). The destruction of β-cells results in a lifelong need for exogenous insulin replacement. Its presentation most commonly occurs during childhood, but age of onset is not a restricting factor for diagnosis. Hallmark symptoms include hyperglycemia, polydipsia, polyphagia, and polyuria (Atkinson et al., 2014).

T2DM is a metabolic disorder caused by a combination of insulin resistance and dysfunction of pancreatic β-cells (ADA, 2016a; Falvo, 2009). Insulin resistance refers to reduced insulin sensitivity and impaired insulin-stimulated glucose uptake in insulin target tissue, such as skeletal muscle, liver, and adipocytes (Abdul-Ghani, 2013). The causes of insulin resistance can be both hereditary and acquired, though the current epidemic of T2DM is strongly linked to obesity, which can interfere with important endocrine and metabolic functions and contribute to insulin resistance (Abdul-Ghani, 2013; Gunawardana, 2014; Selvin, Parrinello, Sacks, & Coresh, 2014). Lifestyle factors, such as physical inactivity, poor diet, cigarette smoking, and insufficient sleep, can also reduce insulin sensitivity (Krentz, 2002). When the body's tight metabolic regulation of fuel is disrupted due to reduced insulin sensitivity, the result is excess blood glucose, or hyperglycemia (Newsholme, Cruzat, Arfuso, & Keane, 2014).

Increased insulin resistance alone, however, is generally not sufficient for causing T2DM (Ashcroft & Rorsman, 2012). The development of diabetes also depends on the degree to which pancreatic β-cells are able to compensate for diminished insulin sensitivity by up-regulating insulin secretion to address excess blood glucose. For people with T2DM, β-cell functioning is significantly compromised, and overall reduction of β-cell mass can occur (Halban et al., 2014). A number of different factors may cause β-cell dysfunction, including insulin resistance and chronic hyperglycemia, lipotoxicity, changes in pancreatic islet cell integrity and organization, inflammation, and oxidative stress (Halban et al., 2014). It is unclear which stressor initially disrupts β-cell functioning, and this is actually likely to vary across individuals. Importantly, though, many of the factors that contribute to β-cell dysfunction may actually initiate or exacerbate additional β-cell stressors, creating a complex process of diabetes progression that is difficult to stop (Ashcroft & Rorsman, 2012).

According to the ADA (2016a), diagnosis of diabetes depends on clinical indicators of metabolic dysfunction and impaired glycemic control. Diabetes may be diagnosed based on glycated hemoglobin (HbA_{1c}) criteria or plasma glucose criteria. Current guidelines specify the following values for diagnosis of diabetes: $HbA_{1c} \geq 6.5\%$, fasting plasma glucose (FPG) $\geq$ 126 mg/dL, or two-hour plasma glucose $\geq$ 200 mg/dL after a 75-g oral glucose tolerance test (OGTT). When available, HbA_{1c} testing has several advantages over the FPG and OGTT, including greater convenience for individuals being tested and greater stability of measurement. Regardless of the chosen method, clinical evidence of impaired blood glucose regulation is required for diagnosing diabetes.

The effects of diabetes on physical health can be profound. Diabetes is associated with increased risk for a number of medical complications, which are often categorized as either macrovascular or microvascular complications (Fowler, 2008; Skyler, 2004; Stolar, 2010). Macrovascular complications generally include multiple forms of cardiovascular disease, including coronary artery disease and cerebrovascular disease (Dokken, 2008). Common microvascular complications include retinopathy, neuropathy, and nephropathy, though small blood vessels throughout the entire body may be affected. Encouragingly, existing data indicates that a number of diabetic complications have become less prevalent in recent years, ostensibly due to earlier detection and improved treatments (Gregg et al., 2014). However, diabetes complications still constitute a significant cause of impairment and disability in the United States.

People with diabetes also frequently experience unpleasant diabetic symptoms on a regular basis. Common symptoms associated with hyperglycemia include polydipsia, polyuria, and fatigue (Grootenhuis, Snoek, Heine, & Bouter, 1994; Whitty et al., 1997). Individuals with T1DM and T2DM treated with insulin also commonly experience hypoglycemic symptoms, including anxiety, palpitations, tremors, diaphoresis, paresthesia, polyphagia, drowsiness, and confusion (Amin, Lau, Crawford, Edwards, & Pacaud, 2014; Cryer, Davis, & Shamoon, 2003).

Psychological Aspects of Diabetes

An individual's personal experience living with a chronic condition like diabetes is often multifaceted and complex (Chan, Gelman, Ditchman, Kim, & Chiu, 2009), and it is essential that both healthcare providers and individuals with diabetes are aware of the psychological aspects of the condition. Diabetes is considered one of the most emotionally and behaviorally demanding chronic health conditions because it affects many areas of a person's life (Chew, Shariff-Ghazali, & Fernandez, 2014; Delamater et al., 2001; Snoek & Skinner, 2006). Healthy psychological functioning is critically important for people with diabetes, as it helps ensure that individuals will possess the motivation and mental fortitude necessary to successfully manage their chronic condition.

Once a person receives a diagnosis of diabetes, the psychological adjustment process begins. Individuals' responses to a diagnosis of diabetes can vary significantly and can include shock and denial, depression, or even a sense of relief upon confirming their suspicion that a problem does indeed exist (Coles, 1996; Peel, Parry, Douglas, & Lawton, 2004). Some people may take an active approach to dealing with the condition, seeking out information or engaging fully in treatment, while others may focus on alleviating emotional distress or avoid dealing with the problem entirely (Duangdao & Roesch, 2008; Grey, 2000). Following the onset of diabetes, the day-to-day experience of living with diabetes can also lead to psychological distress due to the behavioral demands of consistently regulating one's dietary choices, taking medication regularly, and monitoring blood glucose levels. People with diabetes may frequently feel that they have restricted or lost opportunities in life, including limitations in travel and social activities, failed relationships with people who were unsupportive, or interferences with career advancement (Browne, Ventura, Mosely, & Speight, 2013). All of these challenges can contribute to psychological distress.

Research indicates that diabetes is associated with a number of psychological concerns, most notably depression and anxiety. People with diabetes are twice as likely to experience depression as people without diabetes (Anderson, Freedland, Clouse, & Lustman, 2001), and depression may significantly interfere with self-care behaviors and glycemic control (Ciechanowski, Katon, Russo, & Hirsch, 2003; Lustman et al., 2000). Co-occurring depression in individuals with diabetes is commonly believed to be the result of impairment-related stress, but impaired glucose metabolism in the brain may contribute to depressive symptoms as well (Detka et al., 2013). Living with diabetes is also associated with greater risk for anxiety symptoms and impairments that can similarly interfere with critically important self-care behaviors (Penckofer, Ferrans, Velsor-Friedrich, & Savoy, 2007; Smith et al., 2013).

Social Aspects of Diabetes

A person's social environment can also strongly affect the experience of living with diabetes. Often, one of the most influential factors to consider is familial dynamics and support (Mier, Medina, & Ory, 2007; Penn, Moffatt, & White, 2008). The family is the context in which much of diabetes self-management occurs, and, as a result, the behaviors and beliefs of family members are often related to diabetes outcomes (Fisher et al., 2000). Family members can both facilitate healthy behaviors (e.g., encouraging exercise, planning healthy meals together), or sabotage the efforts of individuals with diabetes (e.g., bringing unhealthy food items into the house; Mayberry & Osborn, 2014). It is important to remember that diabetes and associated lifestyle changes may affect family and friends as well as the individual with the condition, and outcomes are typically better when all those affected come together, accept diabetes as a part of life, and adjust their lives accordingly (Coles, 1996; Glasgow & Toobert, 1988).

Neighborhood and community characteristics are also highly influential factors that affect the experience of people with diabetes (Deshpande, Baker, Lovegreen, & Brownson, 2005; Gary et al., 2008; Mier et al., 2007; Penn et al., 2008). Reduced access to exercise facilities and transportation, concerns about neighborhood safety, and poverty are all factors that can limit the ability of people with diabetes to engage in a healthy lifestyle and perform self-care behaviors, while stimulating and aesthetically pleasing environments, access to quality facilities, and available transportation can all promote healthy behaviors. Similarly, access to a large selection of high-quality health foods, including fresh fruits and vegetables and low-fat products, may go a long way in determining health outcomes for people with diabetes (Smalls, Gregory, Zoller, & Egede, 2014). Individuals must learn to effectively deal with complications that arise due to various social and environmental factors, such as eating in restaurants or in others' homes or finding ways to be physically active despite inclement weather or other unfavorable circumstances.

People with diabetes also frequently experience employment-related issues, which can place significant financial strain on these individuals, their families, and society at large. Compared to those without diabetes, people with diabetes are more likely to report work limitations and days of work lost due to impairment, are more likely to retire early and miss out on potential years of earnings, and are more likely to be unemployed (Breton et al., 2013; Herquelot, Guéguen, Bonenfant, & Dray-Spira, 2011; Tunceli et al., 2005; Von Korff et al., 2009). People with diabetes may also have greater occupational safety risks, including risks related to hypoglycemia and hyperglycemia, as well as risks resulting from diabetic complications, such as greater likelihood of infection after cuts (Falvo, 2009). Even in the absence of work impairments or significantly elevated risks, the working lives of people with diabetes may be affected by stereotypes, prejudice, and discrimination simply due to having the condition (McMahon, West, Mansouri, & Belongia, 2005).

Reduced earnings and high medical costs associated with diabetes both contribute to significant economic burden for many people and their families (Zhuo et al., 2014). Individuals with diabetes who are socially and economically disadvantaged may experience inadequate access to quality healthcare services and other resources (e.g., nutritious foods) that are important for improving and maintaining health (Drewnowski, 2009; Hill, Nielsen, & Fox, 2013; Raphael et al., 2012). Other barriers associated with poverty that negatively affect health outcomes include lack of quality health insurance coverage, limited participation in preventative healthcare, inadequate transportation, and social isolation (Hill et al., 2013; Zgibor & Songer, 2001).

Finally, negative societal attitudes toward people with diabetes is important to consider, as these can interfere with the adaptation process (Browne et al., 2013). A qualitative study with individuals with T2DM found that many participants felt stigmatized as a result of their condition or the co-occurring obesity that often accompanies the condition (Browne et al., 2013). Common themes described by individuals with T2DM include being viewed as lazy, being blamed for bringing the condition upon one's self, and being viewed less favorably in social interactions due to physical appearance. Some evidence also suggests that physicians commonly view diabetes as more difficult to treat than other chronic conditions and believe that many individuals lack sufficient motivation or understanding to treat their diabetes. As a result, negative attitudes from healthcare providers may adversely affect the treatment that people receive, as well as subsequent outcomes (Zgibor & Songer, 2001).

DIABETES SELF-MANAGEMENT

Diabetes self-management is the cornerstone of the overall management of diabetes (Lorig, Ritter, Villa, & Armas, 2009; Ruggiero et al., 1997). Healthcare providers can help individuals determine an appropriate medical regimen and provide diabetes education, but the day-to-day management of the condition is primarily the responsibility of the individual with diabetes. Each day, people with diabetes must make numerous decisions to engage in a healthy lifestyle and perform the necessary behaviors to successfully manage their condition. This is critically important, as the severity of diabetic complications and symptoms depends largely on one's ability to successfully perform self-management behaviors (Inzucchi et al., 2012).

Treatment goals for individuals with diabetes typically include improving blood glucose control and reducing risk of diabetic complications (Miller et al., 2015; Inzucchi et al., 2015). To accomplish these goals, lifestyle changes are often necessary to address problematic behaviors and increase health-promoting behaviors. The American Association of Diabetes Educators (AADE) identified a comprehensive list of seven diabetes self-care behaviors (AADE7) to address in diabetes care and diabetes self-management education (Mulcahy et al., 2003). These include (a) being physically active, (b) eating a healthy diet, (c) taking medication, (d) monitoring blood glucose, (e) problem-solving, (f) reducing risk of diabetes complications, and (g) psychosocial adaptation to living with diabetes. A joint position statement recently released by the ADA, the AADE, and the Academy of Nutrition and Dietetics endorsed similar key focus areas for diabetes self-management education and ongoing support (Powers et al., 2015). Comprehensive diabetes self-management education and support has been shown to improve HbA1c levels, reduce the onset and/or advancement of diabetic complications, and improve overall quality of life, suggesting that these behaviors are quite effective when integrated into a consistent self-management regimen (Powers et al., 2015).

However, the reality is that although many individuals are able to initiate short-term healthy lifestyle changes, they often struggle to successfully maintain these lifestyle changes long term (Toobert, Strycker, Barrera, & Glasgow, 2010), at least without ongoing intensive clinical intervention (Look AHEAD Research Group, 2010). Most people with diabetes do not engage in regular physical activity (Morrato, Hill, Wyatt, Ghushchyan, & Sullivan, 2007) and are less likely to engage in regular physical activity than people without diabetes (Zhao, Ford, Li, & Mokdad, 2008). Many people also find it extremely difficult to change their eating habits (Peel, Parry, Douglas, & Lawton, 2005), and the majority of individuals with diabetes do not meet general nutrition recommendations (Resnick, Foster, Bardsley, & Ratner, 2006). For example, one study found that only 26% of people with diabetes ate five or more servings of fruits or vegetables per day (Campbell, Khan, Cone, & Raisch, 2011). Approximately one out of four American adults with diabetes smokes cigarettes, despite evidence that cigarette smoking aggravates insulin resistance and significantly increases risk for cardiovascular disease and other diabetes complications (Clair, Bitton, Meigs, & Rigotti, 2011). Further, many people with diabetes also struggle to follow their diabetic medication regimen (Cramer, 2004). In light of these findings, it may not be surprising that only about 50% of adults with diabetes achieve the recommended goals for HbA_{1c}, blood pressure, and LDL cholesterol, and fewer than 20% meet all three targets (Casagrande, Fradkin, Saydah, Rust, & Cowie, 2013).

DIABETES SELF-MANAGEMENT BEHAVIORS

Effective strategies for helping individuals with diabetes successfully manage their condition are critically important for improving health outcomes. In this section, we review current knowledge and best practices for each of the self-management behaviors identified by the AADE, ADA, and Academy of Nutrition and Dietetics.

Exercise

Exercise is a standard recommendation for individuals with diabetes. For people with T1DM, exercise is recommended due to its numerous health benefits, including gains in physical fitness, improved insulin sensitivity, weight management, and psychological benefits (Chiang, Kirkman, Laffel, & Peters, 2014). The ADA (2016b) currently recommends that adults aim for at least 150 minutes of moderate-intensity aerobic exercise each week, spread over at least three days per week with no more than two consecutive days without exercising. Current guidelines also recommend muscle-strengthening activities involving all major muscle groups at least two days per week. When engaging in exercise, individuals with T1DM must be aware of unique considerations to avoid harmful consequences (Chiang et al., 2014). Risk of hypoglycemia increases during, immediately after, and about 7 to 11 hours postexercise, and individualized strategies must be developed to actively prevent and treat hypoglycemia. For most people with T1DM, it is safest to have a blood glucose level of 100 mg/dL prior to engaging in exercise, which can be achieved by reducing the prandial insulin dose before exercising or consuming additional food. Reducing insulin or consuming additional carbohydrates during prolonged periods of exercise can also help reduce hypoglycemia risk. People with T1DM may also experience hyperglycemia in the presence of insufficient insulin due to excessive hepatic glucose production and limited glucose uptake into skeletal muscles (Chiang et al., 2014). When people with T1DM are ketotic and deprived of insulin for 12 to 48 hours, exercise can worsen hyperglycemia and ketosis, and vigorous exercise should be avoided.

For individuals with T2DM, physical activity is a cornerstone of frontline treatment along with a healthful nutrition plan and antidiabetic medication (Nathan et al., 2009). As with T1DM, the ADA (2016b) currently recommends that individuals with T2DM aim for at least 150 minutes of moderate-intensity aerobic exercise each week and recommends participation in resistance training at least twice per week. The health benefits of physical activity for individuals with T2DM are immense and have been well documented in scientific literature. A recent review summarized a great deal of the existing research, presenting evidence for both acute and long-term effects of exercise on diabetic outcomes (Colberg et al., 2010). Some of the immediate benefits of physical activity include increased glucose uptake during exercise and reduced blood glucose after exercise. For people with T2DM, during moderate exercise, blood glucose utilization by muscles typically increases more than hepatic glucose production, resulting in a decline in blood glucose. Physical activity also improves insulin sensitivity and glucose tolerance, with effects corresponding to exercise duration and intensity. Improved insulin action is perhaps the most significant benefit of exercise for management of T2DM, with positive effects lasting from 2 to 72 hours postexercise (Colberg et al., 2010).

Longer-term health outcomes associated with physical activity are largely positive. Continued performance of physical activity leads to clinically significant improvements in insulin sensitivity, glycemic control, and fat oxidation (Colberg et al., 2010). Further, meta-analyses have found beneficial effects of exercise on key risk factors for cardiovascular disease, including blood pressure, blood lipids, and cardiorespiratory fitness (Boulé, Kenny, Haddad, Wells, & Sigal, 2003; Chudyk & Petrella, 2011; Hayashino, Jackson, Fukumori, Nakamura, & Fukuhara, 2012), although others have suggested that available evidence for the effects of exercise on blood pressure and lipids is still somewhat inconclusive (Colberg et al., 2010). Evidence that exercise promotes weight loss in individuals with diabetes is also limited. The amount of exercise needed to produce weight loss may be greater than the amount required for improvement in glycemic control. In addition, although studies have found little evidence to support an association between exercise and changes in body mass and scale weight (Boulé, Haddad, Kenny, Wells, & Sigal, 2001), such outcomes may not reflect changes in body composition that often result from exercising (i.e., gaining muscle mass while losing body fat; Colberg, 2007). Studies using alternative methods to assess changes in body composition, such as waist circumference and dual-energy X-ray absorptiometry, have shown favorable results from exercise (Church et al., 2010; Ross, Hudson, Stotz, & Lam, 2015).

Specific exercise interventions for diabetes management vary significantly and may range anywhere from a single group educational session (e.g., Polonsky, Zee, Yee, Crosson, & Jackson, 2005) to a full year of structured, supervised exercise sessions twice per week, along with ongoing individualized counseling (e.g., Balducci et al., 2010). Interventions often vary with regard to type, duration, volume, and intensity of exercise, with many different interventions demonstrating positive effects on health outcomes (Kavookjian, Elswick, & Whetsel, 2007). As a result, comprehensive reviews frequently conclude that no one form of exercise intervention is superior to others. Still, some general trends have been observed. Regarding type of exercise, existing evidence indicates that aerobic training, resistance training, and a combination of both aerobic and resistance training all lead to improved glycemic control, insulin sensitivity, and fat oxidation and storage in muscles, with some evidence that combined approaches confer the greatest benefit (Colberg et al., 2010; Kavookjian et al., 2007; Snowling & Hopkins, 2006; Umpierre et al., 2011; Yang, Scott, Mao, Tang, & Farmer, 2014). Interventions with higher intensity physical activity generally produce larger effects on glycemic control and cardiorespiratory fitness compared with lower intensity interventions (Colberg et al., 2010; Kavookjian et al., 2007). Similar results have been found for increasing the volume of exercise, with interventions of more than 150 minutes per week of exercise showing larger effects on HbA1c levels than interventions of fewer than 150 minutes (Umpierre et al., 2011). The duration of exercise interventions also appears to influence outcomes, with interventions lasting a minimum of 12 weeks producing larger effects on glycemic control than interventions lasting fewer than 12 weeks.

Exercise interventions also differ with regard to content, with some interventions including structured, supervised exercise sessions and others offering only counseling, education, and/or advice. Structured, supervised physical training sessions show consistent effects on exercise adherence and blood glucose control, while interventions offering advice and education alone often do not produce such favorable outcomes (Colberg et al., 2010; Kavookjian et al., 2007; Umpierre et al., 2011). This is concerning, as brief education and advice is often much more feasible in today's modern healthcare environments than extensive supervised exercise regimens (Karstoft et al., 2013).

Fortunately, initial evidence does also support behavior change approaches aimed at promoting "free living" physical activity, defined as physical activity performed on a person's own time in one's own environment (Avery, Flynn, van Wersch, Sniehotta, & Trenell, 2012). Further, available literature on exercise interventions for people with diabetes suggests that while many programs are effective at producing short-term behavior changes, long-term maintenance of exercise participation remains elusive. Long-term participation rates for self-management behaviors often decline drastically once the support of highly structured interventions is removed (Norris et al., 2002; Toobert et al., 2010). To facilitate long-term participation in physical activity, interventions will likely need to target psychological aspects of behavior change (e.g., motivation, self-efficacy) and capitalize on available supports in a person's environment (e.g., family, friends, neighborhood resources; Colberg et al., 2010; Praet & van Loon, 2009).

In summary, most reviews of exercise interventions for individuals with diabetes conclude that differences between types of exercises may be negligible, and the primary goal is to find an exercise regimen that the individual will actually perform (Kavookjian et al., 2007; Thomas, Elliot, & Naughton, 2006; Yang et al.,

2013). This means that attention should be given to individual considerations and preferences, such as cost, accessibility, convenience, level of ability, and enjoyment. It is important to note that vigorous exercise may not be appropriate for some people, and some forms of exercise may be contraindicated for some individuals as they may increase risk of injury. Individuals who take insulin and/or insulin secretagogues are at increased risk for hypoglycemia during physical activity and must learn to compensate for the effects of exercise with supplemental carbohydrate consumption or adjustments to insulin dosing. Still, physical activity is recommended for individuals with both T1DM and T2DM for reduced risk of cardiovascular complications, improved insulin sensitivity, weight loss, and improved quality of life (Kavookjian et al., 2007; Yardley, Hay, Abou-Setta, Marks, & McGavock, 2014). Readers are encouraged to see the position statement published by Colberg and associates (2010) for specific recommendations for evaluating individuals with diabetes prior to recommending exercise programs. In the absence of contraindications, individuals should be encouraged to participate in physical activity according to the guidelines put forth by the ADA.

Diet

Determining what to eat is often one of the most difficult aspects of diabetes self-management. Several times each day, individuals with diabetes must make decisions about what to eat, when to eat, and how much to eat, and these decisions are affected by factors such as food availability, family eating patterns, personal preferences, and knowledge of the relationship between nutrition and health (Mulcahy et al., 2003). Due to the complex nature of dietary decisions, as well as a lack of evidence to support one plan over all others, the ADA (2016b) has taken the position that there is no one-size-fits-all eating plan that is appropriate for all people with diabetes. Instead, the ADA recommends that each individual work with his or her healthcare provider to develop an individualized eating plan as part of a comprehensive self-management program.

The current gold standard for dietary intervention in diabetes care is medical nutrition therapy (MNT). MNT is an evidence-based practice provided by registered dietitian nutritionists to assist people with diabetes in developing individualized eating plans and improving diabetes management (Pastors, Franz, Warshaw, Daly, & Arnold, 2003; Franz et al., 2010). The key components of MNT include an individualized nutrition assessment, nutrition diagnosis, intervention and monitoring, and evaluation (Powers et al., 2015). Effective MNT for individuals with diabetes ideally includes a series of at least three to four sessions with a registered dietitian nutritionist lasting from 45 to 90 minutes, which should begin at diagnosis of diabetes or at first referral to a registered dietitian nutritionist, and should be completed within three to six months. At least one follow-up session is recommended annually to reinforce lifestyle changes and determine if changes to the plan are indicated. Goals of MNT for diabetes frequently include improvement in overall glycemic control, improved postprandial glycemic control, prevention of hypoglycemia, achievement of lipid and blood pressure goals, weight management, and management of medical complications and co-occurring impairments (ADA, 2016b; Powers et al., 2015). MNT should be individualized and should aim to address individual nutrition needs while maintaining the pleasure of eating (ADA, 2016b; Franz, 2007).

While existing research indicates that dietary interventions are generally effective for improving diabetic outcomes (Brown, Upchurch, Anding, Winter, & Ramirez, 1996; Padgett, Mumford, Hynes, & Carter, 1988), as noted already, there is no one ideal dietary pattern that is expected to benefit all individuals with diabetes. Available evidence suggests that a number of different eating patterns may potentially lead to improvement in glycemic control and/or cardiovascular risk, including a Mediterranean-style diet, a vegetarian diet, a low-carbohydrate diet, and a low-fat diet, but these eating patterns may be inappropriate for some individuals, and observed effects may depend largely upon a reduction in total energy intake (Evert et al., 2013). One meta-analysis found evidence that low-glycemic index diets may lead to better blood glucose control than high-glycemic index diets (Brand-Miller, Hayne, Petocz, & Colaguiri, 2003), but others caution that research surrounding diets based on glycemic load is inconclusive (Evert et al., 2013). For individuals with T1DM and those with T2DM treated with insulin, training in flexible insulin therapy using the carbohydrate-counting approach is encouraged for optimizing glycemic control (Powers et al., 2015). This approach involves adjusting insulin doses based on planned carbohydrate intake. For individuals using fixed daily insulin doses, carbohydrate intake should remain consistent on a day-to-day basis with respect to time and amount.

Some general strategies that may be of benefit to some individuals with diabetes include reduced energy intake, carbohydrate counting, simplified meal plans, healthful food choices, food exchange lists, and meal planning based on insulin-to-carbohydrate ratios (Evert et al., 2013; Franz, 2007). Still, what may be most important is tailoring interventions to individual treatment goals and personal preferences. A healthful eating plan is only effective if it is actually followed. When assisting an individual with diabetes in developing an eating plan, it is critical that personal, health, cultural, and socioeconomic factors are considered to determine the most appropriate form of intervention.

Medication

For individuals with T1DM, insulin-replacement therapy is the primary pharmacological treatment, and use of other medications for blood-glucose control is rare (Miller et al., 2015; Odegard & Capoccia, 2007). Insulin therapy is typically administered through injections or insulin pumps, depending on individual needs and preferences. As of 2014, approximately 60% of individuals with T1DM used insulin pumps (Miller et al., 2015). A landmark clinical trial demonstrated that intensive insulin therapy aimed at achieving glycemic levels as close to the non-diabetic range as possible can significantly reduce the risk of severe microvascular complications and cardiovascular disease among individuals with T1DM who have had the condition between 1 and 15 years (Nathan & DCCT/EDIC Research Group, 2014).

For many individuals with T2DM, pharmacological therapy is also is a key aspect of treatment for achieving and maintaining glycemic control (Ho et al., 2006; Krapek et al., 2004; Odegard & Capoccia, 2007). Current best practices in diabetes care recommend personalized medication regimens that take into account potential benefits and risks, individual characteristics, adverse effects, cost, and other factors (Inzucchi et al., 2012; Inzucchi et al., 2015). In most cases, metformin is considered the optimal drug for monotherapy, due to its effectiveness for reducing hepatic glucose production, proven safety record, low cost, weight neutrality, and possible benefits on cardiovascular outcomes. In instances when metformin is contraindicated or combination therapy is warranted, a number of other classes of medications may be used in T2DM treatment, including sulfonylureas, thiazolidinediones, glucagon-like peptide-1 receptor agonists, and sodium-glucose cotransporter 2 inhibitors (for a more thorough review of pharmacotherapy for T2DM, see Inzucchi et al., 2012 and Inzucchi et al., 2015). Each class of diabetic medication has unique effects on metabolic processes, as well as associated advantages and disadvantages that must be considered in relation to each individual.

Insulin replacement therapy is also frequently required for people with T2DM due to progressive β-cell dysfunction. The goal of insulin therapy is to create as normal a glycemic profile as possible while avoiding hypoglycemia or unacceptable weight gain. As with other diabetic medications, insulin therapy should ideally be tailored to each individual to match the supply of insulin to dietary and exercise habits and their effects on blood glucose trends (Inzucchi et al., 2012; Inzucchi et al., 2015). Research has demonstrated that achieving glycemic control through intensive treatment with medication and/or insulin may reduce risk of cardiovascular disease and microvascular complications in individuals with newly diagnosed T2DM (Holman, Paul, Bethel, Matthews, & Neil, 2008). For those with more advanced T2DM, intensive pharmacotherapy has not demonstrated clear benefits for reducing cardiovascular disease, and potential beneficial effects on microvascular complications must be weighed against risk of severe hypoglycemia, mortality, and other adverse outcomes (ADVANCE Collaborative Group, 2008; Ismail-Beigi et al., 2010).

For diabetes treatment to be effective, taking medication as prescribed is often required. Unfortunately, it is quite common for adverse outcomes to occur when medication regimens are not followed (Ho et al., 2006; Melikian, White, Vanderplas, Dezii, & Chang, 2002). In published research, the proportion of individuals taking diabetic medication as prescribed varies widely, and ranges anywhere from 31% to 87% (Odegard & Capoccia, 2007). Therefore, to promote effective diabetes self-management practices, individuals with diabetes and healthcare providers must collaborate in the development of medication regimens, and must discuss strategies for ensuring that diabetic medication is taken as prescribed.

Understanding existing barriers to taking medication as prescribed is the first step toward improving outcomes. Odegard and Capoccia (2007) listed commonly reported individual, medication, and provider-related barriers to taking diabetes medication. Individual-related barriers include fears (e.g., weight gain, hypoglycemia), low levels of self-efficacy, lack of confidence in the benefits of the medication, depressive symptoms, and remembering doses and refills. Medication-related barriers include complexity of medication regimen, frequency of dosing, cost of medications, and adverse effects of medications. Provider-related barriers include lack of time or resources to train individuals and follow-up sufficiently and limited knowledge or skills on the part of some providers for treating diabetes effectively. Similar barriers have also been identified specifically for the use of insulin therapy and other injectable medications, including resistance and fear, inconvenience, financial costs, inadequate support and healthcare resources, and physician resistance (i.e., avoiding advancement to insulin therapy in T2DM due to fear that individuals would not be able to use it effectively; Meece, 2006; Polonsky, Fisher, Guzman, Villa-Caballero, & Edelman, 2005; Siminerio, 2006).

Healthcare providers must work with individuals with diabetes to develop strategies for overcoming barriers to taking medication as prescribed (Odegard & Capoccia, 2007). For example, simplifying medication regimens, improving individual motivation and understanding, and addressing psychological barriers like depression may all potentially improve participation in treatment. Unfortunately, few intervention studies are available from which to glean information about best practices. One study found that mailed medication refill reminders and unit-dose packaging may both improve participation rates over standard care, with the combination of these two approaches producing perhaps the greatest benefit (Skaer, Sclar, Markowski, & Won, 1993). Other promising interventions with initial empirical support include brief counseling and follow-up calls from pharmacists after missed refills (Odegard & Christensen, 2012), automated medication monitoring and text message reminders (Vervloet et al., 2012), regular phone calls from health educators every four to six weeks (Walker et al., 2011), and health education interventions enhanced with pictorial images or a "teach back" strategy (Negarandeh, Mahmoodi, Noktehdan, Heshmat, & Shakibazadeh, 2013).

As a general rule, effective communication between healthcare providers and recipients may also be important for addressing concerns of individuals with diabetes and increasing participation in pharmaceutical treatment regimens (Grant, Devita, Singer, & Meigs, 2003). In clinical practice, healthcare providers must work with each individual to identify relevant barriers to taking medication as prescribed and create individualized strategies for addressing each area of concern (Letassy, 2007). It is also important that healthcare providers employ culturally sensitive approaches, seek input from care recipients about their perspectives on taking medication, and remain alert to opportunities to provide further education and clarification (Meece, 2006). Finally, healthcare providers should consider providing ongoing assessment and follow-up to monitor and address participation in treatment regimens over time (Odegard & Capoccia, 2007).

Self-Monitoring of Blood Glucose

Self-monitoring of blood glucose (SMBG) is a key element of treatment for many individuals with diabetes (Funnell, 2007; Mulcahy et al., 2003). The goals of SMBG are to (a) maintain day-to-day glycemic control and enable individuals to make appropriate adjustments to their diet or diabetic medication, (b) equip healthcare providers with information about individuals with diabetes' day-to-day glycemic control that can inform treatment plans, and (c) improve detection of hypoglycemia and hyperglycemia (Benjamin, 2002; Gallichan, 1997). Thus SMBG empowers individuals with diabetes to monitor their own condition and allows both care recipients and providers to assess the effectiveness of the current treatment plan (ADA, 2016c).

SMBG is a critical aspect of self-management for individuals with T1DM. Self-monitoring with glucometers remains the most common approach, with the average person testing about four to six times per day. Continuous glucose monitoring systems are also gaining popularity and may provide additional benefits for improving glycemic control and reducing severe hypoglycemia (Choudhary et al., 2013; Deiss et al., 2006).

SMBG is also widely recognized as a best practice for improving blood glucose control in individuals with T2DM treated with insulin (Funnell, 2007; McAndrew, Schneider, Burns, & Leventhal, 2007). However, recommending SMBG for individuals with T2DM not treated with insulin is more controversial. Some suggest that SMBG can still be an effective method for enhancing diabetes self-efficacy, empowering individuals to take personal responsibility for their health status, and improving glycemic control when used in a structured and intentional manner (Polonsky & Fisher, 2013). Others argue against the use of SMBG for individuals with T2DM not treated with insulin, claiming that there is insufficient evidence for a clinically relevant effect and that the huge costs associated with SMBG materials (e.g., meters, test strips, lancets, lancing devices, batteries) could be better spent on other more effective treatment strategies for this group (Malanda, Bot, & Nijpels, 2013).

For SMBG to be effective, individuals must be competent in the multiple steps of the self-monitoring process and must use the practice in a goal-oriented manner (McAndrew et al., 2007). They must know how to take and understand the reading, connect deviant readings with prior behavior, and create and implement an action plan to adjust behaviors and control blood glucose levels based on the data. When used effectively, SMBG has the potential to improve understanding of how foods, physical activity, and medications affect blood glucose levels, and individuals can use this information to tailor their behaviors and maintain tighter control (AADE, 2009).

Based on a review by McAndrew and colleagues (2007), Funnell (2007) identified several strategies that healthcare providers can use to improve the effectiveness of SMBG. These strategies include (a) emphasizing that SMBG is an important guide for making personal decisions, not just for obtaining information for healthcare providers; (b) reminding individuals that the results are not a judgment of their efforts but simply a number to use in decision-making; (c) helping individuals deal with results that do not reflect their efforts; and (d) helping people develop strategies to obtain necessary support from others and role-play responses to negative comments from family members and healthcare providers. These strategies can be used in addition to individualized goal-setting and addressing potential barriers to create a comprehensive plan for incorporating SMBG into individuals' self-management programs. Healthcare providers should collaborate with people with diabetes to develop a SMBG plan that will fit with each individual's own unique circumstances (McAndrew et al., 2007).

Problem-Solving

Problem-solving refers to the process of identifying a problem, forming a list of potential solutions, selecting and implementing the most appropriate strategy, and evaluating the effectiveness of the strategy (D'Zurilla & Goldfried, 1971). Learning to solve problems is critically important for effective diabetes self-management because it facilitates other self-management behaviors in the presence of obstacles (Mulcahy et al., 2003). To manage blood glucose levels and address fluctuations, people with diabetes frequently must make decisions about food, physical activity, and medication adjustments. Therefore, learning effective strategies for solving problems and making decisions enables individuals with diabetes to more successfully manage their condition.

Hill-Briggs (2003) created a model of problem-solving adapted to diabetes self-management based on cognitive psychology theories and social problem-solving theory. The model identifies four major components of diabetes-specific problem-solving: (a) problem-solving orientation, (b) problem-solving process, (c) transfer of past learning, and (d) diabetes-specific knowledge. Problem-solving orientation refers to a person's attitudes and beliefs about managing the condition, as well as beliefs about one's own capacity for dealing with problems. Problem-solving process refers to how one attempts to solve problems and can be either effective (i.e., rational) or ineffective (i.e., careless or avoidant). Transfer of past learning refers to one's ability to use past experiences to adjust future behavior. Diabetes-specific knowledge refers to the degree to which an individual has sufficient knowledge for addressing a problem and is able to apply that knowledge to manage his or her condition. In a qualitative study examining this model, participants with well-controlled and poorly controlled diabetes identified similar problems but differed in their approaches to problem-solving according to the key dimensions of the model (Hill-Briggs, Cooper, Loman, Brancati, & Cooper, 2003).

There are a number of ways that healthcare providers can assess problem-solving skills, with different instruments designed for a variety of purposes and respondents (Hill-Briggs & Gemmell, 2007). One of the more frequently used approaches is to present vignettes with hypothetical problematic situations and ask participants to describe how they would respond. An example specifically designed for adults with T2DM is the Diabetes Problem-Solving Inventory (Glasgow, Toobert, Barrera, & Strycker, 2004), which allows healthcare providers to evaluate and address ineffective problem-solving strategies. Another example is the Diabetes Numeracy Test (Huizinga et al., 2008), which assesses a respondent's ability to use numeracy skills often required for effective diabetes self-management (e.g., calculating amount of carbohydrates consumed or number of test strips needed for a two-week vacation).

Two systematic reviews have captured much of what is known about the effectiveness of problem-solving interventions for people with diabetes. Hill-Briggs and Gemmell (2007), in a review of studies conducted between 1990 and 2006, found that problem-solving interventions tend to demonstrate significant improvements in problem-solving skills and frequently lead to improvements in isolated self-management behaviors, including diet, exercise, and SMBG. Evidence for effects of problem-solving interventions on glycemic control was less clear, with 50% of studies reporting significant improvements in HbA1c. Hill-Briggs and Gemmell concluded that problem-solving interventions show promising results for facilitating behavior change and alleviating depression. In a more recent review of studies conducted between 2006 and 2012, Fitzpatrick, Schumann, and Hill-Briggs (2013) found similar positive effects of problem-solving interventions on problem-solving ability, but reported more inconsistent effects of problem-solving interventions on self-management behaviors and glycemic control.

Available evidence suggests that interventions may be more effective if they are delivered over multiple sessions instead of a single session. For example, Hill-Briggs and colleagues (2011) compared an intensive problem-solving intervention with eight weekly group sessions to a condensed single group session and found that participants in the intensive intervention group showed greater improvements in problem-solving ability, self-management behaviors, and HbA1c.

Problem-solving skills may be particularly important for people with T1DM and T2DM treated with insulin, as dietary choices, physical activity, and medication can all cause fluctuations in blood glucose levels that may require behavioral responses (Mulcahy et al., 2003). Individuals must develop awareness of their own blood glucose levels, including the effects of lifestyle factors and the physical signs and symptoms associated with blood glucose variations. Individuals with diabetes must also learn how to respond appropriately to the wide variety of challenging situations that can occur. Goals of problem-solving interventions should target both acute concerns (e.g., hypoglycemia recognition and reaction), as well as the bigger picture concern of establishing a lifestyle that minimizes blood glucose fluctuation.

Reducing Risks

As mentioned, diabetic complications may affect numerous body organs (e.g., heart, brain, muscles, skin, and kidneys; ADA, 2016b; Fowler, 2008), and individuals with diabetes are at increased risk for many health problems, including cardiovascular disease, renal impairments, blindness, amputations of the legs and feet, and early death (ADA, 2016b, 2016e). Understanding these risks, as well as actions one can take to mitigate these risks, are crucial aspects of effective diabetes self-management. However, many barriers may interfere with risk-reduction behavior, including financial constraints, lack of awareness, social-environmental influences, and mobility limitations. Therefore, it is important for individuals with diabetes to receive support to overcome barriers and reduce health risks (Boren, Gunlock, Schaefer, & Albright, 2007).

Reducing risks refers to implementing behaviors that prevent or slow the progression of diabetes complications (Boren et al., 2007). This involves having an accurate understanding of complications and their prevalence and seeking appropriate preventive healthcare services to maintain adequate health (Boren et al., 2007; Mulcahy et al., 2003). In their systematic literature review, Boren and colleagues identified seven categories of risk-reducing behaviors: (a) smoking cessation, (b) eye examination, (c) foot care, (d) cardiovascular risk reduction, (e) oral health, (f) vaccination, and (g) combined risk reduction. For example, evidence indicates that individuals with diabetes who smoke cigarettes have significantly greater risk for developing cardiovascular disease (Fagard & Nilsson, 2009; Tonstad, 2009), nephropathy (Gambaro et al., 2001), and peripheral vascular problems (Adler et al., 2002). Healthcare providers should routinely ask individuals with diabetes about their smoking status and advise smokers to quit smoking. Individuals with diabetes are more likely to quit smoking if they receive advice from several healthcare providers on multiple occasions (Hokanson, Anderson, Hennrikus, Lando, & Kendall, 2006).

Diabetic retinopathy is a major cause of visual impairment among adults in the United States (Eye Diseases Prevalence Research Group, 2004). Historically, the majority of individuals with diabetes experienced some form of retinopathy within two decades of living with the condition (Fong et al., 2004). Recent improvements in self-management practices appear to be having a beneficial impact on the incidence and progression of diabetic retinopathy, but retinopathy remains a serious cause of impairment for many people with diabetes (Klein, Knudtson, Lee, Gangnon, & Klein, 2008). Therefore, routine eye examinations constitute a major risk-reducing behavior in comprehensive diabetes self-management (Mulcahy et al., 2003). The ADA (2016e) currently recommends that adults with T1DM have an initial dilated and comprehensive eye examination within five years after onset of diabetes, and individuals with T2DM should have an initial dilated and comprehensive eye examination at the time of diagnosis. If there is no evidence of retinopathy for one or more annual eye exams, then exams every two years may be considered. In the presence of retinopathy, dilated retinal examinations are recommended at least annually, with more frequent examinations if the retinopathy is progressing or sight-threatening (ADA, 2016e).

Foot ulcers and amputations are also common complications among individuals with diabetes that result from diabetic neuropathy and/or peripheral arterial disease (ADA, 2016e) and have a significant adverse impact on health-related quality of life (Tennvall & Apelqvist, 2000; Valensi et al., 2005). Although the risk of developing foot ulcers is high among individuals with diabetes, appropriate screening and intervention measures may reduce this risk (Singh, Armstrong, & Lipsky, 2005). Smoking cessation, intensive podiatric care, optimizing glycemic control, and debridement of calluses are known effective interventions for reducing the risk of foot ulcers (Singh et al., 2005). In addition, daily self-examination may reduce and prevent foot ulcers; therefore, individuals with peripheral neuropathy should examine their feet for ulcers daily (Chin, Huang, & Hsu, 2013). Research has shown that educational interventions can indeed improve foot care knowledge and behavior (Corbett, 2003; Fan, Sidani, Cooper-Brathwaite, & Metcalfe, 2014).

Cardiovascular disease is common among individuals with diabetes, and cardiovascular risk reduction interventions should be considered paramount in diabetes care (Selvin et al., 2004). The ADA (2016d) recommends that all individuals with diabetes be assessed for cardiovascular risk factors at least annually. These risk factors include dyslipidemia, hypertension, smoking, family history of cardiovascular disease, and the presence of albuminuria. Both pharmacological interventions and lifestyle modifications may be beneficial for reducing cardiovascular risks (ADA, 2016d). Treatment approaches vary widely and may incorporate individualized education, counseling, medication management, and telephone contacts to target an assortment of risk-reducing behaviors (Boren et al., 2007). For example, individuals with T2DM in one study who received cardiovascular risk reduction training and counseling reduced their consumption of red meat and fast food, increased water consumption, and increased physical activity levels, all of which may reduce risk of cardiovascular complications (Çevik, Özcan, & Satman, 2015).

Finally, individuals with diabetes often have compromised immune functioning, which increases risk of developing infectious diseases, including serious bacterial infections (Shah & Hux, 2003) and oral infections (Jones et al., 2007). Infections increase risk of mortality and may also exacerbate metabolic dysfunction (Kiran, Arpak, Unsal, & Erdogan, 2005). As a result, individuals with diabetes should engage in routine preventive health practices, including receiving vaccinations and routine dental examinations (Boren et al., 2007). While research in this area is limited, existing evidence suggests that educational interventions can increase performance of preventive behaviors by individuals with diabetes (Latessa, Cummings, Lilley, & Morrissey, 2000).

Coping and Psychosocial Adaptation

Living with a chronic condition like diabetes presents many life challenges. In addition to dealing with the vicissitudes of life, living with diabetes may add several layers of stressors including social stigma, social isolation, unpleasant symptoms, functional limitations, employment problems, and financial burden. These stressors in the lives of people with diabetes can cause anger, frustration, anxiety, depression, and other psychosocial adjustment problems. Recognizing the interconnection among coping, behavior, emotions, and metabolism in diabetes management, the AADE has identified healthy coping as one of seven key diabetes management behaviors that needs to be incorporated in diabetes self-management education programs (Fisher, Thorpe, DeVellis, & DeVellis, 2007). Research has indicated that although complex treatment regimens and the presence of diabetic complications may negatively affect quality of life, psychological characteristics and socioenvironmental factors may have an equivalent or even stronger influence on quality of life than clinical aspects of diabetes (Fisher et al., 2007; Rubin & Peyrot, 1999). External locus of control, avoidance coping, and number of stressful life events are associated with poorer metabolic control, while internal locus of control, problem-solving coping, social support, and positive orientation are associated with better metabolic control (Fisher et al., 2007). In addition, psychosocial research has shown that depression and emotional problems are associated with poorer treatment engagement (Gonzalez et al., 2008). Co-occurring depression is highly prevalent among individuals with diabetes; the age-adjusted prevalence rate of major depression for people with diabetes was estimated to be 8.3% (Li, Ford, Strine, & Mokdad, 2008) and 28% to 44% for self-reported minimal-mild depression (Fisher et al., 2007). Other emotional problems that are common among individuals with diabetes include anxiety and social withdrawal. Individuals with diabetes are also at greater risk for eating disorders (Herpertz et al., 1998) and sexual dysfunction (De Berardis et al., 2002; Enzlin, Mathieu, Van den Bruel, Vanderschueren, & Demyttenaere, 2003). Therefore, helping individuals develop healthy coping skills to deal with the challenges of living with diabetes is critically important, as is encouraging participation in mental health treatment for depression and other psychological concerns when appropriate.

In their systematic review, Fisher and colleagues (2007) concluded that including healthy coping training and mental health treatment in diabetes self-management education may result in decreased psychological distress, improved treatment engagement, and better overall quality of life. Their review provided empirical support for several types of coping and mental health interventions. Cognitive-behavioral therapy has been found to reduce depressive symptoms, increase acceptance of diabetes, and contribute to improvements in HbA1c. Problem-solving interventions have also been shown to enhance self-management outcomes, as described earlier in this chapter. Additionally, antidepressant medication appears to be effective for individuals with diabetes and co-occurring depression for improving mood; it may also facilitate weight loss and increased participation in pharmacotherapy. Additional research is needed before drawing conclusions about whether specific interventions may be indicated for specific groups of people with diabetes. However, when selecting an intervention to facilitate psychosocial adjustment to diabetes, it is critically important that healthcare providers recognize that the need for effective coping strategies is often substantial and ongoing, as individuals frequently contend with a myriad of challenges, including stress and depression, co-occurring medical conditions, relationship issues, and vocational concerns.

STRATEGIES FOR IMPROVING DIABETES SELF-MANAGEMENT

This section discusses methods for enhancing diabetes self-management efforts. These include integrating diabetes self-management interventions into comprehensive, theory-driven education programs and using technological resources to enhance outcomes.

Diabetes Self-Management Education Programs

The key self-management behaviors identified by the AADE and ADA provide a solid foundation for conceptualizing diabetes self-management interventions. These content domains can be used to develop a comprehensive diabetes self-management education program. The importance of motivating individuals with diabetes to develop and use self-management skills to control the effect of diabetes on their lives is well-documented (Lorig et al., 2009). The extent to which individuals manage their condition depends more on what they do for themselves than on what services are provided to them (Funnell & Andereson, 2004). People with diabetes need to engage in health-promoting behaviors, address symptoms and co-occurring conditions, and build working relationships with healthcare providers (Lorig et al., 2009). They also need to learn to perform self-care behaviors using multiple problem-solving and coping strategies (Fisher et al., 2007; Hill-Briggs & Gemmell, 2007). However, making behavior change is notoriously difficult because non-adaptive behaviors are often deeply ingrained and automatic to the individual. Learning and practicing adaptive self-management behaviors may seem unpleasant or overwhelming, and these critical health-promoting behaviors may not occur if the individual is ambivalent or insufficiently motivated. As a result, many self-management interventions for people with chronic health conditions tend to underscore the importance of behavioral interventions based on prominent motivational theories (Lorig et al., 2009; Tulloch et al., 2009).

One of the most recognized intervention programs is the Diabetes Self-Management Program (DSMP) developed by Dr. Kate Lorig at Stanford University. It was developed based on Bandura's (1989, 2004) self-efficacy theory to help people with T2DM learn self-care skills and gain confidence in their ability to manage their health and maintain active and fulfilling lives. It is a six-week course facilitated by two trained leaders, one or both of whom are peer leaders with diabetes themselves. The workshops are held in community settings such as senior centers, churches, libraries, and hospitals. Participants meet weekly for two hours to learn and practice techniques for building a diabetes self-management program tailored to their own needs. Workshops include educational sessions covering five topics: (a) techniques to deal with the symptoms of diabetes, fatigue, pain, hyper/hypoglycemia, stress, and emotional problems, such as depression, anger, fear and frustration; (b) appropriate exercise for maintaining and improving strength and endurance; (c) healthy eating; (d) appropriate use of medication; and (e) working more effectively with healthcare providers. Participants are taught to make weekly action plans, share experiences, and help each other solve problems they encounter in creating and carrying out their self-management programs. Participants also participate in group discussions to obtain feedback and suggestions from their peers about coping with diabetes-related problems and practice suggested approaches at home and report their progress in group discussion. Each participant also receives the *Living a Healthy Life with Chronic Conditions* (4th ed.) text, which contains all of the program content. In a randomized controlled trial to test the efficacy of the DSMP with 345 adults with T2DM, Lorig and colleagues (2009) found that individuals in the treatment group had significant improvements in depression, symptoms of hypoglycemia, communication with physicians, healthy eating, reading food labels, patient activation, and self-efficacy. The CDC also conducted a review and meta-analysis of Stanford's Chronic Disease Self-Management Programs across a variety of chronic health conditions (Brady et al., 2013). The review included 23 studies with 8,688 individuals. Results revealed significant small to moderate effect sizes for improvements in aerobic exercise, stretching/strengthening exercise, cognitive symptom management, and psychological health.

These results highlight the multitude of potential benefits individuals may receive from a comprehensive intervention informed by behavior change theory. The ADA's (2016b) current standards of care emphasize holistic, person-centered services that address the multiple aspects of diabetes self-management while taking into account the individual's values and life circumstances. As described in earlier sections of this chapter, numerous intervention options exist that target a wide range of specific self-management behaviors, and ample resources are available for developing multifaceted, multidisciplinary interventions. While no single intervention will be appropriate for all individuals, the ADA (2016b) guidelines for diabetes self-management education and support and the identified AADE7 diabetes self-management behaviors (Mulcahy et al., 2003) provide a solid foundation from which individualized treatment plans can be developed.

Technology-Based Interventions

In this exciting time of rapid technological innovation and proliferation of digital devices, technology-based interventions may hold enormous promise for augmenting existing diabetes self-management programs. Making multiple behavior changes is complicated and difficult, and individuals must often track and interpret large amounts of data, such as fluctuating blood glucose levels, amount of exercise performed, overall energy consumption, carbohydrate consumption, and medication administered (El-Gayar, Timsina, Nawar, & Eid, 2013). Individuals must also monitor their own behavior, remember to perform self-management tasks, and stay motivated despite setbacks and frustrations (Hunt, 2015). Fortunately, technology-based resources like mobile applications and computer-based tools are being created to address these concerns.

Mobile phones are perhaps the most practical means of increasing individual engagement in healthcare (Boland, 2007). 90% of US adults have access to a cell phone (Forgays, Hyman, & Schreiber, 2014), and 64% own a smartphone (Pew Research Center, 2015). A review of diabetes self-management phone applications (apps) found that apps are currently available to assist users with all of the self-management activities described in this chapter (El-Gayar et al., 2013). The most common features are support for exercise, diet, SMBG, and taking medication. Some apps also offer additional features, like social support, aids for reducing health risks, and assistance with problem-solving and decision-making related to insulin dosing. Future efforts to enhance these technologies (e.g., personalized education and support, automated data upload) should only serve to increase the potential value of these tools (El-Gayar et al., 2013). Text messaging, voice mail, and email functions of mobile phones have also been used to facilitate flow of information between individuals and providers, offer advice and support between clinic visits, and deliver reminders to prompt health behaviors (Krishna & Boren, 2008). The results of existing studies indicate that mobile phones have the potential to enhance diabetes self-management outcomes, with positive results found for self-management self-efficacy, performance of health behaviors, and HbA1c (Krishna & Boren, 2008; Saffari, Ghanizadeh, & Koenig, 2014). There is some evidence that mobile-phone interventions may help individuals with T2DM improve glycemic control and maintain improvements for up to 12 months (Yoon & Kim, 2008). However, others caution that evidence for long-term persistent use and long-term effectiveness of these self-management technologies is currently limited (Garabedian, Ross-Degnan, & Wharam, 2015).

Computer and Internet-based interventions have also been developed to assist individuals with diabetes self-management efforts. Similar to interventions using mobile phones, computer and Internet-based interventions are appealing options because they can be available 24 hours per day, may be cost-effective, and can free healthcare providers to focus on other healthcare priorities (Glasgow et al., 2010). Computer and Internet-based interventions may provide a variety of features, including educational content, goal-setting, behavior tracking, and individualized feedback and support (Hunt, 2015). A recent systematic review and meta-analysis found small, beneficial effects of computer and Internet-based diabetes self-management interventions on HbA1c outcomes (Pal et al., 2014), and some individual studies have found positive effects on specific behavior changes, such as increased physical activity and improved diet (Christian et al., 2008; Glasgow et al., 2010). Some of the most effective aspects of these tools appear to be behavioral tracking, tailored feedback based on performance, and assistance with action planning (Pal et al., 2014).

Overall, both mobile phone and computer and Internet-based interventions appear to be valuable additions to comprehensive diabetes self-management programs. Mobile–phone interventions appear to provide superior benefits, perhaps due to greater convenience and more rapid and frequent contacts (Pal et al., 2014).

It is important to note that current evidence does not support technology-based interventions as stand-alone treatments but rather as supplemental interventions that can provide cost-effective assistance between clinic visits to enhance participation in self-management activities (Hunt, 2015; Krishna & Boren, 2008). As digital devices become increasingly popular and technology-based resources continue to be developed and refined, it is likely that mobile phone and computer-based interventions will become more prominent components of diabetes self-management programs. Still, healthcare providers must consider individual variables, such as literacy, financial resources, and personal preferences when incorporating technology-based strategies into self-management programs.

CONCLUSION

In this chapter, we provided an overview of the biopsychosocial aspects of diabetes, described seven key areas of self-care behaviors, and discussed the current state of diabetes management practices and research. Our review identified numerous interventions that have demonstrated beneficial effects on a wide range of clinical outcomes. This review of the literature also indicated treatment engagement remains problematic for individuals with diabetes. In recent years, healthcare providers and researchers have called for person-centered, comprehensive treatment approaches and have explored interventions guided by behavioral theories and supplemented by technological components. These advances will hopefully lead to improved long-term outcomes for individuals with diabetes. It is essential that diabetes self-management programs encourage and empower people to actively participate in all aspects of managing their chronic health conditions.

REFERENCES

Abdul-Ghani, M. A. (2013). Type 2 diabetes and the evolving paradigm in glucose regulation. *American Journal of Managed Care, 19*(Suppl. 3), S43–S50.

Adler, A. I., Stevens, R. J., Neil, A., Stratton, I. M., Boulton, A. J. M., & Holman, R. R. (2002). UKPDS 59: Hyperglycemia and other potentially modifiable risk factors for peripheral vascular disease in type 2 diabetes. *Diabetes Care, 25,* 894–899.

ADVANCE Collaborative Group. (2008). Intensive blood glucose control and vascular outcomes in patients with type 2 diabetes. *The New England Journal of Medicine, 358,* 2560–2572. doi:10.1056/NEJMoa0802987

American Association of Diabetes Educators. (2009). AADE guidelines for the practice of diabetes self-management education and training (DSME/T). *Diabetes Educator, 35*(Suppl. 3), 85S–107S. doi:10.1177/0145721709352436

American Diabetes Association. (2016a). 2. Classification and diagnosis of diabetes. *Diabetes Care, 39*(Suppl. 1), S13–S22. doi:10.2337/dc16-S005

American Diabetes Association. (2016b). 3. Foundations of care and comprehensive medical evaluation. *Diabetes Care, 39*(Suppl. 1), S23–S35. doi:10.2337/dc16-S006

American Diabetes Association. (2016c). 5. Glycemic targets. *Diabetes Care, 39*(Suppl. 1), S39–S46. doi:10.2337/dc16-S0008

American Diabetes Association. (2016d). 8. Cardiovascular disease and risk management. *Diabetes Care, 39*(Suppl. 1), S60–S71. doi:10.2337/dc16-2011

American Diabetes Association. (2016e). 9. Microvascular complications and foot care. *Diabetes Care, 39*(Suppl. 1), S72–S80. doi:10.2337/dc16-S012

Amin, A., Lau, L., Crawford, S., Edwards, A., & Pacaud, D. (2014). Prospective assessment of hypoglycemia symptoms in children and adults with type 1 diabetes. *Canadian Journal of Diabetes, 38*, 263–268. doi:10.1016/j.jcjd.2014.05.007

Anderson, R. J., Freedland, K. E., Clouse, R. E., & Lustman, P. J. (2001). The prevalence of comorbid depression in adults with diabetes: A meta-analysis. *Diabetes Care, 24*, 1069–1078.

Ashcroft, F. M., & Rorsman, P. (2012). Diabetes mellitus and the beta cell: The last ten years. *Cell, 148*, 1160–1171. doi:10.1016/j.cell.2012.02.010

Atkinson, M. A., Eisenbarth, G. S., & Michels, A. W. (2014). Type 1 diabetes. *The Lancet, 383*(9911), 69–82. doi:10.1016/s0140-6736(13)60591-7

Avery, L., Flynn, D., van Wersch, A., Sniehotta, F. F., & Trenell, M. I. (2012). Changing physical activity behavior in type 2 diabetes: A systematic review and meta-analysis of behavioral interventions. *Diabetes Care, 35*, 2681–2689. doi:10.2337/dc11-2452

Balducci, S., Zanuso, S., Nicolucci, A., De Feo, P., Cavallo, S., Cardelli, P., . . . Pugliese, G. (2010). Effect of an intensive exercise intervention strategy on modifiable cardiovascular risk factors in subjects with type 2 diabetes mellitus: A randomized controlled trial: The Italian Diabetes and Exercise Study (IDES). *Archives of Internal Medicine, 170*, 1794–1803.

Bandura, A. (1989). Human agency in social cognitive theory. *American Psychologist, 44*, 1175–1184.

Bandura, A. (2004). Health promotion by social cognitive means. *Health Education & Behavior, 31*, 143–164. doi:10.1177/1090198104263660

Benjamin, E.M. (2002). Self-monitoring of blood glucose: The basics. *Clinical Diabetes, 20*, 45–47.

Boland, P. (2007). The emerging role of cell phone technology in ambulatory care. *Journal of Ambulatory Care Management, 30*, 126–133. doi:10.1097/01.JAC.0000264602.19629.84

Bonow, R. O., & Gheorghiade, M. (2004). The diabetes epidemic: A national and global crisis. *American Journal of Medicine, 116*(Suppl. 5), 2S–10S. doi:10.1016/j.amjmed.2003.10.014

Boren, S. A., Gunlock, T. L., Schaefer, J., & Albright, A. (2007). Reducing risks in diabetes self-management: A systematic review of the literature. *Diabetes Educator, 33*, 1053–1077. doi:10.1177/0145721707309809

Boulé, N. G., Haddad, E., Kenny, G. P., Wells, G. A., & Sigal, R. J. (2001). Effects of exercise on glycemic control and body mass in type 2 diabetes mellitus: A meta-analysis of controlled clinical trials. *JAMA, 286*, 1218–1227.

Boulé, N. G., Kenny, G. P., Haddad, E., Wells, G. A., & Sigal, R. J. (2003). Meta-analysis of the effect of structured exercise training on cardiorespiratory fitness in type 2 diabetes mellitus. *Diabetologia, 46*, 1071–1081. doi:10.1007/s00125-003-1160-2

Brady, T. J., Murphy, L., O'Colmain, B. J., Beauchesne, D., Daniels, B., Greenberg, M., . . . Chervin, D. (2013). Meta-analysis of health status, health behaviors, and health care utilization outcomes of the Chronic Disease Self-Management Program. *Preventing Chronic Disease: Public Health Research, Practice, and Policy, 10*, 120112. doi:10.5888/pcd10.120112

Brand-Miller, J., Hayne, S., Petocz, P., & Colagiuri, S. (2003). Low-glycemic index diets in the management of diabetes: A meta-analysis of randomized controlled trials. *Diabetes Care, 26*, 2261–2267.

Breton, M. C., Guénette, L., Amiche, M. A., Kayibanda, J. F., Grégoire, J. P., & Moisan, J. (2013). Burden of diabetes on the ability to work: A systematic review. *Diabetes Care, 36*, 740–749. doi:10.2337/dc12-0354

Brown, S. A., Upchurch, S., Anding, R., Winter, M., & Ramirez, G. (1996). Promoting weight loss in type II diabetes. *Diabetes Care, 19*, 613–624.

Browne, J. L., Ventura, A., Mosely, K., & Speight, J. (2013). "I call it the blame and shame disease": A qualitative study about perceptions of social stigma surrounding type 2 diabetes. *BMJ Open, 3*. doi:10.1136/bmjopen-2013-003384

Campbell, H. M., Khan, N., Cone, C., & Raisch, D. W. (2011). Relationship between diet, exercise habits, and health status among patients with diabetes. *Research in Social and Administrative Pharmacy, 7*, 151–161. doi:10.1016/j.sapharm.2010.03.002

Casagrande, S. S., Fradkin, J. E., Saydah, S. H., Rust, K. F., & Cowie, C. C. (2013). The prevalence of meeting A1C, blood pressure, and LDL goals among people with diabetes, 1988–2010. *Diabetes Care, 36*, 2271–2279. doi:10.2337/dc12-2258

Centers for Disease Control and Prevention. (2014). *National diabetes statistics report: Estimates of diabetes and its burden in the United States, 2014*. Atlanta: US Department of Health and Human Services.

Çevik, A. B., Özcan, Ş., & Satman, I. (2015). Reducing the modifiable risks of cardiovascular disease in Turkish patients with type 2 diabetes: The effectiveness of training. *Clinical Nursing Research, 24*, 299–317. doi:10.1177/1054773814531288

Chan, F., Sasson Gelman, J., Ditchman, N., Kim, J.-H., & Chiu, C.-Y. (2009). The World Health Organization ICF Model as a Conceptual Framework of Disability. In F. Chan, E. Da Silva Cardoso, & J. A. Chronister (Eds.), *Understanding psychosocial adjustment to chronic illness and disability: A handbook for evidence-based practitioners in rehabilitation* (pp. 23–50). New York, NY: Springer Publishing Company.

Chew, B. H., Shariff-Ghazali, S., & Fernandez, A. (2014). Psychological aspects of diabetes care: Effecting behavioral change in patients. *World Journal of Diabetes, 5*, 796–808. doi:10.4239/wjd.v5.i6.796

Chiang, J. L., Kirkman, M. S., Laffel, L. M., & Peters, A. L. (2014). Type 1 diabetes through the life span: A position statement of the American Diabetes Association. *Diabetes Care, 37*, 2034–2054. doi:10.2337/dc14-1140

Choudhary, P., Ramasamy, S., Green, L., Gallen, G., Pender, S., Brackenridge, A., . . . Pickup, J. C. (2013). Real-time continuous glucose monitoring significantly reduces severe hypoglycemia in hypoglycemia-unaware patients with type 1 diabetes. *Diabetes Care, 36*, 4160–4162. doi:10.2337/dc13-0939

Christian, J. G., Bessesen, D. H., Byers, T. E., Christian, K. K., Goldstein, M. G., & Bock, B. C. (2008). Clinic-based support to help overweight patients with type 2 diabetes increase physical activity and lose weight. *Archives of Internal Medicine, 28*, 141–146. doi:10.1001/archinternmed.2007.13

Chudyk, A., & Petrella, R. J. (2011). Effects of exercise on cardiovascular risk factors in type 2 diabetes. *Diabetes Care, 34*, 1228–1237. doi:10.2337/dc10-1881

Church, T. S., Blair, S. N., Cocreham, S., Johannsen, N., Johnson, W., Kramer, K., ... Earnest, C. P. (2010). Effects of aerobic and resistance training on hemoglobin A1c levels in patients with type 2 diabetes: A randomized controlled trial. *JAMA, 304,* 2253–2262. doi:10.1001/jama.2010.1710

Ciechanowski, P. S., Katon, W. J., Russo, J. E., & Hirsch, I. B. (2003). The relationship of depressive symptoms to symptom reporting, self-care and glucose control in diabetes. *General Hospital Psychiatry, 25,* 246–252. doi:10.1016/s0163-8343(03)00055-0

Clair, C., Bitton, A., Meigs, J. B., & Rigotti, N. A. (2011). Relationships of cotinine and self-reported cigarette smoking with hemoglobin A1c in the U.S. *Diabetes Care, 34,* 2250–2255. doi:10.2337/dc11-0710

Chin, Y. F., Huang, T. T., & Hsu, B. R. (2013). Impact of action cues, self-efficacy and perceived barriers on daily foot exam practice in type 2 diabetes mellitus patients with peripheral neuropathy. *Journal of Clinical Nursing, 22,* 61–68. doi:10.1111/j.1365-2702.2012.04291.x

Cnop, M., Welsh, N., Jonas, J.-C., Jörns, A., Lenzen, S., & Elzirik, D. L. (2005). Mechanisms of pancreatic β-cell death in type 1 and type 2 diabetes. *Diabetes, 54*(Suppl. 2), S97–S107. doi:10.2337/diabetes.54.suppl_2.S97

Colberg, S. R. (2007). Being active: A commentary. *Diabetes Educator, 33,* 989–990. doi:10.1177/0145721707308479

Colberg, S. R., Sigal, R. J., Fernhall, B., Regensteiner, J. G., Blissmer, B. J., Rubin, R. R., ... Braun, B. (2010). Exercise and type 2 diabetes: The American College of Sports Medicine and the American Diabetes Association: Joint position statement. *Diabetes Care, 33,* e147–e167. doi:10.2337/dc10-9990

Coles, C. (1996). Psychology in diabetes care. *Practical Diabetes International, 13,* 55–57.

Corbett, C. F. (2003). A randomized pilot study of improving foot care in home health patients with diabetes. *Diabetes Educator, 29,* 273–282.

Cramer, J. A. (2004). A systematic review of adherence with medications for diabetes. *Diabetes Care, 2004,* 1218–1224. doi:10.2337/diacare.27.5.1218

Cryer, P. E., Davis, S. N., & Shamoon, H. (2003). Hypoglycemia in diabetes. *Diabetes Care, 26,* 1902–1912.

De Berardis, G., Franciosi, M., Belfiglio, M., Di Nardo, B., Greenfield, S., Kaplan, S. H., ... Nicolucci, A. (2002). Erectile dysfunction and quality of life in type 2 diabetic patients. *Diabetes Care, 25,* 284–291.

Deiss, D., Bolinder, J., Riveline, J. P., Battelino, T., Bosi, E., Tubiana-Rufi, N., ... Phillip, M. (2006). Improved glycemic control in poorly controlled patients with type 1 diabetes using real-time continuous glucose monitoring. *Diabetes Care, 29,* 2730–2732. doi:10.2337/dc06-1134

Delamater, A. M., Jacobson, A. M., Anderson, B., Cox, D., Fisher, L., Lustman, P., ... Wysocki, T. (2001). Psychosocial therapies in diabetes: Report of the psychosocial therapies working group. *Diabetes Care, 24,* 1286–1292.

Deshpande, A. D., Baker, E. A., Lovegreen, S. L., & Brownson, R. C. (2005). Environmental correlates of physical activity among individuals with diabetes in the rural midwest. *Diabetes Care, 28,* 1012–1018.

Detka, J., Kurek, A., Basta-Kaim, A., Kubera, M., Lason, W., & Budziszewska, B. (2013). Neuroendocrine link between stress, depression and diabetes. *Pharmacological Reports, 65,* 1591–1600.

Dokken, B. B. (2008). The pathophysiology of cardiovascular disease and diabetes: Beyond blood pressure and lipids. *Diabetes Spectrum, 21,* 160–165.

Drewnowski, A. (2009). Obesity, diets, and social inequalities. *Nutrition Reviews, 67*(Suppl. 1), S36–S39. doi:10.1111/j.1753-4887.2009.00157.x

Duangdao, K. M., & Roesch, S. C. (2008). Coping with diabetes in adulthood: A meta-analysis. *Journal of Behavioral Medicine, 31,* 291–300. doi:10.1007/s10865-008-9155-6

D'Zurilla, T. J., & Goldfried, M. R. (1971). Problem solving and behavior modification. *Journal of Abnormal Psychology, 78,* 107–126.

El-Gayar, O., Timsina, P., Nawar, N., & Eid, W. (2013). Mobile applications for diabetes self-management: Status and potential. *Journal of Diabetes Science and Technology, 7,* 247–262.

Enzlin, P., Mathieu, C., Van den Bruel, A., Vanderschueren, D., & Demyttenaere, K. (2003). Prevalence and predictors of sexual dysfunction in patients with type 1 diabetes. *Diabetes Care, 26,* 409–414.

Evert, A. B., Boucher, J. L., Cypress, M., Dunbar, S. A., Franz, M. J., Mayer-Davis, E. J., . . . Yancy, W. S. Jr. (2013). Nutrition therapy recommendations for the management of adults with diabetes. *Diabetes Care, 36,* 3821–3842. doi:10.2337/dc13-2042

Eye Diseases Prevalence Research Group. (2004). Causes and prevalence of visual impairment among adults in the United States. *Archives of Ophthalmology, 122,* 477–485. doi:10.1001/archopht.122.4.477

Fagard, R. H., & Nilsson, P. M. (2009). Smoking and diabetes: The double health hazard! *Primary Care Diabetes, 3,* 205–209. doi:10.1016/j.pcd.2009.09.003

Falvo, D. R. (2009). *Medical and psychosocial aspects of chronic illness and disability* (4th ed.). Sudbury, MA: Jones & Bartlett.

Fan, L., Sidani, S., Cooper-Brathwaite, A., & Metcalfe, K. (2014). Improving foot self-care knowledge, self-efficacy, and behaviors in patients with type 2 diabetes at low risk for foot ulceration: A pilot study. *Clinical Nursing Research, 23,* 627–643.

Fisher, E. B., Thorpe, C. T., Devellis, B. M., & Devellis, R. F. (2007). Healthy coping, negative emotions, and diabetes management: A systematic review and appraisal. *Diabetes Educator, 33,* 1080–1103. doi:10.1177/0145721707309808

Fisher, L., Chesla, C. A., Skaff, M. M., Gilliss, C., Mullan, J. T., Bartz, R. J., . . . Lutz, C. P. (2000). The family and disease management in Hispanic and European-American patients with type 2 diabetes. *Diabetes Care, 23,* 267–272.

Fitzpatrick, S. L., Schumann, K. P., & Hill-Briggs, F. (2013). Problem solving interventions for diabetes self-management and control: A systematic review of the literature. *Diabetes Research and Clinical Practice, 100*(2), 145–161. doi:10.1016/j.diabres.2012.12.016

Fong, D. S., Aiello, L., Gardner, T. W., King, G. L., Blankenship, G., Cavallerano, J. D., . . . American Diabetes Association. (2004). Retinopathy in diabetes. *Diabetes Care, 27*(Suppl. 2), S84–S87.

Forgays, D. K., Hyman, I. E., & Schreiber, J. (2014). Texting everywhere for everything: Gender and age differences in cell phone etiquette and use. *Computers in Human Behavior, 31,* 314–321. doi:10.1016/j.chb.2013.10.053

Fowler, M. J. (2008). Microvascular and macrovascular complications of diabetes. *Clinical Diabetes, 26,* 77–82. doi:10.2336/diaclin.26.2.77

Fox, C. S., Pencina, M. J., Meigs, J. B., Vasan, R. S., Levitzky, Y. S., & D'Agostino, R. B., Sr. (2006). Trends in the incidence of type 2 diabetes mellitus from the 1970s to the 1990s: The Framingham Heart Study. *Circulation, 113*, 2914–2918. doi:10.1161/CIRCULATIONAHA.106.613828

Franz, M. J. (2007). Diabetes and healthy eating: A commentary. *Diabetes Educator, 33*, 960–961. doi:10.1177/0145721707308632

Franz, M. J., Powers, M. A., Leontos, C., Holzmeister, L. A., Kulkarni, K., Monk, A., ... Gradwell, E. (2010). The evidence for medical nutrition therapy for type 1 and type 2 diabetes in adults. *Journal of the American Dietetic Association, 110*, 1852–1889. doi:10.1016/j.jada.2010.09.014

Funnell, M. M. (2007). Self-monitoring of blood glucose: A commentary. *Diabetes Educator, 33*, 1012–1013. doi:10.1177/0145721707308630

Funnell, M. M., & Anderson, R. M. (2004). Empowerment and self-management of diabetes. *Clinical Diabetes, 22*, 127–127.

Gallichan, M. (1997). Self monitoring of glucose by people with diabetes: Evidence based practice. *BMJ, 314*, 964–967.

Gambaro, G., Bax, G., Fusaro, M., Normanno, M., Manani, S. M., Zanella, M., ... Favaro, S. (2001). Cigarette smoking is a risk factor for nephropathy and its progression in type 2 diabetes mellitus. *Diabetes, Nutrition & Metabolism, 14*, 337–342.

Garabedian, L. F., Ross-Degnan, D., & Wharam, J. F. (2015). Mobile phone and smartphone technologies for diabetes care and self-management. *Current Diabetes Reports, 15*, 109. doi:10.1007/s11892-015-0680-8

Gary, T. L., Safford, M. M., Gerzoff, R. B., Ettner, S. L., Karter, A. J., Beckles, G. L., & Brown, A. F. (2008). Perception of neighborhood problems, health behaviors, and diabetes outcomes among adults with diabetes in managed care: The Translating Research into Action for Diabetes (TRIAD) Study. *Diabetes Care, 31*, 273–278. doi:10.2337/dc07-1111

Geiss, L. S., Wang, J., Cheng, Y. J., Thompson, T. J., Barker, L., Li, Y., ... Gregg, E. W. (2014). Prevalence and incidence trends for diagnosed diabetes among adults aged 20 to 79 years, United States, 1980–2012. *JAMA, 312*, 1218–1226. doi:10.1001/jama.2014.11494

Glasgow, R. E., Kurz, D., King, D., Dickman, J. M., Faber, A. J., Halterman, E., ... Ritzwoller, D. (2010). Outcomes of minimal and moderate support versions of an internet-based diabetes self-management support program. *Journal of General Internal Medicine, 25*, 1315–1322. doi:10.1007/s11606-010-1480-0

Glasgow, R. E., & Toobert, D. J. (1988). Social environment and regimen adherence among type II diabetic patients. *Diabetes Care, 11*, 377–386.

Glasgow, R. E., Toobert, D. J., Barrera, M. Jr., & Strycker, L. A. (2004). Assessment of problem-solving: A key to successful diabetes self-management. *Journal of Behavioral Medicine, 27*, 477–490.

Gonzalez, J. S., Peyrot, M., McCarl, L. A., Collins, E. M., Serpa, L., Mimiaga, M. J., & Safren, S. A. (2008). Depression and diabetes treatment nonadherence: A meta-analysis. *Diabetes Care, 31*, 2398–2403. doi:10.2337/dc08-1341

Grant, R. W., Devita, N. G., Singer, D. E., & Meigs, J. B. (2003). Polypharmacy and medication adherence in patients with type 2 diabetes. *Diabetes Care, 26*, 1408–1412.

Gregg, E. W., Li, Y., Wang, J., Burrows, N. R., Ali, M. K., Rolka, D., ... Geiss, L. (2014). Changes in diabetes-related complications in the United States, 1990–2010. *The New England Journal of Medicine, 370*, 1514–1523. doi:10.1056/NEJMoa1310799

Grey, M. (2000). Coping and diabetes. *Diabetes Spectrum, 13*, 167–169.

Grootenhuis, P. A., Snoek, F. J., Heine, R. J., & Bouter, L. M. (1994). Development of a type 2 diabetes symptom checklist: A measure of symptom severity. *Diabetic Medicine, 11,* 253–261.

Gunawardana, S. C. (2014). Benefits of healthy adipose tissue in the treatment of diabetes. *World Journal of Diabetes, 5,* 420–430. doi:10.4239/wjd.v5.i4.420

Halban, P. A., Polonsky, K. S., Bowden, D. W., Hawkins, M. A., Ling, C., Mather, K. J., ... Weir, G. C. (2014). B-cell failure in type 2 diabetes: Postulated mechanisms and prospects for prevention and treatment. *Diabetes Care, 37,* 1751–1758. doi:10.2337/dc14-0396

Hayashino, Y., Jackson, J. L., Fukumori, N., Nakamura, F., & Fukuhara, S. (2012). Effects of supervised exercise on lipid profiles and blood pressure control in people with type 2 diabetes mellitus: A meta-analysis of randomized controlled trials. *Diabetes Research and Clinical Practice, 98,* 349–360. doi:10.1016/j.diabres.2012.10.004

Herpertz, S., Albus, C., Wagener, R., Kocnar, M., Wagner, R., Henning, A., ... Senf, W. (1998). Comorbidity of diabetes and eating disorders: Does diabetes control reflect disturbed eating behavior? *Diabetes Care, 21,* 1110–1116.

Herquelot, E., Guéguen, A., Bonenfant, S., & Dray-Spira, R. (2011). Impact of diabetes on work cessation: Data from the GAZEL cohort study. *Diabetes Care, 34,* 1344–1349. doi:10.2337/dc10-2225

Hill, J., Nielsen, M., & Fox, M. H. (2013). Understanding the social factors that contribute to diabetes: A means to informing health care and social policies for the chronically ill. *Permanente Journal, 17,* 67–72. doi:10.7812/TPP/12-099

Hill-Briggs, F. (2003). Problem solving in diabetes self-management: A model of chronic illness self-management behavior. *Annals of Behavioral Medicine, 25,* 182–193.

Hill-Briggs, F., Cooper, D. C., Loman, K., Brancati, F. L., & Cooper, L. A. (2003). A qualitative study of problem solving and diabetes control in type 2 diabetes self-management. *Diabetes Educator, 29,* 1018–1028. doi:10.1177/014572170302900612

Hill-Briggs, F., & Gemmell, L. (2007). Problem solving in diabetes self-management and control: A systematic review of the literature. *Diabetes Educator, 33,* 1032–1050. doi:10.1177/0145721707308412

Hill-Briggs, F., Lazo, M., Peyrot, M., Doswell, A., Chang, Y. T., Hill, M. N., ... Brancati, F. L. (2011). Effect of problem-solving-based diabetes self-management training on diabetes control in a low income patient sample. *Journal of General Internal Medicine, 26,* 972–978. doi:10.1007/s11606-011-1689-6

Ho, P. M., Rumsfeld, J. S., Masoudi, F. A., McClure, D. L., Plomondon, M. E., Steiner, J. F., & Magid, D. J. (2006). Effect of medication nonadherence on hospitalization and mortality among patients with diabetes mellitus. *Archives of Internal Medicine, 166,* 1836–1841. doi:10.1001/archinte.166.17.1836

Hokanson, J. M., Anderson, R. L., Hennrikus, D. J., Lando, H. A., & Kendall, D. M. (2006). Integrated tobacco cessation counseling in a diabetes self-management training program: A randomized trial of diabetes and reduction of tobacco. *Diabetes Educator, 32,* 562–570. doi:10.1177/0145721706289914

Holman, R. R., Paul, S. K., Bethel, M. A., Matthews, D. R., & Neil, H. A. W. (2008). 10-year follow-up of intensive glucose control in type 2 diabetes. *The New England Journal of Medicine, 359,* 1577–1589. doi:10.1056/NEWMoa0806470

Huizinga, M. M., Elasy, T. A., Wallston, K. A., Cavanaugh, K., Davis, D., Gregory, R. P., ... Rothman, R. L. (2008). Development and validation of the Diabetes Numeracy Test (DNT). *BMC Health Services Research, 8*, 96. doi:10.1186/1472-6963-8-96

Hunt, C. W. (2015). Technology and diabetes self-management: An integrative review. *World J Diabetes, 6*, 225–233. doi:10.4239/wjd.v6.i2.225

International Diabetes Federation. (2015). *IDF Diabetes Atlas* (7th ed.). Brussels: Author.

Inzucchi, S. E., Bergenstal, R. M., Buse, J. B., Diamant, M., Ferrannini, E., Nauck, M., ... Matthews, D. R. (2012). Management of hyperglycemia in type 2 diabetes: A patient-centered approach: Position statement of the American Diabetes Association (ADA) and European Association for the Study of Diabetes (EASD). *Diabetes Care, 35*, 1364–1379. doi:10.2337/dc12-0413

Inzucchi, S. E., Bergenstal, R. M., Buse, J. B., Diamant, M., Ferrannini, E., Nauck, M., ... Matthews, D. R. (2015). Management of hyperglycemia in type 2 diabetes, 2015: A patient centered approach: Update to a position statement of the American Diabetes Association and the European Association for the Study of Diabetes. *Diabetes Care, 38*, 140–149. doi:10.2337/dc14-2441

Ismail-Beigi, F., Craven, T., Banerji, M., Basile, J., Calles, J., Cohen, R., ... Hramiak, I. (2010). Effect of intensive treatment of hyperglycemia on microvascular complications of type 2 diabetes in ACCORD: A randomized trial. *The Lancet, 376*, 419–430. doi:10.1016/S0140-6736(10)60576-4

Jones, J. A., Miller, D. R., Wehler, C. J., Rich, S. E., Krall-Kaye, E. A., McCoy, L. C., ... Garcia, R. I. (2007). Does periodontal care improve glycemic control? The Department of Veterans Affairs Dental Diabetes Study. *Journal of Clinical Periodontology, 34*, 46–52. doi:10.1111/j.1600-051X.2006.01002.x

Karstoft, K., Winding, K., Knudsen, S. H., Nielsen, J. S., Thomsen, C., Pedersen, B. K., & Solomon, T. P. (2013). The effects of free-living interval-walking training on glycemic control, body composition, and physical fitness in type 2 diabetic patients: A randomized, controlled trial. *Diabetes Care, 36*, 228–236. doi:10.2337/dc12-0658

Kavookjian, J., Elswick, B. M., & Whetsel, T. (2007). Interventions for being active among individuals with diabetes: A systematic review of the literature. *Diabetes Educator, 33*, 962–988. doi:10.1177/0145721707308411

Kiran, M., Arpak, N., Unsal, E., & Erdoğan, M. F. (2005). The effect of improved periodontal health on metabolic control in type 2 diabetes mellitus. *Journal of Clinical Periodontology, 32*, 266–272. doi:10.1111/j.1600-051X.2005.00658.x

Klein, R., Knudtson, M. D., Lee, K. E., Gangnon, R., & Klein, B. E. K. (2008). The Wisconsin Epidemiologic Study of Diabetic Retinopathy XXII: The twenty-five-year progresion of retinopathy in persons with type 1 diabetes. *Ophthalmology, 115*, 1859–1868.

Kolb, H., & Mandrup-Poulsen, T. (2010). The global diabetes epidemic as a consequence of lifestyle-induced low-grade inflammation. *Diabetologia, 53*, 10–20. doi:10.1007/s00125-009-1573-7

Krapek, K., King, K., Warren, S. S., George, K. G., Caputo, D. A., Mihelich, K., ... Lubowski, T. J. (2004). Medication adherence and associated hemoglobin A1c in type 2 diabetes. *Annals of Pharmacotherapy, 38*, 1357–1362. doi:10.1345/aph.1D612

Krentz, A. J. (2002). *Insulin resistance: A clinical handbook*. Oxford: Blackwell.

Krishna, S., & Boren, S. A. (2008). Diabetes self-management care via cell phone: A systematic review. *Journal of Diabetes Science and Technology, 2*, 509–517. doi:10.1177/193229680800200324

Latessa, R. A., Cummings, D. M., Lilley, S. H., & Morrissey, S. L. (2000). Changing practices in the use of pneumococcal vaccine. *Family Medicine, 32*, 196–200.

Letassy, N. (2007). Medication taking: A commentary. *Diabetes Educator, 33*, 1030–1031. doi:10.1177/0145721707308477

Li, C., Ford, E. S., Strine, T. W., & Mokdad, A. H. (2008). Prevalence of depression among U.S. adults with diabetes: Findings from the 2006 Behavioral Risk Factor Surveillance System. *Diabetes Care, 31*, 105–107. doi:10.2337/dc07-1154

Look AHEAD Research Group. (2010). Long-term effects of a lifestyle intervention on weight and cardiovascular risk factors in individuals with type 2 diabetes mellitus: Four-year results of the Look AHEAD trial. *Archives of Internal Medicine, 170*, 1566–1575. doi:10.1001/archinternmed.2010.334

Lorig, K., Ritter, P. L., Villa, F. J., & Armas, J. (2009). Community-based peer-led diabetes self-management: A randomized trial. *Diabetes Educator, 35*, 641–651. doi:10.1177/0145721709335006

Lustman, P. J., Anderson, R. J., Freedland, K. E., De Groo, M., Carney, R. M., & Clouse, R. E. (2000). Depression and poor glycemic control: A meta-analytic review of the literature. *Diabetes Care, 23*, 934–942.

Malanda, U. L., Bot, S. D., & Nijpels, G. (2013). Self-monitoring of blood glucose in noninsulin-using type 2 diabetic patients: It is time to face the evidence. *Diabetes Care, 36*, 176–178. doi:10.2337/dc12-0831

Mayberry, L. S., & Osborn, C. Y. (2014). Family involvement is helpful and harmful to patients' self-care and glycemic control. *Patient Educaton and Counseling, 97*, 418–425. doi:10.1016/j.pec.2014.09.011

McAndrew, L., Schneider, S. H., Burns, E., & Leventhal, H. (2007). Does patient blood glucose monitoring improve diabetes control? A systematic review of the literature. *Diabetes Educator, 33*, 991–1011. doi:10.1177/0145721707309807

McMahon, B. T., West, S. L., Mansouri, M., & Belongia, L. (2005). Workplace discrimination and diabetes: The EEOC Americans with Disabilities Act research project. *Work, 25*, 9–18.

Meece, J. (2006). Dispelling myths and removing barriers about insulin in type 2 diabetes. *Diabetes Educator, 32* (Suppl.), 9S–18S. doi:10.1177/0145721705285638

Melikian, C., White, T. J., Vanderplas, A., Dezii, C. M., & Chang, E. (2002). Adherence to oral antidiabetic therapy in a managed care organization: A comparison of monotherapy, combination therapy, and fixed-dose combination therapy. *Clinical Therapeutics, 24*, 460–467.

Mier, N., Medina, A. A., & Ory, M. G. (2007). Mexican Americans with type 2 diabetes: Perspectives on definitions, motivators, and programs of physical activity. *Preventing Chronic Disease: Public Health Research, Practice, and Policy, 4*(2), 1–8.

Miller, K. M., Foster, N. C., Beck, R. W., Bergenstal, R. M., DuBose, S. N., DiMeglio, L. A., . . . Tamborlane, W. V. (2015). Current state of type 1 diabetes treatment in the U.S.: Updated data from the T1D Exchange clinic registry. *Diabetes Care, 38*, 971–978. doi:10.2337/dc15-0078

Morrato, E. H., Hill, J. O., Wyatt, H. R., Ghushchyan, V., & Sullivan, P. W. (2007). Physical activity in U.S. adults with diabetes and at risk for developing diabetes, 2003. *Diabetes Care, 30,* 203–209. doi:10.2337/dc06-1128

Mulcahy, K., Maryniuk, M., Peeples, M., Peyrot, M., Tomky, D., Weaver, T., & Yarborough, P. (2003). Diabetes self-management education core outcomes measures. *Diabetes Educator, 29,* 768–770, 773–784, 787-803.

Nathan, D. M., Buse, J. B., Davidson, M. B., Ferrannini, E., Holman, R. R., Sherwin, R., & Zinman, B. (2009). Medical management of hyperglycemia in type 2 diabetes: A consensus algorithm for the initiation and adjustment of therapy: A consensus statement of the American Diabetes Assocation and the European Association for the Study of Diabetes. *Diabetes Care, 32,* 193–203. doi:10.2337/dc08-9025

Nathan, D. M., & DCCT/EDIC Research Group. (2014). The Diabetes Control and Complications Trial/Epidemiology of Diabetes Interventions and Complications study at 30 years: Overview. *Diabetes Care, 37,* 9–16. doi:10.2337/dc13-2112

Negarandeh, R., Mahmoodi, H., Noktehdan, H., Heshmat, R., & Shakibazadeh, E. (2013). Teach back and pictorial image educational strategies on knowledge about diabetes and medication/dietary adherence among low health literate patients with type 2 diabetes. *Primary Care Diabetes, 7,* 111–118. doi:10.1016/j.pcd.2012.11.001

Newsholme, P., Cruzat, V., Arfuso, F., & Keane, K. (2014). Nutrient regulation of insulin secretion and action. *Journal of Endocrinology, 221,* R105–R120. doi:10.1530/JOE-13-0616

Norris, S. L., Lau, J., Smith, S. J., Schmid, C. H., & Engelgau, M. M. (2002). Self-management education for adults wth type 2 diabetes: A meta-analysis of the effect on glycemic control. *Diabetes Care, 25,* 1159–1171.

Odegard, P. S., & Capoccia, K. (2007). Medication taking and diabetes: A systematic review of the literature. *Diabetes Educator, 33,* 1014–1029. doi:10.1177/0145721707308407

Odegard, P. S., & Christensen, D. B. (2012). MAP study: RCT of a mediation adherence program for patients with type 2 diabetes. *Journal of the American Pharmacists Association, 52,* 753–762. doi:10.1331/JAPhA.2012.11001

Padgett, D., Mumford, E., Hynes, M., & Carter, R. (1988). Meta-analysis of the effects of educational and psychosocial interventions on management of diabetes mellitus. *Journal of Clinical Epidemiology, 41,* 1007–1030.

Pal, K., Eastwood, S. V., Michie, S., Farmer, A., Barnard, M. L., Peacock, R., . . . Murray, E. (2014). Computer-based interventions to improve self-management in adults with type 2 diabetes: A systematic review and meta-analysis. *Diabetes Care, 37,* 1759–1766. doi:10.2337/dc13-1386

Pastors, J. G., Franz, M. J., Warshaw, H., Daly, A., & Arnold, M. S. (2003). How effective is medical nutrition therapy in diabetes care? *Journal of the American Dietetic Association, 103,* 827–831. doi:10.1053/jada.2003.50186

Peel, E., Parry, O., Douglas, M., & Lawton, J. (2004). Diagnosis of type 2 diabetes: A qualitative analysis of patients' emotional reactions and views about information provision. *Patient Education and Counseling, 53,* 269–275. doi:10.1016/j.pec.2003.07.010

Peel, E., Parry, O., Douglas, M., & Lawton, J. (2005). Taking the biscuit? A discursive approach to managing diet in type 2 diabetes. *Journal of Health Psychology, 10,* 779–791. doi:10.1177/1359105305057313

Penckofer, S., Ferrans, C. E., Velsor-Friedrich, B., & Savoy, S. (2007). The psychological impact of living with diabetes: Women's day-to-day experiences. *Diabetes Educator, 33,* 680–690. doi:10.1177/0145721707304079

Penn, L., Moffatt, S. M., & White, M. (2008). Participants' perspective on maintaining behaviour change: A qualitative study within the European Diabetes Prevention Study. *BMC Public Health, 8.* doi:10.1186/1471-2458-8-235

Pew Research Center. (2015). U.S. smartphone use in 2015. Retrieved from http://pewinternet.org/2015/04/01.us-smartphone-use-in-2015

Polonsky, W. H., & Fisher, L. (2013). Self-monitoring of blood glucose in noninsulin-using type 2 diabetic patients: Right answer, but wrong question: Self-monitoring of blood glucose can be clinically valuable for noninsulin users. *Diabetes Care, 36,* 179–182. doi:10.2337/dc12-0731

Polonsky, W. H., Fisher, L., Guzman, S., Villa-Caballero, L., & Edelman, S. V. (2005). Psychological insulin resistance in patients with type 2 diabetes: The scope of the problem. *Diabetes Care, 28,* 2543–2545.

Polonsky, W. H., Zee, J., Yee, M. A., Crosson, M. A., & Jackson, R. A. (2005). A community-based program to encourage patients' attention to their own diabetes care: Pilot development and evaluation. *Diabetes Educator, 31,* 691–699. doi:10.1177/0145721705280416

Powers, M. A., Bardsley, J., Cypress, M., Duker, P., Funnell, M. M., Hess Fischl, A., ... Vivian, E. (2015). Diabetes self-management education and support in type 2 diabetes: A joint position statement of the American Diabetes Association, the American Association of Diabetes Educators, and the Academy of Nutrition and Dietetics. *Diabetes Care.* doi:10.2337/dc15-0730

Praet, S. F. E., & van Loon, L. J. C. (2009). Exercise therapy in type 2 diabetes. *Acta Diabetologica, 46,* 263–278. doi:10.1007/s00592-009-0129-0

Tennvall, G. R., & Apelqvist, J. (2000). Health-related quality of life in patients with diabetes mellitus and foot ulcers. *Journal of Diabetes and its Complications, 14,* 235–241. doi:10.1016/S1056-8727(00)00133-1

Raphael, D., Daiski, I., Pilkington, B., Bryant, T., Dinca-Panaitescu, M., & Dinca-Panaitescu, S. (2012). A toxic combination of poor social policies and programmes, unfair economic arrangements and bad politics: The experiences of poor Canadians with type 2 diabetes. *Critical Public Health, 22,* 127–145. doi:10.1080/09581596.2011.607797

Resnick, H. E., Foster, G. L., Bardsley, J., & Ratner, R. E. (2006). Achievement of American Diabetes Association clinical practice recommendations among U.S. adults with diabetes, 1999–2002: The National Health and Nutrition Examination Survey. *Diabetes Care, 29,* 531–537.

Ross, R., Hudson, R., Stotz, P. J., & Lam, M. (2015). Effects of exercise amount and intensity on abdominal obesity and glucose tolerance in obese adults: A randomized trial. *Annals of Internal Medicine, 162,* 325–334. doi:10.7326/M14-1189

Rubin, R. R., & Peyrot, M. (1999). Quality of life and diabetes. *Diabetes/Metabolism Research and Reviews, 15,* 205–218.

Ruggiero, L., Glasgow, R., Dryfoos, J. M., Rossi, J. S., Prochaska, J. O., Orleans, C. T., ... Johnson, S. (1997). Diabetes self-management: Self-reported recommendations and paterns in a large population. *Diabetes Care, 20,* 568–576.

Saffari, M., Ghanizadeh, G., & Koenig, H. G. (2014). Health education via mobile text messaging for glycemic control in adults with type 2 diabetes: A systematic review and meta-analysis. *Primary Care Diabetes, 8,* 275–285. doi:10.1016/j.pcd.2014.03.004

Selvin, E., Marinopoulos, S., Berkenblit, G., Rami, T., Brancati, F. L., Powe, N. R., & Hill Golden, S. (2004). Meta-analysis: Glycosylated hemoglobin and cardiovascular disease in diabetes mellitus. *Annals of Internal Medicine, 141*, 421–431.

Selvin, E., Parrinello, C. M., Sacks, D. B., & Coresh, J. (2014). Trends in prevalence and control of diabetes in the United States, 1988–1994 and 1999–2010. *Annals of Internal Medicine, 160*, 517–525. doi:10.7326/M13-2411

Shah, B. R., & Hux, J. E. (2003). Qualifying the risk of infectious diseases for people with diabetes. *Diabetes Care, 26*, 510–513.

Siminerio, L. (2006). Challenges and strategies for moving patients to injectable medications. *Diabetes Educator, 32* (Suppl. 2), 82S–90S. doi:10.1177/0145721706287653

Singh, N., Armstrong, D. G., & Lipsky, B. A. (2005). Preventing foot ulcers in patients with diabetes. *JAMA, 293*, 217–228. doi:10.1001/jama.293.2.217

Skaer, T. L., Sclar, D. A., Markowski, D. J., & Won, J. K. (1993). Effect of value-added utilities on prescription refill compliance and Medicaid health care expenditures: A study of patients with non-insulin dependent diabetes mellitus. *Journal of Clinical Pharmacy and Therapeuticis, 18*, 295–299.

Skyler, J. S. (2004). Effect of glycemic control on diabetes complications and on the prevention of diabetes. *Clinical Diabetes, 22*, 162–166.

Smalls, B. L., Gregory, C. M., Zoller, J. S., & Egede, L. E. (2014). Effect of neighborhood factors on diabetes self-care behaviors in adults with type 2 diabetes. *Diabetes Research and Clinical Practice, 106*, 435–442. doi:10.1016/j.diabres.2014.09.029

Smith, K. J., Beland, M., Clyde, M., Gariepy, G., Page, V., Badawi, G., . . . Schmitz, N. (2013). Association of diabetes with anxiety: A systematic review and meta-analysis. *Journal of Psychosomatic Research, 74*, 89–99. doi:10.1016/j.jpsychores.2012.11.013

Snoek, F. J., & Skinner, T. C. (2006). Psychological aspects of diabetes management. *Medicine, 34*, 61–62. doi:10.1383/medc.2006.34.2.61

Snowling, N. J., & Hopkins, W. G. (2006). Effects of different modes of exercise training on glucose control and risk factors for complications in type 2 diabetic patients: A meta-analysis. *Diabetes Care, 29*, 2518–2527. doi:10.2337/dc06-1317

Steinbrook, R. (2006). Facing the diabetes epidemic: Mandatory reporting of glycosylated hemoglobin values in New York City. *The New England Journal of Medicine, 354*, 545–548.

Stolar, M. (2010). Glycemic control and complications in type 2 diabetes mellitus. *American Journal of Medicine, 123*(Suppl. 3), S3–S11. doi:10.1016/j.amjmed.2009.12.004

Thomas, D., Elliott, E. J., & Naughton, G. A. (2006). Exercise for type 2 diabetes mellitus. *Cochrane Database of Systematic Reviews, 2006*(3), 1–56. doi:10.1002/14651858.CD002968.pub2

Tonstad, S. (2009). Cigarette smoking, smoking cessation, and diabetes. *Diabetes Research and Clinical Practice, 85*, 4–13. doi:10.1016/j.diabres.2009.04.013

Toobert, D. J., Strycker, L. A., Barrera, M. Jr., & Glasgow, R. E. (2010). Seven-year follow-up of a multiple-health-behavior diabetes intervention. *American Journal of Health Behavior, 34*, 680–694.

Tulloch, H., Reida, R., D'Angeloa, M. S., Plotnikoff, R. C., Morrina, L., Beatona, L., . . . Pipe, A. (2009). Predicting short and long-term exercise intentions and behaviour in patients with coronary artery disease: A test of protection motivation theory. *Psychology & Health, 24*, 255–269. doi:10.1080/08870440701805390

Tunceli, K., Bradley, C. J., Nerenz, D., Williams, L. K., Pladevall, M., & Lafata, J. E. (2005). The impact of diabetes on employment and work productivity. *Diabetes Care, 28*, 2662–2667.

Umpierre, D., Ribeiro, P. A. B., Kramer, C. K., Leitão, C. B., Zucatti, A. T. N., Azevedo, M. J., . . . Schaan, B. D. (2011). Physical activity advice only or structured exercise training and association with HbA1c levels in type 2 diabetes. *JAMA, 305*, 1790–1799.

Valensi, P., Girod, I., Baron, F., Moreau-Defarges, T., & Guillon, P. (2005). Quality of life and clinical correlates in patients with diabetic foot ulcers. *Diabetes & Metabolism, 31*, 263–271.

Vervloet, M., van Dijk, L., van Vlijmen, B., van Wingerden, P., Bouvy, M. L., & de Bakker, D. H. (2012). SMS reminders improve adherence to oral medication in type 2 diabetes patients who are real time electronically monitored. *International Journal of Medical Informatics, 81*, 594–604. doi:10.1016/j.ijmedinf.2012.05.005

Von Korff, M., Katon, W., Lin, E. H. B., Simon, G., Ciechanowski, P., Ludman, E., . . . Young, B. (2009). Work disability among individuals with diabetes. *Diabetes Care, 28*, 1326–1332.

Walker, E. A., Shmukler, C., Ullman, R., Blanco, E., Scollan-Koliopoulus, M., & Cohen, H. W. (2011). Results of a successful telephonic intervention to improve diabetes control in urban adults: A randomized trial. *Diabetes Care, 34*, 2–7. doi:10.2337/dc10-1005

Whitty, P., Steen, M., Eccles, M., McColl, E., Hewison, J., Meadows, K., . . . Hutchinson, A. (1997). A new self-completion outcome measure for diabetes: Is it responsive to change? *Quality of Life Research, 6*, 407–413.

Yang, Z., Scott, C. A., Mao, C., Tang, J., & Farmer, A. J. (2014). Resistance exercise versus aerobic exercise for type 2 diabetes: A systematic review and meta-analysis. *Sports Medicine, 44*, 487–499. doi:10.1007/s40279-013-0128-8

Yardley, J. E., Hay, J., Abou-Setta, A. M., Marks, S. D., & McGavock, J. (2014). A systematic review and meta-analysis of exercise interventions in adults with type 1 diabetes. *Diabetes Research and Clinical Practice, 106*, 393–400. doi:10.1016/j.diabres.2014.09.038

Yoon, K. H., & Kim, H. S. (2008). A short message service by cellular phone in type 2 diabetic patients for 12 months. *Diabetes Research and Clinical Practice, 79*, 256–261. doi:10.1016/j.diabres.2007.09.007

Zgibor, J. C., & Songer, T. J. (2001). External barriers to diabetes care: Addressing personal and health system issues. *Diabetes Spectrum, 14*, 23–28. doi:10.2337/diaspect.14.1.23

Zhao, G., Ford, E. S., Li, C., & Mokdad, A. H. (2008). Compliance with physical activity recommendations in US adults with diabetes. *Diabetic Medicine, 25*, 221–227. doi:10.1111/j.1464-5491.2007.02332.x

Zhuo, X., Zhang, P., Barker, L., Albright, A., Thompson, T. J., & Gregg, E. (2014). The lifetime cost of diabetes and its implications for diabetes prevention. *Diabetes Care, 27*, 2557–2564. doi:10.2337/dc13-2484

13

Self-Management of Epilepsy

JANICE M. BUELOW AND W. HENRY SMITHSON ■

INTRODUCTION

Epilepsy is a chronic health condition that is associated with a wide range of disabilities. Some with epilepsy may have well-controlled seizures and no other consequences, while others may have multiple co-occurring conditions and have many seizures a day. Despite this wide range of disabilities, all people with epilepsy must self-manage their disease. This chapter reviews the concept of self-management in people with epilepsy. It guides readers in beginning to understand the complex nature of self-management in this population.

What Is Epilepsy?

Epilepsy is a frightening word that often elicits negative and stigmatizing reactions. Descriptions of epilepsy go back into antiquity. A "falling disease" caused by possession from a "demon from the desert" can be found in tablets circa 700 BC. In the Gospels, Luke (9:39) wrote about a child afflicted with seizures that occur when "the spirit seizes him" (Kammerman & Wasserman, 2001). Both descriptions leave the impression that epilepsy is a condition outside the control of the individual—something that happens from time to time without warning. This view is understandable, because seizures are often (at least ostensibly) unprovoked and recurrent events. However, the majority of seizures can be controlled, and many people with epilepsy can live their lives without being ruled by the seizures. This chapter attempts to help people live well with epilepsy.

The term "epilepsy" can be unhelpful. It is too general to say merely that someone "has epilepsy." Like other umbrella terms, it is not always understood correctly by many people, including some health professionals. The classification of the epilepsies continues to change as more is known about the various underlying causes of the seizures and the mechanisms involved. Seizures are now classified by mode of onset that can be focal, generalized, or unknown. A seizure can range from a focal seizure that does no more than cause an unusual sensation in a part of a limb to the significant generalized seizure that affects both sides of the brain and results in unconsciousness and sometimes convulsions of all limbs.

The first step in helping individuals manage their epilepsy is to provide a complete diagnosis. This is done on three levels: (a) the cause of the epileptic seizure, (b) the seizure type, and (c) the matching of any associated features with an epilepsy syndrome (though some seizures do not fit into a particular syndrome). A detailed diagnosis can offer a more accurate forecast of outcome (prognosis) and can help healthcare providers choose the most effective form of treatment. This is where the complexity of the condition can overwhelm the individual as well as nurses and doctors. Epilepsy presents in at least six types of generalized seizures, 10 groups of syndromes, and many kinds of focal seizures that are characterized by the affected parts of the brain, including the temporal, frontal, parietal, or occipital lobes (Berg et al., 2010).

Impact

Epilepsy is associated with multiple co-occurring conditions that impact self-management or require a high degree of self-management. These conditions can include physical problems, psychological and mental health problems, social problems, and general health problems.

Physical Impact

Epilepsy is a condition that is associated with recurrent seizures. Seizures are motor or sensory events. They can occur without warning in any setting and can be frightening both for the person experiencing the seizure and those witnessing it. Seizures may be as mild as a localized motor movement with no impairment of awareness (absence seizures or localized motor activity) or as serious as events that cause sudden unconsciousness and tightening and relaxing of the limbs, commonly called "convulsions" (i.e., generalized tonic-clonic seizures). Most, but not all, seizures are associated with some form of altered consciousness. They are often unpredictable and in some people can occur in clusters. The physical manifestations of seizures can affect many areas of a person's life. Those who have frequent episodes of cluster seizures or prolonged difficult-to-treat episodes (status epilepticus) must have a plan for coping. Unfortunately, plans like these are not frequently discussed with healthcare providers (Buelow et al., 2016).

Chronic seizures have been associated with cognition problems, though the reason is not clear (Laxer et al., 2014). Seizures are often associated with cerebral palsy. Those with spastic quadriplegia are 53% more likely to have epilepsy (Delacy & Reid, 2016). While antiseizure medications have improved over time, they are still associated with significant side effects (Beghi, 2016; Keezer, Sisodiya, & Sander, 2016; Laxer et al., 2014) that can both affect the ability to self-manage and require individual and professional management.

General overall health can also be affected by epilepsy. People with epilepsy are more likely to have migraines (Beghi, 2016; Keezer et al., 2016) and heart disease than the general public (Beghi, 2016). People with epilepsy tend to live less healthy lives overall than individuals who do not have the impairment. People with epilepsy are more likely to smoke and less likely to exercise than the general public (Bjorholt, Nakken, Rohme, & Hansen, 1990; Cui, Kobau, Zack, Buelow, & Austin, 2015). However, a study from Canada reported that healthy behavior has improved over time (Roberts et al., 2015). In early studies, lack of activity in people with epilepsy might have been associated with overprotection and understimulation (Bjorholt et al., 1990), but as Roberts et al.'s (2015), research suggests, lifestyle may be improving as there often are more opportunities for those with disabilities.

Psychological and Social Impact

Clinicians have long recognized that quality of life is affected by epilepsy, but research shows quality of life for people with epilepsy has not improved significantly (Buelow, 2001; Elliott & Richardson, 2014). Seizure severity may be the most important factor involved, suggesting that the best means of improving quality of life is to increase seizure control, but other factors may also play a role, like social factors (social isolation) and psychological factors (depression and anxiety; Jacoby, Snape, & Baker, 2009). Anxiety and depression have been closely associated with epilepsy (Buelow, McNelis, Shore, & Austin, 2006; Buelow & Shore, 2010). In one study of adults with epilepsy, depression was the most common problem for people with epilepsy, with 66% of those interviewed displaying symptoms (Tunde-Ayinmode, Abiodun, Ajiboye, Buhari, & Sanya, 2014). In another study, 23% of youth with epilepsy reported depressive symptoms (Guilfoyle et al., 2015). The unpredictable nature of seizures and fear of death for people with epilepsy affect mental health, resulting in anxiety and depression (Novy et al., 2012; Tunde-Ayinmode et al., 2014).

Stigma

Stigma is a contributing factor to psychosocial difficulties associated with epilepsy. Stigma is defined as a "mark or token of infamy, disgrace, or reproach" (Dictionary.com, 2016). People with epilepsy are often singled out as being different because of their lack of control over seizures. The stigma attached to epilepsy has deep historical roots. In the past, people with epilepsy were viewed as having personality defects, criminal tendencies, and even demonic possession (Dwyer, 1992). As recently as the late nineteenth century, neurologists categorized "epileptics" as individuals with strange behaviors, and even in the early twentieth century children with epilepsy were confined to colonies (Dwyer, 1992).

In addition to the actual stigma that society attaches to epilepsy, another difficulty arises from perceived stigma. Distinct from actual stigma acted upon in society, perceived stigma is a feeling in the affected individual of disability or disgrace that is not related to actual factors (Collings, 1990a, 1990b). Early studies of quality of life in epilepsy denoted stigma as a serious problem (Ryan, Kempner,

& Emlen, 1980), and it continues to be a problem today in our supposedly more "enlightened" culture. In sum, stigma attach to epilepsy has not changed greatly over the years (Austin, McNelis, Shore, Dunn, & Musick, 2002; Laxer et al., 2014).

Employment and Social Isolation

According to many studies, employment and social isolation continue to be a problem for people with epilepsy. Employment rates of those with epilepsy are about half those without (Herman & Jacoby, 2009; Holland, Lane, Whitehead, Marson, & Jacoby, 2009). Further, people with epilepsy are twice as likely not to finish school and are more likely to find jobs as unskilled workers (Hermann & Jacoby, 2009; Holland, Lane, Whitehead, Marson, & Jacoby, 2009). One study reported that employment rates did not differ significantly between those with and those without epilepsy, although those with epilepsy were likely to have lower salaries (Puka & Smith, 2016). Several studies associated the likelihood of employment with seizure control (Puka & Smith, 2016; Wo, Lim, Choo, & Tan, 2015). Social isolation for people with epilepsy can be debilitating. Social isolation may be related to the inability to drive, the difficulty procuring meaningful employment, stigma, and poor self-esteem (Kerr, 2012).

Managing the Risk of Living with Epilepsy

Not-for-profit epilepsy organizations can provide print materials and online information on how to reduce risks associated with epilepsy, which depend mostly on the type and frequency of seizures. It is encouraging that the outlook for most people with epilepsy is good, with up to 70% achieving seizure freedom using correct and targeted treatment (Kobau et al. 2008). Getting the most out of life while aiming for seizure freedom requires making informed choices. Each individual situation is different. Making the right choices means obtaining appropriate information from a variety of sources, including the medical team, family, and friends, others with epilepsy, and the aforementioned local, national, and international epilepsy associations and their help-line staff.

For those with active epilepsy, some general advice can help reduce risk for those individuals who experience seizures that impair awareness (Taylor, 2000). At home, it is sensible to work out ways to avoid accidents involving hot water or hot cooking oils. Consider turning handles of pans away while cooking so pans are not knocked over. A cooker guard can prevent accidents. If seizures are frequent, it is best to carry plates to the stove rather than hot food to the table and use a microwave to heat a cup rather than pouring boiling water from a kettle. Taking a bath may be risky, and so others in the house should be informed. The bathroom door should not be locked. Showers may be less risky. Parents with epilepsy should never bathe a baby when alone and may find it safest to use a baby bath on the floor rather than on a table.

Further, according to Taylor (2000), sports should generally be encouraged and restrictions must be sensible. Cycling may be permissible as long as a helmet and high-visibility clothing are worn. Swimming may be reasonable if someone with lifesaving skills is available and informed. Sports like rock-climbing are best avoided.

Employment opportunities are often restricted by epilepsy, which may result in a bar on jobs such as vocational driving or flying and some jobs in the armed forces (Thompson, 1995; www.epilepsy.ie; www.epilepsy.org.uk). Legal rules about driving and guidance about employment may vary from country to country, so advice should be sought from the relevant authorities. When people receive a diagnosis of epilepsy, they need to consider what interventions may help them return to living a life with epilepsy rather than living for epilepsy. Their rehabilitation should not focus on the medical aspects of the condition only but also on the social, psychological, and neuropsychological aspects of the diagnosis (Thompson, 1995). Part of that rehabilitation process involves addressing the factors associated with employment of people with epilepsy. There are a number of complex problems in finding and maintaining employment that are broader than seizure frequency and severity. Stigma and psychosocial variables including low self-esteem and low self-efficacy must be identified and addressed through specific training programs (Smeets et al., 2007).

ACCIDENTS, TRAUMA, AND MORTALITY ASSOCIATED WITH EPILEPSY

While it is true that epilepsy is associated with a higher rate of premature death than among the general population, this risk is in reality quite small for the majority of people with epilepsy. The most common cause of premature death among those with epilepsy is sudden unexpected death in epilepsy (SUDEP). It is difficult to quantify the incidence of SUDEP because of the variable reporting of this cause of death. SUDEP occurs due to autonomic deregulation of cardiorespiratory pathways as a result of seizures (Smithson, Colwell, & Hanna, 2014). It is more common in generalized convulsive events while the person is asleep. It affects males more than females and occurs more in people with abrupt and frequent changes in antiepilepsy drugs (AEDs). The risk of SUDEP can be reduced by good seizure control, and the most effective way to do this is to ensure treatment with targeted AEDs taken as prescribed (Smithson et al., 2014). For individuals to be able to make informed choices, it is important for them to be aware of their personal risks. It may be helpful to collect information about these risks from a trusted source and to assess whether there is a need to consider using personal epilepsy monitoring equipment, such as an epilepsy application for a phone or some form of seizure-detection device.

KNOWLEDGE ABOUT THE IMPAIRMENT THAT AN INDIVIDUAL NEEDS FOR SELF-MANAGEMENT

Because disability associated with epilepsy is highly variable based on syndrome, seizure frequency, and co-occurring conditions, describing what individuals need to know to be good self-managers is complex. Early research suggested that all people with epilepsy needed only to take their medications as ordered and that those who had frequent interactions with their clinicians were more likely to do that

(Cramer, 1991). A plethora of early literature looked at how to help people with epilepsy take their medications as ordered (Cramer, 1991; DiIorio & Manteuffel, 1995; Pryse-Phillips, Jardine, & Bursey, 1982). However, despite research designed to help people do as the doctor ordered, outcomes have not changed. While most of the early literature examined linear mechanisms to help people take their medications as ordered, a few researchers widened the net by addressing the multiple issues that accompanied taking medications. In an extensive qualitative study that included medication management, individuals identified alternative strategies to manage medications different than what the physician ordered and suggested that people taking AEDs purposefully decided how to fit them into their lives (Schneider & Conrad, 1981). DiIorio, Hennessy, and Manteuffel (1996) looked at medication management in conjunction with other factors and proposed a model to help people with epilepsy not only take medications as ordered but also become better self-managers. Buelow and Smith (2004) found that taking medications carried a component of embarrassment, and side effects often influenced how medications were taken. These findings suggest that people make decisions about taking medications that might be influenced by a number of positive and negative factors. The "necessity concerns framework" acknowledges that taking medicines can be a difficult decision for some people and that the decision to take them is a balance between the perceived necessity of medicines and concerns about long-term use (Phillips, Diefenbach, Kronish, Negron, & Horowitz, 2014).

Later research suggested that self-management was far more complex than just medication management and required a high level of skill to navigate everyday life with epilepsy. DiIorio and colleagues proposed that social integration, self-efficacy, and regimen-specific support affected outcome expectations, which in turn impacted self-management (DiIorio et al., 1996; DiIorio, Faherty, & Manteuffel, 1991, 1994). Knowledge alone was not enough to help people with epilepsy become better self-managers. Clark and Nothwehr (1997) suggested that self-management requires mastery of three categories: (a) knowledge of the condition, (b) activities directed at management of the condition, and (c) skills to maintain adequate psychosocial functioning. In Clark and Nothwehr's view, self-management is more than knowledge; it is a complex mixture of knowledge about the epilepsy process and effects and the individual's goals and beliefs. This was a transition away from the idea that people needed only to know enough about their epilepsy and their medications to manage their medicines and their impairment. DiIorio (1997) defined self-management as the sum of steps that people perform to gain seizure control, minimize the impact of having epilepsy, and maximize quality of life. This definition broadened the concept of self-management from only medication control to other skills including life management.

Buelow (2001) conducted a hybrid concept analysis of self-management in people with epilepsy. The analysis included an extensive review of the literature and individual interviews. The end product was a conceptual framework. In that framework, self-management consisted of actions to manage clinicians' prescriptions, seizure-management activities other than those prescribed by a clinician, and life-management activities. The framework was the foundation of a further study where 25 people with poorly controlled epilepsy were interviewed about their understanding of self-management. In that study, Buelow and Johnson (2000) found that those interviewed could be classified as either *proactive* or *reactive* managers; they had to employ techniques to manage medications, seizure events, social relationships, employment and education, and transportation. Unger and Buelow (2009), in an effort to further define self-management in adults newly diagnosed with epilepsy, conducted a concept analysis using both literature reviews and a fieldwork phase. They found interactive themes regarding the participants' self-management experiences that included emotional and physical comfort, functional ability, and self-management actions and behavior.

DiIorio is the most-published epilepsy self-management expert. In several studies, she associated multiple variables with self-management outcomes. Higher levels of perceived stigma were associated with lower levels of self-efficacy in epilepsy management, medication management and taking medicines as ordered, and individual satisfaction (DiIorio et al., 2006). Additionally, people experienced stigma if they experienced poor seizure control, could not drive, or had early onset of seizures and/or recent seizures (DiIorio et al., 2003). She tested a psychosocial model of self-management based on Bandura's social cognitive theory and specifically on his concept of self-efficacy. She found that social support and stigma were related to self-efficacy and depressive symptoms and concluded that self-management including medication management is related to a set of interactions among psychosocial variables. In a later study, she found that self-efficacy, outcome expectancies, depressive symptoms, and social support all related to self-management behaviors. In that study, self-efficacy was associated with lifestyle management (Robinson et al., 2008).

In summary, research into self-management in epilepsy suggests that the person with epilepsy needs to understand both diagnosis and treatment. However, knowledge alone is not sufficient to help individuals with epilepsy become better self-managers. Clinicians need to work with the person with epilepsy to identify barriers to self-management. Clinicians must address not only treatment but also epilepsy in everyday life. Also, people who experience seizures are more likely to be involved in accidental events that can cause harm, and people who have seizures, even those who do not have frequent seizures, may be at risk for SUDEP.

OTHER BARRIERS TO SELF-MANAGEMENT

As in other chronic health conditions, effective self-management in epilepsy faces multiple barriers that are related to not only treatment but also life situations.

Barriers Related to Taking Seizure Medications

Taking seizure medications requires a set of activities that are based on factors beyond the medical model perspective (i.e., treating pathology) and are often not considered by the prescriber. These factors include (a) the cost of the medication and the individual's ability to pay for it; (b) the individual's mobility (or other methods of getting medications when needed), (c) side effects of the medication and the ways in which the individual reacts to those side effects, (d) the individual's understanding of (and agreement with) the importance of the medication in his or her overall treatment plan, and (e) the individual's mental state and likelihood of missing doses of medication. Seizure medications are often expensive. Many individuals with epilepsy do not have high-paying jobs, and some do not have insurance. When diagnosed with epilepsy, most people lose their driver's license. Depending on where they live and with whom they live, they may then lack the means to obtain their medications. Seizure medications can also cause side effects that individuals feel they cannot tolerate, and therefore they self-adjust the treatment regimen (i.e., reduce the dosage or frequency) to control those side effects.

Implementing agreed-on decisions about medicines is a dynamic and variable behavior. Not following the decision can be intentional because it is influenced by peoples' attitudes about their condition, the balance of concerns about taking medicines, and their judgment of the necessity of the treatment (Chapman, Horne, Chater, Hukins, & Smithson, 2014). Even when people merely forget to take their medications, they may not have a plan on how to get back on track. Thus, the individual and the prescriber need to work out a plan to reduce the unintentional non-implementation due to forgetfulness. In summary, individuals with epilepsy and their clinicians should have regular discussions regarding barriers to taking the medications.

Barriers Related to Seizure Management beyond the Clinician's Prescription

People with seizures often identify their own seizure triggers. These might be related to certain foods or diet in general, amount of sleep, stress or stress-related events, or other individualized triggers. Managing these seizure triggers can often be difficult for the person with epilepsy, especially those related to social situations and life events over which they have no control. In some cases, managing seizure triggers becomes the person's preoccupation—sometimes almost an obsession. This can result in decreasing social interactions, increased stress, and increased perceived stigma, eventuating in a vicious cycle from which the person with seizures cannot escape. DiIorio's and colleagues (2006) have shown that all of these can be related to poor self-management and also to poor seizure control.

Barriers Related to Coping

Other management barriers relate to how a person with epilepsy lives or copes with their condition. While public awareness of epilepsy has increased somewhat, there is still a stigma associated with telling others about epilepsy, as we have already discussed. Individuals with epilepsy are often not sure what to tell employers, school officials, friends, and neighbors about their seizures. Their fear of losing a job, having difficulties in school, and being discriminated against are very real. As has been noted, active epilepsy is a guarantee of losing one's driver's license. This alone increases social isolation and dependency on others and exacerbates the perception of stigma.

Barriers Related to Life Management

Finally, for many individuals with epilepsy, managing the impact of having a seizure in public becomes a barrier to life-management. Some people describe how recovering from a seizure takes a long time, even in the case of milder partial seizures. This recovery, of course, interferes with the ability to continue normal activities. Others with epilepsy describe dangerous situations that have happened related to having a seizure in public.

CASE STUDY

The following is a true story. It characterizes some of the issues surrounding self-management. Consider Mr. W. who lives in a rural area in the United States. He is 60 years old and relies on farming for a living. He lives 10 miles out of town, and his nearest neighbors are approximately 2 miles away. He has two grown children who live in a city about 45 minutes away with their families. His wife has had a stroke, and while she is home and recovering, she requires care and frequent therapy visits. Mr. W. began having "spells" that he could not well describe other than that he knew something was happening to him. He might have had an alteration in awareness when he had a spell, but he did not really know. He went to his family doctor who thought he was under a lot of stress because of his wife and told him to take it easy. After Mr. W. complained of this problem for about six months to his primary care physician, he was referred to a neurologist. The neurologist did not think it was anything serious but did an EEG and MRI anyway. Except for some mild white-matter changes, the MRI looked okay, but the EEG was abnormal. In fact, the farmer had an event while having the EEG. This was suggestive of focal epilepsy. The doctor explained what that meant, put him on medication that he was required to take twice a day, and sent him home. As Mr. W. was on his way out the doctor said, "By the way, you can't drive until you have been seizure free for six months."

When thinking about Mr. W., we can see that the idea of self-management can be very complex. Taking his own medication is only one piece of the puzzle facing Mr. W. The doctor hopes he will take his pills as ordered as he traverses this difficult scenario. But if he cannot drive, how will he work his farm? How is he going to get his wife to the doctor and to her therapy appointments? How will he get his medicine and do the grocery shopping? The difficulties that result from this diagnosis unfold like some unwelcome weed blossoming in the garden. Taken together, this situation can be overwhelming for an individual. It becomes clear that self-management is not a one-size-fits-all concept or a one-and-done intervention where individuals learns about their impairment and therapy, gains or regains confidence in themselves, and goes on their way through life. Many individuals need help working through problems such as Mr. W. faces, and they need that help on an ongoing basis. Mr. W. needed someone to sit down with him to explain his epilepsy and his medication and how to take that medication. This kind of discussion would include what to do if he had side effects, forgot a dose, or had a seizure. Finally, on that first visit, he would need help to get home. After that, phone visits (or office visits if transportation can be arranged) should be scheduled to help him identify and "get a handle on" the problems he encounters and to identify his goals and solutions to those problems. This kind of care is individual-centered and seeks solutions that address individuals' needs cooperatively.

Admittedly, Mr. W.'s is a complex situation, but it is not far from that of many people with epilepsy. His story can help to illustrate the types of situations that individuals face as they go home from a doctor's office with a new diagnosis of epilepsy. Unfortunately, little incentive to provide this type of comprehensive care for people with epilepsy exists in the United States, as no insurance or governmental agency provides substantial reimbursement for the individual-centered type of activity described here. Research is necessary to show that frequent interactions with healthcare educators not only improves individual outcomes but also decreases healthcare utilization and costs. This kind of work is currently being considered by the Centers for Disease Control (CDC) and the Epilepsy Foundation in the United States.

EVIDENCE-BASED PRACTICES ON INTERVENTIONS THAT IMPROVE HEALTH OUTCOMES

In examining the range of existing self-management interventions for those with epilepsy, we looked at two types of review articles: Cochrane Database reviews and systematic reviews. In general, Cochrane articles reviewed randomized controlled trials only, while systematic reviews included more varied articles. While they both used rigorous criteria, the second type of reviews yielded a larger number of examined self-management interventions.

Reviews of Self-Management Interventions for Adults

In a Cochrane review, Bradley, Bradley, and Lindsay (2008) examined 16 interventions regarding self-management in adults. They found that all studies had methodological weaknesses and that therefore findings must be approached with caution. However, two intervention types showed promise: epilepsy nurse specialist educational programs and programs that provided self-management education.

A systematic review of 16 articles addressing self-management in adults with epilepsy supported the ability of epilepsy education programs to improve knowledge and self-confidence in managing epilepsy (Edward, Cook, & Giandinoto, 2015). The types of programs presented in the paper were all different, but the components of each intervention might be considered when developing programs to help people manage their epilepsy.

According to reviews such as these, intervention studies had methodological problems, but this should come as no surprise. Behavioral and intervention research is necessarily done with human beings who live in a complex world; therefore such research comes with a special set of challenges. The "lab" is the world, and it is impossible to control all the variables that come into play. However, the evidence suggests that these interventions do help people with epilepsy become better managers and that they should be continued. Second, interventions should be funded and carried out for the populations they were designed to serve. We would not consider an intervention tested for adults to necessarily be appropriate for children. In the same manner, we should consider culturally sensitive interventions, age-appropriate interventions, and topic-specific interventions. When developing programs, however, it makes sense to address the methodological issues identified where possible.

COPING STRATEGIES OR SKILLS TAUGHT FOR IMPAIRMENT

Strategies to manage a life with epilepsy are developed by the individual to cope with the condition and as individuals meet and discuss their experiences, a body of evidence builds. This can then be used as a basis for educational initiatives. Information is available in a number of different forms and can be disseminated in a number of ways.

Anecdotal Reports

Clinicians' interest in self-management in epilepsy is apparent when reading discussions in the literature. Expert opinions about self-management all point to the individual's need for knowledge about epilepsy. Areas of self-management and self-management behavior discussed anecdotally in the literature include the individual's and the caregiver's educational needs in relation to self-management and the impact of stigma and co-occurring impairments on self-management (Legion, 1991; Shafer, 1994). Other topics include the unique self-management needs of special populations, which are also discussed in the literature (Buelow et al., 2000; Shafer, 1998), and potential interventions such as relaxation therapy and complementary and alternative therapies (Noeker, 2004). While not empirically based, these publications raise awareness of the need for programs that improve epilepsy individuals' and their families' ability to manage their epilepsy.

Reported Self-Management Interventions

Many programs designed to improve individual knowledge and address actions that will improve self-management behavior have been reported. Most of these programs aim at improving knowledge, self-management skills, or quality of life, but only a few have been rigorously developed and tested. Many of the reported programs are not empirically based or they have a low degree of evidence because they were not rigorously tested and could not be replicated. Regardless of these difficulties, the studies do support the need for programs that are accessible to people with epilepsy and their families. Programs such as these may help people become better self-managers, decrease medical costs, and improve quality of life.

EDUCATIONAL NEEDS

In 1978, Nelson, Edwards, Roberts, and Keller discussed a comprehensive self-medication program in the hospital meant to help individuals gradually assume responsibility for self-medicating. Individuals completed a four-phase individual program that trained them to take their medications. Outcomes were not reported. Ridsdale, Morgan, and O'Connor (1999) discussed the success of a nurse-run educational clinic. Nurses trained people in one-to-one educational sessions. In that program, people reported being satisfied with speaking to nurses because the nurses had dedicated time to answer their questions. People believed that physicians were too busy to adequately answer their questions. Again, long-term outcomes were not discussed.

Three emergency departments (ED) in London were involved in a comparison study to see if nurse education would decrease unnecessary ED visits. The individuals in the intervention group completed two educational sessions with an epilepsy nurse specialist. The intervention group took place in the ED. Individuals from two other EDs without such a program were the treatment-as-usual (control) group. The authors found no significant difference in number of ED visits between the groups but did find that those most likely to repeat ED visits expressed feelings of stigmatization and had low confidence in managing epilepsy (Noble, Morgan, Virdi, & Ridsdale, 2013).

In a program in Iran, individuals were recruited in neurology clinics and randomly assigned to intervention or control groups. The treatment group received four educational sessions on epilepsy including a self-management plan. The treatment group scored significantly better on self-management scores after one month (Aliasgharpour, Dehgahn Nayeri, Yadegary, & Haghani, 2013). Similarly, a group in India provided four structured health education classes to 90 individuals randomized to the treatment group, which improved modestly in regard to following treatment guidelines (i.e., "adherence"), while the control group did not. In this study, no difference was found in self-efficacy scores (Dash, Sebastian,

Aggarwal, & Tripathi, 2015). In a recent study, individuals ($n = 20$) who attended a clinic-based educational program designed to teach a self-management protocol improved in their self-efficacy and self-management scores (Cole & Gaspar, 2015).

The reported studies had methodological challenges, with these studies including small sample sizes, lack of true or any randomization, and questions regarding intervention fidelity, all of which make replication difficult. Nevertheless, these interventions suggest that providing education to individuals with epilepsy and their caregivers can be beneficial. Overall, while the best and most cost-effective methods for doing this have yet to be discovered or verified, education should be considered an integral part of every hospital or clinic visit.

Telephone and Web-Based Education, Problem-Solving, and Support

Telephone interventions have also been tested. DiIorio, Reisinger, Yeager, and McCarty (2009) conducted a feasibility test of a telephone-based self-management program for adults with epilepsy. The program used motivational interviewing principles for 22 individuals recruited from a hospital clinic. Participants were randomly assigned to the intervention or control group. The intervention group had five sessions with an epilepsy nurse specialist trained in motivational interviewing. The first session was face-to-face, and the remaining sessions were by phone. The authors found that this format was feasible and worthy of continued development and testing.

Web-Based Programs Teaching Coping, Problem-Solving, and Support

With the advent of the Internet and smartphones, telephone interventions have been replaced by web-based programs to address problems seen in face-to-face and telephone programs. For example, an online program for US veterans was tested to both determine the usability of an online community for veterans and the program's efficacy in improving self-management and self-efficacy (Hixson et al., 2015). The results of a within-subject comparison study suggested that self-management skills and self-management self-efficacy improved due to the program and that this type of program was both feasible and usable (Hixson et al., 2015). In another study of an online community of adults with epilepsy in Taiwan, two groups were compared (Koo et al., 2012). One group was a preexisting online community and the second group consisted of adults who attended an epilepsy clinic and comprised the usual-care group. Those who participated in the online community seemed to improve in self-management skills and reported that the program was usable. However, the authors showed that online users tended to have more frequent seizures, more adverse events, and more anxiety and depression than the usual-care group, making the two groups different at baseline (Koo et al., 2012). A different study looked at online use in the US veteran population and found that while veterans reported the need for a distance-based program, only 51% had the ability to be online (Pramuka, Hendrickson, Zinski, & Van Cott, 2007), thus limiting the usability of an online program. Wicks et al. (2012) discussed the usefulness of a virtual "epilepsy community" to share data and information between individuals. Those using the community discussed how important it was to find other individuals who had problems similar to their own.

The interventions and programs discussed here do not provide a unified strategy to address self-management, but they do help to identify successful delivery methods. For example, web use may be one alternative to helping individuals build community where coming together for in-person meetings is difficult. The phone may be an alternative to reaching individuals in need who do not have Internet access and cannot easily attend a clinic-based program. Healthcare professionals should assess the educational needs of individuals that they assist.

Buelow, Johnson, Perkins, Austin, and Dunn (2013) implemented a problem-solving program for parents of children with severe epilepsy. The program was a wait-list controlled pilot study. Three separate groups of 8 to 10 parents attended four sessions providing education, problem-solving, and goal-setting. Parents who attended were especially impressed with working with other parents; some of the groups continued to meet after the completion of the intervention. While parents were satisfied with the program, recruitment was highly problematic. Parents who did not attend cited time constraints.

TESTED TECHNIQUES TO FACILITATE SELF-MANAGEMENT

Some programs have been more broadly tested than the ones described earlier and might be replicated. Several are discussed in this section.

Modular Service Package Epilepsy

The Modular Service Package Epilepsy (MOSES) was developed in Germany as a multidisciplinary effort to educate and support adults and children with epilepsy and their families (May & Pfafflin, 2002;May & Pfafflin, 2005; Wohlrab, Rinnert, Bettendorf, Fischbach, Heinen, Klein (2007)). The purpose of MOSES is to improve individuals' knowledge about epilepsy and its consequences, help them gain a better understanding of psychosocial and occupational problems, and provide them with active coping skills. MOSES has been broadly used and widely tested. It was reported to improve knowledge and coping and to decrease seizure frequency, which the authors related to better self-management skills (May & Pfafflin, 2002).

The Self-Management Education for Adults with Poorly Controlled Epilepsy

This intervention is based on the MOSES program. The Self-Management Education for Adults with Poorly Controlled Epilepsy (SMILE) program was tested in the UK for acceptability and appropriateness of its format in a community setting, how well it improved quality of life, and its cost-effectiveness. The effectiveness testing of this program is ongoing (Kralj-Hans et al., 2014; Magill et al., 2015).

Managing Epilepsy Well Network

The Managing Epilepsy Well (MEW) program was developed in 2007 by the CDC to address priorities listed by both the 2003 Living Well with Epilepsy workshop and the Institute of Medicine's "Epilepsy Across the Spectrum" recommendations of 2012 related to accelerating, promoting, and disseminating epilepsy self-management research. The MEW network is one of CDC's Prevention Center Research Program thematic networks, and information on all programs can be retrieved from the MEW Network (CDC, 2016).The network has produced four available intervention programs. A brief description follows.

WEB EPILEPSY, AWARENESS, SUPPORT, AND EDUCATION
Web Epilepsy, Awareness, Support, and Education (WEBEASE) is an online, theory-based, interactive self-management support and education program. Participants engage in three interactive modules that address medication management, stress, and sleep. An online journal is provided to facilitate monitoring of seizures, medication management, and other related stress and sleep issues. The program was developed with input from both individuals with epilepsy and professionals who work with epilepsy. It has undergone extensive testing and is one of the few programs that has been shown to be sustainable and to improve individual self-management (DiIorio, Bamps, Walker, & Escoffery, 2011; DiIorio, Escoffery, et al., 2009). It has also been translated into Spanish. The program is offered free online through both Emory University and the Epilepsy Foundation.

USING PRACTICE AND LEARNING TO INCREASE FAVORABLE THOUGHTS
Using Practice and Learning to Increase Favorable Thoughts (UPLIFT) is designed to provide treatment for depression in people with epilepsy by delivering mindfulness-based cognitive therapy to groups of six to eight people by telephone or Internet. It uses eight sessions and is conducted by mental health experts. In a randomized controlled trial, UPLIFT was found to decrease the incidence of depression and depressive symptoms and to reduce seizure frequency in adults with epilepsy (Thompson et al., 2015).

MANAGEMENT INFORMATION DECISION SUPPORT EPILEPSY TOOL
The Management Information Decision Support Epilepsy Tool (MINDSET) is a tablet-based program providing real-time self-management assessment identified by the individual with epilepsy and relayed to his or her doctor, thus allowing both individual and clinician to prioritize self-management discussions and plans. MINDSET is still being tested broadly in conjunction with other self-management

strategies. In early testing, individuals and clinicians rated MINDSET favorably on communications and shared decision-making (Begley et al., 2015).

PROGRAM TO ENCOURAGE ACTIVE, REWARDING LIVES FOR SENIORS
The Program to Encourage Active, Rewarding Lives for Seniors (PEARLS) is a program intended to reduce depression in seniors with epilepsy. It incorporates theoretical approaches to teach clients to take action to make life changes. It was developed for both adults and seniors with epilepsy and is delivered in the home utilizing a multidisciplinary approach. It involves problem-solving, behavioral activation, and psychiatric consults. PEARLS has had two randomized controlled trials (Chaytor et al., 2011; Ciechanowski et al., 2010) providing evidence for both the efficacy of the program and the long-term outcomes. In those trials, it was shown to decrease depressive symptoms in up to 50% of those attending the programs, and it improved emotional well-being. These findings were sustained for up to 18 months. Furthermore, this program has been disseminated broadly.

CONCLUSION

More than four decades of work support the need for self-management skills for people who have a diagnosis of epilepsy. Early work was based primarily on a medical model (i.e., a perspective focused only on treating pathology), suggesting that all individuals with epilepsy needed do is take their medications as ordered. That research evolved into a more complex approach to self-management that considered all areas of a person's life. While there are many empirically based interventions available, more research is necessary because we do not really know the long-term effects of the available interventions and there is not good evidence for their usefulness in ethnically and culturally diverse populations or among individuals in the lower socioeconomic strata. Despite these concerns, self-management research has come a long way in understanding individuals' needs regarding self-management.

REFERENCES

Aliasgharpour, M., Dehgahn Nayeri, N., Yadegary, M. A., & Haghani, H. (2013). Effects of an educational program on self-management in patient with epilepsy. *Seizure, 22*(1), 48–52. doi:10.1016/j.seizure.2012.10.005

Austin, J. K., McNelis, A. M., Shore, C. P., Dunn, D. W., & Musick, B. (2002). A feasibility study of a family seizure management program: "Be seizure smart." *Journal of Neuroscience Nursing, 34*(1), 30–37.

Beghi, E. (2016). Addressing the burden of epilepsy: Many unmet needs. *Pharmacological Research, 107*, 79–84. doi:10.1016/j.phrs.2016.03.003

Begley, C., Shegog, R., Harding, A., Goldsmith, C., Hope, O., & Newmark, M. (2015). Longitudinal feasibility of MINDSET: A clinic decision aid for epilepsy self-management. *Epilepsy & Behavior, 44*, 143–150. doi:10.1016/j.yebeh.2014.12.031

Berg, A. T., Berkovic, S. F., Brodie, M. J., Buchhalter, J., Cross, J. H., van Emde Boas, W, & Scheffer, I. E. (2010). Revised terminology and concepts for organization of seizures and epilepsies: Report of the ILAE Commission on Classification and Terminology, 2005-2009. *Epilepsia, 51*(4), 676-685. doi:10.1111/j.1528-1167.2010.02522.x

Bjorholt, P. G., Nakken, K. O., Rohme, K., & Hansen, H. (1990). Leisure time habits and physical fitness in adults with epilepsy. *Epilepsia, 31*(1), 83-87.

Bradley, P. M., & Lindsay, B. (2008). Care delivery and self-management strategies for adults with epilepsy. *Cochrane Database of Systematic Reviews, 1*, CD006244. doi:10.1002/14651858.CD006244.pub2

Buelow, J. M. (2001). Epilepsy management issues and techniques. *Journal of Neuroscience Nursing, 33*(5), 260-269.

Buelow, J. M., & Johnson, J. (2000). Self-management of epilepsy: A review of the concepts and its outcomes. *Disease Management and Health Outcomes, 8*, 327-336.

Buelow, J. M., Johnson, C. S., Perkins, S. M., Austin, J. K., & Dunn, D. W. (2013). Creating Avenues for Parent Partnership (CAPP): An intervention for parents of children with epilepsy and learning problems. *Epilepsy & Behavior, 27*(1), 64-69. doi:10.1016/j.yebeh.2012.12.013

Buelow, J. M., McNelis, A., Shore, C. P., & Austin, J. K. (2006). Stressors of parents of children with epilepsy and intellectual disability. *Journal of Neuroscience Nursing, 38*(3), 147-154, 176.

Buelow, J. M., Shafer, P., Shinnar, R., Austin, J., Dewar, S., Long, L., & Santilli, N. (2016). Perspectives on seizure clusters: Gaps in lexicon, awareness, and treatment. *Epilepsy & Behavior, 57*, 16-22. doi:10.1016/j.yebeh.2016.01.028

Buelow, J. M., & Shore, C. P. (2010). Management challenges in children with both epilepsy and intellectual disability. *Clinical Nurse Specialist, 24*(6), 313-320. doi:10.1097/NUR.0b013e3181f903cb

Buelow, J. M., & Smith, M. C. (2004). Medication management by the person with epilepsy: Perception versus reality. *Epilepsy & Behavior, 5*(3), 401-406. doi:10.1016/j.yebeh.2004.02.002

Chapman, S. C., Horne, R., Chater, A., Hukins, D., & Smithson, W. H. (2014). Patient' perspectives on antiepileptic medication: Relationships between beliefs about medicines and adherence among patients with epilepsy in UK primary care. *Epilepsy & Behavior, 31*, 312-320. doi:10.1016/j.yebeh.2013.10.016

Chaytor, N., Ciechanowski, P., Miller, J. W., Fraser, R., Russo, J., Unutzer, J., & Gilliam, F. (2011). Long-term outcomes from the PEARLS randomized trial for the treatment of depression in patients with epilepsy. *Epilepsy & Behavior, 20*(3), 545-549. doi:10.1016/j.yebeh.2011.01.017

Ciechanowski, P., Chaytor, N., Miller, J., Fraser, R., Russo, J., Unutzer, J., & Gilliam, F. (2010). PEARLS depression treatment for individuals with epilepsy: A randomized controlled trial. *Epilepsy & Behavior, 19*(3), 225-231. doi:10.1016/j.yebeh.2010.06.003

Clark, N. M., & Nothwehr, F. (1997). Self-management of asthma by adult patients. *Patient Education and Counseling, 32*, S5-S20.

Cole, K. A., & Gaspar, P. M. (2015). Implementation of an epilepsy self-management protocol. *Journal of Neuroscience Nursing, 47*(1), 3-9. doi:10.1097/JNN.0000000000000105

Collings, J. A. (1990a). Correlates of wellbeing in a New Zealand epilepsy sample. *New Zealand Medical Journal, 103*(892), 301-303.

Collings, J. A. (1990b). Psychosocial well-being and epilepsy: An empirical study. *Epilepsia, 31*(4), 418–426.

Cramer, J. A. (1991). Medication in epilepsy. *Archives of Internal Medicine, 151*(6), 1236–1237.

Cui, W., Kobau, R., Zack, M. M., Buelow, J. M., & Austin, J. K. (2015). Recent changes in attitudes of US adults toward people with epilepsy: Results from the 2005 SummerStyles and 2013 FallStyles surveys. *Epilepsy & Behavior, 52*(Pt A), 108–118. doi:10.1016/j.yebeh.2015.08.040

Dash, D., Sebastian, T. M., Aggarwal, M., & Tripathi, M. (2015). Impact of health education on drug adherence and self-care in people with epilepsy with low education. *Epilepsy & Behavior, 44*, 213–217. doi:10.1016/j.yebeh.2014.12.030

Delacy, M. J., Reid, S. M., & Australian Cerebral Palsy Register Group. (2016). Profile of associated impairments at age 5 years in Australia by cerebral palsy subtype and Gross Motor Function Classification System level for birth years 1996 to 2005. *Developmental Medicine and Child Neurology, 58*(Suppl. 2), 50–56. doi:10.1111/dmcn.13012

Dictionary.com. (n.d.). Stigma. Retrieved from http://www.dictionary.com/stigma

DiIorio, C. (1997). *Epilepsy self-management.* Handbook of Health Behavior Research II. Springer.

DiIorio, C., Bamps, Y., Walker, E. R., & Escoffery, C. (2011). Results of a research study evaluating WebEase, an online epilepsy self-management program. *Epilepsy & Behavior, 22*(3), 469–474. doi:10.1016/j.yebeh.2011.07.030

DiIorio, C., Escoffery, C., McCarty, F., Yeager, K. A., Henry, T. R., Koganti, A., . . . Wexler, B. (2009). Evaluation of WebEase: An epilepsy self-management web site. *Health Education Research, 24*(2), 185–197. doi:10.1093/her/cyn012

DiIorio, C., Faherty, B., & Manteuffel, B. (1991). Cognitive-perceptual factors associated with antiepileptic medication compliance. *Research in Nursing and Health, 14*(5), 329–338.

DiIorio, C., Faherty, B., & Manteuffel, B. (1994). Epilepsy self-management: Partial replication and extension. *Research in Nursing and Health, 17*(3), 167–174.

DiIorio, C., Hennessy, M., & Manteuffel, B. (1996). Epilepsy self-management: A test of a theoretical model. *Nursing Research, 45*(4), 211–217.

DiIorio, C., & Manteuffel, B. (1995). Preferences concerning epilepsy education: Opinions of nurses, physicians, and persons with epilepsy. *Journal of Neuroscience Nursing, 27*(1), 29–34.

DiIorio, C., Reisinger, E. L., Yeager, K. A., & McCarty, F. (2009). A telephone-based self-management program for people with epilepsy. *Epilepsy & Behavior, 14*(1), 232–236. doi:10.1016/j.yebeh.2008.10.016

DiIorio, C., Shafer, P. O., Letz, R., Henry, T. R., Schomer, D. L., Yeager, K., & Project, E. S. G. (2006). Behavioral, social, and affective factors associated with self-efficacy for self-management among people with epilepsy. *Epilepsy & Behavior, 9*(1), 158–163. doi:10.1016/j.yebeh.2006.05.001

DiIorio, C., Yeager, K., Shafer, P. O., Letz, R., Henry, T., Schomer, D. L., & McCarty, F. (2003). The epilepsy medication and treatment complexity index: Reliability and validity testing. *Journal of Neuroscience Nursing, 35*(3), 155–162.

Dwyer, E. (1992). Stories of epilepsy: 1880–1930. *Hospital Practice, 27*(9A), 65–68, 71–72, 84–86.

Edward, K. L., Cook, M., & Giandinoto, J. A. (2015). An integrative review of the benefits of self-management interventions for adults with epilepsy. *Epilepsy & Behavior*, *45*, 195–204. doi:10.1016/j.yebeh.2015.01.026

Elliott, J. O., & Richardson, V. E. (2014). The biopsychosocial model and quality of life in persons with active epilepsy. *Epilepsy & Behavior*, *41*, 55–65. doi:10.1016/j.yebeh.2014.09.035

Guilfoyle, S. M., Monahan, S., Wesolowski, C., & Modi, A. C. (2015). Depression screening in pediatric epilepsy: Evidence for the benefit of a behavioral medicine service in early detection. *Epilepsy & Behavior*, *44*, 5–10. doi:10.1016/j.yebeh.2014.12.021

Hermann, B., & Jacoby, A. (2009). The psychosocial impact of epilepsy in adults. *Epilepsy & Behavior*, *15* (Suppl. 1), S11–S16. doi:10.1016/j.yebeh.2009.03.029

Hixson, J. D., Barnes, D., Parko, K., Durgin, T., Van Bebber, S., Graham, A., & Wicks, P. (2015). Patients optimizing epilepsy management via an online community: The POEM Study. *Neurology*, *85*(2), 129–136. doi:10.1212/WNL.0000000000001728

Holland, P., Lane, S., Whitehead, M., Marson, A. G., & Jacoby, A. (2009). Labor market participation following onset of seizures and early epilepsy: Findings from a UK cohort. *Epilepsia*, *50*(5), 1030–1039. doi:10.1111/j.1528-1167.2008.01819.x

Jacoby, A., Snape, D., & Baker, G.A. (2009). Determinents of quality of life in people with epilepsy. *Neurologic Clinics*, *27*(5), 843–863.

Kammerman, S., & Wasserman, L. (2001). Seizure disorders: Part 2. Treatment. *Western Journal of Medicine*, *175*(3), 184–188.

Keezer, M. R., Sisodiya, S. M., & Sander, J. W. (2016). Comorbidities of epilepsy: Current concepts and future perspectives. *Lancet Neurology*, *15*(1), 106–115. doi:10.1016/S1474-4422(15)00225-2

Kerr, M. P. (2012). The impact of epilepsy on patients' lives. *Acta Neurologica Scandinavica. Supplementum*, *194*, 1–9. doi:10.1111/ane.12014

Kobau, R., Zahran, H., Thurman, D. J., Zack, M. M., Henry, T. R., Schachter, S. C., & Price, P. H. (2008). Epilepsy surveillance among adults—19 states, behavioral risk factors surveilillance system, 2005. *Morbiity and Mortality Weekly Report*, *57*, 1–20.

Koo, Y. S., Yang, K. S., Seok, H. Y., Lee, S. K., Lee, I. K., Cho, Y. W., & Jung, K. Y. (2012). Characteristics of patients with epilepsy who use a website providing healthcare information about epilepsy in South Korea. *Epilepsy & Behavior*, *25*(2), 156–161. doi:10.1016/j.yebeh.2012.06.002

Kralj-Hans, I., Goldstein, L. H., Noble, A. J., Landau, S., Magill, N., McCrone, P., . . . Ridsdale, L. (2014). Self-Management education for adults with poorly controlled epILEpsy (SMILE (UK)): A randomised controlled trial protocol. *BMC Neurology*, *14*, 69. doi:10.1186/1471-2377-14-69

Laxer, K. D., Trinka, E., Hirsch, L. J., Cendes, F., Langfitt, J., Delanty, N., & Benbadis, S. R. (2014). The consequences of refractory epilepsy and its treatment. *Epilepsy & Behavior*, *37*, 59–70. doi:10.1016/j.yebeh.2014.05.031

Legion, V. (1991). Health education for self-management by people with epilepsy. *Journal of Neuroscience Nursing*, *23*(5), 300–305.

Magill, N., Ridsdale, L., Goldstein, L. H., McCrone, P., Morgan, M., Noble, A. J., & Landau, S. (2015). Self-management education for adults with poorly controlled epilepsy (SMILE (UK)): Statistical, economic and qualitative analysis plan for a randomised controlled trial. *Trials*, *16*, 269. doi:10.1186/s13063-015-0788-9

May, T. W., & Pfafflin, M. (2002). The efficacy of an educational treatment program for patients with epilepsy (MOSES): Results of a controlled, randomized study. Modular Service Package Epilepsy. *Epilepsia, 43*(5), 539–549.

May, T. W., & Pfafflin, M. (2005). Psychoeducational programs for patents with epilepsy. *Dis Manage Health Outcomes, 13*(3), 185–199.

Nelson, W. J., Edwards, S. A., Roberts, A. W., & Keller, R. J. (1978). Comprehensive self-medication program for epileptic patients. *American Journal of Hospital Pharmacy, 35*(7), 798–801.

Noble, A. J., Morgan, M., Virdi, C., & Ridsdale, L. (2013). A nurse-led self-management intervention for people who attend emergency departments with epilepsy: The patients' view. *Journal of Neurology, 260*(4), 1022–1030. doi:10.1007/s00415-012-6749-2

Noeker, M. (2004). Epilepsy—improvement of giving the diagnosis between the demands for standardisation versus individualisation. *Seizure, 13*(2), 95–98.

Novy, J., Castelao, E., Preisig, M., Vidal, P. M., Waeber, G., Vollenweider, P., & Rossetti, A. O. (2012). Psychiatric co-morbidities and cardiovascular risk factors in people with lifetime history of epilepsy of an urban community. *Clinical Neurology and Neurosurgery, 114*(1), 26–30. doi:10.1016/j.clineuro.2011.08.019

Phillips, L. A., Diefenbach, M.A., Kronish, I. A., Negron, R. M., & Horowitz, C. R. (2014). The necessity concnerns framework: A multidimensional theory benefits from multidimensional analysis. *Annals of Behavioral Medicine, 48*(1), 7–16.

Pramuka, M., Hendrickson, R., Zinski, A., & Van Cott, A. C. (2007). A psychosocial self-management program for epilepsy: A randomized pilot study in adults. *Epilepsy & Behavior, 11*(4), 533–545. doi:10.1016/j.yebeh.2007.06.013

Pryse-Phillips, W., Jardine, F., & Bursey, F. (1982). Compliance with drug therapy by epileptic patients. *Epilepsia, 23*(3), 269–274.

Puka, K., & Smith, M. L. (2016). Where are they now? Psychosocial, educational, and vocational outcomes after epilepsy surgery in childhood. *Epilepsia, 57*(4), 574–581. doi:10.1111/epi.13327

Ridsdale, L., Morgan, M., & O'Connor, C. (1999). Promoting self-care in epilepsy: The views of patients on the advice they had received from specialists, family doctors and an epilepsy nurse. *Patientl Education and Counseling, 37*(1), 43–47.

Roberts, J. I., Hrazdil, C., Wiebe, S., Sauro, K., Vautour, M., Wiebe, N., & Jette, N. (2015). Neurologists' knowledge of and attitudes toward epilepsy surgery: A national survey. *Neurology, 84*(2), 159–166. doi:10.1212/WNL.0000000000001127

Roberts, J. I., Patten, S. B., Wiebe, S., Hemmelgarn, B. R., Pringsheim, T., & Jette, N. (2015). Health-related behaviors and comorbidities in people with epilepsy: Changes in the past decade. *Epilepsia, 56*(12), 1973–1981. doi:10.1111/epi.13207

Robinson, E., DiIorio, C., DePadilla, L., McCarty, F., Yeager, K., Henry, T., & Shafer, P. (2008). Psychosocial predictors of lifestyle management in adults with epilepsy. *Epilepsy & Behavior, 13*(3), 523–528. doi:10.1016/j.yebeh.2008.05.015

Ryan, R., Kempner, K., & Emlen, A. C. (1980). The stigma of epilepsy as a self-concept. *Epilepsia, 21*(4), 433–444.

Schneider, J. W., & Conrad, P. (1981). Medical and sociological typologies: The case of epilepsy. *Social Science & Medicine. Part A: Medical Sociology, 15*(3 Pt. 1), 211–219.

Shafer, P. O. (1994). Nursing support of epilepsy self-management. *Clinical Nursing Practice in Epilepsy, 2*(1), 11–12.

Shafer, P. O. (1998). Counseling women with epilepsy. *Epilepsia, 39*(Suppl. 8), S38–S44.

Smeets, V. M. J., van Lierop, B. A. G., Vanhoutvin, J. P. G., Aldenkamp, A. P., & Nijhuis, J. N. (2007) Epilepsy and employment: Literature review. *Epilepsy & Behavior, 10*(3), 354–362.

Smithson, W. H., Colwell, B., & Hanna, J. (2014). Suddent unexpected death in epilepsy: Addressing the challenges. *Currents in Neurology and Neuroscience Reports, 14*(2), 502.

Taylor, D. C. (2000). Cerebral lesions, psychoses, and epilepsy: Disease versus illness. *Advances in Neurology, 84*, 463–477.

Thompson, N. J., Patel, A. H., Selwa, L. M., Stoll, S. C., Begley, C. E., Johnson, E. K., & Fraser, R. T. (2015). Expanding the efficacy of Project UPLIFT: Distance delivery of mindfulness-based depression prevention to people with epilepsy. *Journal of Consulting and Clinical Psychology, 83*(2), 304–313. doi:10.1037/a0038404

Thompson, P. J. (1995). The rebabilitations of people with epilepsy. In A. Hopkins, S. Shorvon, & G. Cascino (Eds.), *Epilepsy* (pp. 573–577). New York: Chapman & Hall Medical.

Tunde-Ayinmode, M. F., Abiodun, O. A., Ajiboye, P. O., Buhari, O. I., & Sanya, E. O. (2014). Prevalence and clinical implications of psychopathology in adults with epilepsy seen in an outpatient clinic in Nigeria. *General Hospital Psychiatry, 36*(6), 703–708. doi:10.1016/j.genhosppsych.2014.08.009

Unger, W. R., & Buelow, J. M. (2009). Hybrid concept analysis of self-management in adults newly diagnosed with epilepsy. *Epilepsy & Behavior, 14*(1), 89–95. doi:10.1016/j.yebeh.2008.09.002

Wicks, P., Keininger, D. L., Massagli, M. P., de la Loge, C., Brownstein, C., Isojarvi, J., & Heywood, J. (2012). Perceived benefits of sharing health data between people with epilepsy on an online platform. *Epilepsy & Behavior, 23*(1), 16–23. doi:10.1016/j.yebeh.2011.09.026

Wo, M. C., Lim, K. S., Choo, W. Y., & Tan, C. T. (2015). Employability in people with epilepsy: A systematic review. *Epilepsy Research, 116*, 67–78. doi:10.1016/j.eplepsyres.2015.06.016

Wohlrab, G. C., Rinnert, S., Bettendorf, U., Fischbach, H., Heinen, G., Klein, P., . . . Famoses Project, G. (2007). Famoses: A modular educational program for children with epilepsy and their parents. *Epilepsy & Behavior, 10*(1), 44–48. doi:10.1016/j.yebeh.2006.10.005

14

Self-Management of Hearing Impairment

LUCY HANDSCOMB, GABRIELLE H. SAUNDERS, AND DEREK J. HOARE ■

HEARING IMPAIRMENT AND TYPICAL FUNCTIONAL LIMITATIONS

Hearing loss is common and increases with age (Lee, Matthews, Dubno, & Mills, 2005). Known associations include genetics factors, viral infections, injury, ototoxic drugs, and excessive noise exposure. In more than 90% of cases, adult hearing loss is sensorineural in origin and affects both ears (Cruickshanks et al., 1998). It can present with other hearing symptoms, such as tinnitus or loudness recruitment (exaggerated sensitivity to noises). All told, hearing loss amounts to a leading cause of disability due to sensory loss (World Health Organization, 2012) and represents a significant healthcare burden because it requires management and a revisiting of intervention decisions over years or decades.

Hearing *impairment* is defined as hearing loss that leads to difficulties in hearing or deafness; it affects an estimated 360 million people worldwide (World Health Organization, 2012). Impairment is distinct from hearing difficulties; audiometric thresholds, as determined by a standard clinical hearing test, do not always reflect the difficulties in communication experienced by the individual. Even with normal hearing thresholds, individuals may report hearing difficulties in situations where there are multiple speakers or competing noise. In fact, about 10% of those who report difficulties hearing have a normal audiogram (Saunders & Haggard, 1989; Tremblay et al., 2015). In the absence of an identifiable hearing loss, hearing impairment may be associated with any number of impaired processes, such as central (cortical) auditory processing disorders, central presbycusis, or hidden hearing loss, to name a few (Humes et al., 2012; Moore 2011; Schaette & McAlpine, 2011). Non-auditory factors, such as lifestyle, emotional state, medical and noise-induced impairments, environment, and cognition, may also play a role in hearing difficulties in those without detectable hearing loss. For example, Sommers et al. (2011) showed a significant association between listening comprehension and processing speed on a range of cognitive tasks and that the association was independent of any hearing loss. The odds of reporting hearing difficulties are also increased in those reporting symptoms of depression, neuropathy, or vision difficulties (Tremblay et al., 2015).

Hearing impairment is generally associated with a number of functional and emotional consequences. Emotional consequences are discussed in detail later. The functional impacts of hearing impairment might best be described according to the World Health Organization's (2001) International Classification of Functioning, Disability, and Health, as activity limitations and participation restrictions. As summarized by Laplante-Lévesque, Hickson, and Worrall (2010), activities that may be limited by hearing impairment include speech comprehension, being able to follow a TV or radio program, or being able to detect or localize important sounds, such as moving cars or a ringing telephone. Even cooking can become "fraught with difficulties as boiling pans and kettles, 'pinging' microwaves, and running taps [become] unheard" (Barlow, Turner, Hammond, & Gailey, 2007, p. 115). Such limitations may lead to strain and fatigue for the individual.

Restrictions on participation might include withdrawal from interactions with individuals or the community (Laplante-Lévesque et al., 2010). For late deafened adults, profound hearing loss is notably restricting in terms of communication where there are multiple speakers or high levels of background noise (e.g., in staff meetings; Scherich, 1996). Older people with hearing impairment too are more likely to have difficulty with activities of daily living, especially those involving venturing beyond their immediate neighbourhood (Gopinath et al., 2012a).

EVIDENCE-BASED PRACTICES ON INTERVENTIONS THAT IMPROVE HEALTH OUTCOMES

The standard intervention for hearing impairment is the provision of hearing aids or in the case of profound hearing loss, a cochlear implant. Alternative interventions include hearing assistance technology, communication programs, and auditory training interventions. While there is evidence that all types of intervention have similar outcomes, their optimization, availability, and acceptability to individuals with a hearing impairment vary (Laplante-Lévesque et al., 2010).

Hearing aids detect and amplify external sounds, delivering an amplified acoustic signal to the ear, although not necessarily restoring hearing function. Frequency response characteristics of hearing aids, distortions, poor clarity, or loudness of speech all impact listening with hearing aids (Dillon, 2012). Hearing aids amplify *all* sounds, so communication difficulties can persist, particularly in situations where there is a noisy background (Picou, Ricketts, & Hornsby, 2013).

In their systematic review, Chisolm et al. (2007) asked whether hearing aids compared to the non-use of hearing aids resulted in improvements in health-related quality of life for adults with sensorineural hearing loss. They concluded that hearing aids improve adult health-related quality of life "by reducing psychological, social, and emotional effects of [hearing impairment]." (p.151). However, only two of the studies included in the review were randomized controlled trials, so the estimate of effect that they report is highly likely to change with further studies. In the absence of robust evidence, it is unsurprising that audiologists can sometimes differ in opinion on the minimum level of hearing loss at which it is appropriate to recommend a hearing aid (Sereda, Hoare, Nicholson, Smith, & Hall, 2015). A Cochrane review of hearing aids for mild to moderate hearing loss (where practice is most variable) has since been developed (see Ferguson, Kitterick, Edmondson-Jones, & Hoare, 2015 for the protocol), so it will be interesting to see how far the field has developed since the review by Chisolm et al. (2007).

Hearing aids may be something of a default when managing hearing impairment. In an interaction analysis, Grenness, Hickson, Laplante-Lévesque, Meyer, and Davidson (2015) observed that it was recommended to 83% of individuals with hearing impairment that they should undergo some form of rehabilitation and that 100% of those were recommended hearing aids. Alternatives to hearing aids such as hearing-assistive technology or communication classes were only recommended in 8% of consultations and only after hearing aids had been recommended and rejected by the individual with hearing impairment. In the same study, it was observed that audiologist-delivered education and information-giving was overly complex and placed a strong emphasis on hearing aids, with limited discussion of diagnoses, communication tactics, or living with hearing impairment. Yet as Henshaw and Ferguson (2013) posit, "Although hearing aids may help people with hearing loss *hear* speech, their ability to *listen to* and *make sense of* speech may still be sub-optimal" (p. 1, emphasis in original), suggesting alternatives or interventions complimentary to hearing aids need due consideration. There is an important role for the clinicians here, in evaluating the evidence, relating that evidence to the individual with hearing impairment, and evaluating the outcome of the process in order to appropriately offer intervention options to the individual with hearing impairment beyond the focus on hearing aids (Hickson, Laplante-Lévesque, & Wong, 2013).

Hearing assistance technology refers to assistive listening devices that can employ visual and tactile stimuli, as well as auditory stimuli. These may include induction loops that allow those with the appropriate receivers to hear microphone-delivered speech or cordless headphones to amplify the TV's auditory signal.

Communication programs involve training people with hearing impairment to improve their speech perception and manage communication more effectively. Such programs might be conducted with individuals or in a group setting and include speech-reading training, auditory training, auditory-visual training, repair strategies (how to deal with missing information during an interaction; Tye-Murray 1991), through to more general topics such as assertiveness, stress management, and personal adjustment (Laplante-Lévesque et al., 2010).

For example, Andersson, Melin, Scott, and Lindberg (1995) applied a behavioral approach to hearing impairment by using treatment that involved individualized coping skills (hearing tactics), posture control, and relaxation skills; participants reported improved coping posttreatment. Only some communication programs have been subjected to systematic review to date. In their broad review of aural rehabilitation interventions for adults and children with hearing impairment, Chisolm and Arnold (2012) found that individual auditory training programs improved speech perception and that counseling-based group programs led to reduced disability (reduced activity limitations and reduced participation restrictions).

Recently, computer-based auditory training has been proposed as an intervention for hearing loss. Data regarding its efficacy or effectiveness are mixed. Specifically, the review by Henshaw and Ferguson (2013) found evidence for improved performance in trained tasks, untrained measures of speech intelligibility, cognition, and self-reported hearing abilities, but they cautioned that the effects were small and the quality of the evidence low. Furthermore, effects were highly variable across individuals. Nevertheless, computer-based or online interventions might be particularly useful to those with hearing impairments; Henshaw, Clark, Kang, and Ferguson (2012) found that slight hearing impairment was associated with greater computer skills and Internet use than having no hearing impairment in their sample of adults ages 50 to 74 years. However, a recent large randomized controlled trial of a computerized auditory training program found no evidence that computerized auditory training resulted in improved outcomes over standard-of-care hearing aid intervention alone (Saunders, Smith, et al., 2016). Secure therapist contact, interactive homework, and text, video, or audio files can all be delivered using this medium (Vlaescu, Carlbring, Lunner, & Andersson, 2015); for example through Internet-based cognitive-behavior therapy/acceptance and commitment therapy for hearing problems (Molander et al., 2015), multimedia educational for first-time hearing aid users (Ferguson, Brandreth, Brassington, Leighton, & Wharrad, 2016), and online rehabilitation for adult hearing aid users (Thorén, Oberg, Wanstrom, Andersson, & Lunner, 2014).

Self-management support interventions, where the objective is to empower and prepare individuals to self-manage their hearing impairment and associated problems, have also been subject to systematic review. Barker, Mackenzie, Elliott, Jones, and de Lusignan (2014) conducted a Cochrane review of interventions to improve hearing aid use in adult auditory rehabilitation, which included a number of self-management support interventions: self-management assessment, education, activation (e.g., behavior change), resources and tools to support self-management (e.g., services and equipment), and shared decision-making. While evidence was generally of low quality, self-management support was observed in a small number of studies to reduce hearing handicap and increase verbal communication strategies in the short and medium term. Studies on the effects of self-management support interventions on optimal use of hearing aids, possible adverse effects, and long-term outcomes have yet to be reported.

RESEARCH ON THE EMOTIONAL IMPACT OF HEARING IMPAIRMENT

There is no doubt that hearing loss can have far-reaching effects on well-being. A number of large population studies have shown that, compared to people without hearing loss, people with impaired hearing are more likely to suffer from symptoms of emotional distress, particularly depression (Keidser, Seeto, Rudner, Hygge, & Ronnberg, 2015, Saito et al., 2010, Tambs, 2004). A detailed questionnaire study was conducted by Kerr and Cowie (1997), which involved adults ages 40 and above with varying degrees of hearing impairment. They found that 40% of respondents felt that their hearing impairment had at least "badly affected" their lives, while 10% felt their lives had been "almost completely destroyed" by it. The same study identified that feelings of abandonment, being held back in life, and being poorly understood by individuals with normal hearing were common among individuals who were deafened. Emotional loneliness has also been identified as a consequence of hearing loss, particularly among those living with a partner (Pronk, Deeg, & Kramer, 2013), suggesting that a person with hearing impairment may be physically close to another person but may not feel emotionally connected to them.

The adverse effect of hearing impairment on relationships with others is likely to be one of the major causes of emotional distress. Difficulties experienced by couples include frustration when communication breaks down, frequent misunderstandings, tension over the volume of the television, and lack of intimacy (Hetu, Jones, & Getty, 1993). A source of sadness for many couples is the loss of chat and banter; when understanding is a struggle, conversation tends to be reduced to essentials (Echalier, 2012). An important consideration is that quality of life has consistently been shown to be adversely affected in hearing partners of people with hearing impairment (Kamil & Lin, 2015); to a large extent, participation restrictions are felt by both parties.

In a longitudinal study, Saito et al. (2010) found that older people with hearing loss were more likely to develop depressive symptoms over three years than their peers with good hearing. However, some studies have indicated that the emotional impact of acquired hearing loss is greater for younger people than older. For example, Keidser et al. (2015) found that the relationship between depression and hearing loss was significantly stronger for those ages 39 to 59 than for those ages 60 to 70. Similarly, Tambs (2004), whose population ranged from 20 to 101 years old, found that the effects of hearing impairment on mental health increased significantly with decreasing age. One possible reason is that working life places considerable demands on hearing. Nachtegaal et al. (2009) found that people with hearing impairment reported a much greater need for recovery after work than those without and that the lack of sufficient recovery can lead to emotional exhaustion or burn-out. Furthermore, older people are more likely to have peers with hearing difficulties and so perhaps feel less alone. However, this does not mean that older people do not perceive any stigma around hearing impairment. An interview study conducted by Wallhagen (2010) found concerns about "looking old" with hearing aids to be a common theme.

A fairly consistent finding is that self-reported hearing difficulty is a better predictor of emotional distress and poor quality of life than measured hearing thresholds (Gopinath et al., 2012b, Tambs 2004), indicating that such factors as lifestyle, personal coping mechanisms, and social support are likely to play a part. Thinking style is also important; Garnefski and Kraaij (2012a) found that both rumination (dwelling on problems) and catastrophizing (overly negative thinking) were positively correlated with depression and anxiety in people with hearing impairment (although causality could be in either direction). Additional symptoms related to hearing impairment can also intensify its negative effects. A Swedish investigation of people with sudden sensorineural hearing loss found that quality of life was rated significantly lower among those who also reported annoying tinnitus or vertigo (Carlsson, Hall, Lind, & Danermark, 2011).

Although the primary focus of research is on emotional difficulties associated with hearing impairment, there is some evidence that there may be a few positive emotional aspects to the experience of losing hearing for some people (see Manchaiah, Baguley, Pyykkö, Kentala, & Levo, 2015 for a review). For example, Kerr and Stephens (1997) asked individuals with hearing impairment attending audiology appointments to list any positive experiences they could think of. While some individuals felt there were none, others listed practical benefits, such as being less bothered by noise at night and being able to get out of disliked tasks. More emotional benefits were feeling an affinity to other people who are deaf or people with other disabilities and a sense of personal growth (more patience, better observation skills, and more awareness of strengths were all listed).

KNOWLEDGE ABOUT HEARING IMPAIRMENT THAT AN INDIVIDUAL NEEDS FOR SELF-MANAGEMENT

Perhaps the most important basic knowledge that an individual needs to have is that there are actually options available for the management of hearing impairment. For example, if people believe that an increasing hearing impairment is directly connected with getting older, they may gradually adapt to the impairment and may not seek help. A study by van Eijken et al. (2004) found that less than half of participants, who self-reported a hearing impairment, had actually spoken to their family doctor about it. In this study, participants received structured guidance to enhance decision-making on self-management and seeking healthcare from their family doctor, but few additional participants had actually spoken to their doctor about their impairment at three-month follow-up. The extent of the issue is captured by Davis, Smith, Ferguson, Stephens, and Gianopoulos (2007), who found that those who were referred for hearing assessment recognized that they had had a hearing problem for about 10 years or even longer, were aged in their mid-70s, and had at that point a substantial hearing problem.

A number of factors may be at play. Individuals with hearing impairment may have psychosocial concerns or fears related to diagnosis or rehabilitation (Grenness et al., 2015) that need to be addressed before any progress can be made. If these concerns or fears are dealt with, then self-efficacy may still be an issue. Self-efficacy beliefs (in this case, judgments about one's own ability to manage hearing impairment) influences choice of activities and motivational engagement, acquisition of knowledge, and refinement of new abilities (Bandura, 1994). For example, in the case of hearing aids, proper device-handling (e.g., inserting them into the ear, changing batteries) and simply adjusting to wearing them is essential; difficulty with either is a common reason for discontinuation of use (West & Smith 2007). Rightly so perhaps that Smith and West (2006) conclude audiologist interventions are more effective when incorporating a self-efficacy framework. The impact of self-efficacy on self-management of hearing loss is further addressed in the "Barriers to Self-Management" section.

Knowledge needs to be sufficient and appropriate to motivate the individual with hearing impairment within realistic expectations. Laplante-Lévesque et al. (2010) propose that it is essential that individuals are able to discuss their perspectives and be genuinely interested in their individual experiences of living with any chronic health condition. Engaging individuals with hearing impairment sufficiently for them to take control of the condition, through their involvement in decision-making and goal-setting and encouraging them to ask questions, is important to the promotion of optimization (e.g., use of hearing aids or communication strategies) for effective longer-term self-management.

Lack of knowledge therefore represents a significant barrier to successful self-management. In the next section, we review barriers to self-management in more detail and specifically in terms of awareness, self-efficacy, social support, communication environment and needs, lack of skill, and co-occurring conditions. We also consider how these barriers might best be overcome.

BARRIERS TO SELF-MANAGEMENT

Barriers to self-management are many and include a individual's lack of awareness of their hearing difficulties, low self-efficacy, inadequate social support, limited personal motivation to communicate in different listening environments, inadequate skill or training to self-manage, and some co-occurring conditions.

Awareness

People with hearing loss are often unaware of its effect on themselves and others. A lack of awareness is a barrier to self-management. Lockey, Jennings, and Shaw (2010) interviewed four older women who were successfully managing their hearing loss noting "Without being aware of their hearing loss these individuals would not think to pursue hearing aids that could improve their participation with others" (p. 546). This comment was made after a participant had stated "as I say, it sort of creeps up on you ... you aren't really aware yourself, as much as other people are" (p. 546).

Becoming aware of a hearing problem can take time. Southall, Gagné, and Leroux (2006) and Southall, Gagné, and Jennings (2010) propose that once individuals recognize that their hearing is compromising participation in a valued activity, there come two critical junctures that motivate behavior change and self-management. The first is when negative stress from the inability to participate becomes unmanageable and leads to an abrupt intensification to seek help. This is followed by the second positive juncture at which individuals begin to feel a sense of community, for example, from involvement in peer-support groups.

Promoting self-awareness of hearing loss is not simple. When others, such as friends and family, intervene, it often leads to conflict, stress, and poor outcomes. Indeed, Ridgway, Hickson, and Lind (2015) determined that autonomous motivation (engaging in an activity with eagerness and will) was positively associated with hearing-aid usage, but controlled motivation (engaging in an activity because of a sense of pressure, demand, or coercion) was not. One approach that has shown some success in promoting self-awareness is motivational interviewing (Miller, 1983). The goal of motivational interviewing is to help individuals with hearing impairment think differently about their behavior and what might be gained through change. It also serves to increase individuals' awareness of the potential problems caused, consequences of, and risks faced from their health condition (Cummings, Cooper, & Cassie, 2009). Several groups of researchers are currently examining applications of motivational interviewing to promote awareness of hearing loss among individuals with hearing impairment (Aazh, 2015; Weineland et al., 2015).

Self-Efficacy

Self-efficacy is a central construct in many health behavior models (e.g., social cognitive theory, health belief model, theory of planned behavior), reflecting its importance in self-management. Several studies have shown relationships between hearing self-management and self-efficacy. For example, Kelly-Campbell and McMillan (2015) found individuals with low hearing aid self-efficacy had lower reported hearing aid satisfaction than those with adequate self-efficacy. Similarly, Meyer, Hickson, Lovelock, Lampert, and Khan (2014) found that more unsuccessful than successful hearing-aid owners in their study had low self-efficacy. Saunders, Frederick, et al. (2016) reported that the odds of using hearing aids decreased by about half for each 1-point decrease in self-efficacy measured using the Hearing Beliefs Questionnaire (Saunders, Frederick, Silverman, & Papesh, 2013).

Self-efficacy is modified by prior experience, such as observation of others engaging in particular tasks, encouragement received from others, and reactions an individual experiences prior to attempting to achieve a goal (Bandura, 1992). As such, self-efficacy for self-management of hearing impairment can be increased where clinicians provide clear, simple, and thorough information that complies with health literacy principals. Providing video examples of older adults using hearing aids and involving family or friends when educating individuals about management of hearing loss are useful strategies (Hickson, Meyer, Lovelock, Lampert, & Khan, 2014).

Social Support

There is considerable evidence that individuals who feel supported in their decisions to manage hearing impairment have better hearing outcomes than those who do not feel supported. For instance, Southall et al. (2006) interviewed 10 older individuals with hearing loss, all of whom owned hearing aids and used two or more forms of other hearing assistance technology (e.g., an amplified telephone, a portable doorbell, an induction loop) about barriers and benefits of device use. All participants noted that a positive family attitude had facilitated their use of technology. The opposite is also true; a lack of support from family was associated with non-use of hearing technology (Southall et al. 2010; Wallhagen, 2010).

Involvement of family members and friends in management of hearing impairment has the potential to change these negative opinions. Indeed, the participants in Kelly et al. (2013) identified reasons why family members should be involved in management. These included being able to help with remembering and/or understanding information provided by the audiologist, understanding the problems that the hearing loss has caused, and learning communication strategies together. There is an ongoing movement to involve communication partners in the rehabilitation process because it is appreciated by both individuals with hearing impairment and their communication partners (Laplante-Lévesque et al., 2010; Poost-Foroosh, Jennings, & Cheesman, 2015) and family members (Ekberg, Meyer, Scarinci, Grenness, & Hickson, 2015).

Communication Environment and Needs

Communication needs and the communication environment can be barriers to self-management of hearing impairment. For example, Pryce and Gooberman-Hill (2012) showed that the communication environment can decrease motivation to communicate. They interviewed residents of a constantly noisy care facility. Many individuals living at the facility said they chose to avoid communication rather than manage it because listening conditions were so adverse. Communication needs, or the perceived lack thereof, led some individuals to say they had no need to manage their hearing impairment (e.g., Kochkin, 2007;

Vuorialho, Karinen, & Sorri, 2006). In other words, without a perceived need to communicate, the motivation to manage hearing loss is absent.

Lack of Skill

Use of assistive technology requires the skill to manage it. Poor instruction in device management is a known barrier to successful self-management. To illustrate this point, research by Kelly et al. (2013) found that when 154 individuals who had been fitted with a hearing aid were asked if they had received enough instruction, practical help, and support during the process, 36% reported feeling that they had not received enough instruction; 48% felt they had received insufficient practical help; 49% felt they received enough support to use the hearing aid after fitting; and 36% reported not feeling confident about using their hearing aids or using the controls on the aid. Surprisingly, these results were consistent across long-term and new users (Kelly et al., 2013). In the words of one participant: "There's lack of information about the pluses and minuses about wearing hearing aids and how they fit or how long it takes you, should you wear these things, how you should clean them, how you should look after them. There's absolutely zilch information" (Kelly et al., 2013, p. 298). Others have identified similar concerns (Campos, Bozza, & Ferrari, 2014; Desjardins & Doherty, 2009; Grenness et al., 2014). While audiologists may feel that they are giving adequate or more than adequate information to individuals with a hearing impairment, the individual may not share this view.

The onus should be on the clinician to provide good instruction, not on the individual with hearing impairment to seek it out. This barrier should be relatively simple to overcome through provision of well-designed materials, sufficient assigned time, use of teach-back (i.e. individuals confirm their understanding of healthcare instructions by repeating back or demonstrating what they were taught), provision of supplemental take-home materials, and involvement of caregivers in the process.

Co-occurring Conditions

In addition to instruction, the ability to self-manage hearing loss can be impacted by the presence of normal age-related conditions. These include presbyopia and decreased tactile sensitivity, as well as impairments common in aging, such as macular degeneration and arthritis—all of which impact an individual's ability to see and manipulate small objects. Unfortunately, the ability to see and handle small objects is required for successful management of hearing technology. The inability to do so likely in part explains so many individuals are irregular users of hearing aids. As found by Bertoli et al. (2009), relative to individuals who report they have good ability to manage their hearing aids, those who report their ability to manage their hearing aids as "bad" or "very bad" are 6.3 and 13.4 times less likely to regularly use their hearing aid, respectively. This form of barrier can be addressed from a couple of angles. First, the need to include communication partners in the rehabilitation process should be emphasized. Second, clinicians need to be aware of and sensitive to the limitations of the individual with hearing impairment when selecting hearing technology. For instance, it makes little sense to provide an individual who has poor eyesight or arthritis a model of a hearing aid that requires tiny batteries.

Co-occurring conditions also indirectly act as barriers to self-management of hearing impairment where priority is given to managing other health conditions and life events. Typically, individuals with hearing impairments consider it to be a lower priority than many other conditions or concerns (e.g., Carson, 2005; Chung, Des Roches, Meunier, & Eavey, 2005; Franks & Beckmann, 1985; Southall et al., 2006). It is often cited as being a part of normal aging and thus not something to be concerned about (Carson, 2005). Overcoming this barrier is a matter of changing public opinion about the importance of communication and hearing.

Recent data showing possible associations between hearing loss and cognitive decline has generated much media attention. Although a recent meta-analysis of published studies cautions that while hearing impairment does seem to be associated with cognitive problems, this conclusion may be premature because studies are small and poorly control for potentially important variables, such as other health factors. Further work in this field is strongly indicated. Figure 14.1 provides our schematic overview of these barriers and the ways in which they may interact. As a whole, there is a need to personalize care when planning and educating individuals about hearing loss and to ensure that they have social support and the necessary tools (e.g. decision aids) to make informed choices and optimize self-management capabilities and motivation.

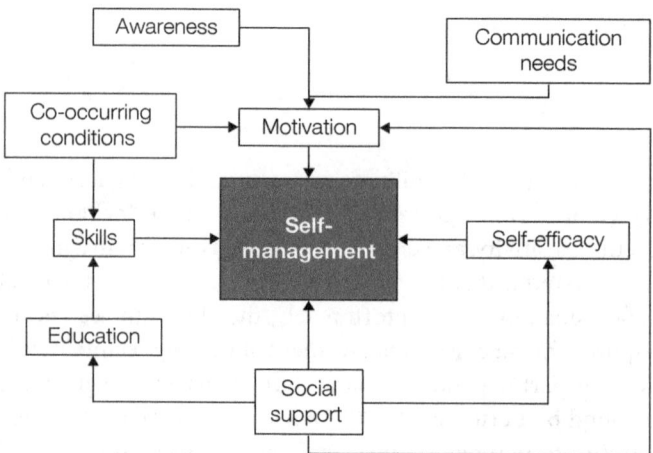

Figure 14.1 Model of interplay between factors impacting self-management.

COPING STRATEGIES OR SKILLS TAUGHT FOR HEARING IMPAIRMENT

The use of coping strategies by individuals with hearing impairment has been the topic of only a small number of studies over many years. In addition to being taught how to use and maintain their hearings aids (if they have them), people with hearing impairments are encouraged to develop good communication strategies in order to cope in difficult listening conditions. These might include asking people to slow down their speech, moving away from background noise, or rearranging seating to give a better view of faces to enable lip reading (Field & Haggard, 1989).

In an attempt to model coping strategies used by 61 individuals with hearing impairment, Gomez and Madey (2001) examined the interactions between strategies, perceived effectiveness of those strategies, hearing loss, hearing impairment, and psychosocial variables. Psychosocial variables in their model included anxiety about aging, personal adjustment to hearing loss, perceived social support, and attitudes and behaviors of others. They used regression analyses to predict the use of adaptive coping strategies (e.g., asking someone to repeat what he or she said) or non-adaptive coping strategies (e.g., pretending to understand the conversation) in their study population. Perhaps not surprisingly, the strongest predictor of using *any* coping strategy was the perceived effectiveness of that strategy as a coping mechanism. Strategy use was not predicted by the degree of hearing loss, hearing impairment, or psychosocial factors. Gomez and Maday (2001) also note that individuals who reported poorer adjustment to hearing loss were more likely to employ non-adaptive coping strategies.

Andersson and Hägnebo (2003) also examined coping strategy use in a sample of 94 individuals with hearing impairment; the types of strategy used more or less often were determined from subscale scores on the Ways of Coping Questionnaire (Folkman & Lazarus 1988). They found that individuals with hearing impairment are more likely to use planful problem-solving (i.e., develop and follow a plan of action) or self-controlling (e.g., trying to keep feelings to themselves) coping strategies. Escape or avoidance strategies (e.g., wishing the situation would go away) were least often used by individuals in their sample.

In terms of coping interventions, rather than simply teaching a list of strategies (which is likely to be ineffective), individual and group rehabilitation programs encourage the development of problem-solving skills. For example, in the Active Communication Education program (ACE; Hickson, Worral, & Scarinci, 2007a, 2015), participants are invited to generate as many solutions as possible to communication problems that are presented within the group. This is done so that, in real-life situations, they are readily able to think of strategies to reduce communication difficulties as they arise.

Even with good use of communication strategies, people may find themselves unable to continue with some aspects of their usual work or social life when they develop hearing impairment. In these cases, flexible thinking may be a useful skill. Garnefski and Kraaij (2012b) found that people who were able to disengage with goals that had become unattainable due to hearing loss and instead were able to direct their attention toward alternative, meaningful goals did not report symptoms of anxiety. They also observed a reduction in depression and anxiety in people following a self-help program involving realistic goal-setting (Garnefski & Kraaij, 2012a).

TESTED TECHNIQUES TO FACILITATE SELF-MANAGEMENT

When individuals with hearing impairment go to see an audiologist, they are usually given some advice about managing their hearing loss. However, as discussed earlier, audiology appointments tend to be information-heavy and to focus on hearing-aid fitting, with little opportunity to discuss wider issues that go along with living with hearing loss (Grenness et al., 2015). Other interventions outside routine audiology appointments may provide better self-management support.

Aural rehabilitation groups bring people with hearing impairment together and often include communication partners. They are usually facilitated by an audiology professional, and the aim is to empower participants to better cope with their hearing impairment in everyday life. Often they involve problem-solving exercises and role-play; for example, participants might practice explaining their hearing loss to a stranger. A review of 13 investigations of aural rehabilitation groups (Hawkins, 2005) concluded that they increase participation and improve quality of life, at least in the short term. Since this review, the ACE program was developed and manualized (Hickson et al., 2007a), which has shown positive effects on participation and well-being in two trials (Hickson, Worral, & Scarinci, 2007b; Oberg, Bohn, & Larsson, 2014). These positive effects were largely maintained after six months, which suggests that successful self-management continues to occur once group sessions are finished.

For many reasons, groups are not accessible to everyone with hearing loss. A more widely available tool is the self-help book or manual. Garnefski and Kraaij (2012a) developed a self-help program comprising a printed manual and computer program. Participants were instructed to spend an hour a day for four days each week over a month on a series of graded exercises designed to help them first relax, then change their irrational thoughts, and finally to identify and work toward a realistic goal. Anxiety and depression scores improved in those following the program but not in a waiting-list control group.

A Swedish self-help book was tested by Thorén et al. (2014). Participants in the study were asked to read through the book and some supplementary material, one section at a time, and complete several weekly tasks related to their reading. The task might be to describe their experience with hearing aids in different situations or to try out particular communication strategies. They were encouraged to discuss their experience weekly with a clinician online. They also could take part in an online peer discussion forum. This forum had a new topic assigned each week by an audiologist (such as "How well have you coped with changes associated with hearing loss?"). The forum was monitored for inappropriate content, but otherwise there was no professional involvement. The authors reported a decrease in anxiety and depression scores and reduced participation restriction after the five-week program. An earlier study (Lundberg, Andersson, & Lunner, 2011) used the same book with weekly telephone support from an audiologist instead of online discussion. Reductions were noted in anxiety, depression, and participation restrictions in that study. A control group who read the book without any additional support improved in these domains to a lesser degree. This suggests that the benefit of written self-help material could be increased with supplementary support. Internet-delivered self-help is likely to be a rich area of future development, although it should be kept in mind that not all individuals attending audiology appointments feel confident using a computer (Ferguson & Henshaw, 2015).

Successful hearing-aid use is an important part of self-management for many people with hearing loss, but there is no clear evidence that either aural rehabilitation groups or self-help manuals help to improve hearing-aid use or satisfaction. In order to manage their hearing aids successfully, people need to learn a number of practical skills such as how to insert the aids, change batteries, clean the tubing, and so on; some people struggle with these tasks (Campos et al., 2014). A potential solution to these problems is a DVD or computer program that individuals using hearing aids can watch at home as they learn to manage hearing aids themselves. In a randomized controlled trial, a group of individuals with hearing impairment who were given access to video clips about using hearing aids after fitting performed significantly better on a free-recall test of hearing aid skills and knowledge than a control group who only had a hearing-aid fitting appointment (Ferguson et al., 2015).

CONCLUSION

Hearing impairment cannot be cured, but its consequences can be reduced with self-management, whereby the individual adopts, refines, and maintains health behaviors, supported through the provision and availability of suitable interventions. The barriers to self-management are many. A knowledge and appreciation of those barriers, understanding whom they typically affect and how, and what approaches might be tried to overcome them are all important factors that should inform decision-making between the clinician and the individual with hearing impairment. Individuals with hearing impairment want the opportunity to self-manage. Ensuring that the conversation occurs within the audiology appointment, therefore, will facilitate self-management that is informed, realistic, and fully accounts for the preferences and values of the individual.

ACKNOWLEDGMENTS

The first author is funded by the British Tinnitus Association.

GS: This work was in part supported by VA Rehabilitation Research and Development grant #C9230C. The views and opinions expressed here do not necessarily reflect the views of the United States Government or the Department of Veterans Affairs.

DJH is funded through the National Institute for Health Research (NIHR) Biomedical Research Unit scheme. The views expressed are those of the authors and not necessarily those of the NIHR, the NHS, or the Department of Health.

REFERENCES

Aazh, H. (2015). Feasibility of conducting a randomized controlled trial to evaluate the effect of motivational interviewing on hearing-aid use. *International Journal of Audiology, 2,* 1–9.

Andersson, G., & Hägnebo, C. (2003). Hearing impairment, coping strategies, and anxiety sensitivity. *Journal of Clinical Psychology in Medical Settings, 10,* 35–39.

Andersson, G., Melin, L., Scott, B., & Lindberg, P. (1995). An evaluation of a behavioral treatment approach to hearing impairment. *Behavior Research and Therapy, 33,* 283–292.

Bandura, A. (1994). Self-efficacy. In V. S. Ramachaudran (Ed.), *Encyclopedia of human behavior* (Vol. 4, pp. 71–81). New York: Academic Press.

Bandura, A. (Ed.). (1992). Self-efficacy mechanism in psychologic functioning. In R. Schwarzer (Ed.), *Self-efficacy: Thought control of action* (pp. 355–394). Washington, DC: Hemisphere.

Barker, F., Mackenzie, E., Elliott, L., Jones, S., & de Lusignan S. (2014). Interventions to improve hearing aid use in adult auditory rehabilitation. *Cochrane Database of Systematic Reviews, 7,* CD010342.

Barlow, J. H., Turner, A. P., Hammond, C. L., & Gailey, L. (2007). Living with late deafness: Insight from between worlds: Viviendo con sordera tardía: introspecci ó n entre dos mundos. *International Journal of Audiology, 46,* 442–448.

Bertoli, S., Staehelin, K., Zemp, E., Schindler, C., Bodmer, D., & Probst, R. (2009). Survey on hearing aid use and satisfaction in Switzerland and their determinants. *International Journal of Audiology, 48,* 183–195.

Campos, P. D., Bozza, A., & Ferrari, D.V. (2014). Hearing aid handling skills: Relationship with satisfaction and benefit. *Codas, 26,* 10–16.

Carlsson, P. I., Hall, M., Lind, K. J., & Danermark, B. (2011). Quality of life, psychosocial consequences, and audiological rehabilitation after sudden sensorineural hearing loss. *International Journal of Audiology, 50,* 139–144.

Carson, A. J. (2005). "What brings you here today?" The role of self-assessment in help-seeking for age-related hearing loss. *Journal of Aging Studies, 19,* 185–200.

Chisolm, T., & Arnold, M. (2012). Evidence about the effectiveness of aural rehabilitation programs for adults. In L. Wong & L. Hickson (Eds.), *Evidence-based practice in audiology: Evaluating interventions for children and adults with hearing impairment* (pp. 237–266). San Diego, CA: Pleural.

Chisolm, T. H., Johnson, C. E., Danhauer, J. L., Portz, L. J., Abrams, H. B., Lesner, S., ... Newman, C. W. (2007). A systematic review of health-related quality of life and hearing aids: Final report of the American Academy of Audiology Task Force on the Health-Related Quality of Life Benefits of Amplification in Adults. *Journal of the American Academy of Audiology, 18,* 151–183.

Cruickshanks, K. J., Wiley, T. L., Tweed, T. S., Klein, B. E. K., Klein, R., Mares-Perlman, J. A., ... Nondahl, D. M. (1998). Prevalence of hearing loss in older adults in Beaver Dam, Wisconsin: The epidemiology of hearing loss study. *American Journal of Epidemiology, 148,* 879–86.

Chung, J. H., Des Roches, C. M., Meunier, J., & Eavey R. D. (2005). Evaluation of noise-induced hearing loss in young people using a web-based survey technique. *Pediatrics, 115,* 861–867.

Cummings, S. M., Cooper, R. L., & Cassie, K. M. (2009). Motivational interviewing to affect behavioral change in older adults. *Research on Social Work Practice, 19,* 195–204.

Davis, A., Smith, P., Ferguson, M., Stephens, D., & Gianopoulos, I. (2007). *Acceptability, benefit and costs of early screening for hearing disability: A study of potential screening tests and models.* Southampton, UK: National Coordinating Centre for Health Technology Assessment, University of Southampton.

Desjardins, J. L., & Doherty, K. A. (2009). Do experienced hearing aid users know how to use their hearing aids correctly? *American Journal of Audiology, 18,* 69–76.

Dillon, H. (2012). *Hearing Aids.* (2nd ed.). New York: Thieme.

Echalier, M. (2012). *In it together: The impact of hearing loss on personal relationships.* London: Action on Hearing Loss.

Ekberg, K., Meyer, C., Scarinci, N., Grenness, C., & Hickson, L. (2015). Family member involvement in audiology appointments with older people with hearing impairment. *International Journal of Audiology, 54,* 70–76.

Ferguson, M. A., Kitterick, P. T., Edmondson-Jones, M., & Hoare, D. J. (2015). Hearing aids for mild to moderate hearing loss in adults (protocol). *Cochrane Database of Systematic Reviews, 12,* CD012023.

Ferguson, M., Brandreth, M., Brassington, W., Leighton, P., & Wharrad, H. (2016). A randomized controlled trial to evaluate the benefits of a multimedia educational program for first-time hearing aid users. *Ear and Hearing.* 37, 123–136.

Ferguson, M., & Henshaw, H. (2015). Computer and Internet interventions to optimise listening and learning for people with hearing loss: Accessibility, use and adherence. *American Journal of Audiology, 24,* 338–343.

Field, D. L., & Haggard, M. P. (1989). Knowledge of hearing tactics 1. Assessment by questionnaire and inventory. *British Journal of Audiology, 23,* 349–354.

Folkman, S., & Lazarus, R. (1988). *Ways of coping questionnaire.* Palo Alto, CA: Consulting Psychologists Press.

Franks, J. R., & Beckmann, N.J. (1985) Rejection of hearing aids: Attitudes of a geriatric sample. *Ear and Hearing, 6,* 161–166

Garnefski, N., & Kraaij, V. (2012a). Cognitive coping and goal adjustment are associated with symptoms of depression and anxiety in people with acquired hearing loss. *International Journal of Audiology, 51,* 545–550.

Garnefski, N., & Kraaij, V. (2012b). Effects of a cognitive behavioral self-help program on emotional problems for people with acquired hearing loss: A randomized controlled trial. *Journal of Deaf Studies and Deaf Education, 17,* 75–84.

Gomez, R. G., & Madey, S. F. (2001). Coping-with-hearing-loss model for older adults. *The Journals of Gerontology Series B: Psychological Sciences and Social Sciences, 56,* 223–225.

Gopinath, B., Schneider, J., Hickson, L., McMahon, C. M., Burlutsky, G., Leeder, S. R., & Mitchell, P. (2012b). Hearing handicap, rather than measured hearing impairment, predicts poorer quality of life over 10 years in older adults. *Maturitas, 72,* 146–151.

Gopinath, B., Schneider, J., McMahon, C. M., Teber, E., Leeder, S. R., & Mitchell, P. (2012a). Severity of age-related hearing loss is associated with impaired activities of daily living. *Age and Ageing, 41,* 195–200.

Grenness, C., Hickson, L., Laplante-Lévesque, A., & Davidson, B. (2014). Patient-centred audiological rehabilitation: Perspectives of older adults who own hearing aids. *International Journal of Audiology, 53*(suppl 1), S68–S75.

Grenness, C., Hickson, L., Laplante-Lévesque, A., Meyer, C., & Davidson, B. (2015). The nature of communication throughout diagnosis and management planning in initial audiologic rehabilitation consultations. *Journal of the American Academy of Audiology, 26,* 36–50.

Hawkins, D. B. (2005). Effectiveness of counseling-based adult group aural rehabilitation programs: A systematic review of the evidence. *Journal of the American Academy of Audiology, 16,* 485–493.

Henshaw, H., Clark, D. P. A., Kang, S., & Ferguson, M. A. (2012). Computer skills and Internet use in adults aged 50-74 years: Influence of hearing difficulties. *Journal of Medical Internet Research, 14,* e113.

Henshaw, H., & Ferguson, M. A. (2013). Efficacy of individual computer-based auditory training for people with hearing loss: A systematic review of the evidence. *PLoS One, 8,* e62836.

Hetu, R., Jones, L., & Getty, L. (1993). The impact of acquired hearing impairment on intimate relationships—implications for rehabilitation. *Audiology, 32,* 363–381.

Hickson, L., Laplante-Lévesque, A., & Wong, L. (2013). Evidence-based practice in audiology: Rehabilitation options for adults with hearing impairment. *American Journal of Audiology, 22,* 329–331.

Hickson, L., Meyer, C., Lovelock, K., Lampert, M., & Khan, A. (2014). Factors associated with success with hearing aids in older adults. *International Journal of Audiology, 53*(Suppl. 1), S18–S27.

Hickson, L., Worral, L., & Scarinci N. (2007a). *Active Communication Education (ACE): A program for older people with hearing impairment,* London: Speechmark.

Hickson, L., Worrall, L., & Scarinci, N. (2007b). A randomized controlled trial evaluating the Active Communication Education program for older people with hearing impairment. *Ear and Hearing, 28,* 212–230.

Humes, L. E., Dubno, J. R., Gordon-Salant, S., Lister, J. J., Cacace, A. T., Cruickshanks, K. J., ... Wingfield, A. (2012). Central presbycusis: A review and evaluation of the evidence. *Journal of the American Academy of Audiology, 23,* 635–666.

Kamil, R. J., & Lin, F. R. (2015). The effects of hearing impairment in older adults on communication partners: A systematic review. *Journal of the American Academy of Audiology, 26,* 155–182.

Keidser, G., Seeto, M., Rudner, M., Hygge, S., & Ronnberg, J. (2015). On the relationship between functional hearing and depression. *International Journal of Audiology, 54*, 653–664.

Kelly, T. B., Tolson, D., Day, T., McColgan, G., Kroll, T., & Maclaren, W. (2013). Older people's views on what they need to successfully adjust to life with a hearing aid. *Health and Social Care in the Community, 21*, 293–302.

Kelly-Campbell, R. J., & McMillan, A. (2015). The relationship between hearing aid self-efficacy and hearing aid satisfaction. *American Journal of Audiology, 24*, 529–535.

Kerr, P. C., & Cowie, R. I. D. (1997). Acquired deafness: A multi-dimensional experience. *British Journal of Audiology, 31*, 177–188.

Kerr, P. C., & Stephens, D. (1997). The use of an open-ended questionnaire to identify positive aspects of acquired hearing loss. *Audiology, 36*, 19–28.

Kochkin, S. (2007). MarkeTrak VII: Obstacles to adult non-user adoption of hearing aids. *The Hearing Journal, 60*, 27–43.

Laplante-Lévesque, A., Hickson, L., & Worrall, L. (2010). Promoting the participation of adults with acquired hearing impairment in their rehabilitation. *Journal of the Academy of Rehabilitative Audiology, 43*, 11–26.

Lee, F. S., Matthews, L. J., Dubno, J. R., & Mills, J. H. (2005). Longitudinal study of pure-tone thresholds in older persons. *Ear and Hearing, 26*, 1–11.

Lockey, K., Jennings, M. B., & Shaw, L. (2010). Exploring hearing aid use in older women through narratives. *International Journal of Audiology, 49*, 542–549.

Lundberg, M., Andersson, G., & Lunner, T. (2011). A randomized, controlled trial of the short-term effects of complementing an educational program for hearing aid users with telephone consultations. *Journal of the American Academy of Audiology, 22*, 654–662.

Manchaiah, V., Baguley, D. M., Pyykkö, I., Kentala, E., & Levo, H. (2015). Positive experiences associated with acquired hearing loss, Ménière's disease, and tinnitus: a review. *International Journal of Audiology, 54*, 1–10.

Meyer, C., Hickson, L., Lovelock, K., Lampert, M., & Khan, A. (2014). An investigation of factors that influence help-seeking for hearing impairment in older adults. *International Journal of Audiology, 53*(Suppl. 1), S3–S17.

Miller, W. R. (1983). Motivational interviewing with problem drinkers. *Behavioral Psychotherapy, 11*, 147–172.

Molander, P., Hesser, H., Weineland, S, Bergwall, K., Buck, S., Hansson-Malmlöf, J., . . . Andersson, G. (2015). Internet-based acceptance and commitment therapy for psychological distress experienced by people with hearing problems: Study protocol for a randomized controlled trial. *American Journal of Audiology, 24*, 307–310.

Moore, D. R. (2011). The diagnosis and management of auditory processing disorder. *Language, Speech, and Hearing Services in Schools, 42*, 303–308.

Nachtegaal, J., Kuik, D. J., Anema, J. R., Goverts, S. T., Festen, J. M., & Kramer, S. E. (2009). Hearing status, need for recovery after work, and psychosocial work characteristics: Results from an Internet-based national survey on hearing. *International Journal of Audiology, 48*, 684–691.

Oberg, M., Bohn, T., & Larsson, U. (2014). Short- and long-term effects of the modified Swedish version of the Active Communication Education (ACE) program for adults with hearing loss. *Journal of the American Academy of Audiology, 25*, 848–858.

Picou, E. M., Ricketts, T. A., & Hornsby, B. W. (2013). How hearing aids, background noise, and visual cues influence objective listening effort. *Ear and Hearing, 34*, e52–e64.

Poost-Foroosh, L., Jennings, M. B., & Cheesman, M. F. (2015). Comparisons of client and clinician views of the importance of factors in client-clinician interaction in hearing aid purchase decisions. *Journal of the American Academy Audiology, 26*, 247–259.

Pronk, M., Deeg, D. J. H., & Kramer, S. E. (2013). Hearing status in older persons: A significant determinant of depression and loneliness? Results from the longitudinal aging study Amsterdam. *American Journal of Audiology, 22*, 316–320.

Pryce, H., & Gooberman-Hill, R. (2012). "There's a hell of a noise": Living with a hearing loss in residential care. *Age and Ageing, 41*, 40–46.

Ridgway, J., Hickson, L., & Lind, C. (2015). Autonomous motivation is associated with hearing aid adoption. *International Journal of Audiology, 54*, 476–484.

Saito, H., Nishiwaki, Y., Michikawa, T., Kikuchi, Y., Mizutari, K., Takebayashi, T., & Ogawa, K. (2010). Hearing handicap predicts the development of depressive symptoms after 3 years in older community-dwelling Japanese. *Journal of the American Geriatrics Society, 58*, 93–97.

Saunders, G. H., Frederick, M. T., Silverman, S. C., Nielsen, C., & Laplante-Lévesque, A. (2016). Health behavior theories as predictors of hearing aid uptake and outcomes. *International Journal of Audiology, 55*(Suppl. 3), S59–S68.

Saunders, G. H., Frederick, M. T., Silverman, S., & Papesh, M. (2013). Application of the health belief model: Development of the Hearing Beliefs Questionnaire (HBQ) and its associations with hearing health behaviors. *International Journal of Audiology, 52*, 558–567.

Saunders, G. H., & Haggard, M. P. (1989). The clinical assessment of obscure auditory dysfunction-1: Auditory and psychological factors. *Ear and Hearing, 10*, 200–208.

Saunders, G. H., Smith, S. L., Chisolm, T. H., Frederick, M. T., McArdle, R. A., & Wilson, R. H. (2016). A randomized control trial: Supplementing hearing aid use with listening and communication enhancement (LACE) auditory training. *Ear and Hearing, 37*(4), 381–396.

Schaette, R., & McAlpine, D. (2011). Tinnitus with a normal audiogram: Physiological evidence for hidden hearing loss and computational model. *The Journal of Neuroscience, 31*, 13452–13457.

Scherich, D. L. (1996). Job accommodations in the workplace for persons who are deaf or hard of hearing: Current practices and recommendations. *Journal of Rehabilitation, 62*, 27.

Sereda, M., Hoare, D. J., Nicholson, R., Smith, S., & Hall, D. A. (2015). Consensus on hearing aid candidature and fitting for mild hearing loss, with and without tinnitus: Delphi review. *Ear and Hearing, 36*, 417.

Smith, S. L., & West, R. L. (2006). The application of self-efficacy principles to audiologic rehabilitation: A tutorial. *American Journal of Audiology, 15*, 46–56.

Sommers, M. S., Hale, S., Myerson, J., Rose, N., Tye-Murray, N., & Spehar B. (2011). Listening comprehension across the adult lifespan. *Ear and Hearing, 32*, 775.

Southall, K., Gagné, J., & Jennings, M. (2010). Stigma: A negative and a positive influence on help-seeking for adults with acquired hearing loss. *International Journal of Audiology, 49*, 804–814.

Southall, K., Gagné, J. P., & Leroux, T. (2006). Factors that influence the use of assistance technologies by older adults who have a hearing loss. *International Journal of Audiology, 45*, 252–259.

Tambs, K. (2004). Moderate effects of hearing loss on mental health and subjective well-being: Results from the Nord-Trondelag hearing loss study. *Psychosomatic Medicine, 66*, 776–782.

Thorén, E. S., Oberg, M., Wanstrom, G., Andersson, G., & Lunner, T. (2014). A randomized controlled trial evaluating the effects of online rehabilitative intervention for adult hearing-aid users. *International Journal of Audiology, 53*, 452–461.

Tremblay, K. L., Pinto, A., Fischer, M. E., Klein, B. E., Klein R, Levy, S. . . . Cruickshanks, K. J. (2015). Self-reported hearing difficulties among adults with normal audiograms: The Beaver Dam offspring study. *Ear and Hearing, 36*, e290–e299.

Tye-Murray, N. (1991). Repair strategy usage by hearing-impaired adults and changes following communication therapy. *Journal of Speech, Language, and Hearing Research, 34*, 921–928.

van Eijken, M., Wensing, M., de Konink, M., Vernooy, M., Zielhuis, G., Lagro, T. . . . Grol, R. 2004. Health education on self-management and seeking health care in older adults: A randomized trial. *Patient Education and Counseling, 55*, 48–54.

Vlaescu, G., Carlbring, P., Lunner, T., & Andersson, G. (2015). An e-platform for rehabilitation of persons with hearing problems. *American Journal of Audiology, 24*, 271–275.

Vuorialho, A., Karinen, P., & Sorri, M. (2006). Counseling of hearing aid users is highly cost-effective. *European Archives of Otorhinolaryngology, 263*, 988–995.

Wallhagen, M. (2010). The stigma of hearing loss. *Gerontologist, 50*, 66–75.

Weineland, S. M., Andersson, G., Lunner, T., Carlbring, P., Hesser, H., Ingo, E. . . . Laplante-Lévesque, A. (2015). Bridging the gap between hearing screening and successful rehabilitation: Research protocol of a randomized controlled trial of motivational interviewing via Internet. *American Journal of Audiology, 24*, 302–306.

West, R. L., & Smith, S. L. (2007). Development of a hearing aid self-efficacy questionnaire. *International Journal of Audiology, 46*, 759–771.

World Health Organization. (2001). *International classification of functioning, disability and health: ICF*. Geneva: World Health Organization.

World Health Organization. (2012). *Facts about deafness*. Retrieved from http://www.who.int/pbd/deafness/facts/en/

15

Self-Management of HIV

FAITH MARTIN ■

The face of human immunodeficiency virus (HIV) has changed dramatically since the early days of the epidemic in the 1980s. No longer seen as a death sentence with the advent of effective life-prolonging medication, HIV has for nearly 15 years been seen as a chronic health condition (Siegal & Lekas, 2002).

This chapter provides an overview of self-management and HIV. The prevalence and treatment of HIV are first outlined. Next the impact of HIV in terms of functional limitations, and distress experienced, are summarized. The link between physical health, mental health, and issues such as poverty are set out to highlight the need for a multidimensional approach to this long-term condition. Evidence-based interventions are described, which illustrate the complexity of self-management for HIV, due to its multidimensional impact. Knowledge needs are discussed, again illustrating the wide range of areas that are important. HIV can have a range of emotional impacts, not least due to the complex social meaning the virus carries in terms of stigma in particular. Barriers to self-management are then considered, including the role of stigma. Given this range of challenges and barriers, coping tasks and strategies are briefly summarized. Finally, important techniques to support self-management are identified, particularly highlighting the importance of peer-based interventions, which can be widely applicable with few resources. This is highly relevant given the multidimensional nature of HIV, particularly the high prevalence of HIV in areas of very limited resources, such as in many areas of sub-Saharan Africa.

GLOBAL OVERVIEW OF HIV

Data from 2015 estimate 2.1 million new HIV infections in that year, leading to a worldwide total of 36.7 million people living with HIV, 19.1 million of which are in eastern and southern Africa (UNAIDS, 2016). Gender remains highly relevant to HIV: adolescent girls and young women account for 20% of new HIV infections globally; however, they represent just 11% of the adult population (UNAIDS, 2016).

Globally, access to (and seeking of) diagnostic testing and then effective medical treatment and monitoring of HIV are variable. While accessibility to medication is high in high-income countries, diagnosis remains problematic with approximately 17% of people with HIV in the UK unaware of their status (Public Health England, 2015). It is important to note, however, that nearly 70% of people with HIV in the world are located in sub-Saharan Africa, with a further 14% living in Asia and the Pacific. In these regions, the percentage of adults accessing medication are 43% and 36%, respectively (UNAIDS, 2015).

FUNCTIONAL LIMITATIONS AND SPECIFIC CHALLENGES PRESENTED BY HIV

The Range of Functional Limitations Related to HIV

Even with effective antiretroviral medication, HIV continues to be associated with and cause functional limitations and health difficulties including neurocognitive impairments of varying severity (Heaton et al., 2010). Functional impairments due to immune activation and inflammation can lead to weight loss and physical weakness, for example, affecting walking (Erlandson et al., 2013). HIV's other functional limitations can be thought of as being related to the conditions and issues experienced by those living with HIV, such as pain, fatigue, association with other infectious conditions (e.g., TB and hepatitis), and greater risks for a number of other conditions caused by both biological factors and associated behavioral factors (e.g., higher rates of smoking among people living with HIV further impact physical health; Reynolds, 2009).

Pain is reported by 54% to 88% of people with HIV (in the last three months) and is best considered within a biopsychosocial framework, because it is often related to variables such as psychological meanings, unhelpful cognitions, vicious behavioral cycles and/or social reinforcers, in addition to biological factors relating to a suppressed immune system and potential opportunistic infections (Parker, Stein, & Jelsma, 2014). Pain has its own functional impacts, often on sleep and energy. Fatigue itself is commonly associated with HIV in relation to the immunological effects, the adverse effects of medication, commonly co-occurring health conditions, and associated low mood (Voss, Dodd, Portillo, & Holzemer, 2006).

Psychological distress is associated with HIV; however, the direction or causality of this relationship remains unclear and is likely to be complex, together with the interrelated issue of lower socioeconomic status, which may mean that people may be more at risk of engaging in transactional sex, being exposed to drug use, and experiencing greater mental health problems, in part due to the situational stressors (Breuer, Myer, Struthers, & Joska, 2011; Sherr, Clucas, Harding, Sibley, & Catalan, 2011). Receiving a HIV diagnosis may itself present a traumatic event and can worsen low mood and anxiety (Basu, Chwastiak, & Bruce, 2005; Boarts,

Buckley-Fischer, Armelie, Bogart, & Delahanty, 2009). All of the functional challenges that are linked to psychological distress then may also impact people with HIV: withdrawal, isolation, sleep disturbances, inactivity, and unhelpful health behaviors, such as smoking, poor diet, or alcohol use (Katon, 2003).

Multidimensional Approach to HIV

HIV also presents a number of emotional challenges, which are discussed in greater detail later in this chapter. There are also important relational challenges—in terms of interpersonal relationships and the social views of HIV. Due to the range of functional limitations, psychological distress, impact on relationships, and social meaning and stigma associated with HIV, it must be thought of in a biopsychosocial and cultural framework. The meanings given to this virus render it more complex, compounding the multifaceted impact HIV has upon physical health, including the neurological impacts that can directly impact mental health from a biological standpoint. The risk factors of acquiring HIV and other difficulties that it is associated with, including a complex bidirectional relationship with mental health and substance use, lead to challenges in understanding causal relationships. The co-occurrence in many situations of structural drivers, such as poverty and gender inequalities, adds further strands to our understanding of HIV (Seeley et al., 2012). The heterogeneity among people with HIV must also be observed—factors like sexuality, mental health, drug use, and poverty have different strength of association to HIV for individuals, and diverse patterns are seen across geographical areas. As such, observations about the functional impairments of HIV, knowledge needs, emotional impacts, coping skills, and suitability and effectiveness of different interventions should always be considered in relation to the specific characteristics of groups.

EVIDENCE-BASED PRACTICES TO IMPROVE HEALTH OUTCOMES WITHIN HIV

The evidence base for self-management interventions in HIV is summarized in this section. It is important to note, as described herein, that there is a lack of high-quality evidence to allow broad claims to be made about effective interventions across the different domains of self-management. Interventions to support medication-taking have perhaps received the most attention, and there are a number of approaches with good evidence. Interventions that more generally aim to improve other elements of self-management, such as maintain a healthy diet, are less well-evidenced. A recent review of self-management interventions identified six relevant interventions and identified short-term improvements in physical, psychosocial, health knowledge, and health behaviors (e.g., taking medications; Millard, Elliott, & Girdler, 2013). A wide range of intervention strategies were included—including peer-based work, focuses on symptom management, training for coping effectiveness, and positive-self management groups that included education, cognitive-behavioral approaches, and problem-solving. There was insufficient evidence to allow conclusions about the longer-term benefits or the optimal content of such interventions.

Interventions to Support Medication-Taking

A fundamentally important element to improving survival of people with HIV is the development of increasingly effective antiretroviral therapy (ART). Understanding factors and developing interventions to improve the extent to which people with HIV take their medication as directed are therefore important to optimize physical health. Since 2010, more than 40 systematic reviews have explored interventions to support medication-taking. One review identified 124 relevant interventions, the majority of which tested multicomponent interventions that included a mix of cognitive-behavioral, education, treatment supporters, direct observation of medication-taking, and technological solutions to act as reminders (Chaiyachati et al., 2014). The review found that combination interventions were similarly effective as compared to single interventions, and the intervention effect varied based on culture and setting, with behavioral interventions (e.g., goal-setting, motivational interviews, and problem-solving approaches to remove barriers to taking medication) being most consistently effective.

Another review identified only 10 studies of high quality that improved medication-taking and clinical outcomes (Mbuagbaw, Sivaramalingam, et al., 2015). Intervention techniques included counseling, simplification of the regimen, text messages, cognitive-behavioral interventions delivered via the web, face-to-face intensive behavioral work, contingency management, direct observation of medication taking, and nurse support in visits and telephone calls. Several reviews have focused on specific interventions (e.g., economic incentives found to have some effectiveness; Galarraga, Genberg, Martin, Barton Laws, & Wilson, 2013) or specific populations (e.g., finding a lack of interventions tailored for children and adolescents; Arrivillaga, Martucci, Hoyos, & Arango, 2013). Focusing specifically on motivational interviewing, a review identified five randomized controlled trials and suggested the approach is promising (Hill & Kavookjian, 2012). Motivational interviewing can be delivered by non-specialists, it has been successfully used outside of HIV research with a wide range of client groups, and it is useful in issues that at times co-occur with HIV, such as substance use/alcohol and mental health difficulties (Miller & Rose, 2009). This renders it particularly useful in resource-constraint settings (Patel et al., 2013).

Examining these reviews, a pattern emerges of a lack of high-quality studies; more research is required to understand which specific intervention components are required for optimal effectiveness and there is a need for longer-term follow-ups. Nevertheless, a range of interventions to improve medication-taking show effectiveness, and the challenge for service planners and practitioners working with people with HIV is now to understand which interventions to suggest when working with people with HIV with different characteristics and in varying sociocultural settings.

Interventions to Support Self-Management beyond Medication

Interventions to support positive health behaviors as part of self-management have some evidence for effectiveness in relation to HIV. Increasing physical exercise has positive effects on physiological measures of health and physical functioning (Gomes-Neto, Conceição, Carvalho, & Brites, 2013; Nixon, O'Brien, Glazier, & Tynan, 2005). How best to help people with HIV to increase and maintain optimal levels of physical activity remains unclear, with research from other populations likely to offer useful insights (Michie, Abraham, Whittington, McAteer, & Gupta, 2009).

Nutrition is important to support the immune system and health generally, including for people with HIV, and some evidence suggests that people with HIV have greater energy consumption needs even when asymptomatic (World Health Organization, 2003). However, interventions that target nutrition have been found to have unclear impacts on mortality, disability, retention in care, and quality of life in resource-limited settings (Tang, Quick, Chung, & Wanke, 2015). Interventions to improve nutritional outcomes have used education and counseling strategies and had some success; however, as ever, the evidence base is somewhat limited in terms of number, quality, and scope of studies (Kaye & Moreno-Leguizamon, 2010). As with other types of interventions, there is a need to tailor to specific groups in relation to nutrition, particularly, while taking the stigma of HIV into account, as this was found to reduce attendance at group sessions (Kaye & Moreno-Leguizamon, 2010).

Education for people with HIV has often focused mainly on medication-taking (Millard et al., 2013; Rueda et al., 2006), like many other approaches designed to facilitate self-management and improve HIV care. The importance of medication-taking is clear. However, research into the broader educational needs of people with HIV is required, as are high-quality studies and reviews of interventions; for example, there is a lack of systematic reviews to provide insight into the most effective strategies for posttest counseling and education.

Peer-support interventions are common in chronic conditions, including HIV. A systematic review of support groups identified significant positive effects (Bateganya, Amanyeiwe, Roxo, & Dong, 2015). This review found that support groups may have positive impacts on mortality, with research taking place in low-income settings, such as Mozambique. Further, support-group participants have been found to have better viral load suppression in some studies, although there is a lack of well-designed controlled trials. This review study observed a moderate impact on quality of life; yet the expected impact on HIV transmission was uncertain with poor-quality evidence. Peer-support interventions are of particular relevance to facilitating self-management as they can be delivered at low cost, use "task-shifting" (movement of healthcare activities from healthcare professionals to non-specialists), can be tailored to fit the local needs, and therefore are implementable in low-income settings (Callaghan, Ford, & Schneider, 2010).

Psychological therapies, with a clear focus on improving mental health, have been tested in a range of settings with promising results (Spies, Asmal, & Seedat, 2013). For example, in Uganda group psychotherapy has been shown to improve not only depression but also role functioning (Nakimuli-Mpungu et al., 2015). In the United States, cognitive-behavioral therapy has improved both medication-taking and depression (Safren et al., 2009). Evidence-based psychological therapy is recommended for depression and anxiety for people with HIV (MedFASH, 2011).

KNOWLEDGE NEEDS AND SELF-MANAGEMENT TASKS

Knowledge needs about HIV and self-management tasks are present from diagnosis and throughout, even when HIV is asymptomatic, owing to stigma, changes in relationships and social life, and psychological distress (Martin et al., 2010). HIV is similar to many other chronic health conditions in terms of managing long-term health difficulties, uncertainty, and changes to functioning. However, there are some elements that are specific to HIV, as Swendeman, Ingram, and Rotheram-Borus (2009) point out: lack of direct self-monitoring for physical health status, stigma and disclosure, and the criminalization, in some nations, of exposing others to HIV. This section therefore provides an overview of knowledge needs and self-management tasks, particularly focusing on these HIV specific elements, while providing brief consideration of other issues.

Knowledge

Knowledge about HIV and medication are key elements of informed self-management. Knowledge and understanding of HIV treatment are lower among those with a lower educational background (Braga Ceccato, Acurcio, Vallano, Comini Cesar, & Crosland Guimaraes, 2009), which is relevant given that HIV is predominately seen in areas of poverty in sub-Saharan Africa, where education levels are often low and resources to provide or access information about HIV are limited.

In relation to HIV itself, important areas of knowledge include an understanding of what HIV is; how it affects the body, with particular reference to CD4 count and viral load; what monitoring is required; and what symptoms to be concerned about. As there is no self-monitoring available for HIV (i.e., blood tests are still required), people with HIV must learn about the meaning of the results of these tests as indicators for health; in addition they must learn how to work with their healthcare provider to understand drug-resistance test results (i.e., development of the virus that renders it resistant to some medication regimes) and potentially the implications for needing to switch to another medication regime. Although this knowledge is crucial, the process of needing to attend appointments for blood tests, waiting for results, and potentially experiencing dissonance between results indicating "ill-health" while feeling physically well (or vice versa) all provide potential sources of stress and uncertainty. Learning how to collaborate with healthcare providers is a general self-management skill of relevance for HIV.

Other key knowledge needs are how to correctly take medication (e.g., what to do if one misses a dose), the medical rationale behind the need to take as directed (e.g., reducing risks of development of resistance), and how to identify and manage adverse effects of medication. Within the adult population, studies continue to identify deficits in knowledge: in a sample from a study in France, 48% felt they had no knowledge of HIV-related health complications (Bouzille et al., 2012).

Of particular relevance is how knowledge is provided to young people with perinatally acquired HIV. Disclosure to young people remains contested—with the minority of those in low-resource settings (predominately sub-Saharan Africa) being made aware of their status (Vreeman, Gramelspacher, Gisore, Scanlon, & Nyandiko, 2013). Disclosure may not take place until the person with HIV is a teen. This chapter focuses on adult population; however, the way HIV status is disclosed to children is likely to have important impacts on their adult life with HIV: disclosure may be important to acceptance and management of HIV in adulthood (Krauss, Letteney, De Baets, Baggaley, & Okero, 2013). Pregnant women must also have knowledge of the risks of transmission to their baby, including preventative treatments and the relative risks of breastfeeding.

Knowledge and support to access and optimally use nutrition is important to HIV self-management. Nutritional supplements may be needed by those people with HIV who may be in situations with fewer resources to access food or who have substance/alcohol use difficulties or mental health problems, which can lead to poorer daily nutrition and can contribute further to the depletion of immune cells, particularly CD4 (Ellis, 2015).

Unlike many other chronic conditions, HIV is transmissible, and knowledge around transmission risks is important to self-management and public health. People with HIV must be made aware of the laws around HIV risk; indeed, in the UK, this is considered, in part, the healthcare professional's responsibility. With successful medical treatment, risks of transmission are very low. Condom use and refraining from drug use or safely injecting drugs are recommended, because of risks of other infections. Nevertheless, in several nations, behaviors that place others are risk of acquiring HIV have been criminalized. These fall into three broad categories: nondisclosure prior to sex, HIV exposure, and HIV transmission (Bernard & Bennett-Carlson, 2012). In the United States, several states legally require disclosure to sexual partners, and some to needle-sharing partners, while other states criminalize behaviors that place others at risk of acquiring HIV, with many of these laws not taking into account the dramatically reduced risk of transmission associated condom use and medication use (Centers for Disease Control and Prevention, 2015). In other nations, a legal evaluation of transmission risks takes into account the viral load and does not criminalize nondisclosure; for example, in the UK, prosecutions have focused on reckless transmission, whereas across Africa there are a range of legal frameworks, with some nations moving to reduce criminalization of disclosure or exposure and instead focusing on establishing intention to do harm (see http://www.aidsmap.com/resources/law/).

Research has suggested that criminalizing nondisclosure will adversely impact attendance for HIV testing and treatment (Patterson et al., 2015), which may further damage public health as the virus may be then less controlled. The UNAIDS report (Joint United Nations Programme on HIV/AIDS, 2013) makes a number of recommendations, calling for a focus on intentional transmission. Attempts made to reduce risks of transmission, disclose, and/or seek consent may be taken into account under some nations' laws.

Managing Medication

Based on studies of medication effectiveness, there have been recent changes to prescribing guidelines, meaning that people with HIV will now be offered ART regardless of their CD4 count (Group, 2015; Lundgren et al., 2015; World Health Organization, 2015). This represents a shift from living without ART if CD4 remains above a set level (set at 350 then changed to 500). Taking medication as suggested is rapidly becoming an essential behavior for all people with HIV, and this is currently a lifelong demand. Long-term medication taking presents challenges to self-management, and there are a number of interventions to improve this (discussed in the "Interventions to Support Medication-Taking" section).

Stigma and Disclosure

Stigma relates to the social threat—the idea that others or oneself will see the condition as negative and socially undesirable. Stigma can be enacted in terms of discrimination; yet, self-stigma is also observed, whereby people view themselves as "bad" due to their view of social norms and beliefs (Ostrom, Serovich, Lim, & Mason, 2006). Because of the stigma of HIV, telling others that one is living with HIV can, for some, be stressful. The use of the term "disclosure" is now contested as implicitly reinforcing the stigma (Obermeyer, Baijal, & Pegurri, 2011), as one does not speak of "disclosing" something neutral or positive. The term "disclosure" is used in this chapter as a term that implies the act of telling another/others the information that one is HIV-positive.

Disclosure is associated with better medication-taking and less depression (Katz et al., 2013). It is typically done with the aim of sharing information for social support or to maintain relationships (Obermeyer et al., 2011). Voluntary disclosure of HIV status involves a number of decisions and processes, not least the decision to disclose in the first place, whom to disclose to, the details of what information will be shared, and where, and how to present the information. Those involved in providing care or testing for people with HIV often offer support around disclosure. However, it is important, in order to ensure self-management, that those involved explore and respect the views of the people with HIV (Obermeyer et al., 2011).

There is a broad range of knowledge needs for people with HIV. Knowledge of the condition itself, understanding medical test results, and managing medication are fundamental, as are topics of living well, including good nutrition and other elements of maintaining physical health. However, HIV has such a complex social meaning that issues of disclosure and how to manage stigma are additional crucial areas where the person may benefit from knowledge. HIV's transmissible nature leads to needs for knowledge of transmission routes and techniques to avoid transmission and the legal issues around responsibility for potential transmission to another person. The knowledge needs are beyond the infection and its medical treatment and extend into wider well-being topics and social issues.

EMOTIONAL IMPACT OF HIV

It is important to note that emotional distress, depression, anxiety, and/or posttraumatic symptoms are by no means inevitable consequences of living with HIV (Steward et al., 2011). Resilience and posttraumatic growth are seen, which in turn are linked with better physical health outcomes (Sherr, Nagra, et al., 2011). Posttraumatic growth may occur when coping succeeds (discussed under the section "Coping Strategies and Skills"). Individuals with HIV, where treatment is available, can live an average lifespan. The emotional impact of HIV may wax and wane over the lifespan– perhaps being strong at diagnosis but then fading, re-emerging around times of disclosure or starting a family, and perhaps also as people become fatigued with treatment.

The context of the person with HIV must also be considered when thinking about the emotional impact of the virus. A study in Uganda found that people with HIV on ART had better quality of life and lower depression than people without a HIV diagnosis (Martin, Russell, & Seeley, 2014b). This finding may make sense when context is considered—access to healthcare and social support, including counseling, may be higher among people with HIV than the general population in Uganda, where HIV care systems are well-embedded. This potentially explains the finding and cautions us to be mindful of context when understanding emotional impact.

Overall, HIV is typically associated with elevated levels of both depression (Nanni, Caruso, Mitchell, Meggiolaro, & Grassi, 2015; Sherr, Clucas, et al., 2011) and anxiety (Kemppainen, MacKain, & Reyes, 2013). Compared to the population without HIV, higher levels of posttraumatic stress disorder also appear to be present, although the estimated prevalence covers a wide range, from 5% to 74% (Sherr, Nagra, et al., 2011). As HIV can be associated with mental health difficulties, substance abuse, sexual assault, or sex work, some of these factors may explain the greater levels of distress seen in among people with HIV. However, this is not to imply that all people with HIV have experienced these difficulties; rather, these covariants complicate our attempts to understand the emotional impact of HIV itself.

HIV may be linked to depression and anxiety, for example, as HIV can represent uncertainty for the future. Although now a chronic health condition in most settings, HIV is a serious threat to health. It also represents a social threat due to its stigmatized nature. Feelings of loss about an imagined future and potentially sorrow for previous actions can promote depression, together with a sense of no longer belonging (Lawrence & Cross, 2013). Together with these psychological and social factors, HIV may create neurobiological changes, which can (a) cause neuroendocrine and inflammatory changes, which may increase the likelihood of depression in light of stress, and (b) create neurocognitive changes, which may lead to depression in terms of changes to functioning (Nanni et al., 2015). A diagnosis of depression, however, is complicated with HIV, as with many other health conditions, because the physical symptoms of depression and some of the cognitive complaints, such as lack of concentration, may be due to either the HIV or the medication (Benton, 2008).

Anxiety is also found to be common in people with HIV (Kemppainen et al., 2013). Concerns and uncertainty about physical health, stigma, and, for some, reduced social support can all create anxiety, which can be experienced physically as nausea and therefore also confused with adverse effects of medication or symptoms of opportunistic infections (Marinho, Amaral, Pereira, Marques, & Bragança, 2016). Further, due to the potential or feared cognitive impairments that can occur with HIV, the cognitive symptoms of anxiety (Kemppainen et al., 2013) that include impaired concentration and memory can then cause further anxiety. These factors complicate the diagnosis of anxiety in a manner similar to depression in the context of HIV.

The emotional distress associated with HIV has a non-trivial impact of functional status. For example, one study with HIV-positive men who have sex with men found that depression and posttraumatic stress accounted for a small but significant amount of variation in general health, pain, and everyday role functioning (e.g., work) when virus and treatment-related variables were taken into account (O'Cleirigh, Skeer, Mayer, & Safren, 2009). A significant amount of the functional impact seen in people with HIV is associated with the psychological factors, which were either present before or resulted from HIV infection, diagnosis, and experiences of living as someone with HIV. Staying active, connecting to a community, and engaging in self-management practices, such as physical activity, are associated with good mental health (Webel et al., 2016), in addition to likely effects on physical well-being.

Since HIV's emergence in the 1980s, huge advances have been made and continue to progress in its treatment. Furthermore, we now have the first group of people with HIV who have used ART long term and the first cohort of babies with perinatally acquired HIV reaching early adulthood, having taken ART for the majority of their lifetimes. The effects of both HIV and ART on these groups have been previously unknown. Uncertainty is present around the virus and its treatment when used in a long-term manner (Solomon, O'Brien, Wilkins, & Gervais,

2014). Additionally, people with HIV must live with uncertainty between medical monitoring about their immune-system status, as no symptoms may present (Madge, Matthews, Singh, & Theobald, 2004). Further, uncertainty is experienced in how other people will react to an individual's disclosure of HIV, due to the stigma that persists. Managing uncertainty then becomes a major aspect for self-management.

Shame as experienced in relation to HIV has recently been reviewed (Bennett, Traub, Mace, Juarascio, & O'Hayer, 2016). Shame is a self-conscious emotion relating to feeling socially defective. Because of the stigma of HIV, shame is also experienced by some people with HIV. It is an emotion that motivates escape, hiding, and avoidance and has a strong link to both depression and anxiety (Gilbert, 2000). Avoidance coping is common with shame. Avoiding shame can be one reason why some stop taking medication or attending appointments: the pain of the reminder of one's shame is experienced as worse than the health consequences of these behaviors.

OTHER BARRIERS TO SELF-MANAGEMENT

Access to care remains a barrier to self-management, particularly in low- or middle-income countries. Access to care in high-income countries may also be limited by health-service structures, stigma, and membership of "hard to reach" groups, such as those who use drugs. There are other "structural drivers" of HIV, such as the interactions between social and cultural norms, structures and institutions, and individual behaviors that affect HIV, in a manner peculiar to each setting (Auerbach, Parkhurst, & Caceres, 2011). For example, poverty can exacerbate the relevance of gender in relation to HIV; poverty may increase transactional sex where protection is not used (to maximize income generation). Thus, women may be vulnerable to acquiring HIV, yet have little funds to travel to obtain testing and/or treatment. Self-management in such settings is hugely challenged by the environment, cultural meanings and customs, and resources available.

Addressing social inequalities can broadly improve self-management in addition to improve self-management for HIV. Stigma is a major structural driver (Mahajan et al., 2008), affecting access to care and use of medications, as are other social norms (e.g., the importance of work for being masculine and social realities, such as the need to earn money to care for family, coupled with the lack of safe ways to effectively achieve this; Seeley et al., 2012). People living with HIV also often are socially marginalized for many reasons, such as sexuality, poverty, race, or ethnicity (Earnshaw, Bogart, Dovidio, & Williams, 2013; Portillo et al., 2005), which can lead to social isolation, poorer employment, and, therefore, greater insecurity and higher levels of perceived stress. All of this may contribute to depression and suicidality (Kalichman, Heckman, Kochman, Sikkema, & Bergholte, 2000). The stigma of HIV can worsen such marginalization.

The stigma of HIV is a barrier to accessing testing, treatment, medication, and social support. It undermines self-management behaviors and coping by diminishing adaptive cognitions about HIV, reducing social support (Katz et al., 2013), and forcing people to hide their status to avoid being treated as "other." Stigma, commonly linked to depression and anxiety, is commonly experienced, with a literature review finding that 52% of people with HIV had experienced stigma in the previous year (Lowther, Selman, Harding, & Higginson, 2014). The social aspects cannot be divorced from the physical and psychological factors, least of all not in relation to HIV. The experience of stigma, due to the social meaning of HIV, can create social isolation and depression and in turn impact health behaviors, such as medication-taking, particularly among women (Turan et al., 2016).

COPING STRATEGIES OR SKILLS

Skills for self-management for people with HIV include interpreting and acting on symptoms, taking medication consistently, and managing side effects. These skills can be improved using health education groups, whereby information and skills practice are delivered, with a focus on improving motivation and self-efficacy (Gifford, Laurent, Gonzales, Chesney, & Lorig, 1998), based on the well-known "positive self-management program" (Lorig et al., 1999).

A wide range of coping styles may be used, with most shown to be beneficial. For example, spiritual coping was found to be used among 72% of study participants over a 10-year longitudinal study and was typically positive; however, for some, it may lead to HIV being viewed negatively and fatalistically (Kremer & Ironson, 2014). Coping styles and strategies may be initially developed around the time of diagnosis. However, as life with HIV moves forward, such strategies may be further developed and redeployed at times of stress (Lawrence & Cross, 2013). Much-researched coping styles are all evident in people with HIV, including problem-focused and emotion-focused coping. Avoidant strategies, including social isolation, are associated with poor outcomes, while spiritual coping, social engagement, positive reappraisal strategies, and other problem-focused coping predicted better outcomes (McIntosh & Rosselli, 2012).

Posttraumatic growth appears to be linked to disclosure and receipt of emotional support (Kamen et al., 2015). Emotion-focused coping, often used with support-seeking strategies, can lead to higher coping self-efficacy, which itself is associated with lower psychological distress and higher posttraumatic growth (Evans, Williams, & Leu, 2013). However, problem-focused coping was also highly associated with self-efficacy of coping and growth. It appears that no coping strategy is associated with greater posttraumatic growth (Sherr, Nagra, et al., 2011).

Adjustment to HIV includes social, cognitive, and behavioral changes, and, as such, it is challenging to distinguish this concept from coping and indeed the very work of "self-management" itself (Martin, Russell, & Seeley, 2014a). Reframing the meaning of HIV and the appraisal of one's ability to manage any associated stress are core elements of the adjustment. People with HIV can be supported with this reframing and reappraisal, using workshops with peer interventions, for example (Bova, Burwick, & Quinones, 2008).

Management of uncertainty is a key coping skill for people with HIV. The fast-moving advances in HIV medication, the lack of legacy of lifelong ART and its effects, the absence of self-monitoring of the virus, and the asymptomatic presentation or experience of adverse medication effects that mimic other health difficulties all contribute to significant uncertainty about HIV. Learning to "negotiate uncertainty" is a key task for self-management and may include reframing, seeking optimism, and habituation to the anxiety as a new normal (Perrett & Biley, 2013). Interventions to manage uncertainty can include sharing techniques and rehearsal of disclosure, maintenance of social networks, and improvements to health literacy to promote location and comprehension of health-related information (Brashers, Basinger, Rintamaki, Caughlin, & Para, 2016).

TESTED TECHNIQUES TO FACILITATE SELF-MANAGEMENT

Support groups and peer support are "low technology" but potentially highly effective techniques that allow the self-management of HIV to thrive, as these groups are easily set up and demand few resources. For example, research focusing on women's use of peer support has found that discrimination, internalized stigma, and psychological distress, such as loneliness and low mood, decrease with support group attendance, while elements of emotion-focused and problem-focused coping, such as emotional support and sharing of strategies for managing disclosure, increase (Paudel & Baral, 2015).

Support groups focusing on relationships have been found to be as good at reducing depression as group interventions designed specifically to improve coping (Heckman et al., 2011). Yet, other studies find no impact of peer-led support over standard care for measures of taking medication as prescribed or depression (Simoni, Pantalone, Plummer, & Huang, 2007). There are inconsistent results between studies, pointing to the need to carefully specify the ingredients of interventions and the control condition to better understand the differences between the interventions, the intended aims, and the characteristics about the population or setting that may impact on the success or failure of the intervention to achieve its aims. For example, support groups may be more beneficial when other sources of support are lacking or when individuals are experiencing isolation. Nevertheless, peer-support and support groups are typically easy to set up and can be readily initiated and managed by people with HIV, supporting their empowerment. The function of these groups can extend beyond clear, clinical outcomes and include important elements of providing a sense of identity, occupation and activity, and advocacy and campaigning.

"Technological" approaches, in terms of using information and communication technology of various types, are common. Simple approaches include setting reminders to take medications (Goldstein, 2010). More sophisticated approaches have been developed. Some of these take into account common co-occurring conditions globally. For example, a review highlighted the effective use of mobile phones to provide education, collect data, and offer monitoring and support for medication-taking for both HIV and tuberculosis (Devi et al., 2015). Text messaging interventions have improved medication-taking and attendance at appointments (Mbuagbaw, Mursleen, et al., 2015). Indeed, thanks to the global proliferation of mobile phones, including smartphones, such technology is offering valuable avenues for interventions in high-, middle-, and low-income settings.

As with many other intervention strategies and therapeutic approaches in HIV, the primary focus has been on using technology to increase medication-taking (Pellowski & Kalichman, 2012). We are now beginning to see the development of broader interventions, to provide information, psychosocial support, and therapy (Mo & Coulson, 2009). However, the design of such technologies does not yet meet the stated needs and desires of people with HIV (Schnall et al., 2015). Greater co-design of interventions between researchers/businesses and people with HIV is required.

Service design can impact on the extent to which people self-manage. One service approach is case management, whereby following diagnosis people with HIV meet with their "case manager" who offers support to identify needs and strengths and to facilitate contact with the HIV clinic. This intervention can reduce the extent to which people do not return to healthcare services following diagnosis (Gardner et al., 2005). Involving a partner of people with HIV can also impact self-management: a two-hour intervention demonstrated potential to improve stress management and medication-taking (Fife, Scott, Fineberg, & Zwickl, 2008).

Broader social interventions may also facilitate self-management by attempting to change public knowledge and attitudes toward HIV and thereby addressing the self-management challenges that arise from ignorance and stigma. Widespread media campaigns and other community-level interventions may reduce stigma, alongside more targeted interventions with particular communities or using more intensive education (Kerr et al., 2015; Stangl, Lloyd, Brady, Holland, & Baral, 2013).

CONCLUSION

This chapter has provided an outline of the issues surrounding HIV self-management. The functional impacts and emotional impacts are of course highly individualized and evolving, as both medical science and the social factors around HIV advance and shift. The knowledge needs are broad, covering not just condition-based knowledge but also strategies to live well, including following good nutrition, managing stigma and disclosure, and avoiding onwards transmission, including the legal knowledge needed around this. Interventions, coping strategies, and techniques to facilitate self-management are necessarily broad in range also, from motivational interviewing to help people take medication, to peer-support groups to tackle stigma and maintain mental health.

The identified challenges to self-management and strategies to manage these arise from a range of life areas: from physical health including medication-taking and nutrition; from mental health, including potential impacts of pain on mental health and the anxiety and depression that can arise from living with a long-term condition; and from social health, particularly due to the stigma that remains around HIV and the complex interrelationships between poverty, gender, mental health, and HIV. The response to these challenges to self-management then must also occur at this range of levels. This can include social interventions to address stigma and to help create the conditions for self-management, for example by reducing the need to hide medication and increasing disclosure and therefore social support.

Many interventions have been designed to facilitate self-management for people with HIV. Many have focused on taking medication in isolation. The relationships between medication-taking, stigma, onward transmission, and mental health have been briefly outlined herein and call now for the important next steps in greater research for self-management interventions that are more holistic. The evidence base for HIV-focused interventions suggests an urgent need for studies with longer-term follow-up that examine in detail what works for whom and when and how these can be delivered with limited resources, as often demanded by the environments in which most people with HIV live. The existing evidence is highly promising, as are encouraging data on prevalence and treatment. The future for self-management in HIV is bright: alongside the need for greater investment in science to optimize interventions there is also a huge amount of current progress and knowledge. Much HIV self-management work is carried out by nongovernmental organizations, and therefore, an important task for people affected by HIV and their healthcare professionals is to engage with these other agencies to share knowledge.

REFERENCES

Arrivillaga, M., Martucci, V., Hoyos, P. A., & Arango, A. (2013). Adherence among children and young people living with HIV/AIDS: A systematic review of medication and comprehensive interventions. *Vulnerable Children and Youth Studies, 8*(4), 321–337.

Auerbach, J. D., Parkhurst, J. O., & Caceres, C. F. (2011). Addressing social drivers of HIV/AIDS for the long-term response: Conceptual and methodological considerations. *Glob Public Health, 6*(Suppl. 3), S293–S309. doi:10.1080/17441692.2011.594451

Basu, S., Chwastiak, L. A., & Bruce, R. D. (2005). Clinical management of depression and anxiety in HIV-infected adults. *AIDS, 19*(18), 2057–2067.

Bateganya, M. H., Amanyeiwe, U., Roxo, U., & Dong, M. (2015). Impact of support groups for people living with HIV on clinical outcomes: A systematic review of the literature. *JAIDS: Journal of Acquired Immune Deficiency Syndromes, 68*(Suppl 3), S368–S374.

Bennett, D. S., Traub, K., Mace, L., Juarascio, A., & O'Hayer, C. V. (2016). Shame among people living with HIV: A literature review. *AIDS Care, 28*(1), 87–91. doi:10.1080/09540121.2015.1066749

Benton, T. D. (2008). Depression and HIV/AIDS. *Current Psychiatry Reports 10*(3), 280–285.

Bernard, E., & Bennett-Carlson, R. (2012). *Criminalization of HIV non-disclosure, exposure and transmission: Background and current landscape*. Geneva: UNAIDS.

Boarts, J. M., Buckley-Fischer, B. A., Armelie, A. P., Bogart, L. M., & Delahanty, D. L. (2009). The impact of HIV diagnosis-related vs. non-diagnosis related trauma on PTSD, depression, medication adherence, and HIV disease markers. *Journal of Evidence-Based Social Work*, 6(1), 4–16. doi:10.1080/15433710802633247

Bouzille, G., Brunet, C., Fialaire, P., Lemonnier, R., Gagnayre, R., & Fanello, S. (2012). [The needs and expectations of HIV patients before starting a therapeutic patient education program]. *Sante Publique*, 24(6), 483–496.

Bova, C. A., Burwick, T. N., & Quinones, M. (2008). Improving women's adjustment to HIV infection: Results of the positive life skills workshop project. *Journal of the Association of Nurses in AIDS Care*, 19(1), 58–65.

Braga Ceccato, M., Acurcio, F., Vallano, A., Comini Cesar, C., & Crosland Guimaraes, M. D. (2009). [Assessment of factors associated with patients' comprehension of treatment at the start of antiretroviral therapy]. *Enfermedades infecciosas y microbiología clínica*, 27(1), 7–13.

Brashers, D. E., Basinger, E. D., Rintamaki, L. S., Caughlin, J. P., & Para, M. (2016). Taking control: The efficacy and durability of a peer-led uncertainty management intervention for people recently diagnosed with HIV. *Health Communication* 32(1), 11–21. doi:10.1080/10410236.2015.1089469

Breuer, E., Myer, L., Struthers, H., & Joska, J. A. (2011). HIV/AIDS and mental health research in sub-Saharan Africa: A systematic review. *African Journal of AIDS Research*, 10(2), 101–122. doi:10.2989/16085906.2011.593373

Callaghan, M., Ford, N., & Schneider, H. (2010). A systematic review of task-shifting for HIV treatment and care in Africa. *Human Resources for Health*, 8(8). doi:10.1186/1478-4491-8-8

Centers for Disease Control and Prevention. (2015). HIV-specific criminal laws. Retrieved from http://www.cdc.gov/hiv/policies/law/states/exposure.html

Chaiyachati, K. H., Ogbuoji, O., Price, M., Suthar, A. B., Negussie, E. K., & Barnighausen, T. (2014). Interventions to improve adherence to antiretroviral therapy: A rapid systematic review. *AIDS*, 28(Suppl. 2), S187–S204. doi:http://dx.doi.org/10.1097/QAD.0000000000000252

Devi, B. R., Syed-Abdul, S., Kumar, A., Iqbal, U., Nguyen, P. A., Li, Y. C. J., & Jian, W. S. (2015). MHealth: An updated systematic review with a focus on HIV/AIDS and tuberculosis long term management using mobile phones. *Computer Methods and Programs in Biomedicine*, 122(2), 257–265. doi:http://dx.doi.org/10.1016/j.cmpb.2015.08.003

Earnshaw, V. A., Bogart, L. M., Dovidio, J. F., & Williams, D. R. (2013). Stigma and racial/ethnic HIV disparities: Moving toward resilience. *American Psychologist*, 68(4), 225–236.

Ellis, W. L. (2015). A self-management framework to assess the need for nutritional supplementation in people living with HIV/AIDS A2. In Ronald Ross Watson (Ed.), *Health of HIV infected people* (pp. 99–115). Boston: Academic Press.

Erlandson, K. M., Allshouse, A. A., Jankowski, C. M., Lee, E. J., Rufner, K. M., Palmer, B. E., . . . Campbell, T. B. (2013). Association of functional impairment with inflammation and immune activation in HIV type 1–infected adults receiving effective antiretroviral therapy. *Journal of Infectious Diseases*, 208(2), 249–259. doi:10.1093/infdis/jit147

Ceccato, M. G. B., Acurcio, F. A., Vallano, A., César, C. C., & Guimarães, M. D. C. (2008). Evaluacion de factores asociados a la comprension del tratamiento en pacientes que inician la terapia antirretroviral. *Enfermedades Infecciosas y Microbiologia Clinica, 27*(1), 7-13.
Evans, S. D., Williams, B. E., & Leu, C. S. (2013). Correlates of posttraumatic growth among African Americans living with HIV/AIDS in Mississippi. *Online Journal of Rural and Urban Research, 3*(1).
Fife, B. L., Scott, L. L., Fineberg, N. S., & Zwickl, B. E. (2008). Promoting adaptive coping by persons with HIV disease: Evaluation of a patient/partner intervention model. *Journal of the Association of Nurses in AIDS Care, 19*(1), 75-84. doi:10.1016/j.jana.2007.11.002
Galarraga, O., Genberg, B. L., Martin, R. A., Barton Laws, M., & Wilson, I. B. (2013). Conditional economic incentives to improve HIV treatment adherence: Literature review and theoretical considerations. *AIDS & Behavior, 17*(7), 2283-2292.
Gardner, L. I., Metsch, L. R., Anderson-Mahoney, P., Loughlin, A. M., del Rio, C., Strathdee, S., . . . Holmberg, S. D. (2005). Efficacy of a brief case management intervention to link recently diagnosed HIV-infected persons to care. *AIDS, 19*(4), 423-431.
Gifford, A. L., Laurent, D., Gonzales, V., Chesney, M., & Lorig, K. R. (1998). Pilot randomized trial of education to improve self-management skills of men with symptomatic HIV/AIDS. *Journal of Acquired Immune Deficiency Syndromes and Humanretrovirology, 18*(2), 136-144.
Gilbert, P. (2000). The relationship of shame, social anxiety and depression: The role of the evaluation of social rank. *Clinical Psychology & Psychotherapy, 7*(3), 174-189.
Goldstein, K. M. (2010). Adherence in the treatment of HIV and other infectious diseases. In H. B. Bosworth (Ed.), *Improving patient treatment adherence: A clinician's guide* (pp. 259-288). New York: Springer.
Gomes-Neto, M., Conceição, C. S., Carvalho, V. O., & Brites, C. (2013). A systematic review of the effects of different types of therapeutic exercise on physiologic and functional measurements in patients with HIV/AIDS. *Clinics, 68*(8), 1157-1167. doi:10.6061/clinics/2013(08)16
Group, T. I. S. S. (2015). Initiation of antiretroviral therapy in early asymptomatic HIV infection. *The New England Journal of Medicine, 373*(9), 795-807. doi:doi:10.1056/NEJMoa1506816
Heaton, R. K., Clifford, D. B., Franklin, D. R., Woods, S. P., Ake, C., Vaida, F., . . . Rivera-Mindt, M. (2010). HIV-associated neurocognitive disorders persist in the era of potent antiretroviral therapy CHARTER study. *Neurology, 75*(23), 2087-2096.
Heckman, T. G., Sikkema, K. J., Hansen, N., Kochman, A., Heh, V., Neufeld, S., . . . Group, A. R. (2011). A randomized clinical trial of a coping improvement group intervention for HIV-infected older adults. *Journal of Behavioral Medicine, 34*(2), 102-111.
Hill, S., & Kavookjian, J. (2012). Motivational interviewing as a behavioral intervention to increase HAART adherence in patients who are HIV-positive: A systematic review of the literature. *AIDS Care, 24*(5), 583-592.
Joint United Nations Programme on HIV/AIDS. (2013). Ending overly broad criminalisation of HIV non-disclosure, exposure and transmission: critical scientific, medical and legal considerations. Geneva: Author.

Kalichman, S. C., Heckman, T., Kochman, A., Sikkema, K., & Bergholte, J. (2000). Depression and thoughts of suicide among middle-aged and older persons living with HIV-AIDS. *Psychiatric Services, 51*(7), 903–907. doi:10.1176/appi.ps.51.7.903

Kamen, C., Vorasarun, C., Canning, T., Kienitz, E., Weiss, C., Flores, S., . . . Gore-Felton, C. (2015). The impact of stigma and social support on development of post-traumatic growth among persons living with HIV. *Journal of Clinical Psychology in Medical Settings, 23*, 126. doi:10.1007/s10880-015-9447-2

Katon, W. J. (2003). Clinical and health services relationships between major depression, depressive symptoms, and general medical illness. *Biological Psychiatry, 54*(3), 216–226. doi:http://dx.doi.org/10.1016/S0006-3223(03)00273-7

Katz, I. T., Ryu, A. E., Onuegbu, A. G., Psaros, C., Weiser, S. D., Bangsberg, D. R., & Tsai, A. C. (2013). Impact of HIV-related stigma on treatment adherence: Systematic review and meta-synthesis. *Journal of the International AIDS Society, 16*(Suppl. 2),18640.

Kaye, H. L., & Moreno-Leguizamon, C. J. (2010). Nutrition education and counselling as strategic interventions to improvehealth outcomes in adult outpatients with HIV: A literature review. *African Journal of AIDS Research, 9*(3), 271–283. doi:10.2989/16085906.2010.530183

Kemppainen, J. K., MacKain, S., & Reyes, D. (2013). Anxiety symptoms in HIV-infected individuals. *Journal of the Association of Nurses in AIDS Care, 24*(1, Suppl.), S29–S39. doi:http://dx.doi.org/10.1016/j.jana.2012.08.011

Kerr, J. C., Valois, R. F., DiClemente, R. J., Carey, M. P., Stanton, B., Romer, D., . . . Fortune, T. (2015). The effects of a mass media HIV-risk reduction strategy on HIV-related stigma and knowledge among African American adolescents. *AIDS Patient Care and STDs, 29*(3), 150–156. doi:10.1089/apc.2014.0207

Krauss, B. J., Letteney, S., De Baets, A. J., Baggaley, R., & Okero, F. A. (2013). Caregiver's HIV disclosure to children 12 years and under: A review and analysis of the evidence. *AIDS Care, 25*(4), 415–429. doi:10.1080/09540121.2012.712664

Kremer, H., & Ironson, G. (2014). Longitudinal spiritual coping with trauma in people with HIV: Implications for health care. *AIDS Patient Care and STDs, 28*(3), 144–154. doi:10.1089/apc.2013.0280

Lawrence, S., & Cross, M. (2013). Life transition with HIV: Some observations of the phenomenon of growing older with the infection. *Counselling Psychology Review, 1*, 25–36.

Lorig, K. R., Sobel, D., Stewart, A. L., Brown, B. W., Bandura, A., Ritter, P., . . . Holman, H. R. (1999). Evidence suggesting that a chronic disease self-management program can improve health status while reducing hospitalization: A randomized trial. *Medical Care, 37*(1), 5–14.

Lowther, K., Selman, L., Harding, R., & Higginson, I. J. (2014). Experience of persistent psychological symptoms and perceived stigma among people with HIV on antiretroviral therapy (ART): A systematic review. *International Journal of Nursing Studies, 51*(8), 1171–1189. doi:10.1016/j.ijnurstu.2014.01.015

Lundgren, J. D., Babiker, A. G., Gordin, F., Emery, S., Grund, B., Sharma, S., . . . Neaton, J. D. (2015). Initiation of antiretroviral therapy in early asymptomatic HIV infection. *The New England Journal of Medicine, 373*(9), 795–807. doi:10.1056/NEJMoa1506816

Madge, S., Matthews, P., Singh, S., & Theobald, N. (2004). *HIV in primary care: Medical foundation for AIDS and sexual health*. London: Medical Foundation for AIDS & Sexual Health.

Mahajan, A. P., Sayles, J. N., Patel, V. A., Remien, R. H., Ortiz, D., Szekeres, G., & Coates, T. J. (2008). Stigma in the HIV/AIDS epidemic: A review of the literature and recommendations for the way forward. *AIDS, 22*(Suppl. 2), S67–S79. doi:10.1097/01.aids.0000327438.13291.62

Marinho, M., Amaral, A., Pereira, E., Marques, J., & Bragança, M. (2016). Anxiety among HIV-infected patients—when anxiety is a disorder and not simply a natural reaction to a life-threatening illness. *European Psychiatry, 33*(Suppl.), S657. doi:10.1016/j.eurpsy.2016.01.1949

Martin, F., Caramlau, I. O., Sutcliffe, P., Martin, S., Choudhry, K., & Bayley, J. (2010). Self management interventions for people living with HIV/AIDS: Protocol stage. *Cochrane Database of Systematic Reviews, 10*, CD008731.

Martin, F., Russell, S., & Seeley, J. (2014a). Adjustment as process and outcome: Measuring adjustment to HIV in Uganda. *Journal of Health Psychology, 21*(5), 872–883. doi:10.1177/1359105314541313

Martin, F., Russell, S., & Seeley, J. (2014b). Higher quality of life and lower depression for people on ART in Uganda as compared to a community control group. *PLoS ONE, 9*(8), e105154.

Mbuagbaw, L., Mursleen, S., Lytvyn, L., Smieja, M., Dolovich, L., & Thabane, L. (2015). Mobile phone text messaging interventions for HIV and other chronic diseases: An overview of systematic reviews and framework for evidence transfer. *BMC Health Services Research, 15*(33).

Mbuagbaw, L., Sivaramalingam, B., Navarro, T., Hobson, N., Keepanasseril, A., Wilczynski, N. J., & Haynes, R. B. (2015). Interventions for enhancing adherence to antiretroviral therapy (ART): A systematic review of high quality studies. *AIDS Patient Care and STDs, 29*(5), 248–266. doi:10.1089/apc.2014.0308

McIntosh, R. C., & Rosselli, M. (2012). Stress and coping in women living with HIV: A meta-analytic review. *Aids and Behavior, 16*(8), 2144–2159. doi:10.1007/s10461-012-0166-5

MedFASH. (2011). *Standards for psychological support for adults living with HIV.* London: British Psychological Society, British HIV Association, and Medical Foundation for AIDS & Sexual Health.

Michie, S., Abraham, C., Whittington, C., McAteer, J., & Gupta, S. (2009). Effective techniques in healthy eating and physical activity interventions: A meta-regression. *Health Psychology, 28*(6), 690–701.

Millard, T., Elliott, J., & Girdler, S. (2013). Self-management education programs for people living with HIV/AIDS: A systematic review. *AIDS Patient Care and STDs, 27*(2), 103–113.

Miller, W. R., & Rose, G. S. (2009). Toward a theory of motivational interviewing. *American Psychologist, 64*(6), 527.

Mo, P. K. H., & Coulson, N. S. (2009). Living with HIV/AIDS and use of online support groups. *Journal of Health Psychology, 15*(3), 339–350.

Nakimuli-Mpungu, E., Wamala, K., Okello, J., Alderman, S., Odokonyero, R., Mojtabai, R., . . . Musisi, S. (2015). Group support psychotherapy for depression treatment in people with HIV/AIDS in northern Uganda: A single-centre randomised controlled trial. *The Lancet HIV, 2*(5), e190–e199. doi:10.1016/S2352-3018(15)00041-7

Nanni, M. G., Caruso, R., Mitchell, A. J., Meggiolaro, E., & Grassi, L. (2015). Depression in HIV infected patients: A review. *Current Psychiatry Reports, 17*(1), 1–11.

Nixon, S., O'Brien, K., Glazier, R., & Tynan, A.-M. (2005). Aerobic exercise interventions for adults living with HIV/AIDS. *Cochrane Database of Systematic Reviews, 2*, CD001796.

O'Cleirigh, C., Skeer, M., Mayer, K. H., & Safren, S. A. (2009). Functional impairment and health care utilization among HIV-infected men who have sex with men: The relationship with depression and post-traumatic stress. *Journal of Behavioral Medicine, 32*(5), 466–477. doi:10.1007/s10865-009-9217-4

Obermeyer, C. M., Baijal, P., & Pegurri, E. (2011). Facilitating HIV disclosure across diverse settings: A review. *American Journal of Public Health, 101*(6), 1011–1023. doi:10.2105/AJPH.2010.300102

Ostrom, R. A., Serovich, J. M., Lim, J. Y., & Mason, T. L. (2006). The role of stigma in reasons for HIV disclosure and non-disclosure to children. *AIDS Care, 18*(1), 60–65. doi:10.1080/09540120500161769

Parker, R., Stein, D. J., & Jelsma, J. (2014). Pain in people living with HIV/AIDS: A systematic review. *Journal of the International AIDS Society, 17*(1), 1–15.

Patel, V., Belkin, G. S., Chockalingam, A., Cooper, J., Saxena, S., & Unützer, J. (2013). Grand challenges: Integrating mental health services into priority health care platforms. *PLoS Medicine, 10*(5), e1001448. doi:10.1371/journal.pmed.1001448

Patterson, S. E., Milloy, M. J., Ogilvie, G., Greene, S., Nicholson, V., Vonn, M., . . . Kaida, A. (2015). The impact of criminalization of HIV non-disclosure on the healthcare engagement of women living with HIV in Canada: A comprehensive review of the evidence. *Journal of the International AIDS Society, 18*(1), 20572. doi:10.7448/IAS.18.1.20572

Paudel, V., & Baral, K. P. (2015). Women living with HIV/AIDS (WLHA), battling stigma, discrimination and denial and the role of support groups as a coping strategy: A review of literature. *Reproductive Health, 12*(1), 1–9. doi:10.1186/s12978-015-0032-9

Pellowski, J. A., & Kalichman, S. C. (2012). Recent advances (2011-2012) in technology-delivered interventions for people living with HIV. *Current HIV/AIDS Reports, 9*(4), 326–334. doi:http://dx.doi.org/10.1007/s11904-012-0133-9

Perrett, S. E., & Biley, F. C. (2013). Negotiating uncertainty: The transitional process of adapting to life with HIV. *Journal of the Association of Nurses in AIDS Care, 24*(3), 207–218. doi:http://dx.doi.org/10.1016/j.jana.2012.06.007

Portillo, C. J., Mãndez, M. R., Holzemer, W. L., Corless, I. B., Nicholas, P. K., Coleman, C., . . . Canaval, G. E. (2005). Quality of life of ethnic minority persons living with HIV/AIDS. *Journal of Multicultural Nursing & Health, 11*(1), 31–37.

Public Health England. (2015). *HIV in the UK—Situation report 2015: Incidence, prevalence and prevention*. London: Author Retrieved from https://www.gov.uk/government/uploads/system/uploads/attachment_data/file/477702/HIV_in_the_UK_2015_report.pdf

Reynolds, N. (2009). Cigarette smoking and HIV: More evidence for action. *AIDS Education & Prevention, 21*(Suppl. 1), 106–121.

Rueda, S., Park-Wyllie, L. Y., Bayoumi, A. M., Tynan, A. M., Antoniou, T. A., Rourke, S. B., & Glazier, R. H. (2006). Patient support and education for promoting adherence to highly active antiretroviral therapy for HIV/AIDS. *Cochrane Database of Systematic Reviews, 3*, CD001442.

Safren, S. A., O'Cleirigh, C., Tan, J. Y., Raminani, S. R., Reilly, L. C., Otto, M. W., & Mayer, K. H. (2009). A randomized controlled trial of cognitive behavioral therapy for adherence and depression (CBT-AD) in HIV-infected individuals. *Health Psychology*, *28*(1), 1–10.

Schnall, R., Mosley, J. P., Iribarren, S. J., Bakken, S., Carballo-Dieguez, A., & Brown Iii, W. (2015). Comparison of a user-centered design, self-management app to existing mHealth apps for persons living with HIV. *JMIR mHealth and uHealth*, *3*(3), e91. doi:10.2196/mhealth.4882

Seeley, J., Watts, C. H., Kippax, S., Russell, S., Heise, L., & Whiteside, A. (2012). Addressing the structural drivers of HIV: A luxury or necessity for programmes? *Journal of the International AIDS Society*, *15*(Suppl. 1), 17397. doi:10.7448/IAS.15.3.17397

Sherr, L., Clucas, C., Harding, R., Sibley, E., & Catalan, J. (2011). HIV and depression: A systematic review of interventions. *Psychology, Health & Medicine*, *16*(5), 493–527. doi:10.1080/13548506.2011.579990

Sherr, L., Nagra, N., Kulubya, G., Catalan, J., Clucas, C., & Harding, R. (2011). HIV infection associated post-traumatic stress disorder and post-traumatic growth—a systematic review. *Psychology, Health & Medicine*, *16*(5), 612–629.

Siegal, K., & Lekas, H. (2002). AIDS as a chronic illness: Psychosocial implications. *AIDS*, *16*, S69–S76.

Simoni, J. M., Pantalone, D. W., Plummer, M. D., & Huang, B. (2007). A randomized controlled trial of a peer support intervention targeting antiretroviral medication adherence and depressive symptomatology in HIV-positive men and women. *Health Psychology*, *26*(4), 488–495. doi:10.1037/0278-6133.26.4.488

Solomon, P., O'Brien, K., Wilkins, S., & Gervais, N. (2014). Aging with HIV and disability: The role of uncertainty. *AIDS Care*, *26*(2), 240–245. doi:10.1080/09540121.2013.811209

Spies, G., Asmal, L., & Seedat, S. (2013). Cognitive-behavioural interventions for mood and anxiety disorders in HIV: A systematic review. *Journal of Affective Disorders*, *150*(2), 171–180.

Stangl, A. L., Lloyd, J. K., Brady, L. M., Holland, C. E., & Baral, S. (2013). A systematic review of interventions to reduce HIV-related stigma and discrimination from 2002 to 2013: How far have we come? *Journal of the International AIDS Society*, *16*(3 Suppl. 2), 18734. doi:10.7448/IAS.16.3.18734

Steward, W. T., Chandy, S., Singh, G., Panicker, S. T., Osmand, T. A., Heylen, E., & Ekstrand, M. L. (2011). Depression is not an inevitable outcome of disclosure avoidance: HIV stigma and mental health in a cohort of HIV-infected individuals from Southern India. *Psychology, Health & Medicine*, *16*(1), 74–85. doi:10.1080/13548506.2010.521568

Swendeman, D., Ingram, B. L., & Rotheram-Borus, M. J. (2009). Common elements in self-management of HIV and other chronic illnesses: An integrative framework. *AIDS Care*, *21*(10), 1321–1334. doi:10.1080/09540120902803158

Tang, A. M., Quick, T., Chung, M., & Wanke, C. A. (2015). Nutrition assessment, counseling, and support interventions to improve health-related outcomes in people living with HIV/AIDS: A systematic review of the literature. *JAIDS: Journal of Acquired Immune Deficiency Syndromes*, *68*, S340–S349. doi:10.1097/qai.0000000000000521

Turan, B., Smith, W., Cohen, M. H., Wilson, T. E., Adimora, A. A., Merenstein, D., . . . Turan, J. M. (2016). Mechanisms for the negative effects of internalized hiv-related stigma on art adherence in women: The mediating roles of social isolation and depression. *JAIDS: Journal of Acquired Immune Deficiency Syndromes*, *72*(2), 198–205.

UNAIDS. (2015). Factsheet: 2014 statistics. Geneva: UNAIDS. Retrieved from http://www.unaids.org/sites/default/files/media_asset/20150714_FS_MDG6_Report_en.pdf

UNAIDS. (2016). Global AIDS update. Geneva: World Health Organization. Retrieved from http://www.who.int/hiv/pub/arv/global-AIDS-update-2016_en.pdf?ua=1.

Voss, J. G., Dodd, M., Portillo, C., & Holzemer, W. (2006). Theories of fatigue: Application in HIV/AIDS. *Journal of the Association of Nurses in AIDS Care, 17*(1), 37–50. doi:http://dx.doi.org/10.1016/j.jana.2005.11.004

Vreeman, R. C., Gramelspacher, A. M., Gisore, P. O., Scanlon, M. L., & Nyandiko, W. M. (2013). Disclosure of HIV status to children in resource-limited settings: A systematic review. *Journal of the International AIDS Society, 16*, 18466.

Webel, A. R., Sattar, A., Schreiner, N., Kinley, B., Moore, S. M., & Salata, R. A. (2016). The impact of mental wellness on HIV self-management. *Journal of the Association of Nurses in AIDS Care, 27*(4), 468–475.

World Health Organization. (2003). *Nutrient requirements for people living with HIV/AIDS. Report of a technical consultation*. Geneva: Author.

World Health Organization. (2015). Guideline on when to start antiretroviral therapy and on pre-exposure prophylaxis for HIV. Geneva: Author. Retrieved from http://www.who.int/hiv/pub/guidelines/earlyrelease-arv/en/

16

Self-Management of Multiple Sclerosis

MALACHY BISHOP AND MICHAEL FRAIN ■

Self-management is a key strategy for improving the physical and psychological health and quality of life of individuals living with chronic health conditions (Bycroft & Tracey, 2006; Lorig & Holman, 2003; Osborne, Elsworth, & Whitfield, 2007). There is no universally accepted definition of self-management, and, in fact, there is a great deal of diversity in the components and program foci in the self-management literature (Barlow, Wright, Sheasby, Turner, & Hainsworth, 2002). Self-management is defined as a multidimensional construct, with the central or unifying philosophy being that the responsibility for day-to-day health and symptom management lies with the person, rather than medical providers (Lorig & Holman, 2003).

Lorig and Holman (2003) described self-management tasks as falling into three categories, including medical management, which incorporates such tasks as understanding and effectively using medication, following a diet or exercise program, and monitoring and managing medical aspects of one's health; role management, including, for example, managing the changes associated with domestic, social, and vocational role changes and maintaining, developing, or modifying social and familial relationships; and emotional management, including coping with the emotional changes associated with living with a chronic condition. In this model, six core self-management skills facilitate the accomplishment of self-management tasks, including problem-solving, decision-making, taking action, using resources, communicating with healthcare providers, and self-tailoring (Lorig & Holman, 2003). Battersby and colleagues, in the Flinders model, proposed a set of key principles of self-management: (a) to know and understand one's condition; (b) to monitor and manage signs and symptoms of one's condition; (c) to actively share in decision-making with health professionals; (d) to adopt lifestyles that promote health; (e) to manage the impact of the condition on one's physical, emotional, and social life; and (f) to follow a treatment plan (care plan) agreed on with one's healthcare providers (Flinders Human Behavior and Health Research Unit, 2006).

Self-management is an important component of person-centered multiple sclerosis (MS) care (Bishop & Frain, 2011; Fraser et al., 2013). Although it has been observed that, relative to other chronic health conditions, self-management has received less attention in the MS literature (Bishop & Frain, 2011; Devins & Shnek, 2000; Rae-Grant et al., 2011), a notable increase in research and self-management program development has occurred over the past several years.

Self-management of MS involves a complex, individual, and ongoing process. For people with MS, self-management includes the elements of the general self-management frameworks described previously, as well as MS-specific considerations that are unique to the experience of living with the disease. Generally, MS self-management, as for other chronic conditions, involves learning specific skills and applying those skills to accomplish certain tasks (Lorig & Holman, 2003). More specifically, MS self-management may involve such tasks as learning about and staying knowledgeable about the disease, its symptoms, and its treatments; monitoring health status; making healthy lifestyle choices with respect to nutrition, exercise, and self-care; maintaining psychological health; establishing and maintaining effective and supportive social networks; managing changing personal, familial, vocational and community participation roles; managing healthcare relationships and coordinating multiple healthcare services; managing fatigue, pain, and changes in cognitive functioning; and generally coping with living with MS (Bishop & Frain, 2011; Ghahari, Khoshbin, & Forwell, 2014).

In this chapter, we first provide an overview of MS and the experiences frequently encountered by people living with and managing this complex chronic condition. We then review the knowledge that people with MS want about managing their condition, present research on the emotional impact of MS, and describe evidence-based research on interventions that have been associated with improved health outcomes and coping. We conclude the chapter by describing frequently experienced barriers to self-management of MS and techniques and strategies that facilitate self-management

MS OVERVIEW

MS is a chronic demyelinating condition of the central nervous system (CNS), currently thought to be mediated by the immune system, characterized by intermittent and recurrent episodes of inflammation that result in damage to CNS myelin and underlying gray matter (Lee & Dunn, 2013; van den Elsen et al., 2014). The demyelination causes disruption and slowing in the conduction of electrical impulses, which can affect physical, sensory, mental, and emotional activity (Schapiro, 2003). CNS damage accrues as patches of myelin deteriorate and are replaced by hardened scar tissue, further interrupting the conduction of nerve impulses (DeLuca & Nocentini, 2011). Although MS has historically been viewed as affecting only CNS white matter, recent advances in MRI technology have enabled recognition that damage to the underlying gray matter is common, especially in progressive MS (Hulst & Geurts, 2011; Multiple Sclerosis Coalition, 2014). There is also evidence that MS has a neurodegenerative component, in that neuronal and axonal loss occurs outside the periods of acute inflammation (van den Elsen et al., 2014).

MS is one of the most common neurological diseases in the world, affecting an estimated 2.5 million people, and is the most common non-traumatic disabling neurologic disorder of young adults (van den Elsen et al., 2014). Although MS may be diagnosed at any age, diagnosis is typically made between the ages of 20 and 50 (Kalb, 2012; Schapiro, 2003). The prevalence of MS among females is approximately three times that among males, and there is evidence that this ratio may be increasing (Dunn & Steinman, 2013; National Multiple Sclerosis Society [NMSS], 2014b). Although MS occurs most frequently among Caucasians in Western Europe and North America, it is seen in most ethnic groups (DeLuca & Nocentini, 2011; NMSS, 2014b). Countries that have particularly high rates of MS include the United Kingdom, Canada, Germany, Denmark, Norway, Sweden, Finland, and the United States (Smith & Schapiro, 2004). MS is much less prevalent in Asia and in tropical and subtropical regions (DeLuca & Nocentini, 2011).

The cause of MS is currently thought to be multifactorial and includes both genetic and environmental factors (Mandia et al., 2014; van den Elsen et al., 2014). Genetic factors appear to have a significant role in the development of MS (NMSS, 2014a), but research also suggests that environmental factors may trigger the autoimmune response in genetically susceptible individuals and influence the evolution of symptoms (Mandia et al., 2014). Among the various environmental risk factors that have been proposed those that have received strong supporting evidence include infection with Epstein-Barr virus, ultraviolet light exposure, vitamin D status, and cigarette smoking (NMSS, 2016c; Wingerchuk, 2011).

The Clinical Courses of MS

Currently, MS is associated with three different courses, including (a) relapsing-remitting MS, (b) primary-progressive MS, and (c) secondary progressive MS. The previously identified course, progressive-relapsing MS, is no longer used in the classification of MS courses. The clinical classification of the courses of MS was recently updated by the International Advisory Committee on Clinical Trials in MS (Lublin et al., 2014). Important changes were made, including the addition of the Clinically Isolated Syndrome (CIS), and the elimination of the identification of a progressive relapsing course of MS. According to the National Multiple Sclerosis Society (2016a), CIS refers to an initial episode of neurologic symptoms, lasting at least 24 hours, caused by CNS inflammation or demyelination. The CIS episode is typically followed by a complete or partial recovery. Individuals who experience CIS may or may not develop MS (NMSS, 2016a).

Relapsing-remitting MS is the initial diagnosis for approximately 85% of people with MS and is characterized by clearly defined flare-ups (i.e., relapses, exacerbations, or attacks) that may last from days to weeks, with or without asymptomatic periods, and that are followed by partial or complete recovery periods, or remissions, during which no disease progression occurs (Lublin et al., 2014; NMSS, 2016a).

The majority of people initially diagnosed with relapsing-remitting MS eventually transition to the secondary progressive course. This course is characterized by a steady progressive course associated with worsening of neurological functioning and accumulation of disability over time (NMSS, 2016b). Primary-progressive MS is diagnosed among approximately 15% of people with MS and is characterized by a slow decline in neurologic function from the onset, with a variable rate of progression and without distinct relapses or remissions but with occasional periods of stability and temporary minor improvements (Lublin et al., 2014; NMSS, 2016b).

Symptoms and Typical Functional Limitations Associated with MS

The symptoms associated with MS vary widely depending upon the location and size of the CNS lesions, resulting in significant interindividual variability in symptom presentation (Bishop, Rumrill, & Timblin, 2016). For example, whereas frontal and parietal lobe lesions often result in cognitive and emotional effects, lesions in the cerebrum, brain stem, and spinal cord may affect physical functioning of the extremities (Fraser, Clemmons, & Bennett, 2002). Visual impairments may result from damage to the optic nerves or the occipital lobe. The most frequently reported symptoms of MS include fatigue (which affects approximately 90% of people with MS; MS Coalition, 2014), balance and coordination problems, bladder and bowel dysfunction, vision problems, dizziness and vertigo, sexual dysfunction, hypersensitivity to heat, pain, cognitive dysfunction, emotional changes, depression, and spasticity (Antao et al., 2013).

Most people with MS eventually experience mobility limitations. Within 10 to 15 years of onset, approximately 80% of individuals with MS develop gait problems due to muscle weakness, spasticity, fatigue, and balance impairments; approximately 50% use an assistive walking device within 15 years of diagnosis and 83% within 30 years (Munschauer & Weinstock-Guttman, 2005; Souza et al., 2010).

In recent years, there has been increased awareness of and attention to the issues of cognitive functioning, energy and fatigue, and mood among individuals living with MS. Current estimates of the prevalence of cognitive impairment range from 43% to 70% (Chiaravalloti & DeLuca, 2008). Cognitive impairment is most frequently seen in the areas of information-processing speed and efficiency, long-term memory retrieval, complex attention, executive functioning, and visual perceptual skills (Chiaravalloti & DeLuca, 2008; Pakenham, 2012). Simple attention and verbal skills are usually not affected (DeLuca and Nocentini, 2011). The severity and type of cognitive impairment vary significantly between individuals and are not strongly correlated with the degree of physical involvement (DeLuca & Nocentini, 2011). Approximately 20% to 30% of people with MS have already experienced cognitive changes before they have their first exacerbation, and some research suggests that cognitive deficits may precede the onset of MS by more than a year (MS Coalition, 2014). Those who present with cognitive impairments early in the course of the disease appear to be at greater risk for decline over time (DeLuca & Nocentini, 2011).

In addition to the primary symptoms associated with MS, people with MS appear to experience relatively higher rates of certain co-occurring and secondary conditions. These conditions include depression, anxiety, hypertension, hypercholesterolemia, chronic lung disease, thyroid disease, and psoriasis (Marrie et al., 2015).

Treatment of MS

Current treatments in MS are aimed at modifying the MS course, managing relapses, and managing ongoing symptoms. Symptom management is addressed with various symptom-specific medications and treatments. Currently, disease-modifying therapies (DMTs) form the basis of treatment for relapsing-remitting and secondary-progressive MS (Pakenham, 2012). These medications have been shown in clinical trials to reduce the number and severity of attacks, reduce disease activity, and delay the onset of disability (Johnson et al., 2006). There are currently 16 US Food and Drug Administration–approved DMTs, including seven injectable medications, three oral medications, and three infused medications (MS Coalition, 2014).

In order to achieve the maximum benefit from DMTs, individuals with MS must follow the prescribed treatment plan and continue treatment throughout their lives (Munschauer & Weinstock-Guttman, 2005). Research suggests that only 50% of Americans with MS, and 60% of those with relapsing-remitting MS, are using DMTs, and many people who initiate therapy discontinue after a brief duration (Johnson et al., 2006). Barriers to maintaining DMT treatment have been associated with the requirement for self-injection, self-injection anxiety, and injection-site reactions. The recent introduction of oral forms of DMTs will help to eliminate these barriers for many, but other barriers have also been identified, including lack of understanding about the purpose and action of DMT, concerns about the cost-effectiveness of treatment, lack of visible improvement in functional status, low treatment self-efficacy, and cognitive or physical impairment (Johnson et al., 2006; Munschauer & Weinstock-Guttman, 2005).

KNOWLEDGE ABOUT MS THAT AN INDIVIDUAL NEEDS FOR SELF-MANAGEMENT

Given the range of ways that MS may affect physical, cognitive, and psychosocial functioning, self-management in MS may require a broad range of knowledge and resources. There are a number of approaches that may be taken to identifying the knowledge, skills, tasks, and activities necessary for MS self-management. One approach is to explore the perspectives and needs of people with MS. Another is to examine the research literature and explore the various ways in which MS self-management outcomes have been defined. We briefly examine each of these perspectives next. We then describe and present a summary of the results of an analysis by the NMSS that directly addressed the knowledge people with MS need for wellness and effective MS management.

The Perspectives of People with MS

Seeking and incorporating the perspectives of people living with MS is a critical component in the development of valid, responsive, and effective MS self-management programs and interventions. Actively incorporating the perspectives of people with MS was one of the key recommendations emerging from a recent international, multidisciplinary consensus conference on self-management for people with MS (Fraser et al., 2013). Specific recommendations from the conference included using participatory action research to guide intervention development and research design, reviewing the existing literature on the qualitative life experience of those with MS, conducting focus groups to determine appropriate self-management techniques and delivery methods specific to the MS population, and investigating the roles of significant others and caregivers in the success of MS self-management interventions (Fraser et al., 2013).

Although there is little evidence of the broad adoption of these recommendations to date, recently researchers have increasingly sought the perspectives of people with MS about the most effective approaches to self-management (e.g., Ghahari et al., 2014; Knaster, Yorkston, Johnson, McMullen, & Ehde, 2011; Mulligan, Wilkinson, & Snowdon, 2016; Ploughman et al., 2012). For example, Knaster and colleagues conducted focus-group research specifically exploring the perspectives of adults with MS on self-management support. Participants described the need for self-management support that recognizes the uniquely individual experience of living with MS and the complex set of symptoms they manage, and programs and information that are motivating and that provide learning resources for use during and after the intervention. Ideally, such active explorations of the perspectives of those living with MS will continue and increase in the development of future self-management programs.

Perspectives Based on the Existing Research

In order to identify the knowledge needed for effective self-management of MS, it is also important to consider the ways that MS self-management has been operationalized in the research. MS self-management research outcomes have generally been defined and measured either in terms of broad outcomes, including primarily self-efficacy, well-being, and quality of life, or in terms of the more specific elements of self-management under focus in a particular study. Examples of specific dimensions of self-management frequently included in the MS research include fatigue management and energy conservation (Finlayson, 2005; Finlayson & Holberg, 2007; Ghahari, Leigh Packer, & Passmore, 2010; Sauter, Zebenholzer, Hisakawa, Zeitlhofer, & Vass, 2008), exercise (McAuley et al., 2007; Plow, Mathiowetz, & Resnik, 2008; Turner, Kivlahan, & Haselkorn, 2009), health-promoting behavior participation (Ennis, Thain, Boggild, Baker, & Young, 2006), medication self-management (Carder, Vuckovic, & Green, 2003; Turner, Williams, Sloan, & Haselkorn, 2009), and relationships with healthcare providers (Heesen, Köpke, Richter, & Kasper, 2007).

The Multiple Sclerosis Self-Management Scale was developed to provide a comprehensive and psychometrically sound assessment of self-management knowledge and behavior among adults with MS and is currently the only MS-specific self-management scale (Bishop & Frain, 2011). The scale was initially developed in 2007 based on a comprehensive review of the self-management literature and existing self-management instruments, to identify common elements typically included in self-management definitions and measures, and consultation with healthcare professionals (Bishop & Frain, 2007) and was revised in 2011. We discuss it here because the factors included in the scale inform the consideration of the knowledge involved or required in MS self-management. Five domains are included in the 24-item revised version, including: (a) Treatment Adherence/Barriers, which addresses attitudes toward medication and medical care, barriers to treatment maintenance, and understanding the purpose of treatments; (b) Healthcare Provider Relationship/Communication, which addresses elements of communication with healthcare providers and the degree of participation in treatment decision-making; (c) Social/Family Support, which includes feelings about self and support from family members and others; (d) MS Knowledge and Information, which addresses the individual's active information-seeking behavior; and (e) Health Maintenance Behavior, including awareness of and participation in positive health behaviors.

Knowledge People with MS Want about Managing Their Condition

In 2015, the NMSS convened a meeting during which clinicians, researchers, and people with MS identified key questions to be answered related to wellness in MS (Dunn, Bhargava, & Kalb, 2015). Based on a review of frequently identified topics and frequently asked questions in the traditional media, social media, website traffic, and calls to the NMSS's Information Resource Center, the participants identified areas of special interest to people with MS. These included (a) managing MS with diet, (b) managing MS through exercise, and (c) managing mood changes, particularly depression (Dunn et al., 2015).

The recommended strategies for promoting wellness with respect to diet, based on current understanding of the role of diet in overall health, included limiting sugar and processed foods, increasing fruit and vegetable consumption, selecting lean sources of protein and healthy fats, and ensuring adequate fiber and fluids intake. The participants also emphasized that people with MS should be provided unbiased information about popular "MS diets," in order to promote educated and informed decision-making. Finally, the participants emphasized the importance of reducing obesity, as obesity may be associated with an increased risk for MS and for other health conditions that can affect the impact of MS (Dunn et al., 2015).

With respect to physical exercise and activity, the symptoms of MS frequently lead to physical inactivity and a sedentary lifestyle, and people with MS have consistently been found to be less physically active than individuals without MS (e.g., Motl et al, 2011; Plow et al. 2012). As a consequence, there has recently been an increased focus on wellness and health promotion both among people with MS and among health professionals (Dunn, Bhargava, & Kalb, 2015), along with a growing recognition that physical activity has a variety of health and psychosocial benefits for individuals with MS. Recommendations concerning exercise emerging from the NMSS meeting included providing clear recommendations about the positive impact of exercise on overall health, MS symptoms, and quality of life and partnering with community organizations to provide exercise programs for people with MS (Dunn et al., 2015). It should be noted that people with MS have been found to experience a wide range of personal, social, and environmental barriers to physical activity and health promotion (e.g., Hebert, Corboy, Manago, & Schenkman, 2011; Morrison & Stuifbergen, 2014; Rietberg, Brooks, Uitdehaag, & Kwakkel, 2004). As a result, it is critical to identify and address individually specific barriers and to work with the individual to identify solutions that will be effective.

Finally, with respect to emotional self-management, recommendations from the NMSS meeting included developing strategies and tools to increase conversations with healthcare providers about the emotional effects of MS, beginning at the time of diagnosis. Potential strategies included developing and providing informational tips and tools to identify and talk with providers about mood changes and identifying proactive strategies to promote emotional health and prevent significant mood disruption, particularly with those newly diagnosed with MS (Dunn et al., 2015).

RESEARCH ON THE EMOTIONAL IMPACT OF MS

People with MS may face a constellation of medical and psychological symptoms, social and psychosocial barriers, and strained family relationships that can increase as the condition progresses, as well as an unpredictable and varied progression of symptoms that make uncertainty and perceived loss of control hallmark characteristics of MS (Alschuler & Beier, 2015; Frain, Bishop, Frain,

Frain, & Tansey, 2015; Rigby, Thornton, & Young, 2008). The psychological distress, fatigue, prolonged medical treatment, and interference in the performance of daily activities may affect participation across a range of roles and social relationships. The often-accompanying experience of reduced control, along with the related concept of uncertainty, has frequently been associated with such outcomes as depressed mood and hopelessness, reduced quality of life, and poor psychosocial adjustment (Bishop, Frain, Espinosa, & Stenhoff, 2009; Devins & Shnek, 2000; McNulty et al., 2004; Wineman, Schwetz, Goodkin, & Rudick, 1996; Wineman, O'Brien, Nealon, & Kaskel, 1993).

Depression and anxiety are the most frequently reported mental health problems among adults with MS (Pakenham, 2012). According to the Multiple Sclerosis Coalition (2014), between 36% and 54% of people with MS will experience a major depressive disorder. The lifetime risk for anxiety disorders, such as panic disorder, generalized anxiety disorder, and obsessive-compulsive disorder, is approximately three times higher than the rate in the general population (DeLuca & Nocentini, 2011). Self-management interventions that appear to promote effective coping and emotional management include educational interventions addressing the impact of MS on mood and emotion, stress management techniques, education about effective therapeutic techniques and supports, and effective management of depression and anxiety.

MS can have a significant, enduring, and complex impact on the emotional life of families (Frain et al., 2015). Incomplete or inconsistent information from healthcare professionals and limited communication between family members can lead to family members being emotionally unprepared for relapse or deterioration. Relationships within the family may undergo substantial changes as the individual with MS responds to the diagnosis and living with the condition. Adaptive changes in the beliefs, values, activities, and outlook of the family member with MS can affect previously established relationships and significantly alter modes of relating with family members (Bowen, MacLehose, & Beaumont, 2011). As the MS progresses, family members have been found to be at high risk for stress resulting from role changes, and this may be particularly true for partners who may take on the added role of caregiver (Bowen et al., 2011).

A variety of self-management intervention strategies may promote the maintenance of existing family roles and help family members adapt to ongoing role changes. These strategies are generally aimed at developing effective communication strategies, teaching effective decision-making and problem-solving skills, developing social support, promoting effective coping strategies, and providing education about the impact of MS on sexuality and intimacy. Family members and caregivers may also have to cope with role changes associated with living with a family member with MS. The importance of addressing the emotional impact of MS on family members and significant others, in addition to the individual with MS, has been identified as an important focus (Fraser et al., 2013).

EVIDENCE-BASED RESEARCH ON INTERVENTIONS THAT IMPROVE HEALTH OUTCOMES

In this section, we review the literature concerning evidence-based self-management interventions related to health outcomes. Unfortunately, as is evident throughout this section, self-management research in MS is still a developing research focus, and the quantity of evidence that can contribute to decisions about the evidence for self-management interventions is very limited relative to other prevalent chronic conditions (Fraser, Johnson, Ehde, & Bishop, 2009). Although the research base is rapidly expanding, there are as yet relatively few meta-analyses or systematic review studies specific to self-management interventions to draw from. In addition to the limited quantity, this issue is compounded by the diversity and heterogeneity of the MS self-management research, as well as methodological limitations in the existing research. Two recent systematic reviews of the MS self-management research (Plow, Finlayson, & Rezac, 2011; Rae-Grant et al., 2011) are reviewed in this section, and both demonstrate the limitations of the current evidence base.

In their 2011 review of MS self-management interventions, Plow et al. (2011) comprehensively searched research on MS self-management interventions between 1980 and 2008. Exclusion of case studies, single-case design studies, and studies providing inadequate description of the intervention resulted in 27 self-management interventions being identified from 34 articles. The interventions were classified using the Lorig and Holman self-management framework. This comprehensive and methodical approach provides a useful perspective on the types of interventions that have been defined as MS self-management interventions, as opposed, for example, to "traditional clinical patient education interventions" (p. 254). Self-management tasks were classified in terms of three categories (medical management, role management, and emotional management) and six core self-management skills that facilitate the accomplishment of self-management tasks (problem-solving, decision-making, using resources, communicating with healthcare providers, taking action, and self-tailoring; Lorig & Holman, 2003, cited in Plow et al., 2011).

Many of the studies reviewed incorporated multiple self-management interventions. The most frequently evaluated interventions were fatigue management ($n = 12$); coping, depression, and stress management ($n = 10$); and medication management ($n = 6$). Also included were topics such as symptom management, nutrition, intimacy, sexuality, marital communication, and cognitive impairment. The medical management tasks generally focused on managing MS-related symptoms. The emotional-management tasks were primarily aimed at addressing depression, reducing stress, and improving coping skills through the use of cognitive and behavioral techniques. The role-management tasks generally focused on increasing effectiveness in communicating health needs.

In terms of the self-management tasks, all 27 interventions provided the opportunity to develop decision-making skills, skills related to taking action, and skills related to self-tailoring information. The majority of interventions ($n = 23$) also taught problem-solving skills, generally related to managing fatigue, coping with depression, or alleviating cognitive impairments.

The most commonly used delivery formats were group or individual face-to-face, in-person contacts. The length of interventions ranged from two weeks to one year, and the total duration of intervention contacts ranged from 4 to 24 hours. Health professionals who delivered the interventions were primarily occupational therapists, nurses, and psychologists (Plow et al., 2011). The most commonly reported outcomes were quality of life and fatigue. In all the studies, positive effects were reported for the intervention between groups or over time; however, only 13 self-management interventions were evaluated using a randomized controlled trial (RCT), and 6 of the 13 used a control group but did not randomize the participants.

Rae-Grant et al. (2011) conducted a comprehensive systematic review of self-management literature in neurological disorders published between 1990 and 2009. Over 500 articles were evaluated in terms of the intervention implementation methods, outcomes measures, and intervention outcomes. Articles were included for review based on reporting a self-management intervention in neurological disorders. Single-case reports, commentaries, editorials, and articles that focused exclusively on caregivers were excluded.

Out of the more than 500 studies reviewed by Rae-Grant et al. (2011), only 23 focused on self-management in MS or, in one case, MS and other conditions. Self-management interventions that were associated with positive outcomes for individuals with MS were generally group-based interventions that focused on providing education and information and that lasted for several weeks. Successful programs included both professional- and lay-led group interventions. The interventions and formats included self-managed exercise programs, motivational interviewing and goal-setting exercises with phone-based follow-up, group and individual self-management sessions, Internet-based self-management strategies, telephone prompting strategies, lay-led self-management programs, and self-managed wellness programs (Rae-Grant et al., 2011). Targets for intervention identified as "promising" included diet, exercise, medication maintenance, smoking cessation, reducing alcohol use, and ongoing management of fatigue, stress, pain, mood, and cognitive issues (Rae-Grant et al., 2011, p. 1096).

The Rae-Grant et al. (2011) review highlighted two important limitations of the current MS self-management research. First, the review demonstrated the limited extent to which MS self-management research has provided evidence-based support for self-management interventions. According to the Institute of Medicine (2001), "evidence-based practice is the integration of best research evidence with clinical expertise and patient values" (p. 147). "Best research evidence" is generally defined as evidence from experimental studies that include randomization, as RCTs are regarded as having the highest level of internal validity and are least subject to bias (Prendergast, 2011). Only 8 of the 23 MS self-management studies in the 19-year period of the Rae-Grant et al. review used a RCT design. The majority of the studies were characterized by a range of methodologies (e.g., focus groups, workshops, surveys, Delphi studies) that may provide preliminary data or describe potentially useful models but that do not provide the level of evidence necessary to support implementation or use of a specific intervention.

Second, the review demonstrates the diversity of self-management interventions and outcomes. Both Rae-Grant et al. (2011) and Plow et al. (2011) noted the wide variation in self-management interventions and outcomes and suggested that this variety, along with the relatively limited number of published studies, makes it difficult to compare the efficacy of different self-management strategies.

COPING STRATEGIES OR SKILLS TAUGHT IN MS SELF-MANAGEMENT

In this section, we review specific strategies and skills that are taught or developed in MS self-management. MS self-management has been found to be associated with a wide range of coping-related outcomes, for example, improved coping with MS symptoms (Shevil & Finlayson, 2009); enhanced decision-making autonomy (Kopke, Kasper, Muhlhauser, Nubling, & Heesen, 2009); increased medication self-maintenance (Berger, Liang, Hudmon, 2005); increased health-promoting behaviors (Bombardier et al., 2008; Ennis, Thain, Boggild, Baker, & Young, 2006); increased perceived control over both illness and non-illness aspects of life (Bishop et al., 2008; Devins & Shnek, 2000); reduced fatigue (Finlayson, 2005; Navipour et al., 2006); reduced depression (Mohr et al., 2000, 2005); increased ability to manage cognitive changes (Shevil & Finlayson, 2009); and reduced psychosocial role limitations (Schwartz, 1999). Thus, many of the interventions or skills described in this section are directly or indirectly related to improving coping. In this section, we focus our discussion particularly on interventions related to stress-management and fatigue-management interventions.

Stress-Management Interventions

Reynard, Sullivan, and Rae-Grant (2014) conducted a systematic analysis of the literature on stress-management interventions in MS. Their search of the literature published through 2013 identified 117 publications, of which only 8 met the criteria for review. The authors noted limitations in both the range of interventions and outcome measures, and in the methodological quality of the studies, and suggested that these limitations made it difficult to draw broad conclusions about the efficacy of stress-management interventions for people with MS.

The most frequently evaluated stress-management interventions were cognitive-behavioral techniques, including self-monitoring of daily stress, cognitive restructuring, and the development of problem-solving skills. The majority of studies included some form of relaxation training, and most were delivered over several weeks. For example, Artemiadis et al. (2012) conducted an eight-week relaxation training for participants with relapsing-remitting MS, administered via a guided audio CD of relaxation breathing and progressive muscle relaxation. Ghahari et al. (2009) evaluated the effects of daily progressive muscle relaxation, completed at home using an instructional audio CD. Hughes et al. (2006) evaluated a six-week group stress self-management intervention for women that incorporated psychoeducation on stress management, time-management strategies, pain-management strategies, relaxation training, social support, relationship issues, and physical self-care. Crawford and McIvor (1987) conducted a 13-week group program of relaxation and cognitive-behavioral stress-management techniques for hospitalized patients with MS. The measured outcomes primarily included quality of life, anxiety, and depression, and in each case, differences were found in favor of the intervention group.

Fatigue Management

Fatigue is one of the most frequently reported symptoms of MS, affecting approximately 90% of people with MS (MS Coalition, 2014). Fatigue is one of the most frequently reported reasons for loss of employment among people with MS (Schiavolin et al., 2013) and can significantly impact a person's ability to function and participate fully in the home and community. With growing awareness of the potential psychosocial impact of MS-related fatigue, fatigue is increasingly becoming a focus in MS self-management research.

In their meta-analysis Cochrane review of exercise therapy for fatigue in self-management, Heine, van de Port, Rietberg, van Wegen, and Kwakkel (2015) evaluated 45 trials (36 of which were included in the meta-analysis), including 69 exercise interventions. The exercise interventions included endurance training, muscle power training, task-oriented training, mixed training, and "other" interventions, including, for example, yoga. These authors found a significant effect on fatigue in favor of exercise therapy and concluded that exercise therapy for fatigue can be used by people with MS without harm. In particular, endurance, mixed, or "other" training may reduce self-reported fatigue, but the authors noted important methodological limitations in the studies in this area of research.

In a recent systematic review of occupational therapy-related interventions for people with MS, Yu and Mathiowetz (2014) reviewed face-to-face and distance-delivered fatigue management courses. They reported that there was strong evidence from high-quality studies supporting face-to-face fatigue management programs, specifically identifying studies (e.g., Mathiowetz, Finlayson, Matuska, Chen, & Luo, 2005; Sauter et al., 2008) that used the Managing Fatigue program (Packer, Brink, & Sauriol, 1995) and the Fatigue: Take Control course (Hugos et al., 2010). There was limited evidence from high-quality studies supporting the use of the Managing Fatigue course delivered in a long-distance teleconference format (Finlayson, 2005; Finlayson & Holberg, 2007). Yu and Mathiowetz concluded from the research that people with MS may benefit from participation in face-to-face courses in terms of improved fatigue impact, self-efficacy, and quality of life and from participation in long-distance courses in terms of improved fatigue impact and quality of life.

BARRIERS TO SELF-MANAGEMENT

Although there has been relatively limited research specific to MS self-management barriers, people with MS, like people with other chronic conditions, may face a wide range of personal, condition-related, social, and environmental barriers. Barriers reported in the broader chronic health condition literature include such factors as inadequate social or family support, difficulties with time management, emotional issues, low self-efficacy, conflicting health beliefs, physical barriers and limitations, lack of knowledge or understanding about one's health condition and the presence of co-occurring conditions (Bayliss, Ellis, & Steiner, 2007). Personal barriers associated with MS may include psychological barriers, such as low self-efficacy beliefs, low expectations for success; and health literacy barriers, related to education level, literacy, or language learning, that make it difficult to obtain and understand and use self-management information.

MS-related barriers may result from the symptoms of MS, including depression, which has been associated with reduced capacity for self-management (Garcia de Alba Garcia et al., 2006), pain and fatigue (Fraser et al., 2013), and the variable and fluctuating nature of symptoms and functional limitations in MS. When no MS symptoms are present, it is easy to forget or move away from stringent or challenging diet plans or exercise regimens (Hancock, Bruce, & Lynch, 2011).

Economic barriers also present a significant barrier for many with MS, as income and financial status may present a variety of access barriers, including barriers to healthcare and transportation. Wilski, Tasiemski, and Kocur (2015) examined the demographic, socioeconomic, and clinical correlates of self-management in MS and found that lower self-management participation was associated with low level of received social support, low socioeconomic resources, and receiving low monthly income.

People with MS generally require comprehensive, life-long healthcare and health management to support and maintain their health, function, and well-being. However, many people with MS also face significant barriers to accessing healthcare, related to barriers to physical access, transportation, economic situation, rural residence, and insurance limitations.

In their US population-based analysis among adults with MS, Minden et al. (2007) found that although the majority of people with MS have healthcare insurance, even among the insured 17.5% of participants reported that their plans did not cover prescription medication, 10.5% had difficulty obtaining prescription medication, 4.1% had obstacles accessing medical care, and 2.4% could not obtain mental health services. Additionally, MS is associated with a high rate of co-occurring health conditions. In a recent analysis of 8,983 individuals with MS, about 77.1% had one or more co-occurring physical and mental conditions, such as hyperlipidemia, hypertension, depression, and anxiety (Marrie & Hanwell,

2013). Self-management of the medical aspects of living with MS promotes taking actions that maintain and enhance physical health and function and prevent the onset of secondary or co-occurring conditions, reducing the need for and cost of medical care, and ameliorating or reducing the extent of healthcare barriers.

TECHNIQUES TO FACILITATE SELF-MANAGEMENT

The self-management information needs of people with MS, and the best means of providing this information, have been the focus of considerable research attention. Access to information about such topics as diagnosis, prognosis, treatment, clinical trials, healthy living, employment rights and protections, and self-care is critical to facilitating effective self-management. Access to self-management information has been associated with enhanced sense of personal control and more informed communication with healthcare professionals and others (Bishop et al., 2009; Marrie, Salter, Tyry, Fox, & Cutter, 2013). In this section, therefore, we focus on effective techniques and methods for delivering self-management information.

Information and Self-Management

Because the course and symptoms of MS are highly variable, the information needs of people with MS may vary widely. Further, different people prefer to receive information from different sources and through different media (Bishop et al., 2009). Education and information resources may be provided in formats such as printed materials, educational programs, websites, social media, and in discussions with healthcare providers and other professionals. The type of information required by individuals with MS has been found to vary over its trajectory and by personal variables, such as age, ethnicity, and socioeconomic status.

In a recent Cochrane systematic review, Köpke, Solari, Khan, Heesen, and Giordano (2014) evaluated informational interventions that provided MS-specific information with the intention of improving health-related outcomes for individuals with MS, including self-management relevant outcomes. Primary outcomes considered included MS-related knowledge and measures of shared-decision making. Secondary outcomes included quality of life, measures of informed choice, psychological status measures, treatment choices, treatment implementation, satisfaction with the information received, hospital admissions and use of healthcare services, measures of activities of daily living, coping, disability, role preferences, and adverse events.

The review included 10 RCTs with a total of 1,314 participants. The information topics included DMT, relapse management, self-care strategies, fatigue management, coping, family planning, and health promotion. The interventions included decision aids, educational programs, self-care interventions, and personal interviews with physicians and the number and extent of the interventions differed between studies. In the four studies assessing MS-related knowledge, significant differences were observed between groups as a result of the interventions, suggesting that information provision may successfully increase participants' knowledge. Four studies evaluating the effects of interventions on decision-making, and five studies assessing quality of life showed mixed results. In summary, the authors concluded that the results provided some evidence that information can increase MS-related knowledge and may have a positive impact on MS-making and quality of life. Importantly, there were no apparent negative effects from providing information. The heterogeneity of the interventions and outcome measures precluded a clear recommendation for specific methods of providing information.

Telehealth and Telerehabilitation

Telehealth and telerehabilitation approaches, also referred to as telemedicine, telehealthcare, e-health, and e-medicine, involve providing healthcare, self-management, health promotion, rehabilitation, and educational programs to people distant from the provider through the use of information and communication technologies (Khan, Amatya, Kesselring, & Galea, 2015). The technology through which telehealth is delivered may include telephones, video technology, and Internet-based applications. Telehealth approaches provide learning and communication opportunities for those living in rural areas, with mobility or transportation barriers, or with other barriers to accessing face-to-face and group-based, in-person interactions. The model can be economical for both providers and users.

Several recent studies have specifically evaluated online and telehealth self-management programs (e.g., Bombadier et al., 2013; Brennan, Mawson, & Brownell, 2009; Finlayson, Preissner, Cho, & Plow, 2011; Ghahari, Leigh Packer, & Passmore, 2010; Miller et al., 2011; Moss-Morris et al., 2012), and many have evaluated online and telehealth interventions that include one or more components of self-management, such as fatigue management, coping, depression or anxiety, stress management, and medication management. The comparative effectiveness of telehealth delivery of self-management, however, is still something of an open question, and conclusions based on the existing comparative studies remain limited by considerable heterogeneity in focus, interventions, delivery approaches, and outcome measures. There are, however, several examples of well-designed studies employing RCTs and some form of telehealth delivery.

For example, Bombardier et al. (2008) conducted a prospective RCT in which the treatment group participated in a single in-person motivational interview, followed by five telephone counseling sessions over 12 weeks in order to facilitate improvement in six health promotion areas (exercise, fatigue management, communication and/or social support, anxiety and/or stress management, and reducing alcohol or other drug use). The primary outcome was the effect of the intervention on health-promotion activities. Members of the treatment group reported significantly greater improvement in physical activity, spiritual growth, stress management, fatigue impact, and mental health compared with the control group members, who remained stable.

In a recent Cochrane review of telehealth interventions, not specific to but inclusive of self-management interventions, Khan et al., (2015) reviewed nine RCTs, including a total of 469 participants. All of the included studies were classified as "low" in the methodological quality assessment. The reviewers found low-level evidence for telerehabilitation interventions in reducing short-term disability and symptoms such as fatigue and low-level evidence supporting telerehabilitation in the longer term for improved functional activities and impairments such as fatigue and pain (Khan et al., 2015). Process evaluation was limited and no data were available for cost effectiveness. There were no adverse events reported as a result of telerehabilitation interventions. The authors concluded that there currently is limited evidence on the efficacy of telerehabilitation in improving functional activities, fatigue, and quality of life in adults with MS. Importantly, they suggested that telehealth provides a range of alternative methods of delivering services but that there is insufficient evidence to support what types of telerehabilitation interventions are effective and in which setting (Khan et al., 2015). As noted by Plow et al. (2011), it remains for the efficacy and effectiveness of different delivery formats to be demonstrated, and then directly compared, in order to determine which format is most cost effective and which format is most likely to be widely disseminated.

CONCLUSION

MS is a complex and multidimensional condition that can impact one's health and functioning, role participation, and quality of life in a variety of ways. The nature of MS makes self-management both critically important and, like the condition itself, multifaceted and highly individualized. Historically, research and clinical attention to MS self-management has received less attention than is the case with more prevalent conditions; however, in recent years an active and rapidly developing focus on MS self-management has emerged. As a result, there is now a well-established, consumer-driven, and interdisciplinary drive to identify effective, research-supported self-management knowledge and practice and knowledge dissemination.

It was frequently highlighted in this chapter that MS self-management research is still a developing research focus and that the quantity and quality of the nascent evidence to inform self-management interventions remains somewhat limited. Equally clear, however, is that significant progress has been made in the development, evaluation, and translation of MS self-management knowledge and interventions. In the present, the refinement and careful evaluation of advances should include increased attention to research methodologies that promote evidence-based practice. Even more important, however, to the further development of effective and successful self-management is that the experiences and perspectives of those living with and affected MS are the primary source for information and understanding about what works, for whom, and why.

REFERENCES

Alschuler, K.N., & Beier, M.L. (2015). Intolerance of uncertainty: Shaping an agenda for research on coping with multiple sclerosis. *International Journal of MS Care, 17*, 153–158.

Antao, L., Shaw, L., Ollson, K., Reen, K., To, F., Bossus, A., & Cooper, L. (2013). Chronic pain in episodic illness and its influence on work occupations. *Work, 44*(1), 11–36.

Artemiadis, A.K., Vervainioti, A.A., Alexopoulos, E.C., Rombos, A., Anagnostouli, M.C., & Darviri, C. (2012). Stress management and multiple sclerosis: A randomized controlled trial. *Archives of Clinical Neuropsychology, 27*, 406–416.

Barlow, J., Wright, C., Sheasby, J., Turner, A., & Hainsworth, J. (2002). Self-management approaches for people with chronic conditions: A review. *Patient Education and Counseling, 48*(2), 177–187.

Bayliss, E. A., Ellis, J. L., & Steiner, J. F. (2007). Barriers to self-management and quality-of-life outcomes in seniors with multimorbidities. *Annals of Family Medicine, 5*(5), 395–402.

Berger, B.A., Liang, H., & Hudmon, K.S. (2005). Evaluation of software-based telephone counseling to enhance medication persistency among patients with multiple sclerosis. *Journal of the American Pharmacology Association, 45*, 466–472.

Bishop, M., & Frain, M. (2007). Development and initial analysis of the Multiple Sclerosis Self-Management Scale. *International Journal of Multiple Sclerosis Care, 9*, 35–42.

Bishop, M., & Frain, M. P. (2011). The Multiple Sclerosis Self-Management Scale: Revision and psychometric analysis. *Rehabilitation Psychology, 56*(2), 150–159.

Bishop, M., Frain, M. P., Espinosa, C. T., & Stenhoff, D. M. (2009). Sources of information about multiple sclerosis: Information seeking and personal, demographic, and MS variables. *Journal of Vocational Rehabilitation, 31*(2), 107–118.

Bishop, M., Frain, M., & Tschopp, M.K. (2008). Self-management, perceived control, and subjective quality of life in multiple sclerosis: An exploratory study. *Rehabilitation Counseling Bulletin, 51*(1), 45–56.

Bishop, M., Rumrill, P. D., & Timblin, R. I. (2016). Medical, psychosocial, and vocational aspects of multiple sclerosis: Implications for rehabilitation professionals. *Journal of Rehabilitation, 82*(2), 6–13.

Bombardier, C. H., Cunniffe, M., Wadhwani, R., Gibbons, L. E., Blake, K. D., & Kraft, G. H. (2008). The efficacy of telephone counseling for health promotion in people with multiple sclerosis: A randomized controlled trial. *Archives of Physical Medicine and Rehabilitation, 89*, 1849–1856.

Bombardier, C. H., Ehde, D. M., Gibbons, L. E., Wadhwani, R., Sullivan, M. D., Rosenberg, D. E. . . . Kraft, G. H. (2013). Telephone-based physical activity counseling for major depression in people with multiple sclerosis. *Journal of Consulting and Clinical Psychology, 81*(1), 89–99.

Bowen, C., MacLehose, A., & Beaumont, J.G. (2011). Advanced multiple sclerosis and the psychosocial impact on families. *Psychology and Health, 26*(1), 113–127.

Brennan, D. M., Mawson, S., & Brownsell, S. (2009). Telerehabilitation: Enabling the remote delivery of healthcare, rehabilitation, and self management. *Studies in Health Technology and Informatics, 145*, 231–248.

Bycroft, J., J., & Tracey, J. (2006). Self-management support: A win-win solution for the 21st century. *New Zealand Family Practitioner, 33*(4), 243–248.

Carder, P. C., Vuckovic, N., & Green, C. A. (2003). Negotiating medications: Patient perceptions of long-term medication use. *Journal of Clinical Pharmacy and Therapeutics, 28*(5), 409–417.

Chiaravalloti, N. D., & DeLuca, J. (2008). Cognitive impairment in multiple sclerosis. *Lancet Neurology, 7,* 1139–1151.

Crawford, J. D., & McIvor, G. P. (1987). Stress management for multiple sclerosis patients. *Psychological Reports, 61,* 423–429.

DeLuca, J., & Nocentini, U. (2011). Neurological, medical, and rehabilitative management in persons with multiple sclerosis. *NeuroRehabilitation, 29,* 197–219.

Devins, G. M., & Shnek, Z. M. (2000). Multiple sclerosis. In R. G. Frank & T. R. Elliott (Eds.), *Handbook of rehabilitation psychology* (pp. 163–184). Washington, DC: American Psychological Association.

Dunn, M., Bhargava, P., & Kalb, R. (2015). Your patients with multiple sclerosis have set wellness as a high priority-and the National Multiple Sclerosis Society is responding. *US Neurology, 11*(2), 80–86.

Dunn, S. E., & Steinman, L. (2013). The gender gap in multiple sclerosis: Intersection of science and society. *JAMA Neurology, 70*(5), 634–635.

Ennis, M., Thain, J., Boggild, M., Baker, G. A., & Young, C.A. (2006). A randomized controlled trial of a health promotion education programme for people with multiple sclerosis. *Clinical Rehabilitation, 20,* 783–792.

Finlayson, M. (2005). Pilot study of an energy conservation education program delivered by telephone conference call to people with multiple sclerosis. *NeuroRehabilitation, 20,* 267–277.

Finlayson, M., & Holberg, C. (2007). Evaluation of a teleconference-delivered energy conservation education program for people with multiple sclerosis. *Canadian Journal of Occupational Therapy, 74*(4), 337–347.

Finlayson, M., Preissner, K., Cho, C., & Plow, M. (2011). Randomized trial of a teleconference-delivered fatigue management program for people with multiple sclerosis. *Multiple Sclerosis, 17*(9), 1130–1140.

Flinders Human Behaviour & Health Research Unit. (2006). *The "Flinders Model" of chronic condition self-management.* Retrieved from: http://www.flinders.edu.au/medicine/fms/sites/FHBHRU/documents/Flinders Program Information Paper_M.pdf

Frain, M., Bishop, M., Frain, J., Frain, J., Tansey, T., & Tschopp, M. K. (2015). The family role in progressive illness. In M. Millington & I. Marini (Eds.), *Families in rehabilitation counseling: A community-based rehabilitation approach* (pp. 171–191). New York: Springer.

Fraser, R., Clemmons, D., & Bennett, F. (2002). *Multiple sclerosis: Psychosocial issues and interventions.* New York: Demos.

Fraser, R., Ehde, D., Amtmann, D., Verrall, A., Johnson, K. L., Johnson, E., & Kraft, G. H. (2013). Self-management for people with multiple sclerosis. *International Journal of MS Care, 15*(2), 99–106.

Fraser, R., Johnson, E., Ehde, D., & Bishop, M. (2009). *Patient self-management in multiple sclerosis.* Hackensack, NJ: Consortium of Multiple Sclerosis Centers.

Garcia de Alba Garcia, J. E., Dallo, F. J., Salcedo Rocha, A. L., Colunga Rodriguez, C., Perez, N., Baer, R. D., & Weller, S. C. (2006). The relative effect of self-management practices on glycaemic control in type 2 diabetic patients in Mexico. *Chronic Illness, 2,* 77–85.

Ghahari, S., Ahmadi, F., Nabavi, M., Anoshirvan, K., Memarian, R., & Rafatbakhsh, M. (2009). Effectiveness of applying progressive muscle relaxation technique on quality of life of patients with multiple sclerosis. *Journal of Clinical Nursing, 18,* 2171–2179.

Ghahari, S., Khoshbin, L. S., & Forwell, S. J. (2014). The Multiple Sclerosis Self-Management Scale: Clinicometric testing. *International Journal of MS Care, 16,* 61–67.

Ghahari, S., Packer, T. L., & Passmore, A. E. (2010). Effectiveness of an online fatigue self-management programme for people with chronic neurological conditions: A randomized controlled trial. *Clinical Rehabilitation, 24*(8), 727–744.

Ghahari, S., Packer, T. L., & Passmore, A. E. (2014). Effectiveness of an online fatigue self-management programme for people with chronic neurological conditions: A randomized controlled trial. *Clinical Rehabilitation, 24*(8), 727–744.

Hancock, L. M., Bruce, J. M., & Lynch, S. G. (2011). Exacerbation history is associated with medication and appointment adherence in MS. *Journal of Behavioral Medicine, 34*(5), 330–338.

Hebert, J. R., Corboy, J. R., Manago, M. M., & Schenkman, M. (2011). Effects of vestibular rehabilitation on multiple sclerosis-related fatigue and upright postural control: A randomized controlled trial. *Physical Therapy, 91*(8), 1166–1183.

Heesen, C., Köpke, S., Richter, T., & Kasper, J. (2007). Shared decision making and self management in multiple sclerosis—A consequence of evidence. *Journal of Neurology, 254 Suppl 2*(S2), 116–121.

Heine, M., van de Port, I., Rietberg, M. B., van Wegen, E. E. H., & Kwakkel, G. (2015). Exercise therapy for fatigue in multiple sclerosis. *Cochrane Database of Systematic Reviews, 9,* CD009956.

Hughes, R. B., Robinson-Whelen, S., Taylor, H. B., & Hall, J. W. (2006). Stress self-management: An intervention for women with physical disabilities. *Women's Health Issues, 16,* 389–399.

Hugos, C. L., Copperman, L. F., Fuller, B. E., Yadev, V., Lovera, J., & Bourdette, D. N. (2010). Clinical trial of a formal group fatigue program in multiple sclerosis. *Multiple Sclerosis, 16*(6), 724–732.

Hulst, H. E., & Geurts, J. J. (2011). Gray matter imaging in multiple sclerosis: What have we learned? *BMC Neurology, 11,* 153. http://doi.org/10.1186/1471-2377-11-153

Institute of Medicine. (2001). *Crossing the quality chasm: A new health system for the 21st Century.* Washington, DC: National Academy Press.

Johnson, K. L., Kuehn, C. M., Yorkston, K. M., Kraft, G. H., Klasner, E., & Amtmann, D. (2006). Patient perspectives on disease-modifying therapy in multiple sclerosis. *International Journal of MS Care, 8,* 11–18.

Kalb, R. (2012). *Multiple sclerosis: The questions you have, the answers you need.* New York: Demos.

Khan, F., Amatya, B., Kesselring, J., & Galea, M. (2015). Telerehabilitation for persons with multiple sclerosis. *Cochrane Database of Systematic Reviews, 4,* CD010508. doi:10.1002/14651858.CD010508.pub2

Knaster, E. S., Yorkston, K. M., Johnson, K., McMullen, K. A., & Ehde, D. M. (2011). Perspectives on self-management in multiple sclerosis: A focus group study. *International Journal of MS Care, 13,* 146–152.

Köpke, S., Kasper, J., Muhlhauser, I., Nubling, M., & Heesen, C. (2009). Patient education program to enhance decision autonomy in multiple sclerosis relapse management: A randomized-controlled trial. *Multiple Sclerosis, 15*, 96–104.

Köpke, S., Solari, A., Khan, F., Heesen, C., & Giordano, A. (2014). Information provision for people with multiple sclerosis. *Cochrane Database of Systematic Reviews, 4*, CD008757. doi:10.1002/14651858.CD008757.pub2

Lee, J.-M., & Dunn, J. (2013). Mobility concerns in multiple sclerosis: Studies and surveys on US patient populations of relevance to nurses. *US Neurology, 9*(1), 17–23.

Lorig, K. R., & Holman, H. R. (2003). Self-management education: History, definition, outcomes, and mechanisms. *Annals of Behavioral Medicine, 26*, 1–7.

Lublin, F. D., Reingold, S. C., Cohen, J. A., Cutter, G. R., Sørensen, P. S., Thompson, A. J., ... Polman, C. H. (2014). Defining the clinical course of multiple sclerosis: The 2013 revisions. *Neurology, 83*(3), 278–286.

Mandia, D., Ferraro, O. E., Nosari, G., Montomoli, C., Zardini, E., & Bergamaschi, E. (2014). Environmental factors and multiple sclerosis severity: A descriptive study. *International Journal of Environmental Research in Public Health, 11*, 6417–6432.

Marrie, R. A., Cohen, J., Stuve, O., Trojano, M., Sørensen, P. S., Reingold, S., ... Reider, N. (2015). A systematic review of the incidence and prevalence of comorbidity in multiple sclerosis. *Multiple Sclerosis Journal, 21*(3), 261–262.

Marrie, R. A., & Hanwell, H. (2013). General health issues in multiple sclerosis: Comorbidities, secondary conditions, and health behaviors. *CONTINUUM: Lifelong Learning in Neurology, 19*(4), 1046–1057.

Marrie, R. A., Salter, A. R., Tyry, T., Fox, R. J., & Cutter, G. R. (2013). Preferred sources of health information in persons with multiple sclerosis: Degree of trust and information sought. *Journal of Medical Internet Research, 15*(4), e67.

Mathiowetz, V., Finlayson, M., Matuska, K., Chen, H. Y., & Luo, P. (2005). A randomized trial of energy conservation for persons with multiple sclerosis. *Multiple Sclerosis, 11*, 592–601.

McAuley, E., Motl, R. W., Morris, K. S., Hu, L., Doerksen, S. E., Elavsky, S., & Konopack, J. F. (2007). Enhancing physical activity adherence and well-being in multiple sclerosis: A randomised controlled trial. *Multiple Sclerosis, 13*(5), 652–659.

McNulty, K., Livneh, H., & Wilson, L. M. (2004). Perceived uncertainty, spiritual well-being, and psychosocial adaptation in individuals with multiple sclerosis. *Rehabilitation Psychology, 49*(2), 91–99.

Miller, D. M., Moore, S. M., Fox, R. J., Atreja, A., Fu, A. Z., Lee, J. C., ... Rudick, R. A. (2011). Web-based self-management for patients with multiple sclerosis: A practical, randomized trial. *Telemedicine Journal and e-Health, 17*(1), 5–13.

Minden, S. L., Frankel, D., Hadden, L., & Hoaglin, D. C. (2007). Access to health care for people with multiple sclerosis. *Multiple Sclerosis, 13*(4), 547–558.

Mohr, D.C., Hart, S.L., Julian, L., Catledge, C., Honos-Webb, L., Vella, L., & Tasch, E. T. (2005). Telephone-administered psychotherapy for depression. *Archives of General Psychiatry, 62*, 1007–1014.

Mohr, D. C., Likosky, W., Bertagnolli, A., Goodkin, D. E., Van Der Wende, J., Dwyer, P., & Dick, L. P. (2000). Telephone-administered cognitive-behavioral therapy for the treatment of depressive symptoms in multiple sclerosis. *Journal of Consulting and Clinical Psychology, 68*, 356–361.

Morrison, J. D., & Stuifbergen, A. K. (2014). Outcome expectations and physical activity in persons with longstanding multiple sclerosis. *Journal of Neuroscience Nursing, 46*(3), 171–179.

Moss-Morris, R., McCrone, P., Yardley, L., Van Kessel, K., Wills, G., & Dennison, L. (2012). A pilot randomised controlled trial of an Internet-based cognitive behavioural therapy self-management programme (MS Invigor8) for multiple sclerosis fatigue. *Behaviour Research and Therapy, 50*(6), 415–421.

Motl, R. W., Dlugonski, D., Wojcicki, T. R., McAuley, E. &, Mohr, D. C. (2011). Internet intervention for increasing physical activity in persons with multiple sclerosis. *Multiple Sclerosis, 17*(1), 116–128.

Mulligan, H., Wilkinson, A., & Snowdon, J. (2016). Perceived impact of a self-management program for fatigue in multiple sclerosis: A qualitative study. *International Journal of MS Care, 18*, 27–32.

Munschauer, F. E., & Weinstock-Guttman, B. (2005). Importance of adherence to and persistence with prescribed treatments in patients with multiple sclerosis. *US Neurology Review* (July), 61–63.

National Multiple Sclerosis Society. (2014a). Genetics. Retrieved from http://www.nationalmssociety.org/For-Professionals/Clinical-Care/About-MS/Interaction-of-Genetics-and-the-Environment/Genetics

National Multiple Sclerosis Society. (2014b). Who gets MS? (Epidemiology). Retrieved from http://www.nationalmssociety.org/What-is-MS/Who-Gets-MS

National Multiple Sclerosis Society. (2016a). Relapsing-remitting MS. Retrieved from http://www.nationalmssociety.org/What-is-MS/Types-of-MS/Relapsing-remitting-MS

National Multiple Sclerosis Society. (2016b). Secondary progressive MS. Retrieved from http://www.nationalmssociety.org/What-is-MS/Types-of-MS/Secondary-progressive-MS

National Multiple Sclerosis Society. (2016c). What causes MS? Retrieved from http://www.nationalmssociety.org/What-is-MS/What-Causes-MS

Navipour, H., Madani, H., Mohebbi, M. R., Navipour, R., Roozbayani, P., & Paydar, A. (2006). Improved fatigue in individuals with multiple sclerosis after participating in a short-term self-care programme. *NeuroRehabilitation, 21*, 37–41.

Osborne, R. H., Elsworth, G. R., & Whitfield, K. (2007). The Health Education Impact Questionnaire (heiQ): An outcomes and evaluation measure for patient education and self-management interventions for people with chronic conditions. *Patient Education and Counseling, 66*, 192–201.

Packer, T. L., Brink, N., & Sauriol, A. (1995). *Managing fatigue: A six-week course for energy conservation*. Tucson, AZ: Therapy Skill Builders.

Pakenham, K. I. (2012). Multiple sclerosis. In P. Kennedy (Ed.), *The oxford handbook of rehabilitation psychology* (pp. 211–234). New York: Oxford University Press.

Ploughman, M., Austin, M. W., Murdoch, M., Kearney, A., Godwin, M., & Stefanelli, M. (2012). The path to self-management: A qualitative study involving older people with multiple sclerosis. *Physiotherapy Canada, 64*, 6–17.

Plow, M., Finlayson, M., & Rezac, M. (2011). A scoping review of self-management interventions for adults with multiple sclerosis. *Physical Medicine and Rehabilitation, 3*(3), 251–262.

Plow, M. A., Mathiowetz, V., & Resnik, L. (2008). Multiple sclerosis: Impact of physical activity on psychosocial constructs. *American Journal of Health Behavior, 32*(6), 614–626

Prendergast, M. L. (2011). Issues in defining and applying evidence-based practices criteria for treatment of criminal-justice involved clients. *Journal of Psychoactive Drugs* (Suppl. 7), 10–18.

Rae-Grant, A. D., Turner, A. P., Sloan, A., Miller, D., Hunziker, J., & Haselkorn, J. K. (2011). Self-management in neurological disorders: Systematic review of the literature and potential interventions in multiple sclerosis care. *Journal of Rehabilitation Research and Development, 48*(9), 1087–1100. DOI:10.1682/JRRD.2010.08.0159

Reynard, A. K., Sullivan, A. B., & Rae-Grant, A. (2014). A systematic review of stress-management interventions for multiple sclerosis patients. *International Journal of MS Care, 16*, 140–144.

Rietberg, M. B., Brooks, D., Uitdehaag, B. M. J., & Kwakkel, G. (2004). Exercise therapy for multiple sclerosis. *Cochrane Database of Systematic Reviews, 3*, CD003980.

Rigby, S. A., Thornton, E. W., & Young, C. A. (2008). A randomized group intervention trial to enhance mood and self-efficacy in people with multiple sclerosis. *British Journal of Health Psychology, 13*(4), 619–631.

Sauter, C., Zebenholzer, K., Hisakawa, J., Zeitlhofer, J., & Vass, K. (2008). A longitudinal study on effects of a six-week course for energy conservation for multiple sclerosis patients. *Multiple Sclerosis, 14*(4), 500–505.

Schapiro, R. T. (2003). *Managing the symptoms of multiple sclerosis* (4th ed.). New York: Demos.

Schiavolin, S., Leonardi, M., Giovannetti, A. M., Antozzi, B., Brambilla, L., Confalonieri, P., Mantegazza, R., & Raggi, A. (2013). Factors related to difficulties with employment in patients with multiple sclerosis: A review of 2002–2011 literature. *International Journal of Rehabilitation Research, 36*, 105–111.

Schwartz, C. E. (1999). Teaching coping skills enhances quality of life more than peer support: Results of a randomized trial with multiple sclerosis patients. *Health Psychology, 18*, 211–220.

Shevil, E., & Finlayson, M. (2009). Process evaluation of a self-management cognitive program for persons with multiple sclerosis. *Patient Education and Counseling, 76*, 77–83.

Smith, C. R., & Schapiro, R. T. (2004). Neurology. In R. C. Kalb (Ed.), *Multiple sclerosis: The questions you have the answers you need* (3rd ed., pp. 7–42). New York: Demos.

Souza, A., Kelleher, A., Cooper, R., Cooper, R. A., Iezzoni, L. I., & Collins, D. M. (2010). Multiple sclerosis and mobility-related assistive technology: Systematic review of literature. *Journal of Rehabilitation Research & Development 47*(3), 213–224.

Turner, A. P., Kivlahan, D. R., & Haselkorn, J. K. (2009). Exercise and quality of life among people with multiple sclerosis: Looking beyond physical functioning to mental health and participation in life. *Archives of Physical Medicine and Rehabilitation, 90*(3), 420–428.

Turner, A. P., Williams, R. M., Sloan, A. P., & Haselkorn, J. K. (2009). Injection anxiety remains a long-term barrier to medication adherence in multiple sclerosis. *Rehabilitation Psychology, 54*(1), 116–121.

van den Elsen, P. J., vanEggermond, M. C. J. A., Puentes, F., vander Valk, P., Baker, D., & Amora, S. (2014). The epigenetics of multiple sclerosis and other related disorders. *Multiple Sclerosis and Related Disorders, 3*, 163–175.

Wilski, M., Tasiemski, T., & Kocur, P. (2015). Demographic, socioeconomic and clinical correlates of self-management in multiple sclerosis. *Disability & Rehabilitation, 37*(21), 1970–1975.

Wineman, N. M., O'Brien, R. A., Nealon, N. R., & Kaskel, B. (1993). Congruence in uncertainty between individuals with multiple sclerosis and their spouses. *Journal of Neuroscience Nursing, 25*, 356–361.

Wineman, N. M., Schwetz, K. M., Goodkin, D. E., & Rudick, R. A. (1996). Relationships among illness uncertainty, stress, coping, and emotional well-being at entry into a clinical drug trial. *Applied Nursing Research,9*, 53–60.

Wingerchuk, D. M. (2011). Environmental factors in multiple sclerosis: Epstein-Barr virus, vitamin D, and cigarette smoking. *Mount Sinai Journal of Medicine, 78*(2), 221–230.

Yu, C.-H., & Mathiowetz, V. (2014). Systematic review of occupational therapy–related interventions for people with multiple sclerosis: Part 1. Activity and participation. *American Journal of Occupational Therapy, 68*, 27–32.

17

Self-Management of Pain

THOMAS HADJISTAVROPOULOS ■

PAIN AND FUNCTIONAL LIMITATIONS

Pain is ubiquitous and a source of human distress. Prevalence estimates for persistent pain range between 10.1% to 55.2%, depending on research method used and population studied (Schopflocher & Harstall, 2008). The International Association for the Study of Pain defines pain as "an unpleasant sensory and emotional experience associated with actual or potential tissue damage, or described in terms of such damage" (Merskey & Bogduk, 1994, p. 210). Pain that is of relatively short duration is considered to be acute, whereas pain that persists beyond the expected healing period is referred to as chronic (Turk & Okifuji, 2001). Chronic pain is often operationalized as pain that has persisted for more than three months (Turk & Okifuji, 2001).

The self-management of pain literature focuses primarily on chronic pain, which can have a profound impact on an individual's physical, social, and psychological functioning. Chronic pain results in work-time loss and difficulty in performing daily chores (e.g., van den Heuvel, Ijmker, Blatter, & de Korte, 2007). Moreover, pain-related disability extends in the areas of socialization, recreation, sexual activity, self-care, as well as life-supporting activities such as eating and sleeping (Rosenbaum, 2010; Scudds & Ostbye, 2001). Given the wide-ranging negative impact on people's functioning, it is not surprising that chronic pain is frequently co-occurring with anxiety, depression, and substance abuse (Tegethoff, Belardi, Stalujanis, & Meinlschmidt, 2015). While pharmacological and other biocentric treatments of pain are often helpful, they are frequently incapable of addressing the multitude of psychosocial and psychological effects of pain. Self-management programs, designed to supplement routine treatments, are usually designed with a focus not only on health education but also on addressing the psychosocial consequences of pain.

SELF-MANAGEMENT AND EVIDENCE-BASED APPROACHES TO CHRONIC PAIN MANAGEMENT

Although a wide range of treatment approaches are used for chronic pain management (e.g., medications, surgery, physical therapy, chiropractic manipulation, exercise, massage, cognitive-behavioral therapy), multidisciplinary approaches, combining several of these modalities, tend to lead to the best outcomes. According to a ground-breaking systematic review of the literature, individuals treated in a multidisciplinary clinic were almost twice as likely to return to work as individuals who were either untreated or who underwent a single modality therapy (Flor, Fydrich, & Turk, 1992). Since the Flor et al. (1992) review was published, evidence favoring multimodality treatment as the best practice in the management of persistent pain continued to mount (Gatchel, McGeary, McGeary, & Lippe, 2014; Kamper et al., 2014). Unfortunately, this type of treatment is not often available to individuals who live in North America and elsewhere, due to a variety of barriers such as location (e.g., not offered in many rural areas) and cost (e.g., unwillingness of many insurance providers to cover the relatively higher short-term costs of such treatment; e.g., Gatchel et al., 2014).

Perhaps due to the inadequate availability of comprehensive multidisciplinary programs, self-management programs have been developed to help sufferers. Coster and Norman (2009) reviewed 30 Cochrane systematic reviews of educational and self-management interventions that were led by nurses or other health professionals. These authors concluded that the evidence for these types of interventions was not overwhelming for most health conditions and that the most promising findings were associated with the management of diabetes and asthma. There was evidence in support of the efficacy of pain self-management, but the findings were not consistent across studies.

In general, the evidence shows small to medium effects of pain self-management programs, although this may vary as a function of pain-related condition (Du et al., 2011; Oliveira et al., 2012). Several meta-analyses and reviews, specifically focusing on the effectiveness of pain self-management, are available. Oliveira et al. conducted a review of meta-analyses on the effectiveness of self-management for low back pain. The authors characterized the evidence as being of moderate quality and concluded that self-management improves pain and disability in low back pain, when compared to minimal intervention, although the effect sizes were small. Du et al. conducted a meta-analysis and examined a broader range of musculoskeletal pain conditions than did Oliveira et al. Du and colleagues concluded that self-management programs for arthritis have small to moderate effects in improving pain and disability in the long-term (over 26 weeks), although the medium-term (13–26 weeks) effect for disability was not significant.

Given recent technological advances, a systematic review of technology-assisted self-management for chronic pain was of special interest (Heapy, Stroud, Higgins, & Sellinger, 2006). A variety of technologies were considered (e.g., telephone, Internet, interactive voice response, mobile smartphones); cognitive-behavioral and other expert-led interventions were also included in the review if they were delivered with the aid of technology. The inclusion of such therapist-led interventions might have resulted in more favorable conclusions about self-management. Nonetheless, Heapy et al. (2006) concluded that the interventions that they reviewed were, generally, efficacious with no evidence of difference as a function of type of technology that was used to deliver the intervention. Effect sizes were small to moderate. Nonetheless, the authors acknowledged the need for further study in this area, including investigations that directly compare different technologies designed for the delivery of interventions.

In conclusion, multidisciplinary treatments are typically best suited for the management of chronic pain. Self-management programs for pain can supplement health professional-administered treatments and show some promise, although the effects tend to be small to moderate. Regardless of the demonstrated effect sizes, however, individuals report that they find participation in such programs to be highly worthwhile and rewarding (Barefoot, Hadjistavropoulos, Carleton, & Henry, 2012), perhaps suggesting that measures used to evaluate outcomes of self-help programs may lack the sensitivity to identify some of the meaningful effects that may be occurring.

KNOWLEDGE NEEDED FOR EFFECTIVE SELF-MANAGEMENT

Understanding that it is possible to improve the quality of one's life despite the presence of pain is critical for the success of self-management. Most often, people consider their chronic pain problem to be entirely physical and firmly hold the belief that a self-management program, with a heavy focus on psychosocial functioning, may be irrelevant given their physical condition. As such, the most important fundamental knowledge to impart to individuals taking part in self-management of pain is that pain is not purely a physical phenomenon but one that incorporates major psychosocial components. Moreover, people can improve their quality of life, despite the pain.

The very definition of pain indicates that pain is a sensory and emotional experience (Merskey & Bogduk, 1994). Emotions that often accompany pain include anger, fear, and disgust (e.g., Hale & Hadjistavropoulos, 1997). If individuals can learn to attenuate such emotions, the experience of pain can become more tolerable. Helping people recognize the psychological components of pain can make pain both easier to manage and more susceptible to a wider range of self-management interventions. A variety of psychological factors (e.g., presence of depression, anxiety, excessive avoidance of activity due to fear of pain) are predictors of long-term disability (Ericsson et al., 2002). The management of these psychological factors improves the probability of successful rehabilitation (e.g., Teh, Zaslavsky, Reynolds, & Cleary, 2010). Quality of life and many negative psychological sequalae of chronic pain can be improved with increased socialization, pleasant activities scheduling, challenging of negative (e.g., catastrophic thoughts about pain), and improved coping with the pain condition (e.g., an active approach to coping tends to lead to more favorable outcomes than passive approaches, such as heavy reliance on hope that the pain will be ameliorated as a result of the actions of others; Ashby & Lenhart, 1994; Boothby, Thorn, Stroud, & Jensen, 1999; DeGood & Cook, 2011; Jensen, Turner, & Romano, 1992; Keefe, Porter, Somers, Shelby, & Wren, 2013).

Similarly, teaching individuals that certain lifestyle changes can facilitate recovery from painful injury is also important. Smoking, for example, has been associated with increased pain and may delay postsurgical healing (Behrend et al., 2014; Boogaard et al., 2015). Similarly, weight loss in individuals who are overweight can ameliorate knee pain (Christensen et al., 2015). Excessive inactivity can also serve to prolong pain problems (Picavet & Schuit, 2003). As such, assisting self-management participants learn how to make lifestyle changes would be an important component of a self-management program.

Although the general core of psychological techniques used in chronic pain self-management bears remarkable similarities across a variety of painful conditions, education about one's specific pain-related ailment can also be a key element of self-management (e.g., treatment options, consequences of non-participation in prescribed regiments, potential exacerbating factors). In sum, general knowledge about the various dimensions of pain, pain-condition information (e.g., the potential negative consequences of excessive inactivity on musculoskeletal pain, common triggers of migraine headaches), treatment options (e.g., medications that may be effective for many types of musculoskeletal injury may be ineffective for neuropathic pain), and healthy lifestyle education are important to impart prior to a focus on specific techniques and coping strategies that comprise the bulk of many self-management interventions. Specific research groups or organizations offering pain self-management sometimes develop leader manuals to guide group facilitators (e.g., see Ersek, Turner, Cain & Kemp, 2004), but often facilitators generate their material from self-help manuals developed for people with pain (e.g., Hadjistavropoulos & Hadjistavropoulos, 2008; Lorig & Fries, 2006).

BARRIERS TO PAIN SELF-MANAGEMENT

Barriers to the self-management of pain could be both practical and psychological (Bair et al., 2009; Rodriguez, 2013). From a practical standpoint, many pain problems limit mobility and, thus, the ability to attend various self-management group meetings. Geographic factors can also limit access to such groups. Moreover, limited access to computers can be a barrier to participation in self-management programs that are available online. Time constraints, due to participants' varied responsibilities (e.g., family and work demands), can be another added practicality that can interfere with effective self-management.

At the personal, psychological level, limited motivation can be a barrier to self-management. Oftentimes, people hold firm beliefs that their pain problem is due to an undiscovered or inadequately understood medical issue and that, unless their issue is diagnosed properly, self-management would be pointless. Similarly, as mentioned earlier, an inadequate understanding of the importance of psychological factors in pain would be a barrier to self-management. Research has demonstrated that strongly-held beliefs about organic factors being the most important in chronic pain are associated with greater disability and more catastrophic thoughts about the consequences of pain (Sloan, Gupta, Zhang, & Walsh, 2008; Walsh & Radcliffe, 2002).

Depression that often accompanies chronic pain (e.g., Tegethoff et al., 2015) can serve as a motivational barrier to taking the actions necessary to better cope with or overcome a pain problem. In addition the aforementioned clinical observations, some empirical research on barriers to pain self-management is available. Specifically, Bair et al. (2009) investigated barriers and facilitators to pain self-management in people with chronic pain and co-occurring depression and identified a variety of barriers including inadequate support from family and friends, financial and related resources (e.g., access to transportation), time constraints, physical limitations, self-management strategies that are not experienced as being effective, and communication barriers with health-care personnel. In contrast, encouragement from health professionals and family and improving both depression and the availability of variety in self-management options were viewed as facilitators. This finding has clear implications for health professionals who wish to encourage self-management options for individuals who are suffering from pain, as well as for their family members.

RESEARCH ON THE EMOTIONAL IMPACT OF PAIN

Pain is an emotional experience (Merskey & Bogduk, 1994) and, as such, has considerable impact on overall emotional functioning. Acute pain is accompanied by emotions, such as fear and anxiety (Brandt, Zvolensky, Daumas, Grover, & Gonzalez, 2015; Hale & Hadjistavropoulos, 1997). Chronic pain is also accompanied by similar emotions and is highly co-occurring with depression and anxiety (Kroenke et al., 2013). In fact, as many as 85% of people with chronic pain suffer from depression, although lower estimates have also been found (depending on study methodology and setting; Bair, Robinson, Katon, & Kroenke, 2003). Other conditions, such as anxiety disorders (e.g., posttraumatic stress disorder) and substance-use disorders, are also seen commonly in individuals with chronic pain (Tegethoff et al., 2015). While there are cases where mental health conditions preceded the onset of the chronic pain condition (Polatin, Kinney, Gatchel, Lillo, & Mayer, 1993), it is recognized that chronic pain and physical injury can play a causal role (Gatchel, 2004) in the onset of emotional disorders. This makes good sense from a psychological standpoint. That is, chronic pain can cause reductions in pleasant and social activities (e.g., as people are less able to participate in sports and attend social events). Reductions in pleasant activities have been associated with depression (Lewinsohn & Graf, 1973; Rider, Thompson & Gallagher-Thompson, 2016; Takano, Sakamoto & Tanno, 2013). Pain also causes disruptions in social relationships, as well as income reductions (through lost work), all of which have the potential of affecting a person's mood and well-being. For these reasons, it is important for pain self-management programs to address the emotional toll that pain takes, as well as co-occurring emotional disorders.

COPING STRATEGIES/SKILLS IN CHRONIC PAIN SELF-MANAGEMENT

In addition to the aforementioned general psychoeducational information (e.g., information about the nature of specific pain conditions and treatment options) offered through self-management programs, there tends to be a focus on specific skills and coping strategies (e.g., Hadjistavropoulos & Hadjistavropoulos, 2008). These skills and coping strategies have much in common with elements incorporated within well-established, cognitive-behavioral psychological therapies for pain (Hadjistavropoulos, 2012) and include, but are not necessarily limited to the following.

Use of Pain Diaries

Learning to use a pain diary to monitor pain levels, as well as the antecedents of pain and consequences of pain exacerbations, can provide useful information for self-management. Pain exacerbations, for example, often have specific triggers (e.g., sitting on a certain chair or couch, stress). Becoming better aware of such triggers would allow an individual to better manage a pain problem by making environmental and/or lifestyle modifications.

Optimization of Participation in Treatment

Discussion of and helping the individual problem-solve about optimization of participation in prescribed regimens (e.g., physiotherapy exercises, appropriate use of medication) can improve outcomes. Education about all available treatment options is always desirable and of importance when it comes to the optimization of treatment participation.

Relaxation Procedures

A variety of relaxation procedures (e.g., progressive muscle relaxation, imagery-based relaxation) can be practiced as part of self-management programs. Often imagery or breathing-based relaxation procedures are preferred, because the applied tension required for progressive muscle relaxation can be discomforting for some individuals with musculoskeletal pain. Relaxation procedures can have several benefits. For example, certain types of pain, such as tension headache and musculoskeletal pain, can be increased by muscle tension, which can be reduced with relaxation training. Moreover, most kinds of pain tend to increase general stress; tension and relaxation procedures can be helpful under such circumstances.

Pacing of Activity

People with chronic pain often experience distress because of difficulty completing certain tasks. Some people, for example, have difficulty completing housework, because chores, such as vacuuming, may result in increased pain. Through pacing, they may learn to break down the task into smaller, more manageable components. Targeting one small component at a time, rather than the whole project at once, may allow people to complete projects with minimal pain exacerbations (i.e., if it takes about 10 minutes of vacuuming before a pain exacerbation occurs, for example, a person may be asked to only vacuum for 5 minutes at a time in order to dissociate the activity/task from the pain).

Problem-Solving

Often people with chronic pain present with problems that either stand in the way of treatment optimization and/or are the direct result of chronic pain. For example, some individuals may have difficulty effectively communicating with their healthcare professional regarding treatment options and potential side effects of treatment. Under such circumstances, they may engage in problem-solving (as part of self-management) and come up with manageable solutions (e.g., sufferers may be encouraged to consider and discuss the preparation of specific questions that they can ask to their healthcare professional). A dialectic Socratic approach can be used to facilitate problem-solving (e.g., asking the participant if there are alternative ways of approaching a challenging situation). Moreover, role-plays involving the facilitator, the participant, and/or other members of a self-management group could facilitate the practice and development of effective communication strategies that can be used with health professionals, family members, or other contacts.

Cognitive Strategies

Participants may be introduced to ways of monitoring and challenging catastrophic or otherwise inaccurate negative beliefs about their pain experience. They may also be encouraged to substitute such beliefs with more adaptive ones. For example, the belief "I cannot do anything because of my pain" could be substituted with "although the pain prevents me from doing certain things that I used to do before my injury, there are many worthwhile activities that I can still do, despite the pain." Catastrophic beliefs about pain could interfere with treatment success (e.g., Rosenberg, Schultz, Duarte, Rosen, & Raza, 2015). Self-management programs should provide guidance as to how such beliefs can be tested (i.e., evaluated by the individual for their accuracy) and potentially can be substituted with more accurate beliefs about one's condition.

Other Cognitive Coping Strategies

In addition to examining specific thoughts about pain, a review of coping strategies would be important to pursue. As mentioned earlier, active coping strategies (e.g., emotional regulation by reinterpreting the pain experience) tend to be more beneficial than passive strategies (e.g., hoping that pain will be relieved as a result of actions of others; avoidance of problem-solving; Covic, Adamson & Hough, 2000; Snow-Turek, Norris, & Tan, 1996).

Increased Engagement in Social and Other Pleasant Activities

Insufficient engagement in pleasant and social activities can predispose individuals with pain to negative emotional consequences. Self-management programs provide a forum to plan and problem-solve around ways of increasing such engagement.

Complimentary Approaches

A variety of complimentary approaches (e.g., meditation) has also been found to be helpful in pain management (e.g., Cheung, Park, & Wyman, 2015) and could be incorporated in self-management programs.

Support

Self-help programs that involve groups of people with chronic pain can be sources of social support for participants. This is important because social support can help people become more resilient to the effects of stress associated with the condition (Ozbay et al., 2007).

TESTED APPROACHES THAT FACILITATE SELF-MANAGEMENT

A variety of formats have been used to facilitate pain self-management. These formats include support groups (usually with a facilitator), telehealth, self-help books, web-based programs, as well as use of smartphone apps (e.g., Appel, Bleiberg, & Noiseux, 2002; Barefoot et al., 2012; Lalloo, Jibb, Rivera, Agarwal, & Stinson, 2015). Nonetheless, more research is needed before the efficacy of some of these formats can be determined with confidence.

Perhaps the most traditional format of delivering a self-management intervention involves the use of groups. Often led by a facilitator, such groups provide a forum for pain sufferers to support one another, exchange ideas, and problem-solve together. Educational information is typically provided and materials (e.g., diary sheets, readings are shared). These groups are most often time-limited (i.e., they run for a set number of weeks) and involve weekly meetings. In a well-controlled investigation, using a group format involving a facilitator, LeFort, Gray-Donald, Rowat, and Jeans (1998) reported encouraging findings with young-adult participants. Ersek, Turner, Cain, and Kemp (2008), focusing on older adult participants, found improvements in coping but no effects on pain and functional outcomes, when compared with a bibliotherapy (i.e., use of a self-help book without the aid of a therapist) control group. As indicated earlier, meta-analytic research has also demonstrated inconsistent effects across studies with small to moderate effect sizes found (e.g., Du et al., 2011).

Pain self-management information can also be shared through self-help books or manuals, although more research is needed in this domain. An evaluation of a bibliotherapy pain self-management program for older adults was conducted by Barefoot et al. (2012). Contrary to expectations, these authors did not identify any differences in outcomes between the bibliotherapy group and a control group. Interestingly, however, bibliotherapy participants expressed a great deal of satisfaction with the self-help program, suggesting that there might have been effects that were not captured by outcome measures used in the study.

Self-management programs administered through the use of technology show considerable promise with no technological modality demonstrating clear superiority (Heapy et al., 2015). Appel et al. (2002) compared self-management training that was delivered in-person, via closed circuit television, or via telephone and found all formats to be comparably effective. The Appel et al. study did not include a no-treatment control group. Similarly, the results from investigations of Internet-based pain self-management show considerable promise. Ruehlman, Karoly, and Enders (2012) conducted a large-scale trial involving use of a web-based, self-directed, and self-paced system that integrated social-networking features and self-management tools. They found that self-management participants, as compared to a wait-list control group, showed significant decreases in pain severity, pain interference, perceived disability, emotional responses, and catastrophizing. Despite the promise shown by web-based self-management programs, it is important for people with pain to be cautious when they seek pain-management information on the Internet because much of the available information may be incomplete or inaccurate, as demonstrated in an evaluation of chronic-pain related information available on the Internet (Bailey, LaChapelle, LeFort, Gordon, & Hadjistavropoulos, 2013).

With the increased popularity of smartphones, there have been a growing number of apps designed to facilitate the self-management of pain. These apps generally require more testing and evaluation before they can be recommended with confidence (Lalloo et al., 2015). Lalloo et al. identified 279 apps providing pain self-care skill support (77%), pain education (45.9%), monitoring (19%), goal setting (.72%), and social support (3.6%). However, the overwhelming majority of these apps were deemed to be simplistic (i.e., serving only a single function), did not involve a health professional facilitator, and were untested. In fact, Lalloo et al. (2015) concluded that only one of the apps that they found (CatchMyPain) was described as being involved in a scientific investigation (i.e., a large-scale descriptive study focusing on the multidimensionality of the pain experience).

CONCLUSION

Despite considerable promise for several pain self-management programs for chronic pain, effect sizes tend to be small to moderate and there are inconsistencies across studies. The inconsistencies are not difficult to understand, given that there is lack of standardization across self-management programs. That is, programs differ from one another in both methodology and content, and such differences can lead to inconsistent results. Once the field reaches a consensus on one or more standardized self-management approaches, it will become easier to better study and understand self-management across different pain groups, as programs would become more consistent and comparable to one another.

Regarding technology-assisted self-management, Heapy et al. (2015) reviewed the literature and concluded that the research has limitations. Specifically, there is a lack of in-person comparison groups, an insufficient number of direct comparisons among modalities, as well as heterogeneity of interventions and research approaches that limit our ability to compare across studies. These limitations should be addressed in future research.

Future research could pave the way for the optimization of self-management programs (e.g., by identifying self-management approaches and components that are most likely to be effective). When combined with the addition of technological advances that facilitate participation in self-management programs for larger numbers of people, optimized self-management interventions could improve quality of life for large numbers of chronic pain sufferers.

REFERENCES

Appel, P. R., Bleiberg, J., & Noiseux, J. (2002). Self-regulation training for chronic pain: Can it be done effectively by telemedicine? *Telemedicine Journal and e-Health, 8*, 361–368. doi:10.1089/15305620260507495

Ashby, J. S., & Lenhart, R. S. (1994). Prayer as a coping strategy for chronic pain patients. *Rehabilitation Psychology, 39*, 205–209. doi:10.1037

Bailey, S. J., LaChapelle, D. L., LeFort, S. M., Gordon, A., & Hadjistavropoulos, T. (2013). Evaluation of chronic pain-related information available to consumers on the internet. *Pain Medicine, 14*, 855–864. doi:10.1111/pme.12087

Bair, M. J., Matthias, M. S., Nyland, K. A., Huffman, M. A., Stubbs, D. L., Kroenke, K., & Damush, T. M. (2009). Barriers and facilitators to chronic pain self-management: A qualitative study of primary care patients with comorbid musculoskeletal pain and depression. *Pain Medicine, 10*, 1280–1290. doi:10.1111/j.1526-4637.2009.00707.x

Bair, M. J., Robinson, R. L., Katon, W., & Kroenke, K. (2003). Depression and pain comorbidity: A literature review. *Archives of Internal Medicine, 163*, 2433–2445. doi:10.1001/archinte.163.20.2433

Barefoot, C., Hadjistavropoulos, T., Carleton, R. N., & Henry, J. (2012). A brief report on the evaluation of a pain self-management program for older adults. *Journal of Cognitive Psychotherapy, 26*, 157–168. doi:10.1891/0889-8391.26.2.157

Behrend, C., Schonbach, E., Coombs, A., Coyne, E., Prasarn, M., & Rechtine, G. (2014). Smoking cessation related to improved patient-reported pain scores following spinal care in geriatric patients. *Geriatric Orthopaedic Surgery & Rehabilitation, 5*, 191–194. doi:10.1177/2151458514550479

Boogaard, S., Heymans, M. W., de Vet, H. C., Peters, M. L., Loer, S. A., Zuurmond, W. W., & Perez, R. S. (2015). Predictors of persistent neuropathic pain: A systematic review. *Pain Physician, 18*(5), 433–457.

Boothby, J. L., Thorn, B. E., Stroud, M. W., & Jensen, M. P. (1999). Coping with pain. In R. J. Gatchel, & D. C. Turk (Eds.), *Psychosocial factors in pain: Critical perspectives* (pp. 343–359). New York: Guilford Press.

Brandt, C. P., Zvolensky, M. J., Daumas, S. D., Grover, K. W., & Gonzalez, A. (2015). Pain-related anxiety in relation to anxiety and depression among persons living with HIV/AIDS. *AIDS Care*, 1–4. doi:10.1080/09540121.2015.1100704

Cheung, C., Park, J., & Wyman, J. F. (2015). Effects of yoga on symptoms, physical function, and psychosocial outcomes in adults with osteoarthritis: A focused review. *American Journal of Physical Medicine & Rehabilitation, 95*(2), 139–151. doi:10.1097/PHM.0000000000000408

Christensen, R., Henriksen, M., Leeds, A. R., Gudbergsen, H., Christensen, P., Sorensen, T. J., . . . Bliddal, H. (2015). Effect of weight maintenance on symptoms of knee osteoarthritis in obese patients: A twelve-month randomized controlled trial. *Arthritis Care & Research, 67*, 640–650. doi:10.1002/acr.22504

Coster, S., & Norman, I. (2009). Cochrane reviews of educational and self-management interventions to guide nursing practice: A review. *International Journal of Nursing Studies, 46*, 508–528. doi:10.1016/j.ijnurstu.2008.09.009

Covic, T., Adamson, B., & Hough, M. (2000). The impact of passive coping on rheumatoid arthritis pain. *Rheumatology, 39*, 1027–1030.

DeGood, D. E., & Cook, A. J. (2011). Psychological assessment: Comprehensive measures specific to pain beliefs and coping. In D. C. Turk, & R. Melzack (Eds.), *Handbook of pain assessment* (2nd ed., pp. 67–97). New York: Guilford Press.

Du, S., Yuan, C., Xiao, X., Chu, J., Qiu, Y., & Qian, H. (2011). Self-management programs for chronic musculoskeletal pain conditions: A systematic review and meta-analysis. *Patient Education and Counseling, 85*, e299–e310. doi:10.1016/j.pec.2011.02.021

Ericsson, M., Poston, W. S., Linder, J., Taylor, J. E., Haddock, C. K., & Foreyt, J. P. (2002). Depression predicts disability in long-term chronic pain patients. *Disability and Rehabilitation, 24*, 334–340.

Ersek, M., Turner, J. A., Cain, K. C., & Kemp, C. A. (2004). Chronic pain self-management for older adults: A randomized controlled trial. *BMC Geriatrics, 4, 7.* doi:10.1186/1471-2318-4-7

Ersek, M., Turner, J. A., Cain, K. C., & Kemp, C. A. (2008). Results of a randomized controlled trial to examine the efficacy of a chronic pain self-management group for older adults. *Pain, 138*, 29–40. doi:S0304-3959(07)00653-7

Flor, H., Fydrich, T., & Turk, D. C. (1992). Efficacy of multidisciplinary pain treatment centers: A meta-analytic review. *Pain, 49*(2), 221–230.

Gatchel, R. J. (2004). Comorbidity of chronic pain and mental health disorders: The biopsychosocial perspective. *The American Psychologist, 59*, 795–805. doi:2004-20395-026

Gatchel, R. J., McGeary, D. D., McGeary, C. A., & Lippe, B. (2014). Interdisciplinary chronic pain management: Past, present, and future. *The American Psychologist, 69*, 119–130. doi:10.1037/a0035514

Hadjistavropoulos, T. (2012). Self-management of pain in older persons: Helping people help themselves. *Pain Medicine, 13*(Suppl. 2), S67–S71. doi:10.1111/j.1526-4637.2011.01272.x

Hadjistavropoulos, T., & Hadjistavropoulos, H. D. (Eds.). (2008). *Pain management for older adults: A self-help guide.* Seattle: IASP Press.

Hale, C., & Hadjistavropoulos, T. (1997). Emotional components of pain. *Pain Research and Management, 2*, 217–225.

Heapy, A. A., Higgins, D. M., Cervone, D., Wandner, L., Fenton, B. T., & Kerns, R. D. (2015). A systematic review of technology-assisted self-management interventions for chronic pain: Looking across treatment modalities. *The Clinical Journal of Pain, 31*, 470–492. doi:10.1097/AJP.0000000000000185

Heapy, A. A., Stroud, M. W., Higgins, D. M., & Sellinger, J. J. (2006). Tailoring cognitive-behavioral therapy for chronic pain: A case example. *Journal of Clinical Psychology, 62*, 1345–1354. doi:10.1002/jclp.20314

Jensen, M. P., Turner, J. A., & Romano, J. M. (1992). Chronic pain coping measures: Individual vs. composite scores. *Pain, 51*(3), 273–280.

Kamper, S. J., Apeldoorn, A. T., Chiarotto, A., Smeets, R. J. E. M., Ostelo, R. W. J. G., Guzman, J., & van Tulder, M. W. (2014). Multidisciplinary biopsychosocial rehabilitation for chronic low back pain. *Cochrane Database of Systematic Reviews, 9*, CD000963. doi:10.1002/14651858.CD000963.pub3

Keefe, F. J., Porter, L., Somers, T., Shelby, R., & Wren, A. V. (2013). Psychosocial interventions for managing pain in older adults: Outcomes and clinical implications. *British Journal of Anaesthesia, 111*, 89–94. doi:10.1093/bja/aet129

Kroenke, K., Outcalt, S., Krebs, E., Bair, M. J., Wu, J., Chumbler, N., & Yu, Z. (2013). Association between anxiety, health-related quality of life and functional impairment in primary care patients with chronic pain. *General Hospital Psychiatry, 35*, 359–365. doi:10.1016/j.genhosppsych.2013.03.020

Lalloo, C., Jibb, L. A., Rivera, J., Agarwal, A., & Stinson, J. N. (2015). "There's a pain app for that": Review of patient-targeted smartphone applications for pain management. *The Clinical Journal of Pain, 31*, 557–563. doi:10.1097/AJP.0000000000000171

LeFort, S. M., Gray-Donald, K., Rowat, K. M., & Jeans, M. E. (1998). Randomized controlled trial of a community-based psychoeducation program for the self-management of chronic pain. *Pain, 74*(2-3), 297–306.

Lewinsohn, P. M., & Graf, M. (1973). Pleasant activities and depression. *Journal of Consulting and Clinical Psychology, 41*(2), 261–268.

Lorig, K.R., & Fries, J.F. (2006). *The arthritis helpbook.* Cambridge, MA: Perseus Books.

Merskey, H., & Bogduk, N. (Eds.). (1994). *Classification of chronic pain* (2nd ed.). Seattle: IASP Press.

Oliveira, V. C., Ferreira, P. H., Maher, C. G., Pinto, R. Z., Refshauge, K. M., & Ferreira, M. L. (2012). Effectiveness of self-management of low back pain: Systematic review with meta-analysis. *Arthritis Care & Research, 64*, 1739–1748. doi:10.1002/acr.21737

Ozbay, F., Johnson, D. C., Dimoulas, E., Morgan, C. A., Charney, D., & Southwick, S. (2007). Social support and resilience to stress: From neurobiology to clinical practice. *Psychiatry, 4*(5), 35–40.

Picavet, H. S., & Schuit, A. J. (2003). Physical inactivity: A risk factor for low back pain in the general population? *Journal of Epidemiology and Community Health, 57*(7), 517–518.

Polatin, P. B., Kinney, R. K., Gatchel, R. J., Lillo, E., & Mayer, T. G. (1993). Psychiatric illness and chronic low-back pain. the mind and the spine—which goes first? *Spine, 18*(1), 66–71.

Rider, K.L., Thompson, L.W., Gallagher-Thompson, D. (2016). California older persons pleasant events scale: A tool to help older adults increase positive experiences. *Clinical Gerontologist, 39*, 64–83.

Rodriguez, K. M. (2013). Intrinsic and extrinsic factors affecting patient engagement in diabetes self-management: Perspectives of a certified diabetes educator. *Clinical Therapeutics, 35*, 170–178. doi:10.1016/j.clinthera.2013.01.002

Rosenbaum, T. Y. (2010). Musculoskeletal pain and sexual function in women. *The Journal of Sexual Medicine, 7*, 645–653. doi:10.1111/j.1743-6109.2009.01490.x

Rosenberg, J. C., Schultz, D. M., Duarte, L. E., Rosen, S. M., & Raza, A. (2015). Increased pain catastrophizing associated with lower pain relief during spinal cord stimulation: Results from a large post-market study. *Neuromodulation, 18*, 277–284. doi:10.1111/ner.12287

Ruehlman, L. S., Karoly, P., & Enders, C. (2012). A randomized controlled evaluation of an online chronic pain self management program. *Pain, 153*, 319–330. doi:10.1016/j.pain.2011.10.025

Schopflocher, D., & Harstall, C. (2008). The descriptive epidemiology of chronic pain. In S. Rashiq, D. Schopflocher, P. Taenzer, & E. Jonsson (Eds.), *Chronic pain a health policy perspective* (pp. 29–40). Weinheim, Germany: Wiley-Blackwell.

Scudds, R. J., & Ostbye, T. (2001). Pain and pain-related interference with function in older canadians: The Canadian study of health and aging. *Disability and Rehabilitation, 23*(15), 654–664.

Sloan, T. J., Gupta, R., Zhang, W., & Walsh, D. A. (2008). Beliefs about the causes and consequences of pain in patients with chronic inflammatory or noninflammatory low back pain and in pain-free individuals. *Spine, 33*, 966–972. doi:10.1097/BRS.0b013e31816c8ab4

Snow-Turek, A. L., Norris, M. P., & Tan, G. (1996). Active and passive coping strategies in chronic pain patients. *Pain, 64*, 455–462.

Takano, K., Sakamoto, S., & Tanno, Y. (2013). Ruminative focus in daily life: Association with daily activities and depressive symptoms. *Emotion, 13,* 657–667.

Tegethoff, M., Belardi, A., Stalujanis, E., & Meinlschmidt, G. (2015). Comorbidity of mental disorders and chronic pain: Chronology of onset in adolescents of a national representative cohort. *The Journal of Pain, 16,* 1054–1064. doi:10.1016/j.jpain.2015.06.009

Teh, C. F., Zaslavsky, A. M., Reynolds, C. F. 3rd, & Cleary, P. D. (2010). Effect of depression treatment on chronic pain outcomes. *Psychosomatic Medicine, 72,* 61–67. doi:10.1097/PSY.0b013e3181c2a7a8

Turk, D. C., & Okifuji, A. (2001). Pain terms and taxonomies. In D. Loeser, S. H. Butler, J. J. Chapman, & D. C. Turk (Eds.), *Bonica's management of pain* (3rd ed., pp. 18–25). Philadelphia, PA: Lippincott Williams & Wilkins.

van den Heuvel, S. G., Ijmker, S., Blatter, B. M., & de Korte, E. M. (2007). Loss of productivity due to neck/shoulder symptoms and hand/arm symptoms: Results from the PROMO-study. *Journal of Occupational Rehabilitation, 17,* 370–382. doi:10.1007/s10926-007-9095-y

Walsh, D. A., & Radcliffe, J. C. (2002). Pain beliefs and perceived physical disability of patients with chronic low back pain. *Pain, 97,* 23–31.

18
Self-Management of Tinnitus

ERIN MARTZ ■

Tinnitus is the perception of sound without external acoustic stimuli (Møller, Langguth, DeRidder, & Kleinjung, 2010). Tinnitus can be experienced as a "ringing in the ears," and/or as a hissing, sizzling, buzzing or other noise that may be rhythmical or pulsatile; it may be constant or intermittent and may occur in one or both ears (Baguley, McFerran, & Hall, 2013; Phillips & McFerran, 2010). Individuals report experiencing the sound of tinnitus in a variety of locations in their heads (Baguley et al., 2013). Objective tinnitus can be attributed to an internal sound source (e.g., a pulsating blood vessel adjacent to the auditory nerve) and can generally be ameliorated by surgery, whereas subjective tinnitus is a "phantom sensation" that has no corresponding external sound and cannot be cured by surgery (Eggermont, 2012). Further, objective tinnitus can be detected by an examiner, while subjective tinnitus cannot be detected by an observer (Hobson, Chisholm, & El Refaie, 2012).

Tunkel and colleagues (2014) reported that often individuals with tinnitus are told by clinicians that "little or nothing can be done to help them" (p. S18), although management strategies for tinnitus exist that can help individuals' symptoms and distress decrease. Given that at the present time there is no cure for most forms of tinnitus, it must be self-managed as a chronic health condition. Healthcare professionals can assist individuals in navigating the range of functional and psychosocial effects triggered by tinnitus in order to help reduce the potential for it having a significant negative impact on their lives. This chapter begins with a discussion about the prevalence and functional limitations of tinnitus, followed by a discussion of evidence-based approaches to tinnitus, the types of knowledge needed to help with tinnitus self-management, research on the emotional impact of tinnitus, and the coping strategies and other approaches that facilitate self-management of tinnitus.

PREVALENCE AND FUNCTIONAL LIMITATIONS OF TINNITUS

Tinnitus is a common impairment in the general population. In the United States, 21.4 million people (about 10% of the population) reported experiencing tinnitus in the past year and, of that group, 27% indicated that they have had symptoms for more than 15 years and 36% experienced nearly constant symptoms of tinnitus (Bhatt, Lin, & Bhattacharyya, 2016). A report for the World Health Organization estimated the global prevalence of tinnitus as ranging from 3% to 36%, depending on the study design and definition used (Deshaies et al., 2005). Other research (primarily from Western Europe or the United States) indicated that a range of 10% to 15% of the adult population experienced tinnitus (Baguley et al., 2013). Some researchers (Henry et al., 2007) noted that of individuals with chronic tinnitus, about 20% have symptoms that are "clinically significant," which the researchers depicted as needing clinical intervention due to tinnitus interfering with their lives. Other researchers (Bhatt, Lin, et al., 2016) found that 7.2% described their tinnitus as a big or a very big problem.

The neural pathways of the central auditory system are deemed as having a primary role in the maintenance of tinnitus (Langguth, Kreuzer, Kleinjung, & De Ridder, 2013; Phillips & McFerran, 2010). Noise exposure (Bhatt, Lin, et al., 2016) and occupational injuries, such as blast exposure in a war zone (Fausti, Wilmington, Gallun, Myers, & Henry, 2009), may trigger tinnitus. A traumatic brain injury (TBI) may have concomitant tinnitus (Cave, Cornish, & Chandler, 2007; Kreuzer, Vielsmeier, & Langguth, 2013; Yurgil et al., 2016). Research among active military indicated that having history of TBI increases the risk of postdeployment tinnitus (Yurgil et al., 2016). There are also cases in which head and neck injury, ear infections, and related health conditions are the main factors behind tinnitus onset (Eggermont, 2012).

Tinnitus is different than hearing loss, although tinnitus and hearing loss co-occur in a majority of individuals (Eggermont, 2012). Individuals may confuse the limitations created by hearing loss with the limitations created by tinnitus. The typical functional limitations of tinnitus may include difficulties in concentration or a disruption of sleep patterns, which can create issues with fatigue and thus can further exacerbate concentration problems (Langguth et al., 2013; Tunkel et al., 2014). Emotional distress about having tinnitus often occurs (more details are provided in the "Research on the Emotional Impact of Tinnitus" section in this chapter). Individuals also may withdraw from their social activities, due to a range of issues that can include fatigue and psychological reactions to tinnitus, such as anger, depression, and anxiety.

SELF-MANAGEMENT AND EVIDENCE-BASED APPROACHES TO TINNITUS

A multidisciplinary approach to tinnitus treatment, which includes education and counseling components (Langguth et al., 2013; Ruth & Hamill-Ruth, 2001; Tunkel et al., 2014), is suggested for the management of tinnitus. After ruling out treatable auditory issues, the standard treatment includes an explanation of the tinnitus phenomenon using audiological education, teaching individuals how to use sound therapy (i.e., sound enrichment devices, such as sound machines, ear-level sound generators, and, if needed, sound amplification devices like hearing aids), and providing some form of counseling to assist with stress reduction (Baguley et al., 2013).

Several stepped-care approaches have been developed for tinnitus (Cima et al., 2009; Cima et al., 2012; Henry et al., 2005; Henry, Zaugg, Myers, & Kendall, 2010; Maes et al., 2014). Stepped-care approaches have been used in healthcare settings for decades and provide increasing levels of interventions based on the individual's response to treatment. A stepped-care approach may involve multidisciplinary treatment if the individual does not experience the desired outcome (e.g., symptom relief or reduction in depression). One stepped-care approach is called Progressive Tinnitus Management (Henry et al., 2005; Henry et al., 2010) and involves five steps: (a) referral, (b) audiological evaluation, (c) skills education (both psychoeducation and audiological education), (d) interdisciplinary evaluation, and (e) individualized support. Langguth and colleagues (2013) developed a stepwise decision-tree approach for professionals who provide tinnitus management. They asserted that a multidisciplinary approach is needed for tinnitus.

A multidisciplinary approach and its cost-effectiveness were studied by Maes and colleagues (2014). The first step in their stepped-care approach included audiological assessment, counseling, hearing aids and/or sound generator, a tinnitus educational session, and an individual consultation with a psychologist. If individuals needed further treatment, they were provided group counseling sessions that contained a range of psychological approaches from cognitive-behavioral therapy (CBT) to Tinnitus Retraining Therapy (TRT).

Audiological Education about Tinnitus

Most healthcare professionals with tinnitus expertise would agree that audiological education should be provided to individuals with tinnitus. This education should include basic information about what may cause tinnitus, why it cannot be cured at this time, and what can be done about it (e.g., sound enrichment, use of sound therapy). The clinical practice guidelines for tinnitus (Tunkel et al., 2014) recommend that individuals be educated about strategies on how to manage their tinnitus.

Tinnitus interventions that provide psychoeducation that targets tinnitus-related stress often include one or more sessions of audiological education about tinnitus (Henry et al., 2005; Henry et al., 2010; Kroner-Herwig, Frenzel, Fritsche, Schilkowsky, & Esser, 2003; Zachriat & Kroner-Herwig, 2004). Yet, the content and the extent of the audiological education about tinnitus vary among interventions. For example, one intervention, TRT (Jastreboff & Jastreboff, 2000), provides both education and "directive" counseling. TRT's audiological education involves extensive teaching on the neurophysiological model of tinnitus and includes detailed explanations about the limbic and autonomic nervous systems, which is provided to help individuals "reclassify" tinnitus as a neutral stimulus instead of a threat (Jastreboff, 2011).

Sound Therapy

Sound therapy interventions can include the use of noise-generating devices or hearing aids that provide sound enrichment to help individuals pay less attention to tinnitus. Hobson et al. (2012) conducted a Cochrane review of six studies using sound therapy for tinnitus. They pointed out that there are two approaches to managing tinnitus: (a) habituating to reactions about having tinnitus (i.e., modifying individuals' psychological reactions about having tinnitus) and (b) habituating to the perception or sensation of "hearing" tinnitus. The researchers' analysis of six studies suggested that the use of sound therapy helped with the second approach; that is, it helped the process of habituation to the perception of tinnitus but it did not demonstrate a significant change in the perceived loudness or severity of tinnitus. These researchers proposed that the differences may be due to the lack of quality research or due to combining multiple strategies in interventions (e.g., sound therapy along with counseling), and they noted that the lack of strong scientific evidence is not the same as clinical evidence that suggests that sound therapy helps individuals manage their tinnitus.

Another group of researchers had similar conclusions as Hobson and colleagues (2012) about the use of sound therapy. Pichora-Fuller and colleagues (2013) conducted a comparative effectiveness review of scientific studies on treatments for tinnitus that included four categories of interventions (pharmacological or food supplements, medical, use of sound technology, and psychological/behavioral). They indicated that, at this time, the available information on sound technology interventions (e.g., hearing aids; sound generators; long-term, low-level white noise; and noise generators) was insufficient to provide a summary of the overall strength of evidence of sound-therapy interventions, due to issues such as small sample sizes and biases in the research studies. They suggested that while multiple studies demonstrated benefits from sound therapy and no drop-outs were mentioned in these reports as arising from adverse effects, significant differences between comparative therapies were not observed; thus, drawing conclusions about its effectiveness cannot be made without further research.

The two aforementioned studies suggest that while positive effects of the use of sound therapy may be observed clinically, the overall strength of evidence is weak at this time. More research is needed, especially studies that compare use sound therapy interventions without bundling sound therapy with other forms of intervention, such as education and counseling, in order to clarify the effects of sound-therapy interventions on the perception of tinnitus.

Counseling Interventions

The clinical practice guidelines for tinnitus (Tunkel et al., 2014) recommend that counseling be used as part of the strategies taught to individuals for better management of their tinnitus. Various forms of counseling have been assessed by numerous researchers in the context of tinnitus. As previously mentioned, TRT (Jastreboff & Jastreboff, 2000) was created to promote habituation to tinnitus by use of directive or structured counseling to help individuals reclassify tinnitus as a "neutral stimuli" and to reduce the perceived strength of tinnitus by the use of sound therapy. A Cochrane review of TRT (Phillips & McFerran, 2010) included only one study. That study, by Henry and colleagues (2006), compared TRT to tinnitus masking (TM); TM consisted of informal counseling and use of wearable devices that may include noise generators, hearing aids, or a combination of both types of devices. The results indicated that both TM and TRT were effective in improving outcomes among individuals with tinnitus over 18 months of treatment, with TM showing better results at 3 months and TRT showing better results at 12 and 18 months of treatment. Yet, Phillips and McFerran cautioned that because this particular study had issues related to subject allocation, the study needs replication before firm conclusions can be drawn.

Langguth and colleagues (2013) noted that psychoeducation, provided as a counseling intervention, is an essential part of the clinical treatment for tinnitus. They suggested that counseling can provide individuals with information, recommendations, and empowerment. See the section "Meta-analyses of Psychological Interventions" for a review of other psychological interventions that have been studied in the context of tinnitus.

KNOWLEDGE NEEDED BY INDIVIDUALS WITH TINNITUS FOR EFFECTIVE SELF-MANAGEMENT

In view of numerous misleading advertisements about curing tinnitus (e.g., on the Internet), individuals need accurate information about what evidence-based medical, pharmacological, audiological, and other treatment options are available. The types of knowledge that individuals with tinnitus need for self-management include auditory-based information about tinnitus and hearing loss, information about how to use sound technology (e.g., hearing aids, sound generators, or environmental enrichment devices), and psychological skills for stress management and reduction (e.g., relaxation, handling negative emotions). The clinical practice guidelines for tinnitus (Tunkel et al., 2014) lists seven areas as "discussion points" for individuals with tinnitus (see Table 10 in Tunkel et al., 2014), including definitions of tinnitus and transient ear noise, tinnitus and hearing loss, temporary tinnitus, drug-induced tinnitus, the lack of a cure, and the current theory on the origins of tinnitus. Yet, the two main components involving information and skills that individuals with tinnitus can be taught are auditory knowledge and psychological knowledge.

Auditory Knowledge

The clinical practice guidelines for tinnitus (Tunkel et al., 2014) recommend that individuals be taught about the associations of tinnitus and hearing loss, and about the need for hearing protection, in view of noise-induced tinnitus.

Individuals can be taught to add noise to their hearing environment (i.e., sound therapy or sound enrichment) in order to draw their attention or focus away from their tinnitus. Henry, Zaugg, Myers, and Schechter (2008) proposed teaching individuals with tinnitus about using three different types of therapeutic sound: (a) soothing sounds, to provide a sense of reprieve from tinnitus-associated stress; (b) background sound to passively divert attention away from tinnitus; and (c) interesting sound to actively divert attention away from tinnitus. Hoare, Edmondson-Jones, Sereda, Akeroyd, and Hall (2014) provided an extensive description of a variety of sound therapy approaches. The rationale behind sound therapy was to blend the internally experienced sound (tinnitus) with an intentionally produced external sound while not attempting to totally "mask" (i.e., cover up) the tinnitus.

For many years, audiologists have observed that the use of hearing aids can help individuals with tinnitus. Reasons for this can include that hearing aids provide a stimulation of regions of the auditory system deprived of auditory input (Henry et al., 2008), as well as that hearing aids can provide more auditory stimuli to the brain, which can draw one's attention away from tinnitus. According to some researchers, the evidence for hearing aids as a stand-alone intervention for tinnitus is not strong (Baguley et al., 2013). However, other researchers indicate that hearing aids can provide noticeable reductions in tinnitus-related distress (Henry, Frederick, Sell, Griest, & Abrams, 2015).

Psychological Knowledge

The often incurable nature of tinnitus itself necessitates individuals with tinnitus to find or learn new coping skills. Many individuals naturally or intuitively use coping strategies to reduce their stress. Yet, teaching coping skills can be helpful to individuals with tinnitus, such as by using "cognitive coping skills training" (Henry & Wilson, 1996), tinnitus coping training (TCT; Kroner-Herwig et al., 1995), or Coping Effectiveness Training (CET; Chesney, Chambers, Taylor, Johnson, & Folkman, 2003). (For more information, see the section "Coping Strategies/Skills in Self-Management of Tinnitus" in this chapter.)

Stress management and reduction are typically major components of tinnitus-based self-management programs. These components can help with insomnia issues that individuals with tinnitus may experience. Some of the psychological knowledge and skills that can be taught to individuals with tinnitus include how to alter negative thinking or non-functional behaviors (CBT) or how to manage a range of unpleasant internal experiences (Acceptance and Commitment Therapy

[ACT]). Some interventions (e.g., CET, CBT, and ACT) encourage individuals to get involved in interesting, pleasant, and/or meaningful tasks, hobbies, activities, or work, which can provide different kinds of stimuli to the brain (other than auditory) and thus, can help to draw individuals' attention away from their tinnitus.

RESEARCH ON THE EMOTIONAL IMPACT OF TINNITUS

A variety of studies have examined the psychosocial sequalae associated with tinnitus. The primary affective constructs that have been studied in the context of tinnitus are anxiety and depression. Decades ago, Harrop-Griffiths, Katon, Dobie, Sakai, and Russo (1987) noted that a group of individuals with tinnitus had significantly higher current and lifetime prevalence of depression than a group of individuals with hearing loss. Sullivan, Katon, Russo, Dobie, and Sakai (1988) replicated their findings, and, since that time, other studies have been published on psychiatric conditions associated with tinnitus. Sullivan, Katon, Russo, Dobie, and Sakai (1993) noted that that the association between tinnitus and depression can be viewed as bidirectional, in that "[t]innitus (like pain) may prompt a depressive episode that may impede habituation to the aversive sensation and thereby increase the severity of the tinnitus experienced" (p. 2258).

Erlandsson and Hallberg (2000) examined 13 predictors of tinnitus-related quality of life among 122 individuals with tinnitus and found that three psychological distress variables (i.e., impaired concentration, depression, and interpersonally related emotional problems) were the strongest predictors of quality of life. Bartels and colleagues (2008) noted that depression and anxiety had an additive effect on the quality of life among 265 individuals with tinnitus.

Krog, Engdahl, and Tambs (2010) examined tinnitus and depression, anxiety, self-esteem, and subjective well-being from 1995 to 1997 among 51,574 Norwegians with hearing loss. They divided the data into four "symptom-level" categories: low, intermediate, or high symptom severity or no tinnitus. They found that after adjusting for age, individuals with tinnitus (all symptom levels) had significantly higher scores on anxiety and depression than individuals without tinnitus.

In an epidemiological study ($N = 3,267$) in the United States, researchers (Nondahl et al., 2011) found that there was an increased risk of having depressive symptoms among individuals with tinnitus. Langguth and colleagues (2011) examined the relation between tinnitus and depression and suggested that neurobiological factors may influence whether tinnitus affects individuals' quality of life. These researchers noted that multiple symptoms related to tinnitus (e.g., insomnia, irritability, concentration problems, fatigue, social withdrawal) were similar to symptoms of depression and thereby may confound the understanding of psychological reactions to tinnitus. This research team proposed that depressive symptoms may not always represent a diagnosis of depression but instead may reflect more general psychological distress.

Geocze and colleagues (2013) conducted a systematic review of depression and tinnitus and provided three possible associations: (a) depression affects tinnitus, (b) tinnitus predisposes individuals to experiencing depression, or (c) tinnitus co-occurs in individuals with depression. Recently, Pinto et al. (2014) conducted a systemic review on psychiatric disorders that accompany tinnitus. They found that both anxiety and depression have been found to be high among individuals with tinnitus across 15 studies. McCormack et al. (2014) investigated anxiety and depression among 171,728 individuals and found that individuals with tinnitus were at increased risk for depression and anxiety, as compared to individuals without tinnitus. A population-based study (Bhatt, Bhattacharyya, & Lin, 2016) analyzed tinnitus-related data gathered by the 2007 National Health Interview Series; 21.4 million individuals reported experiencing tinnitus, while 26.1% of that group reported having problems with depression and anxiety. Compared to individuals without tinnitus, those with tinnitus were significantly more likely to report depression and anxiety in that study.

Clinicians have noted an association between tinnitus and suicide (Harrop-Griffiths et al., 1987; Jacobson & McCaslin, 2001; Lewis, 2002; Pridmore, Walter, & Friedland, 2012; Sullivan et al., 1988). Jacobson and McCaslin suggested that the primary psychiatric issue among individuals who had tinnitus and who committed suicide was depression, and thus clinicians should be aware of the possible risk of suicide among individuals who are clinically depressed and who have tinnitus. Yet, few researchers have done epidemiological studies to examine the possible association between tinnitus and suicide. Seo, Kang, Hwang, Han, and Joo (2016) conducted an epidemiological study that investigated suicidal ideation and attempts in a sample of 17,446 Koreans who took part in the Korean National Health and Nutrition Examination Survey. A chi-square analysis indicated a significant difference among suicidal ideation and suicidal attempts according to tinnitus existence: 20.9% of individuals with tinnitus reported suicidal ideation, compared to 12.2% of individuals without tinnitus, while 1.2% of individuals with tinnitus reported suicide attempts, compared to 0.6% of individuals without tinnitus. However, according to recent research (Martz et al., in preparation), having a tinnitus diagnosis was found to *decrease* the likelihood of suicide among US veterans with a tinnitus diagnosis compared to individuals without tinnitus. One possible explanation for Martz and colleagues' findings of the decreased likelihood of suicide among individuals with tinnitus compared to individuals without tinnitus was that individuals had learned some coping strategies to deal with their tinnitus, and thus, they may have utilized those coping strategies to help them manage other types of stress in their lives.

COPING STRATEGIES/SKILLS IN SELF-MANAGEMENT OF TINNITUS

One teachable aspect of managing tinnitus is coping. Lazarus and Folkman (1984) defined coping as the "constantly changing cognitive and behavioral efforts to manage specific external and/or internal demands that are appraised as taxing or exceeding the resources of the person" (p. 141). People intuitively use coping strategies without having to be taught them: they are natural responses to dealing with stress. However, some coping strategies (e.g., problem-solving, seeking social support, stress-reduction strategies) are more healthy or adaptive than other coping strategies (e.g., avoidance, disengagement, excessive drinking) for dealing with stress. These types of coping skills for tinnitus can be taught in psychoeducation groups, individual counseling, or by means of online interventions.

Interventions That Assessed Coping with Tinnitus

Among research studies that specifically assessed coping outcomes, several older studies indicated the following associations of coping in the context of tinnitus: (a) individuals with depression used significantly less problem-focused coping strategies among than those without depression (Sullivan et al., 1988); (b) non-adaptive and passive coping factors were significantly and positively correlated with anxiety, depression, and self-reported tinnitus severity, while the effective coping factor was significantly and inversely correlated with anxiety (Budd & Pugh, 1996); and (c) non-adaptive coping showed significant differences among four groups (depression-only, anxiety-only, anxiety-plus-depression, or no symptoms; Bartels et al., 2008), with the anxiety-plus-depression group exhibiting the highest level of non-adaptive coping.

Kröner-Herwig and colleagues (1995) created TCT, a CBT-based intervention, which included progressive relaxation training, diverting attention from tinnitus, and non-adaptive changing thoughts. While they called it a coping intervention, they did not specifically assess coping in their first study using TCT. In subsequent research, Kröner-Herwig et al. (2003) revised the TCT and assessed coping by using four items taken from Frenzel's Tinnitus Coping Questionnaire (TCQ) (Frenzel & Kröner-Herwig, 1997). The results indicated that the TCT group had significantly greater improvement of coping compared to two minimal contact groups and a wait-list control group. In a different study using TCT, Zachriat and Kröner-Herwig (2004) conducted a longitudinal study that compared two treatment groups (an 11-session TCT group or a 5-session habituation group) and a control group (receiving one session containing only education). Coping was again measured by Frenzel's (1997) TCQ. The two treatment groups reported significantly less tinnitus-related disability than the control group. When comparing the two treatment groups on coping outcomes, the TCT group reported a significantly greater use of coping strategies than the habituation group.

Henry and Wilson (1996) conducted a randomized controlled trial (RCT) on coping among 60 individuals with tinnitus. They compared three groups: (a) a treatment group involving a psychoeducational program that they called "cognitive coping skills training" (including CBT skills, such as attention diversion, imagery training, and thought-management skills) plus tinnitus education; (b) an education-only treatment group; and (c) a wait-list control group. They used their Tinnitus Coping Strategy Questionnaire (TCSQ) instrument to assess coping outcomes. The results indicated that there were no significant differences on coping when comparing the two treatment groups, but the two treatment groups had significant improvements on coping compared to the control group. A 12-month follow-up study indicated that the findings between the two treatments and the control group were no longer significantly different on coping.

CET (Chesney et al., 2003) is a coping intervention that evolved out of Lazarus and Folkman's (1984) model on stress and coping. CET teaches individuals to distinguish between changeable and unchangeable stress and how to select the most appropriate type of coping strategy according to the type of stress. CET has been adapted for tinnitus (Martz et al., in preparation). CET for tinnitus provides three psychoeducational sessions in which individuals learn how to distinguish between what is modifiable (e.g., their sound environments), what tinnitus-related issues are unmodifiable (e.g., the fact of having tinnitus), and how to choose coping strategies (e.g., problem-solving or stress-reduction strategies) that are appropriate for the type of stressor. Martz's CET for tinnitus protocol included the three core self-management components: (a) education about the health condition (tinnitus) and its treatment (e.g., effective sound enrichment techniques), (b) teaching problem-solving skills, and (c) teaching stress-management skills.

Other Stress-Management Interventions

Numerous clinical interventions have been created to help individuals adapt better to their tinnitus. Some studies do not assess coping outcomes, that is, the coping skills that are typically defined as coping by the scientific literature (Martz & Livneh, 2007; Zeidner & Endler, 1996). CBT has been one of the most frequently studied psychological approaches for tinnitus (Henry & Wilson, 2001; Martinez Devesa, Waddell, Perera, & Theodoulou, 2010). CBT interventions focus on helping individuals to identify and modify unhelpful thoughts and beliefs about tinnitus and to use relaxation techniques to alter their emotional states. While CBT helps individuals manage their tinnitus-related and general distress by teaching relaxation techniques, one of the main focal points of CBT is on changing the content of one's "distorted" thinking.

Another type of psychological intervention, ACT, has been used to help individuals manage their reactions to tinnitus. ACT is categorized as a mindfulness-based intervention for tinnitus (see the next section for a meta-analysis of mindfulness-based approaches for tinnitus). ACT is an approach that teaches "psychological flexibility" (Hayes, Levin, Plumb-Vilardaga, Villatte, & Pistorello, 2013; Hayes, Strosahl, & Wilson, 2011). ACT uses mindfulness approaches to teach individuals how to reduce their avoidance of distressing thoughts and emotions. The mindfulness techniques are taught in a way to help individuals increase their acceptance of their internal experiences, which can include thoughts, emotions, and even tinnitus. ACT differs from CBT in that ACT focuses on teaching a *process* of managing internal experiences, while CBT focuses on helping individuals change the *content* of their thoughts.

Westin et al. (2011) compared ACT to TRT and a wait-list control group. Their findings indicated that at 18 months posttreatment, participants in the ACT group had lower tinnitus-related distress than the TRT group. A different research study (Hesser et al., 2012) compared two self-help Internet treatments based on ACT and CBT. At 8-weeks, both ACT and CBT groups exhibited significant decreases in tinnitus distress (as measured by the Tinnitus Handicap Inventory) when compared to a control group. Based on their findings, the researchers suggested that an ACT intervention may be a "viable alternative" to CBT for helping individuals to manage their tinnitus. However, the clinical practice guidelines for tinnitus (Tunkel et al., 2014) lists CBT as the recommended psychological intervention for tinnitus at this time.

META-ANALYSES OF PSYCHOLOGICAL INTERVENTIONS

Numerous meta-analyses have been conducted on the efficacy of psychological interventions for tinnitus. One of the first meta-analyses was conducted by Andersson and Lyttkens (1999). These researchers examined the results of 18 empirical studies that included CBT, relaxation, hypnosis, biofeedback, educational sessions, and problem-solving interventions. They concluded that CBT was more effective in reducing participants' ratings of tinnitus annoyance than tinnitus loudness. In this meta-analysis, a medium effect size was found for CBT on negative affect (i.e., depression and anxiety).

A second meta-analysis was conducted by Martinez-Devesa and colleagues (2010), who provided a Cochrane review and meta-analysis on eight CBT interventions for tinnitus. They found that across the studies that they analyzed, CBT decreased tinnitus severity (i.e., subjective loudness of tinnitus) and depression while increasing quality of life.

A third meta-analysis was conducted by Hesser, Weise, Westin, and Andersson (2011), who conducted a meta-analysis of 15 studies of CBT interventions for tinnitus. Their meta-analysis indicated that there were statistically significant mean effect sizes for CBT interventions when compared to passive control groups (Hedges's $g = .70$) and active control groups (Hedges's $g = .44$) on tinnitus measures. Further, they found that CBT was moderately effective in reducing mood (i.e., anxiety and depression) and that the effects of 10 CBT interventions were robust over a 3- to 18-month time period. Hesser and colleagues cautioned that if CBT was delivered by audiologists, new research would be required to determine the efficacy of audiologist-delivered CBT programs for tinnitus.

A fourth meta-analysis was conducted by Hoare, Kowalkowski, Kang, and Hall (2011). Their systematic review included 28 RCTs for management for adults with tinnitus. According to the authors, only CBT RCTs were comparable and thus, 11 CBT RCTs were included in the meta-analysis. Their findings indicated that across the CBT studies, CBT did not appear to be effective in reducing depression and anxiety among individuals with tinnitus; however, CBT was associated with reductions in self-reported tinnitus severity. Hoare and colleagues (2011) noted that one problem in their meta-analysis of CBT interventions was that these studies utilized an assortment of procedures and techniques that were provided under the auspices of CBT.

A fifth meta-analysis was conducted by Nyenhuis, Golm, and Kröner-Herwig (2013), which focused on self-help interventions that had little or no therapist interaction. It analyzed data from 10 self-help CBT interventions for tinnitus, including Internet-based interventions and bibliotherapy (i.e., self-help book or manual). The self-help interventions were compared to face-to-face group interventions (involving therapist contact) and "passive" controls, which included wait-list or information-only groups or discussion forums. The results indicated that the self-help groups exhibited lower tinnitus distress (moderate effect) and lower depression (small effect) compared to the passive control groups. Further, there were no differences between the self-help groups and face-to-face group interventions on tinnitus distress or depression, suggesting that "self-help interventions with little or no therapist contact are as efficacious as face-to-face interventions" (Nyenhuis et al., 2013, p. 165), which is similar to findings of other meta-analyses comparing self-help versus therapist-led interventions.

Two more meta-analyses are noteworthy, and even though neither focused solely on tinnitus studies, they can help inform researchers on what kinds of interventions influence mental health outcomes. A sixth meta-analysis contained 16 studies (Ruiz, 2012). The researchers examined the outcomes and change processes in both ACT and CBT. According to these researchers, the mean effect sizes indicated that ACT was significantly more efficacious than CBT on primary outcome measures of depression and quality of life but not anxiety.

A seventh meta-analysis (Spijkerman, Pots, & Bohlmeijer, 2016) consisted of an examination of 15 mindfulness-based interventions, including ACT, Dialectical Behavior Therapy, and mindfulness-based stress reduction (one intervention was for individuals with tinnitus). The results indicated that mindfulness-based interventions exhibited significant effects on the primary outcomes of depression (small effect), anxiety (small effect), well-being (small effect), and stress (moderate effect).

A comparative effectiveness review of scientific studies on treatments for tinnitus (Pichora-Fuller et al., 2013) stated that it was difficult to make conclusions about psychological interventions for tinnitus because of the use of different populations and treatment components, length of study and of follow-up assessments, and outcome measures. The researchers concluded that there was insufficient research to provide summaries of the overall strength of evidence for psychological interventions for tinnitus. This conclusion should *not* be viewed as a statement that psychological interventions do not help individuals with tinnitus; on the contrary, there is evidence that these interventions are effective in reducing distressing reactions to tinnitus. However, more research is required before conclusions can be made about what kind of psychological intervention is the best for helping which kinds of individuals to manage their reactions to tinnitus.

BARRIERS TO SELF-MANAGEMENT OF TINNITUS

Social and environmental factors that may impede an individual in his or her self-management efforts with tinnitus can include issues related to personal resources and social support. Individuals with tinnitus may not have the individual resources (e.g., they may lack transportation or finances to pay for medical care) to obtain tinnitus-related assessment and treatment. Further, lack of personal resources may inhibit individuals from seeking peer support (e.g., in-person, peer-support groups or online support groups through forums or chat rooms). Further, family members may not understand tinnitus or know how to help their family member who has tinnitus. Yet advances in mobile technology (see next section) may help to circumvent some of the barriers that individuals experience when trying to access help for tinnitus.

Individuals with tinnitus may receive disability compensation. For example, tinnitus is currently is the most prevalent service-connected disability in the US Veterans Administration; most of these veterans receive monthly compensation (Veterans Benefits Administration, 2015). While disability compensation can provide some financial relief to individuals with tinnitus, they may not receive needed rehabilitation support, which may could them return to work or to reintegrate into the community (e.g., after returning from a warzone). Further, disability compensation may decrease recipients' motivation in returning to work or may reinforce their perspective that they cannot work while experiencing tinnitus.

OTHER TESTED APPROACHES THAT FACILITATE SELF-MANAGEMENT OF TINNITUS

Research indicates that Internet-based interventions, also known as "e-Health" interventions (Eysenbach, 2004; Strecher, 2007), can be effective means of intervening on health behaviors and can be as efficacious as in-person tinnitus interventions (Nyenhuis et al., 2013). Numerous studies have been conducted using e-Health programs to encourage the self-management of a variety of health conditions (Lorig et al., 2013).

In a systematic review of self-help (i.e., at one's own time and pace), Beatty and Lambert (2013) found that Internet-based interventions, including ones for tinnitus, provided clear indications of improvements in reducing indices of stress. They also reviewed evidence that suggested that therapist-moderated forums are not necessary, although these are commonly used.

E-health interventions have many advantages over in-person visits, including less clinicians' time required, alleviating transportation and travel time for individuals receiving the treatment at specialized centers, permitting individuals to work at their own pace and at times most convenient for them, and eliminating the need to schedule appointments (Brief et al., 2013; Cuijpers, Van Straten, & Andersson, 2008). Other advantages include reducing long waiting lists and increasing the convenience and ease of treatment access, increasing a sense of confidentiality, and reducing perceived stigma related to going to treatment centers (Marks, Cavanagh, & Gega, 2007). Brief and colleagues (2013) noted that Internet interventions can circumvent the problem of living in remote or rural areas and the problem of not having access to specialized treatment centers (e.g., in this case, to a tinnitus specialty clinic, which can occur even in urban areas).

Further, for individuals with auditory-related issues (e.g., tinnitus with hearing loss), web-based interventions that use written or transcribed oral materials with accompanying visuals can help to provide information more understandably and efficiently than what can be provided at an in-person meeting. The broad accessibility of computer-assisted therapies (Kiluk et al., 2011) can facilitate the availability of resources that otherwise may be difficult to access if a person has tinnitus plus other health issues that restrict mobility. Some research noted that e-Health interventions are more cost-effective than in-person treatment (Beatty & Lambert, 2013). Greenwell, Featherstone, and Hoare (2015) suggested that self-help interventions (i.e., self-guided without therapist intervention) provide some benefits over face-to-face psychological therapy in that self-help interventions can allow individuals work through therapeutic materials at their own pace and chosen time. Greenwell and colleagues also noted that Internet-based health interventions can reach a much larger audience compared to face-to-face psychotherapeutic interventions.

Numerous tinnitus interventions, such as Hesser's (2012) previously mentioned study, have been conducted using Internet-based interventions. Andersson (2015) conducted meta-analyses to examine six controlled trials that utilized an Internet-based psychological treatment for tinnitus. When compared against a control condition, Internet-based treatments exhibited a moderate effect size. Further, when compared against in-person group treatments, the Internet-based treatments reflected a small, non-significant difference in effect size, suggesting that both modalities may be effective in helping people with their reactions to tinnitus.

None of the research published to date on tinnitus interventions, however, examines a self-management program that is delivered by using mobile health (known as "m-Health"; Istepanian, Laxminarayan, & Pattichis, 2006). Research on m-Health interventions is emerging, although it is behind the rapid advances in technology (Istepanian et al., 2006; Olff, 2015; Price et al., 2014). Numerous m-Health applications have been created to help individuals with sound therapy for tinnitus, tinnitus matching, or masking (Paglialonga, Tognola, & Pinciroli, 2015), but, to date, none are presented as a multicomponent self-management program.

Two sets of researchers commented on the usefulness of e-Health, which is also applicable to m-Health. Reger and Gahm (2009) emphasized that e-Health therapy can be used in stepped-care models, providing the first line of care to individuals who need assistance with their health impairments. Beatty and Lambert (2013) concluded that online therapeutic interventions "should form the entry-level first step that can be accessed by the majority therefore freeing up face-to-face services for those requiring more intensive assistance" (p. 621). A tinnitus m-Health or e-Health self-management program can serve as a front-line intervention that could be broadly distributed to individuals who are seeking immediate help and relief for their tinnitus.

CONCLUSION

The research on treatments for tinnitus has been rapidly expanding in the past few decades. While the professional consensus is that the evidence for tinnitus treatment options is limited (Landgrebe et al., 2012; Tunkel et al., 2014), healthcare professionals and researchers have been advocating for better quality clinical trials to provide stronger evidence. As better empirical studies are published, information can be provided on what types of interventions help individuals to better adapt and function with tinnitus. Further, better scientific evidence will help to improve interdisciplinary interventions, such as those containing audiological education, use of sound enrichment and sound therapy, and psychoeducational interventions, in order to encourage self-management of tinnitus. Finally, research is compiling that indicates that e-Health and m-Health interventions are as efficacious as in-person interventions, suggesting that effective tinnitus interventions may soon be more accessible to those who have barriers to accessing in-person healthcare.

ACKNOWLEDGEMENT

Thanks are due to Gerhard Andersson for providing feedback on earlier versions of this chapter.

REFERENCES

Andersson, G. (2015). Clinician-supported Internet-delivered psychological treatment of tinnitus. *American Journal of Audiology, 24*(3), 299–301.

Andersson, G., & Lyttkens, L. (1999). A meta-analytic review of psychological treatments for tinnitus. *British Journal of Audiology, 33*, 201–210.

Baguley, D., McFerran, D., & Hall, D. (2013). Tinnitus. *The Lancet, 382*(9904), 1600–1607.

Bartels, H., Middel, B. L., van der Laan, B. F., Staal, M. J., & Albers, F. W. (2008). The additive effect of co-occurring anxiety and depression on health status, quality of life and coping strategies in help-seeking tinnitus sufferers. *Ear and Hearing, 29*(6), 947–956.

Beatty, L., & Lambert, S. (2013). A systematic review of Internet-based self-help therapeutic interventions to improve distress and disease-control among adults with chronic health conditions. *Clinical Psychology Review, 33*(4), 609–622.

Bhatt, J. M., Bhattacharyya, N., & Lin, H. W. (2016). Relationships between tinnitus and the prevalence of anxiety and depression. *The Laryngoscope, 127*(2), 466–469.

Bhatt, J. M., Lin, H. W., & Bhattacharyya, N. (2016). Prevalence, severity, exposures, and treatment patterns of tinnitus in the United States. *JAMA Otolaryngology—Head & Neck Surgery, 142*(10), 959–965.

Brief, D. J., Rubin, A., Keane, T. M., Enggasser, J. L., Roy, M., Helmuth, E., . . . Rosenbloom, D. (2013). Web intervention for OEF/OIF veterans with problem drinking and PTSD symptoms: A randomized clinical trial. *Journal of Consulting and Clinical Psychology, 81*(5), 890–900.

Budd, R. J., & Pugh, R. (1996). Tinnitus coping style and its relationship to tinnitus severity and emotional distress. *Journal of Psychosomatic Research, 41*(4), 327–335.

Cave, K., Cornish, E., & Chandler, D. (2007). Blast injury of the ear: Clinical update from the global war on terror. *Military Medicine, 172*(7), 726–730.

Chesney, M., Chambers, D., Taylor, J., Johnson, L., & Folkman, S. (2003). Coping effectiveness training for men living with HIV: Results from a randomized clinical trial testing a group-based intervention. *Psychosomatic Medicine, 65*(6), 1038–1046.

Cima, R., Joore, M., Maes, I., Scheyen, D., Refaie, A., Baguley, D., . . . Anteunis, L. (2009). Cost-effectiveness of multidisciplinary management of tinnitus at a specialized tinnitus centre. *BMC Health Services Research, 9*(1), 1–8.

Cima, R., Maes, I., Joore, M., Scheyen, D., El Refaie, A., Baguley, D., . . . Vlaeyen, J. (2012). Specialised treatment based on cognitive behaviour therapy versus usual care for tinnitus: A randomised controlled trial. *The Lancet, 379*(9830), 1951–1959.

Cuijpers, P., Van Straten, A., & Andersson, G. (2008). Internet-administered cognitive behavior therapy for health problems: A systematic review. *Journal of Behavioral Medicine, 31*(2), 169–177.

Deshaies, P., Gonzales, Z., Zenner, H., Plontke, S., Paré, L., Hébert, S., . . . Zalaman, I. (2005). *Quantifying burden of disease from environmental noise: Second technical meeting report*. Geneva: World Health Organization.

Eggermont, J. J. (2012). Tinnitus. In A. Palmer & A. Rees (Eds.), *oxford handbook of auditory science* (pp. 543–560). Oxford: Oxford University Press.

Erlandsson, S., & Hallberg, L. R. (2000). Prediction of quality of life in patients with tinnitus. *British Journal of Audiology, 34*(1), 11–19.

Eysenbach, G. (2004). Improving the quality of web surveys: The Checklist for Reporting Results of Internet E-Surveys (CHERRIES). *Journal of Medical Internet Research, 6*(3), e34.

Fausti, S. A., Wilmington, D. J., Gallun, F. J., Myers, P. J., & Henry, J. A. (2009). Auditory and vestibular dysfunction associated with blast-related traumatic brain injury. *Journal of Rehabilitation Research and Development, 46*(6), 797–810.

Frenzel, A., & Kröner-Herwig, B. (1997). Die Behandlung von chronischem Tinnitus mit psychologisch fundierten Verfahren: Ein Überblick. In *Psychologische Behandlung des chronischen Tinnitus: Psychologie Verlags Union, Weinheim* (pp. 22–31). Berlin: Deutschland.

Geocze, L., Mucci, S., Abranches, D. C., de Marco, M. A., & de Oliveira Penido, N. (2013). Systematic review on the evidences of an association between tinnitus and depression. *Brazilian Journal of Otorhinolaryngology, 79*(1), 106–111.

Greenwell, K., Featherstone, D., & Hoare, D. J. (2015). The application of intervention coding methodology to describe the Tinnitus E-Programme, an Internet-delivered self-help intervention for tinnitus. *American Journal of Audiology, 24*(3), 311–315.

Harrop-Griffiths, J., Katon, W., Dobie, R., Sakai, C., & Russo, J. (1987). Chronic tinnitus: Association with psychiatric diagnoses. *Journal of Psychosomatic Research, 31*(5), 613–621.

Hayes, S., Levin, M., Plumb-Vilardaga, J., Villatte, J., & Pistorello, J. (2013). Acceptance and commitment therapy and contextual behavioral science: Examining the progress of a distinctive model of behavioral and cognitive therapy. *Behavior Therapy, 44*(2), 180–198.

Hayes, S., Strosahl, K., & Wilson, K. (2011). *Acceptance and commitment therapy: The process and practice of mindful change.* New York: Guilford Press.

Henry, J., Frederick, M., Sell, S., Griest, S., & Abrams, H. (2015). Validation of a novel combination hearing aid and tinnitus therapy device. *Ear and Hearing, 36*(1), 42–52.

Henry, J., Schechter, M., Zaugg, T., Griest, S., Jastreboff, P., Vernon, J., . . . Stewart, B. (2006). Clinical trial to compare tinnitus masking and tinnitus retraining therapy. *Acta Oto-Laryngologica, 556,* 64–69.

Henry, J. A., Loovis, C., Montero, M., Kaelin, C., Anselmi, K. A., Coombs, R., . . . James, K. (2007). Randomized clinical trial: Group counseling based on tinnitus retraining therapy. *Journal of Rehabilitation Research and Development, 44*(1), 21–32.

Henry, J. A., Schechter, M., Loovis, C., Zaugg, T., Kaelin, C., & Montero, M. (2005). Clinical management of tinnitus using a "progressive intervention" approach. *Journal of Rehabilitation Research and Development, 42*(4 Suppl. 2), 95–116.

Henry, J. A., Zaugg, T. L., Myers, P. M., & Kendall, C. J. (2010). *Progressive tinnitus management: Clinical handbook for audiologists.* San Diego, CA: Plural Publishing.

Henry, J. A., Zaugg, T. L., Myers, P. J., & Schechter, M. A. (2008). Using therapeutic sound with progressive audiologic tinnitus management. *Trends in Amplification, 12*(3), 185–206.

Henry, J. L., & Wilson, P. H. (1996). The psychological management of tinnitus: Comparison of a combined cognitive educational program, education alone and a waiting-list control. *International Tinnitus Journal, 2,* 9–20.

Henry, J. L., & Wilson, P. H. (2001). *The psychological management of chronic tinnitus.* Needham Heights, MA: Allyn & Bacon.

Hesser, H., Gustafsson, T., Lundén, C., Henrikson, O., Fattahi, K., Johnsson, E., . . . Kaldo, V. (2012). A randomized controlled trial of Internet-delivered cognitive behavior therapy and acceptance and commitment therapy in the treatment of tinnitus. *Journal of Consulting and Clinical Psychology, 80*(4), 649–661.

Hesser, H., Weise, C., Westin, V. Z., & Andersson, G. (2011). A systematic review and meta-analysis of randomized controlled trials of cognitive–behavioral therapy for tinnitus distress. *Clinical Psychology Review, 31*(4), 545–553.

Hoare, D., Edmondson-Jones, M., Sereda, M., Akeroyd, M., & Hall, D. (2014). Amplification with hearing aids for patients with tinnitus and co-existing hearing loss. *Cochrane Database of Systematic Reviews, 1,* CD010151. doi:10.1002/14651858.CD010151.pub2

Hoare, D., Kowalkowski, V., Kang, S., & Hall, D. (2011). Systematic review and meta-analyses of randomized controlled trials examining tinnitus management. *The Laryngoscope, 121*(7), 1555–1564.

Hobson, J., Chisholm, E., & El Refaie, A. (2012). Sound therapy (masking) in the management of tinnitus in adults. *Cochrane Database of Systematic Reviews, 11,* CD006371.

Istepanian, R., Laxminarayan, S., & Pattichis, C. S. (2006). *M-health.* New York: Springer.

Jacobson, G. P., & McCaslin, D. L. (2001). A search for evidence of a direct relationship between tinnitus and suicide. *Journal of the American Academy of Audiology, 12*(10), 493–496.

Jastreboff, P. (2011). Tinnitus retraining therapy. In *Textbook of tinnitus*. Edited by A. R. Møller, B. Langguth, D. Ridder, & T. Kleinjung (pp. 575–596). New York: Springer.

Jastreboff, P., & Jastreboff, M. (2000). Tinnitus retraining therapy (TRT) as a method for treatment of tinnitus and hyperacusis patients. *Journal of the American Academy of Audiology, 11*, 162–177.

Kiluk, B. D., Sugarman, D. E., Nich, C., Gibbons, C. J., Martino, S., Rounsaville, B. J., & Carroll, K. M. (2011). A methodological analysis of randomized clinical trials of computer-assisted therapies for psychiatric disorders: Toward improved standards for an emerging field. *The American Journal of Psychiatry, 168*(8), 790–799.

Kreuzer, P. M., Vielsmeier, V., & Langguth, B. (2013). Chronic tinnitus: An interdisciplinary challenge. *Deutsches Ärzteblatt International, 110*(16), 278–284.

Krog, N., Engdahl, B., & Tambs, K. (2010). The association between tinnitus and mental health in a general population sample: Results from the HUNT Study. *Journal of Psychosomatic Research, 69*(3), 289–298.

Kroner-Herwig, B., Frenzel, A., Fritsche, G., Schilkowsky, G., & Esser, G. (2003). The management of chronic tinnitus: Comparison of an outpatient cognitive-behavioral group training to minimal-contact interventions. *Journal of Psychosomatic Research, 54*(4), 381–389.

Kroner-Herwig, B., Hebing, G., van Rijn-Kalkmann, U., Frenzel, A., Schilkowsky, G., & Esser, G. (1995). The management of chronic tinnitus: Comparison of a cognitive-behavioural group training with yoga. *Journal of Psychosomatic Research, 39*(2), 153–165.

Landgrebe, M., Azevedo, A., Baguley, D., Bauer, C., Cacace, A., Coelho, C., . . . Hajak, G. (2012). Methodological aspects of clinical trials in tinnitus: A proposal for an international standard. *Journal of Psychosomatic Research, 73*(2), 112–121.

Langguth, B., Kreuzer, P. M., Kleinjung, T., & De Ridder, D. (2013). Tinnitus: Causes and clinical management. *The Lancet Neurology, 12*(9), 920–930.

Langguth, B., Landgrebe, M., Kleinjung, T., Sand, G. P., & Hajak, G. (2011). Tinnitus and depression. *The World Journal of Biological Psychiatry, 12*(7), 489–500.

Lazarus, R., & Folkman, S. (1984). *Stress, coping, and adaptation*. New York: Springer.

Lewis, J. (2002). Tinnitus and suicide. *Journal of the American Academy of Audiology, 13*(6), 339–341.

Lorig, K., Ritter, P. L., Plant, K., Laurent, D. D., Kelly, P., & Rowe, S. (2013). The South Australia health chronic disease self-management Internet trial. *Health Education & Behavior, 40*(1), 67–77.

Maes, I., Cima, R., Anteunis, L., Scheijen, D., Baguley, D., El Refaie, A., . . . Joore, M. (2014). Cost-effectiveness of specialized treatment based on cognitive behavioral therapy versus usual care for tinnitus. *Otology & Neurotology, 35*(5), 787–795.

Marks, I., Cavanagh, K., & Gega, L. (2007). Computer-aided psychotherapy: Revolution or bubble? *The British Journal of Psychiatry, 191*(6), 471–473.

Martinez Devesa, P., Waddell, A., Perera, R., & Theodoulou, M. (2010). Cognitive behavioural therapy for tinnitus. *Cochrane Database of Systematic Reviews, 9*, CD005233.

Martz, E., Jelleberg, C. E., Chesney, M., Livneh, H., Fuller, B., & Henry, J. (in preparation). A randomized clinical trial comparing three psychoeducational group interventions for individuals with tinnitus.

Martz, E., & Livneh, H. (2007). *Coping with chronic illness and disability*. New York: Springer.

McCormack, A., Edmondson-Jones, M., Fortnum, H., Dawes, P., Middleton, H., Munro, K., & Moore, D. (2014). Investigating the association between tinnitus severity and symptoms of depression and anxiety, while controlling for neuroticism, in a large middle-aged UK population. *International Journal of Audiology, 54*(9), 599–604.

Møller, A. R., Langguth, B., DeRidder, D., & Kleinjung, T. (2010). *Textbook of tinnitus*: New York: Springer.

Nondahl, D., Cruickshanks, K., Huang, G., Klein, B., Klein, R., Nieto, & Tweed, T. (2011). Tinnitus and its risk factors in the Beaver Dam Offspring Study. *International Journal of Audiology, 50*(5), 313–320. doi:10.3109/14992027.2010.551220

Nyenhuis, N., Golm, D., & Kröner-Herwig, B. (2013). A systematic review and meta-analysis on the efficacy of self-help interventions in tinnitus. *Cognitive Behaviour Therapy, 42*(2), 159–169.

Olff, M. (2015). Mobile mental health: A challenging research agenda. *European Journal of Psychotraumatology, 6*, 27882.

Paglialonga, A., Tognola, G., & Pinciroli, F. (2015). Apps for hearing science and care. *American Journal of Audiology, 24*(3), 293–298.

Phillips, J., & McFerran, D. (2010). Tinnitus retraining therapy (TRT) for tinnitus. *Cochrane Database of Systematic Reviews, 3*. doi:10.1002/14651858.CD007330.pub2

Pichora-Fuller, M., Santaguida, P., Hammill, A., Oremus, M., Westerberg, B., Ali, U., . . . Raina, P. (2013). *Evaluation and treatment of tinnitus: Comparative effectiveness*. Retrieved from http://www.ncbi.nlm.nih.gov/books/NBK158963/

Pinto, P., Marcelos, C., Mezzasalma, M., Osterne, F., de Lima, M. D. M. T., & Nardi, A. (2014). Tinnitus and its association with psychiatric disorders: Systematic review. *The Journal of Laryngology & Otology, 128*(8), 660–664.

Price, M., Yuen, E. K., Goetter, E. M., Herbert, J. D., Forman, E. M., Acierno, R., & Ruggiero, K. J. (2014). mHealth: A mechanism to deliver more accessible, more effective mental health care. *Clinical Psychology & Psychotherapy, 21*(5), 427–436.

Pridmore, S., Walter, G., & Friedland, P. (2012). Tinnitus and suicide recent cases on the public record give cause for reconsideration. *Otolaryngology—Head and Neck Surgery, 147*(2), 193–195.

Reger, M. A., & Gahm, G. A. (2009). A meta-analysis of the effects of Internet-and computer-based cognitive-behavioral treatments for anxiety. *Journal of Clinical Psychology, 65*(1), 53–75.

Ruiz, F. (2012). Acceptance and commitment therapy versus traditional cognitive behavioral therapy: A systematic review and meta-analysis of current empirical evidence. *International Journal of Psychology & Psychological Therapy, 12*(2), 333–357.

Ruth, R., & Hamill-Ruth, R. (2001). A multidisciplinary approach to management of tinnitus and hyperacusis. *The Hearing Journal, 54*(11), 26–33.

Seo, J. H., Kang, J. M., Hwang, S. H., Han, K. D., & Joo, Y. H. (2016). Relationship between tinnitus and suicidal behaviour in Korean men and women: A cross-sectional study. *Clinical Otolaryngology, 41*(3), 222–227. doi: 10.1111/coa.12500

Spijkerman, M. P. J., Pots, W. T. M., & Bohlmeijer, E. T. (2016). Effectiveness of online mindfulness-based interventions in improving mental health: A review and meta-analysis of randomised controlled trials. *Clinical Psychology Review, 45*, 102–114.

Strecher, V. (2007). Internet methods for delivering behavioral and health-related interventions (eHealth). *Annual Review of Clinical Psychology, 3,* 53–76.

Sullivan, M., Katon, W., Dobie, R., Sakai, C., Russo, J., & Harrop-Griffiths, J. (1988). Disabling tinnitus: Association with affective disorder. *General Hospital Psychiatry, 10,* 285–291.

Sullivan, M., Katon, W., Russo, J., Dobie, R., & Sakai, C. (1993). A randomized trial of nortriptyline for severe chronic tinnitus: Effects on depression, disability, and tinnitus symptoms. *Archives of Internal Medicine, 153*(19), 2251–2259.

Tunkel, D. E., Bauer, C. A., Sun, G. H., Rosenfeld, R. M., Chandrasekhar, S. S., Cunningham, E. R. Jr., ... Whamond, E. J. (2014). Clinical practice guideline: Tinnitus. *Otolaryngology—Head and Neck Surgery, 151*(2 Suppl.), S1–S40. doi:10.1177/0194599814545325

Veterans Benefits Administration. (2015). *VBA annual report.* Washington, DC: Author.

Westin, V. Z., Schulin, M., Hesser, H., Karlsson, M., Noe, R. Z., Olofsson, U., ... Andersson, G. (2011). Acceptance and commitment therapy versus tinnitus retraining therapy in the treatment of tinnitus: A randomised controlled trial. *Behaviour Research and Therapy, 49*(11), 737–747.

Yurgil, K., Clifford, R., Risbrough, V., Geyer, M., Huang, M., Barkauskas, D., ... Team, M. (2016). Prospective associations between traumatic brain injury and postdeployment tinnitus in active-duty Marines. *The Journal of Head Trauma Rehabilitation, 31*(1), 30–39.

Zachriat, C., & Kroner-Herwig, B. (2004). Treating chronic tinnitus: Comparison of cognitive-behavioural and habituation-based treatments. *Cognitive and Behavioral Therapy, 33*(4), 187–198.

Zeidner, M., & Endler, N. S. (Eds.). (1996). *Handbook of coping: Theory, research, applications* (Vol. 195). New York: John Wiley.

19

Self-Management of Vision Impairments

VICKI BLAIR DRURY, AI TEE AW, AND PRISCILLA SHIOW HUEY LIM ■

INTRODUCTION

Changes in population demographics globally have resulted in aging communities, and non-infectious conditions, particularly long-term conditions, have become major public health challenges. Vision impairments are often neglected in contemporary discussions about long-term conditions, which tend to focus on cardiovascular conditions, cancers, and neurological disorders. In common with other neglected chronic conditions, vision impairment is a condition that is often associated with the elderly, is not obvious to others, and may be associated with poorer overall health status (Centers for Disease Control and Prevention, 2011).

With vision loss cited as being among the top 10 disabilities and often underreported prevalence rates (Bourne et al., 2013; Dandona & Dandona, 2006), it is indeed an issue of concern and a challenge for healthcare professionals. Saaddine et al. (2003) has proposed five criteria that support vision impairment being a public health issue (Table 19.1). There is a plethora of evidence to support these criteria as clearly demonstrating that vision impairment is a public health issue that should be addressed at a community and public health level.

It has been suggested that refractive correction and screening of older adults may minimize risks associated with vision impairment due to eye conditions (Chou et al., 2013); however, with aging populations and increasing longevity, the global prevalence of vision impairment will only increase.

Visual Impairment and Low Vision

Classifications of visual impairment and low vision are less well defined than that of blindness. The terms are often used interchangeably, resulting in confusion. Low

Table 19.1. Functional Limitations of People with Low Vision with Common Everyday Examples

Functional Limitation	Practical Examples
Personal grooming	Difficulty with • matching clothes • tying shoelaces/doing up shoes • shaving • doing hair • applying make-up • discriminating between shampoo/conditioner/body wash
Reading	Challenges reading • mail • the numbers on a telephone • labels when shopping • numbers on banknotes or coins • the temperature on the oven or the markers on the stove
Writing	Difficulty signing forms, writing letters, or addressing envelopes
Walking	Difficulties • seeing traffic properly • reading street signs or house number • identifying obstacles, such as surface changes in footpaths or small branches
Driving	Some, but not all, countries allow driving with bioptic telescopic lens (Owsley, 2012). The loss of a driver's licence may affect a person's independence and may result in difficulties such as • shopping • getting to medical appointments • socializing
Space perception: difficulty with depth perception making movement and orientation to the environment challenging	For example, may • feel unsafe when driving • have trouble navigating new routes • forget where they left their keys or parked the car
Form perception: difficulty distinguishing differences in sizes and shapes of objects	• Difficulties distinguishing faces or facial features • Difficulty recognizing objects when they are in a different orientation or format

(*continued*)

Table 19.1. Continued

Functional Limitation	Practical Examples
Depth perception: inability to view the world in three dimensions and determine the distance of an object	Difficulties with • stairs and uneven ground • determining distances between objects and seeing the world in three dimensions • performing normal tasks, such as driving or reading • learning difficulties (in children)
Color discrimination: inability to distinguish and differentiate colors	May not • know if food is properly cooked • know if fruit is ripe • be able to read LED displays • be able to work in some professions (pilots, electricians)
Visual field loss: certain areas within the normal visual field are loss and are either blank or fuzzy	• May bump into objects • Car accidents • Knocking an object over when reaching for something • Difficulty reading • Inability to recognize faces
Night vision deficit The inability to see in low light environments.	• Light distortion • Halos around lights • Difficulty with driving at night • Slow adaptation from bright to darker conditions

vision has often been classified according to the severity of loss of visual acuity, that is, the clarity of vision. However, in certain conditions, such as glaucoma and macular degeneration, the clarity of remaining vision may be good but the loss of vision in the visual field limits the person's ability to function. Individuals with low vision have some residual vision and light perception, but their vision cannot be improved by refraction and glasses or medical or surgical treatment. For these people, appropriate low-vision services have the potential to maximize remaining functional vision.

Globally, visual impairment is classified according to the criteria specified in the International Classification of Diseases (ICD) 10th revision (1st and 2nd editions). The ICD-10 classification defines low vision as corresponding to visual acuity of less than 6/18 (20/60), but equal to or better than 3/60 (20/400), and/or a visual field of less than 20 degrees in the best eye with correction. In addition, the ICD-10 describes four levels of visual functioning:

I. Normal vision
II. Moderate visual impairment
III. Severe visual impairment
IV. Blindness

Levels II and III are grouped together as low vision and together with Level IV represent all visual impairment (World Health Organization, 2012). Therefore, "low vision" is a term that is used to describe functionality rather than a numerical test result (e.g., Snellen or LogMar results).

The Global Burden of Vision Impairment

A systematic review of surveys across 39 countries estimated that there are 285 million people visually impaired with 39 million of these meeting the criteria for legally blind; 65% of all people with a visual impairment are over the age of 50 years, and more than 80% of those classified as blind are over the age of 50 (Royal National Institue for the Blind, 2015). Of major concern is the finding that preventable causes, such as uncorrected refractive errors and cataracts, are responsible for as many as 80% of all visual impairments. Although it is not surprising, countries with lower socioeconomic profiles, such as India, China, and Indonesia, have larger numbers of people with visual impairments. Other studies have found that low vision or blindness affects 1 in 28 people in the United States (Eye Diseases Prevalence Research Group, 2004), with similar statistics evident in Australia (Wang, Foran, & Mitchell, 2000) and the United Kingdom (Royal National Institue for the Blind, 2015).

Vision impairments can occur in children (Schurink, Cox, Cillessen, van Rens, & Boonstra, 2011); however, the likelihood of experiencing low vision drastically increases with age (Ko et al., 2012). Many older people will have other co-occurring conditions (e.g., diabetes) requiring complex case management.

EYE CONDITIONS THAT LEAD TO VISION IMPAIRMENT

The most frequent causes of vision impairment are macular degeneration, diabetic retinopathy, glaucoma, retinitis pigmentosa, pathological myopia, and retinal dystrophy (Ryan, 2014). Even though these eye conditions cause a decline in vision, many of the cases do not result in blindness; rather, they may cause poor contrast perception, reduced color, or changes in brightness of an object. This chapter describes the most common chronic eye conditions that lead to vision impairment in adults, that is, uncorrected refracted errors, cataracts, age-related macular degeneration (AMD), diabetic retinopathy (DR), and glaucoma.

Normal vision means that a person can see a line on a chart clearly from a distance of 6 meters (20 feet). Images should be sharp and clear, with no loss of contrast sensitivity or color.

Uncorrected Refracted Errors

Uncorrected refracted errors remain the leading cause of vision impairment globally (Resnikoff, Pascolini, Mariotti, & Pokharel, 2008). The launch of Vision 2020 by the World Health Organization in 1997 aimed to eliminate avoidable blindness by 2020 with two of the main priority areas being refractive errors and cataracts (McCarty, 2006).

Uncorrected refractive errors, such as myopia (short-sightedness) or hyperopia (long-sightedness), result in a blurred retinal image. The higher the degree of error, the greater the impact has on the image. The most common and least expensive method of correcting refractive error is eyeglasses. Other options include contact lens and a laser procedure called Lasik surgery.

Reducing refractive error globally is confronted with two main challenges: the rapidly increasing incidence of myopia especially among children in Asia and the "silver tsunami" or global aging. It is estimated that in Asia and some other countries, 60% of children ages 5 to 15 years do not have access to refractive services or eyeglasses (Resnikoff et al., 2004). In lower socioeconomic countries, it has been estimated that up to 90% of older people do not have the correct eyeglasses (Holden et al., 2008).

Numerous strategies have been successful in reducing uncorrected refractive errors. For example, in India, the LV Prasad Eye Institute has initiated a program whereby a small team of staff including an optometrist or vision technician work from a vision clinic providing services for up to 50,000 people (Ricard, 2010). Other strategies include partnerships with organizations, such as Standard Chartered Bank, to establish or expand locally delivered services and the availability of affordable, good-quality lenses and ready-made eyeglasses.

Cataracts

Cataract remains a leading cause of vision impairment globally (Congdon, Friedman, & Lietman, 2003; Group, 2004). Cataracts form in the lens of the eye, a structure behind the pupil that focuses light onto the retina. Cataracts develop when the lens in the eye becomes less flexible and less transparent and thickens. The physiological changes in the lens result in light scattering as it passes through the lens, preventing a sharp image reaching the retina, resulting in a blurred image. As the cataract progresses, the clouding becomes more severe (Agarwal, Agarwal, Buratto, Apple, & Ali, 2002; Gupta & Deepak, 2008).

Although most cataracts are related to age (most people over the age of 80 can expect to develop cataracts), they can also be due to injury to the lens or may be congenital (often related to a maternal infection, such as rubella). Although a cataract may form in one eye only, it is more common for them to be in both eyes. With cataracts people will describe their blurred vision as being similar to looking through a curtain. Other symptoms include seeing "halos" around lights, colors becoming less vibrant, and sensitivity to light and glare.

Age-Related Macular Degeneration

AMD is an eye condition whereby the macula or central area of the retina is damaged, resulting in central vision loss. AMD is associated with aging in the retinal pigment epithelial cells, photoreceptors, and choroid. There are two forms of AMD: wet AMD, which accounts for 10% of AMD cases, and dry AMD, which accounts for 90% of all diagnosed cases. The wet form of AMD develops suddenly from a leakage of blood vessels under the retina and leads to more serious vision loss. Dry AMD progresses slowly and is characterized by the presence of yellow crystalline deposits with the macula (drusen) and atrophy or thinning of the macula (Stuen & Faye, 2003).

In AMD, the person will have difficulty focusing on near tasks, for instance reading the newspaper or using a phone, and is unable to distinguish facial features. As macular degeneration mainly affects the central vision, it results in blind spots in the center of the visual field. As the condition progresses, more blind spots occur, often leaving the person with limited central vision.

Diabetic Retinopathy

DR affects the vision of people who have type I and II diabetes and is a leading cause of visual impairment among working adults (Congdon et al., 2003; Ko et al., 2012). Prolonged hyperglycemia causes capillary breakdown and progressive retinal ischemia with compensatory intraretinal neovascularization (Hazin, Colyer, Lum, & Barazi, 2011). This results in blood vessels leaking into the eye, causing retinal scarring that distorts vision or creates blind spots. An individual with DR may have visual field defects and/ or loss of central vision. Vision may appear splotchy and can vary daily from normal to blurred, distorted, or partially blocked (Fong et al., 2004).

Clinically, diabetic retinal lesions are usually divided into nonproliferative and proliferative phases. Non-proliferative retinopathy is common when diabetes has been present for some years, while proliferative DR is a vision-threatening response to retinal ischemia. The risk factors for developing retinopathy are the level of glycaemic (blood sugar) control and the length of time the person has had diabetes. The prevalence of diabetes and associated retinopathy is growing rapidly in developed countries, making this a global vision problem. The most effective way to minimize the progression of diabetic retinopathy is to control the diabetes.

Glaucoma

Glaucoma is a group of eye conditions caused by damages to the optic nerve head from increased intraocular pressure (Congdon et al., 2003; Torpy, Lynm, & Glass, 2003). In a healthy eye, the amount of aqueous fluid produced is equal to the amount drained daily. For a person with glaucoma, the amount of fluid produced does not drain, leading to a build-up of intraocular pressure and resulting in peripheral and central vision loss (Gupta & Deepak, 2008). In long-standing glaucoma, numerous ocular structures may undergo alteration due to the elevated intraocular pressure.

Glaucoma is classified as being either open-angle or angle-closure glaucoma. Open-angle glaucoma is the most common type and is caused by a blockage in the trabecular meshwork (the aqueous drainage system), causing the pressure in the eye to gradually increase and resulting in damage to the optic nerve. Angle closure glaucoma, on the other hand, is caused by the iris (colored portion of the eye) protruding forward and narrowing the drainage angle formed by the cornea and the iris.

Glaucoma is asymptomatic in the early stages, which means the condition may go unnoticed. Often when the individual with a vision impairment is seen by a healthcare specialist, the damage to the eye has already resulted in loss of peripheral vision, deficits in color vision and contrast sensitivity, and permanent vision impairment (Glen, Crabb, & Garway-Heath, 2011; Quek et al., 2011). The visual loss in glaucoma differs to that of AMD or DR as the vision loss is peripheral. As the damage to the optic nerve increases, the peripheral field becomes smaller and may even result in pinhole vision.

FUNCTIONAL LIMITATIONS AND VISION LOSS

Functional limitations are those tasks a person is unable to perform due to the impact of the visual impairment. Vision loss impacts across all areas of a person's life. While the inability to read mail or pay bills is a significant challenge, everyday activities, such as grooming, dressing, and meal preparation are equally affected (Table 19.1). Functional loss is not only associated with the degree and type of visual impairment but is also dependent on the individual, as it relates to personal perception of the loss and the effect it has on the person's ability to continue to do what he or she wants to do. It is important when assessing individuals with a vision impairment that not only the visual loss is assessed but also the associated functional loss.

Vision impairment is often a hidden impairment. Individuals with a vision impairment may not disclose vision loss due to fear of activity restrictions or because of limited insight about the deficit. Most eye disabilities are not obvious, and therefore others may be unaware that a person has vision impairment. Vision impairment is a complex phenomenon, and it may be difficult for others to fully comprehend the impact it has on a person's life.

EVIDENCE-BASED PRACTICES OR INTERVENTIONS THAT IMPROVE HEALTH OUTCOMES FOR PEOPLE WITH VISUAL IMPAIRMENTS

Vision rehabilitation remains a relatively new field and draws on the expertise of a multidisciplinary team (Markowitz, 2006). Historically, non-government organizations have provided rehabilitation support for people with vision impairments and vision impairments. However, in the past decade there has been an acknowledgment that many chronic eye conditions are disabling and lead to vision impairments that require people to learn new skills to manage their everyday activities. Scientists and clinicians have collaborated on projects to design feasible and acceptable group-based, low-vision programs in Australia (Girdler, Boldy, Dhaliwal, Crowley, & Packer, 2010; Packer, Girdler, Boldy, Dhaliwal, & Crowley, 2009; Rees, Keeffe, Hassell, Larizza, & Lamoureux, 2010; Rees et al., 2015) and Singapore (Drury, Mackey, & Tay, 2012). The results of these studies revealed overall improvements in mood, understanding their condition, accessing services, and managing the consequences of the condition.

Motivational Interviewing

Motivational interviewing (MI) is a form of counseling that has been used for decades in addiction health and psychiatry (Miller & Rollnick, 2012). In recent times, it has been adapted and used to help individuals with long-term conditions explore ambivalence in relation to changing behaviors (Chen, Creedy, Lin, & Wollin, 2012; McCarley, 2009). Indeed, MI has become an important strategy in healthcare that can be used in diverse situations (Lawn & Schoo, 2010). There have been numerous variations to the initial MI process described by Rollnick and Miller (1995). Despite this, the inherent philosophy behind MI remains true, and that is that MI is a collaborative person-centered approach, in which individual autonomy is respected and the clinician prompts the individual to reflect on his or her intrinsic resources that can facilitate change. Within this philosophy, the clinician is seen as being a facilitator rather than an expert, consistent with the philosophy of self-management. For more information on motivational interviewing see chapter 6 of this volume.

Common Elements in Vision Self-Management Programs

The literature highlights common elements in vision self-management programs, including understanding self-management and both individual and clinician roles (Chiang, Drury, Lim, & Tin, 2013), understanding vision loss, use of assistive devices, managing activities of daily living, coping strategies, problem-solving, maintaining personal interests, and mobility and safety (Chiang et al., 2013; Drury et al., 2012; Liu, Brost, Horton, Kenyon, & Mears, 2013; Packer et al., 2009; Rees et al., 2015).

Systematic reviews of low-vision rehabilitation and AMD (Hooper, Jutai, Strong, & Russell-Minda, 2008) and the effectiveness of assistive technologies in low-vision rehabilitation (Jutai, Strong, & Russell-Minda, 2009) have been undertaken. These reviews identified that matching the requirements of individuals with a vision impairment with appropriate assistive technologies and establishing the most effective assistive devices and orientation and mobility programs were areas of unmet need. The reviews also highlight that outcomes are both subjective, for example, how a person feels about a program or device, and objective, for example, a noticeable improvement in ability to perform the activities of daily living. The self-management programs developed by Packer, Girdler, Boldy, Dhaliwal, and Crowley (2009), Rees, Keeffe, Hassell, Larizza, and Lamoureux (2010), and Drury, Mackey, and Peter (2012) all include sessions on the use of assistive technologies and other equipment, acknowledging the valuable role equipment may play in assisting a person to live independently with a vision impairment.

The literature on use of assistive devices and their effectiveness is extensive (Cook & Polgar, 2014; Fok, Polgar, Shaw, & Jutai, 2011; Jutai et al., 2009; Kelly & Smith, 2011; Rabello, Gasparetto, Alves, Monteiro, & Carvalho, 2014) with results emphasizing that success with using assistive devices is related to the performance of the device and individual satisfaction with the device. Therefore, it is essential that individuals with vision impairments are provided with ongoing support as they learn to use new technologies.

It is essential that any program is developed based on evidence. Although the available evidence is limited to four studies, certain elements have been included in all programs. With the recent completion of a randomized controlled trial examining the effectiveness of a self-management low-vision program in Singapore (ClinicalTrials.gov Identifier: NCT01879501), there is further evidence that supports self-management as an effective process for people with vision impairments.

RESEARCH ON THE EMOTIONAL IMPACT OF VISION IMPAIRMENT

Living with a vision impairment not only imposes a serious burden on individuals and their families but also has a negative impact on their individual psychosocial well-being (Percival, 2011). For the person with a vision impairment, an inability to cope with normal daily visual demands can be profoundly damaging to self-esteem and personal dignity (Drury, Mackey & Tay, 2012). Support from family members is critical to successful adaptation to vision loss (Bambara et al., 2009).

Vision Impairment and Mental Wellness

It is also acknowledged that vision impairment may result in feelings of hopelessness and despair and may lead to clinical depression and anxiety, especially among older adults (Evans, Fletcher, & Wormald, 2007; Kempen, Ballemans, Ranchor, van Rens, & Zijlstra, 2012; Rees, Tee, et al., 2010). For most people, the psychosocial impact of vision loss is profound (Nyman, Dibb, Victor, & Gosney, 2012).

Livneh and Antonak (2005), in their model of adaptation to chronic health conditions and disability, argue that individuals progress through eight phases of adaptation. Individuals in the proximal phase may experience shock and denial, while intermediate reactions include anger and depression. Acknowledgement and adjustment occur in the distal phase (Martz & Livneh, 2007). And throughout these phases, individuals use personal knowledge and coping strategies to manage the implications of the loss in their life. Once people are in the adjustment phase, they have accepted the loss and make efforts to adapt to the new impairment. For individuals to effectively self-manage their condition, they must first accept and acknowledge the loss has occurred.

Loneliness and depression may transpire due to a withdrawal from family and social activities. These emotions may go unnoticed during brief medical encounters (Mitchell, Rao, & Vaze, 2011; Mitchell, Vaze, & Rao, 2009). Some vision rehabilitation programs have included sessions on managing emotions (Chiang, Drury, Lim, & Tin, 2013), and all the aforementioned self-management programs included sessions on developing coping behaviors.

It has been found that the severity of loneliness affects the individual's ability to adapt to and manage the consequences of the vision loss (Verstraten, Brinkmann, Stevens, & Schouten, 2005). However, Alma et al. (2011) assert that loneliness may be mitigated by self-management programs as the individual develops self-efficacy and improved coping and adaptation skills. The prevalence of depression in people with vision loss has been acknowledged (Morse, 2013; O'Donnell, 2005; Zhang et al., 2013). Recent studies have found that people with low vision experience higher levels of anxiety and depression and poorer levels of functioning than other older people in society (Kempen et al., 2012). Current research argues that the depression may be mediated by functional limitations and social support networks (Nispen, Vreeken, Comijs, Deeg, & Rens, 2015), therefore highlighting the significance of supporting individuals with vision impairments to manage these factors.

Vision Impairment and Quality of Life

The impact of vision impairment has also been found to adversely affect quality of life. The failure to provide adequate low-vision services has been attributed to depriving people of the rights to social inclusion and divesting society of the contributions they may have been able to make (Tay, Drury & Mackey, 2014). The impact that this has on a person's emotional well-being is significant. Barriers to self-management may include communication challenges as the individual is unable to read or may be unable to recognize faces. This means that all information needs to be verbally produced instead of using information sheets and booklets. Even then, many people with vision impairments find it preferable to communicate on a one-to-one basis due to the lack of ability to perceive nonverbal cues.

Research clearly shows that a person with a vision impairment is more at risk of falls (Lamoureux et al., 2010; Lord, Smith, & Menant, 2010). The fear of falling and being anxious in unknown environments may prevent the person with a vision impairment from attending social events or even showing up for appointments, thus impacting quality of life.

Vision Impairment and Leisure Activities

Vision impairment inhibits a person's ability to participate in some recreation and relaxation activities, and other forms of recreation may not be as enjoyable (Dunning, 2009). A study by Berger (2012) reported that vision loss results in people's inability to engage in out-of-home activities particularly when they are unfamiliar with the environment. This may result in the person becoming withdrawn from social events, further compounding the risks of a depressive episode.

Social support through family members and friends has been found to be integral to adaptation for the person with a vision impairment (Hodge & Eccles, 2014). However, family and friends need to have a sufficient understanding of the degree of impairment and what support they can provide, so that they reinforce self-management and independence and do not encourage helplessness.

The loss of sight is considered to be similar to a bereavement, with people transitioning through similar stages of grief (Percival, 2011). Clark (2005) argued that, for most people, receiving a diagnosis of a chronic health condition is the beginning of a journey into the unknown; therefore, it is imperative to prepare individuals for the journey and help them understand what to expect along the way. Everyone responds to a chronic disability differently. How a person responds to, and manages, the disability is dependent on personal knowledge and coping skills.

KNOWLEDGE ABOUT THE IMPAIRMENT THAT AN INDIVIDUAL NEEDS FOR SELF-MANAGEMENT

In order to effectively self-manage their condition, people with a vision impairment need to know that their condition will not improve over time and may in fact deteriorate further—in other words, they must come to a point whereby they accept their condition. If individuals do not accept their condition, it is difficult for them to leverage on self-management principles to gain independence. People must also accept that they may need to make necessary changes to their lifestyles and activities and may not be able to do all the things they previously did, due to their loss of vision. This acceptance and willingness to make changes to their lifestyle is crucial for self-management to be successful.

Unlike people with visible physical disabilities, it is not obvious that a person has vision impairment. People with vision impairment need to be able to explain their condition to a layperson, describing clearly what they are able/not able to see and what kind of help they may need. Often, people around them would like to help but are not sure how they can assist. However, there are also times when people are too helpful, and thus, it is also important for the person with a vision impairment to know when and how to say no. Being assertive is having the confidence to tell others what is needed and is important in the maintenance of self-esteem and independence.

Understanding how to navigate the healthcare system, the social welfare system (if relevant), what resources are available, and ways to access them are crucial to effective self-management. Being familiar with the treating team and the resources available are only small components of being able to navigate the healthcare system. For some, especially the elderly, the ability to navigate the system on their own will be limited, and this is where the role of the healthcare professional becomes fundamental to success.

THE ROLE OF THE HEALTHCARE PROFESSIONAL

In self-management, the role of the healthcare professional is to support and empower individuals with vision impairments to achieve their goals while working collaboratively within a person-centered model. The 5As model of self-management support provides healthcare professionals with a sequential set of actions applicable to primary healthcare settings when working with individuals with vision impairment (Figure 19.1; Glasgow, Emont, & Miller, 2006). Using these guiding principles, healthcare professionals are able to collaboratively develop a treatment plan with the individual with a vision impairment, focus on individual concerns and challenges, prioritize what is important for the individual, provide support that helps to develop self-management skills, link the individual to relevant resources, involve appropriate healthcare professionals, and organize follow-up care. This ensures continuity of person-centered care. The 5As approach enables healthcare professionals to assist the individual with a vision impairment to become a better self-manager. Acknowledging that these roles are

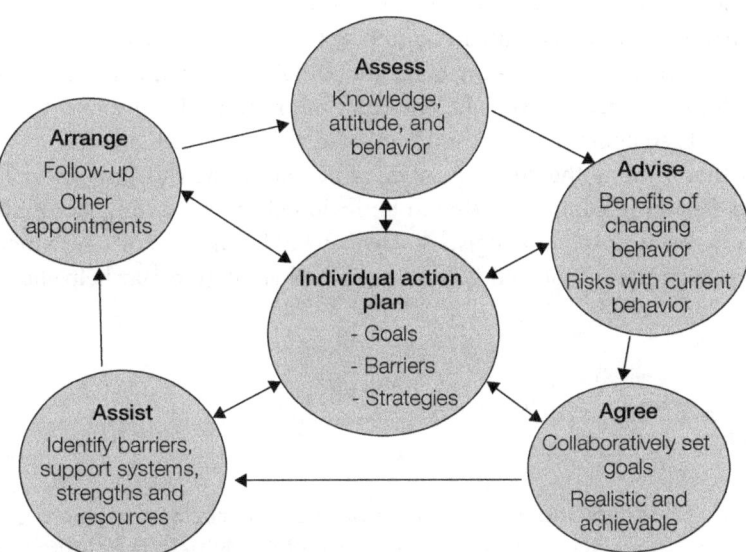

Figure 19.1 Self-management support roles for health-care professionals. Adapted from Glasgow, Emont & Miller, 2006.

healthcare professional roles and educating professionals in the roles is essential for effective self-management support. The term "self-management" may also be perceived by individuals and caregivers as unsupported self-care, so it is important that both individuals and caregivers are provided with adequate explanations of their own roles and those of the healthcare staff.

BARRIERS AND CHALLENGES TO SELF-MANAGEMENT

Managing a long-term vision impairment, especially one that will result in a continued decline in vision, may be both frustrating and frightening. The success of self-management interventions for people with vision impairment depends on individual's ability to effectively sustain the self-management behaviors: follow medication regimens (often eye drops need to be applied a few times a day), coping with the emotional consequences of living with a vision impairment, and adapting behaviors. Many individuals with vision impairments are confronted with multiple barriers to effective self-management, including a lack of knowledge about their condition, low self-efficacy, a lack of financial security, and co-occurring impairments. For some people, an additional barrier is the lack of support from family and friends who may not understand the challenges associated with the vision impairment.

Individuals with vision impairments living independently are not always referred for low-vision rehabilitation (Overbury & Wittich, 2011). A reason for this may be the assumption that if the person is living independently, then he or she does not need rehabilitation services. Alternatively, knowledge of, or access to, services may be difficult. Low-vision rehabilitation services are specialist services and may not be located within general ophthalmology departments, resulting in anxiety for the individual who may have to travel to a different location and an unfamiliar environment (Wittich, Canuto, & Overbury, 2013). Changes in service delivery, for example co-locating general ophthalmic outpatients and low-vision rehabilitation services on specific days each month, has been found to improve the usage of rehabilitation services (Wittich et al., 2013).

A further issue is the small number of people trained to provide low-vision services. Vision rehabilitation should be included in all training for ophthalmic personnel, from ophthalmologists through to ophthalmic assistants. Increasing professional awareness of, and skills in, vision rehabilitation may help alleviate the current challenges.

COPING STRATEGIES OR SKILLS TAUGHT FOR IMPAIRMENT

The ability to understand and identify a problem is crucial if people with vision impairments are to be independent in their daily activities. The ability to recognize and acknowledge a problem enables the person to use skills learned in self-management programs to help solve the problem.

Table 19.2. POWER Problem-Solving Process

Acronym	Process Step	Applying the Process
P	Plan ahead	What do I want to do? How can I do it? What do I need to do it?
O	Organize required resources	Organize resources (e.g., book train tickets and alert station that I need assistance)
W	Weigh the options	What are the different ways I could do this? How confident am I on a scale of 1 to 10 that I will achieve my goal using this plan?
E	Execute the plan	Do the activity
R	Review for improvement	How did it go? What could I do better next time and how could it be done better? What worked well? What didn't work so well?

Reprinted with permission from Chiang, P. P., Drury, V., Lim, P. S. H., & Tin, Y. M. (2013). *ADAPT lah! The Singapore living successfully with low vision program: Facilitator and operation manual.* Singapore: Singapore Eye Research Institute.

The importance of being able to plan activities beforehand cannot be overemphasized, as people with vision impairments need to make sure they have whatever assistive technologies they require. This planning may include details, such as lighting, sighted guides, or tactile markers. A problem-solving tool, developed in Singapore, provides a structured process for the person with a vision impairment to systematically plan to solve a problem (Table 19.2, Chiang et al., 2013). This tool may be used by people with other disabilities as it is a generic, rather than vision-specific, problem-solving tool. The acronym POWER can be used to remember the steps in the problem-solving process (Chiang et al., 2013).

Self-Talk

Self-talk is the inner voice in one's mind that provides opinions and inner discussions about events that are occurring. Self-talk can be negative or positive and has a significant influence on a person's mood, feelings, and behavior. Self-talk is an important tool that enables people to examine their feelings. In particular, positive self-talk boosts self-confidence and may encourage people to explore and push their boundaries (Hardy, 2006; Hatzigeorgiadis, Zourbanos, Mpoumpaki, & Theodorakis, 2009). Negative self-talk, on the other hand, may paralyze people with fear and doubt, discourage them, and cause them to retreat and be withdrawn, which may lead to depression.

It is important that negative self-talk is changed to positive self-talk. This can be done by first learning to listen to one's thoughts and realizing how these thoughts influence individual mood and behavior. The next step is to change these thoughts into helpful or constructive self-talk (Bandura, 2001, 2004).

Relaxation Techniques

Relaxation techniques can be used to help to release tension when the person with a vision impairment is feeling anxious, stressed, or angry, and it will result in the person feeling calmer and more in control of stressful situations (Smith, Hancock, Blake-Mortimer, & Eckert, 2007). Relaxation techniques include mindfulness meditation, deep breathing techniques, and progressive muscle relaxation (Hassett & Gevirtz, 2009).

Social Support

Support of family and friends play an important role in helping people with chronic conditions and/or disabilities to accept the consequences of the condition, adapt to their new circumstances, and maintain their independence. It is important that caregivers understand what the person with the visual impairment can and cannot see, so they can provide support when necessary. It is also crucial that caregivers understand that they should not be overprotective of people with vision impairments, but rather help them to maintain and improve their independence as much as possible.

Knowing what resources are available in the local community and how to access them is also important. Such resources help the person remain independent in the community. Resource may include support groups, recreation and leisure activities, help with seeking employment, learning new skills, orientation and mobility, and volunteer transportation.

Peer-Support Programs

The person with a vision impairment may seek out vision-support groups in healthcare or community settings. These groups aim to help the person with a vision impairment cope and live independently. Peer support from people with the same chronic health condition has been found to provide significant benefits in reducing depression, alleviating anxiety, and improving self-management behaviors (Heisler, 2007). Additionally, often clinicians are involved in facilitating the groups—organizing meeting times and venues, initially helping to get groups running, and so forth. Clinicians may learn a lot from these sessions as the individuals share strategies they have found useful and help each other problem-solve challenges. For example, during one session a participant described how he used his smartphone in the shops instead of a magnifier. By taking a photo of the label and then zooming in, the phone operated as a mini-magnifier.

Group dynamics in a support group are a crucial element that determines whether the group is successful (Cartwright, 2008). Group dynamics reinforce positive behaviors and encourage those who are not as confident to make similar changes when others in the group show progress. It also helps in changing negative self-talk (e.g., "I don't think I can do it") to positive self-talk (e.g., "If he can do it, I think I can too"; Toseland & Rivas, 2005).

STRATEGIES THAT FACILITATE SELF-MANAGEMENT

Self-management acknowledges the central role played by the individual in the effective management of a long-term condition. There is a plethora of literature that clearly demonstrates that self-management improves outcomes (Bodenheimer, Lorig, Holman, & Grumbach, 2002; Bourbeau & Van Der Palen, 2009; Coleman & Newton, 2005; Lorig et al., 2001). In the past, many of the self-management programs focused on the major long-term conditions affecting first-world populations, such as diabetes and cardiovascular conditions. However, more recently the same principles have been effectively applied to programs for people with low vision (Brody, Roch-Levecq, Thomas, Kaplan, & Brown, 2005; Drury, et al. 2012; Girdler et al., 2010; Rees, Keeffe, et al., 2010).

Assessment

The first step in facilitating self-management in the individual with a vision impairment is to assess the person. The following factors should be considered when planning self-management programs for individuals with vision impairments:

1. Degree and type of the vision impairment (central or peripheral vision loss).
2. Underlying cause of the impairment and prognosis.
3. The age of the individual and developmental and cognitive level.
4. Overall health status and any co-occurring conditions.
5. Other sensory or mobility issues.
6. Individual's acceptance of vision loss and readiness for change.
7. Available support systems.

It is not the purpose of this chapter to describe the numerous tests and assessments that may be performed to determine the first five of these factors. However, it is important that clinicians are cognizant of the factors and take these into consideration when assessing a person for inclusion in a self-management program.

Assessing Readiness and Motivation for Change

It is essential that people being encouraged to self-manage their conditions are willing to consider changes that may assist them in adapting to their vision loss. Some individuals will already have made changes and adapted to the vision loss; however, many individuals lack the knowledge and skills to make adaptive changes on their own. The first step in the process of self-management is acceptance of the vision impairment and acknowledgment that the loss is impacting on one's life and preventing the individual from involvement in chosen activities (Drury, Chiang, Tey, Soon, & Aw, 2014). Intrinsic motivation, that is being motivated from within without external rewards, has also been found to influence behavior in low-vision rehabilitation (Tay, Drury, & Mackey, 2013).

Often individuals are simply channeled into programs without assessing whether they are ready and/or motivated to make changes to their current lives. There are many tools available that can be used to help clinicians assess readiness to change; however, a comprehensive assessment should include exploring an individual's beliefs and attitudes, self-efficacy, and the perceived need for change. Using MI strategies, clinicians are able to shift from a care paradigm of advice giving and providing instructions to one of collaborative, person-centered care. A person will be assessed as either ready and motivated to make changes that facilitate adaptation to their condition or not ready.

Interventions for Individuals Not in a State of Readiness

It is important that those individuals not ready to make changes are supported through their decision-making. These people may be in denial of their condition, or they may have a degree of depression; whatever the reason for their lack of readiness, the individual needs to be gently guided through the process to acceptance. Once again, assessment is critical at this stage to ensure a thorough understanding of the individual's state of readiness.

MI strategies involve two phases: building motivation to change and strengthening a person's commitment to change (Hall, Gibbie, & Lubman, 2012). The focus of MI is on getting individuals to a point where they decide that they want to change and then work with them to resolve ambivalence and increase self-efficacy. In the initial phase of MI, the acronym OARS (open-ended questions, affirmations, reflections, summarizing) describes the basic counseling strategies that facilitate this exploration (Miller & Rollnick, 2012).

Strengthening commitment to change involves setting goals and negotiating an action plan for change. To do this, individuals can be asked a series of focused questions that help them highlight where they are now and where they want to be.

Self-Management Interventions for Individuals in a State of Readiness

It is suggested that a multidisciplinary approach to care be considered for individuals with vision impairments. The key elements of this approach are (Integrating the Healthcare Enterprise, 2006):

- All members of the healthcare team working collaboratively as a team, with a case manager in charge.
- Regular communication among team members, keeping all members informed of the individual's progress.
- Ability to access required resources to provide the care described.
- Provision of evidence-based care.
- Individuals are actively involved in their care.

Specifically, involvement of a social worker, nurse, occupational therapist, and low-vision optometrist is recommended. Each of these clinicians brings a different type of professional expertise, facilitating a holistic and person-centered approach. Collaboration in the multidisciplinary team ensures the person with a vision impairment receives the most relevant professional expertise from the appropriate expert, at the appropriate time, and individual care is coordinated among the experts by the case manager to obtain maximum benefit.

An established care-path for vision-impaired individuals is integral to the success of a multidisciplinary approach. The care-path defines the care and interventions required along the care continuum from medical on one end to the community at the other end. The transition from healthcare to community setting is crucial if the vision-impaired individual is to gain independence. The long-term objective is for the person with a vision impairment to be independent in the community and to be able to contribute actively in the community. The limited evidence available (Drury, Mackey, & Tay, 2012; Girdler et al., 2010; Packer et al., 2009; Rees, Keeffe, et al., 2010) highlights specific elements that have, to date, been included in successful self-management programs. These are:

- Information on eye conditions and low vision.
- Strategies to help maximize remaining vision.
- Psychosocial strategies and support.
- Managing activities of daily living and household tasks.
- Working with healthcare workers.
- Strategies to enhance mobility and safety.
- Strategies to maintain relationships and leisure activities.

Low-vision self-management programs help people manage one or more of the following:

- The low vision itself—managing the symptoms of their underlying condition.
- Preventing new symptoms or complications and reducing risk factors.
- The emotional consequences of low vision—this includes depression, feelings of loss, and grief and coping strategies.
- The impact of low vision on daily life—how to change work, family, and leisure activities to meet expectations, how to set personal goals, and how to remain independent.

Low-vision self-management programs can be run in many different ways including group programs, individual programs, or online programs; however, most commonly they are group-based (Drury et al., 2012; Girdler et al., 2010; Rees, Keeffe, et al., 2010). Low-vision self-management programs are not simply peer support groups or educational groups. The advantages of a group-based program are that it facilitates self-efficacy, reduces the sense of isolation many people with low-vision experience, and empowers participants.

Technology—Phone Applications

Although it is acknowledged that not everyone, especially the elderly, has a mobile phone these days, they have significant advantages for the person with a vision impairment. For example, a free smartphone application (app) has been developed to remind individuals when to apply eye drops (Glaucoma Research Foundation, 2012). Singapore National Eye Center has developed a free eye-drop regimen app as well as an app that provides comprehensive health education information on a wide range of eye conditions, their symptoms, and management (Singapore National Eye Center 2013).

Telehealth

"Telehealth" is an umbrella term that is often used to describe any type of medical service provided via telephone or the Internet; for example, a specialist may be sitting in an office in the city and be assessing an individual with a vision impairment in a clinic in a remote area. Telemedicine may also be used to deliver group self-management programs and one-to-one self-management programs and for peer-support groups. For example, Vision Australia has a program called Connecting with Others that includes online forums and telelink support groups, which improves accessibility for individuals with vision impairments (Vision Australia, 2012).

CONCLUSION

Self-management focuses on ability rather than disability, encouraging the individual to consider strategies that may be useful in reframing how specific activities are performed. Low-vision services in combination with a self-management approach empower individuals to continue their lives and maintain their independence. The ability to perform activities of daily living and undertake routine home, leisure, and work-related activities with confidence are the keys to living well with vision loss.

Although vision impairment may have a profound impact on the biopsychosocial aspects of a person's life, creative solutions and positive thinking enable individuals to live independently and continue with favorite activities. Vision rehabilitation services, including self-management programs, play a pivotal role in empowering and supporting individuals to self-manage their condition and maintain independence. The development of new services, fully integrated with current services and delivered in an accessible manner by health professionals trained in self-management, will ensure long-term sustainability of services. Collaboration between all members of the healthcare team and the individual and family will enable care that is responsive to the needs of the individual and family, thus improving individual outcomes.

REFERENCES

Agarwal, S., Agarwal, A., Buratto, L., Apple, D. J., & Ali, J. L. (2002). *Textbook of ophthalmology.* New Delhi: Jaypee Brothers.

Alma, M. A., Van der Mei, S. F., Feitsma, W. N., Groothoff, J. W., Van Tilburg, T. G., & Suurmeijer, T. P. (2011). Loneliness and self-management abilities in the visually impaired elderly. *Journal of Aging and Health, 23*(5), 843–861.

Bambara, J. K., Wadley, V., Owsley, C., Martin, R. C., Porter, C., & Dreer, L. E. (2009). Family functioning and low vision: A systematic review. *Journal of Visual Impairment & Blindness, 103*(3), 137–149.

Bandura, A. (2001). Social cognitive theory: An agentic perspective. *Annual Review of Psychology, 52*(1), 1–26.

Bandura, A. (2004). Health promotion by social cognitive means. *Health Education & Behavior, 31*(2), 143–164.

Berger, S. (2012). Is my world getting smaller? The challenges of living with vision loss. *Journal of Visual Impairment & Blindness, 106*(1), 5–16.

Bodenheimer, T., Lorig, K., Holman, H., & Grumbach, K. (2002). Patient self-management of chronic disease in primary care. *JAMA, 288*(19), 2469–2475.

Bourbeau, J., & Van Der Palen, J. (2009). Promoting effective self-management programmes to improve COPD. *European Respiratory Journal, 33*(3), 461–463.

Bourne, R. R., Stevens, G. A., White, R. A., Smith, J. L., Flaxman, S. R., Price, H., . . . Naidoo, K. (2013). Causes of vision loss worldwide, 1990–2010: A systematic analysis. *The Lancet Global Health, 1*(6), e339–e349.

Brody, B. L., Roch-Levecq, A.-C., Thomas, R. G., Kaplan, R. M., & Brown, S. I. (2005). Self-management of age-related macular degeneration at the 6-month follow-up: A randomized controlled trial. *Archives of Ophthalmology, 123*(1), 46–53.

Cartwright, D. (2008). Achieving change in people: Some applications of group dynamics theory. *Group Facilitation*(9), 59.

Centers for Disease Control and Prevention. (2011). The state of vision, aging, and public health in America. Retrieved from https://www.cdc.gov/visionhealth/pdf/vision_brief.pdf

Chen, S. M., Creedy, D., Lin, H.-S., & Wollin, J. (2012). Effects of motivational interviewing intervention on self-management, psychological and glycemic outcomes in type 2 diabetes: A randomized controlled trial. *International Journal of Nursing Studies, 49*(6), 637–644.

Chiang, P. P., Drury, V., Lim, P. S. H., & Tin, Y. M. (2013). *ADAPT lah! The Singapore Living Successfully with Low Vision program: Facilitator and operation manual.* Singapore: Singapore Eye Research Institute.

Chou, C.-F., Cotch, M. F., Vitale, S., Zhang, X., Klein, R., Friedman, D. S., . . . Saaddine, J. B. (2013). Age-related eye diseases and visual impairment among US adults. *American Journal of Preventive Medicine, 45*(1), 29–35.

Clark, M. (2005). Managing psychosocial impacts of diabetes. *Practice Nursing, 16*(7), 334–339.

Coleman, M. T., & Newton, K. S. (2005). Supporting self-management in patients with chronic illness. *Amerian Family Physician, 72*(8), 1503–1510.

Congdon, N. G., Friedman, D. S., & Lietman, T. (2003). Important causes of visual impairment in the world today. *JAMA, 290*(15), 2057–2060.

Cook, A. M., & Polgar, J. M. (2014). *Assistive technologies: Principles and practice*: St. Louis, MO: Elsevier Health Sciences.

Dandona, L., & Dandona, R. (2006). What is the global burden of visual impairment? *BMC Medicine, 4*(1), 1.

Drury, V., Chiang, P. P., Tey, C. S., Soon, H. J., & Aw, A. T. (2014). Assessing the willingness to change: Optimising behaviour change in the management of chronic eye conditions. *International Journal of Ophthalmic Practice, 5*(5), 182–188.

Drury, V., Mackey, S., & Tay, P. (2012). The feasibility and acceptability of a low vision self-management programme for older Singaporeans: A pilot study. *International Journal of Ophthalmic Practice, 3*(5), 189–193.

Dunning, T. (2009). Low vision and blindness technology. *Activities Adaptation and Aging, 33*(2), 120–121.

Evans, J. R., Fletcher, A. E., & Wormald, R. P. (2007). Depression and anxiety in visually impaired older people. *Ophthalmology, 114*(2), 283–288.

Eye Diseases Prevalence Research Group. (2004). Causes and prevalence of visual impairment among adults in the United States. *Archives of Ophthalmology, 122*(4), 477–485.

Fok, D., Polgar, J. M., Shaw, L., & Jutai, J. W. (2011). Low vision assistive technology device usage and importance in daily occupations. *Work, 39*(1), 37–48.

Fong, D. S., Aiello, L., Gardner, T. W., King, G. L., Blankenship, G., Cavallerano, J. D., . . . Klein, R. (2004). Retinopathy in diabetes. *Diabetes Care, 27*(Suppl. 1), s84–s87.

Girdler, S. J., Boldy, D. P., Dhaliwal, S. S., Crowley, M., & Packer, T. L. (2010). Vision self-management for older adults: a randomised controlled trial. *British Journal of Ophthalmology, 94*(2), 223–228.

Glasgow, R. E., Emont, S., & Miller, D. C. (2006). Assessing delivery of the five "As" for patient-centered counseling. *Health Promotion International*, *21*(3), 245–255.

Glaucoma Research Foundation. (2012). *Free smartphone app helps patients manage eye medications*. Retrieved from http://www.glaucoma.org/news/free-smartphone-app-helps-patients-manage-eye-medications.php

Glen, F. C., Crabb, D. P., & Garway-Heath, D. F. (2011). The direction of research into visual disability and quality of life in glaucoma. *BMC Ophthalmology*, *11*(1), 19.

Group, E. D. P. R. (2004). Causes and prevalence of visual impairment among adults in the United States. *Archives of Ophthalmology*, *122*(4), 477–485.

Gupta, M., & Deepak, P. (2008). Principles and practice of ophthalmology. In D. M. Albert & F. A. Jakobiec (Eds.), *Principles and practice of ophthalmology* (Vol. 1, pp. 3725–3735). Philadelphia: W. B. Saunders.

Hall, K., Gibbie, T., & Lubman, D. I. (2012). Motivational interviewing techniques: Facilitating behaviour change in the general practice setting. *Australian Family Physician*, *41*(9), 660–667.

Hardy, J. (2006). Speaking clearly: A critical review of the self-talk literature. *Psychology of Sport and Exercise*, *7*(1), 81–97.

Hassett, A. L., & Gevirtz, R. N. (2009). Nonpharmacologic treatment for fibromyalgia: Patient education, cognitive-behavioral therapy, relaxation techniques, and complementary and alternative medicine. *Rheumatic Disease Clinics of North America*, *35*(2), 393–407.

Hatzigeorgiadis, A., Zourbanos, N., Mpoumpaki, S., & Theodorakis, Y. (2009). Mechanisms underlying the self-talk–performance relationship: The effects of motivational self-talk on self-confidence and anxiety. *Psychology of Sport and exercise*, *10*(1), 186–192.

Hazin, R., Colyer, M., Lum, F., & Barazi, M. K. (2011). Revisiting diabetes 2000: Challenges in establishing nationwide diabetic retinopathy prevention programs. *American Journal of Ophthalmology*, *152*(5), 723–729.

Heisler, M. (2007). Overview of peer support models to improve diabetes self-management and clinical outcomes. *Diabetes Spectrum*, *20*(4), 214.

Hodge, S., & Eccles, F. (2014). *Loneliness, social isolation and sight loss*. London: Thomas Pocklington Trust.

Holden, B. A., Fricke, T. R., Ho, S. M., Wong, R., Schlenther, G., Cronjé, S., . . . Frick, K. D. (2008). Global vision impairment due to uncorrected presbyopia. *Archives of Ophthalmology*, *126*(12), 1731–1739.

Hooper, P., Jutai, J. W., Strong, G., & Russell-Minda, E. (2008). Age-related macular degeneration and low-vision rehabilitation: A systematic review. *Canadian Journal of Ophthalmology/Journal Canadien d'Ophtalmologie*, *43*(2), 180–187.

Integrating the Healthcare Enterprise. (2006). *Multidisciplinary healthcare*. Retrieved from http://www.ihe-online.com/fileadmin/artimg/multidisciplinary-healthcare.pdf

Jutai, J. W., Strong, J. G., & Russell-Minda, E. (2009). Effectiveness of assistive technologies for low vision rehabilitation: A systematic review. *Journal of Visual Impairment & Blindness*, *103*(4), 210.

Kelly, S. M., & Smith, D. W. (2011). The impact of assistive technology on the educational performance of students with visual impairments: A synthesis of the research. *Journal of Visual Impairment & Blindness*, *105*(2), 73.

Kempen, G. I., Ballemans, J., Ranchor, A. V., van Rens, G. H., & Zijlstra, G. R. (2012). The impact of low vision on activities of daily living, symptoms of depression, feelings of anxiety and social support in community-living older adults seeking vision rehabilitation services. *Quality of Life Research, 21*(8), 1405–1411.

Ko, F., Vitale, S., Chou, C.-F., Cotch, M. F., Saaddine, J., & Friedman, D. S. (2012). Prevalence of nonrefractive visual impairment in US adults and associated risk factors, 1999–2002 and 2005–2008. *JAMA, 308*(22), 2361–2368.

Lamoureux, E., Gadgil, S., Pesudovs, K., Keeffe, J., Fenwick, E., Dirani, M., . . . Rees, G. (2010). The relationship between visual function, duration and main causes of vision loss and falls in older people with low vision. *Graefe's Archive for Clinical and Experimental Ophthalmology, 248*(4), 527–533.

Lawn, S., & Schoo, A. (2010). Supporting self-management of chronic health conditions: Common approaches. *Patient Education and Counseling, 80*(2), 205–211.

Liu, C.-J., Brost, M. A., Horton, V. E., Kenyon, S. B., & Mears, K. E. (2013). Occupational therapy interventions to improve performance of daily activities at home for older adults with low vision: A systematic review. *American Journal of Occupational Therapy, 67*(3), 279–287.

Livneh, H., & Antonak, R. F. (2005). Psychosocial adaptation to chronic illness and disability: A primer for counselors. *Journal of Counseling & Development, 83*(1), 12–20.

Lord, S. R., Smith, S. T., & Menant, J. C. (2010). Vision and falls in older people: Risk factors and intervention strategies. *Clinics in Geriatric Medicine, 26*(4), 569–581.

Lorig, K. R., Ritter, P., Stewart, A. L., Sobel, D. S., Brown, B. W. Jr., Bandura, A., . . . Holman, H. R. (2001). Chronic disease self-management program: 2-year health status and health care utilization outcomes. *Medical Care, 39*(11), 1217–1223.

Markowitz, S. N. (2006). Principles of modern low vision rehabilitation. *Canadian Journal of Ophthalmology/Journal Canadien d'Ophtalmologie, 41*(3), 289–312.

Martz, E., & Livneh, H. (Eds.). (2007). *Coping with chronic illness and disability*. New York: Springer.

McCarley, P. (2009). Patient empowerment and motivational interviewing: Engaging patients to self-manage their own care. *Nephrology Nursing Journal, 36*(4), 409–413.

McCarty, C. (2006). Uncorrected refractive error. *British Journal of Ophthalmology, 90*(5), 521–522.

Miller, W. R., & Rollnick, S. (2012). *Motivational interviewing: Helping people change*: N ew York: Guilford Press.

Mitchell, A. J., Rao, S., & Vaze, A. (2011). Can general practitioners identify people with distress and mild depression? A meta-analysis of clinical accuracy. *Journal of Affective Disorders, 130*(1), 26–36.

Mitchell, A. J., Vaze, A., & Rao, S. (2009). Clinical diagnosis of depression in primary care: a meta-analysis. *The Lancet, 374*(9690), 609–619.

Morse, A. R. (2013). Vision function, functional vision, and depression. *JAMA Ophthalmology, 131*(5), 667–668.

Nispen, R., Vreeken, H. L., Comijs, H. C., Deeg, D. J., & Rens, G. H. (2015). Role of vision loss, functional limitations and the supporting network in depression in a general population. *Acta Ophthalmologica, 94*(1), 76–82.

Nyman, S. R., Dibb, B., Victor, C. R., & Gosney, M. A. (2012). Emotional well-being and adjustment to vision loss in later life: A meta-synthesis of qualitative studies. *Disability and Rehabilitation, 34*(12), 971–981.

O'Donnell, C. (2005). The greatest generation meets its greatest challenge: Vision loss and depression in older adults. *Journal of Visual Impairment & Blindness, 99*(4).

Overbury, O., & Wittich, W. (2011). Barriers to low vision rehabilitation: The Montreal Barriers Study. *Investigative Ophthalmology & Visual Science, 52*(12), 8933–8938.

Owsley, C. (2012). Driving with bioptic telescopes: Organizing a research agenda. *Optometry and Vision Science, 89*(9), 1249–1256.

Packer, T. L., Girdler, S., Boldy, D. P., Dhaliwal, S. S., & Crowley, M. (2009). Vision self-management for older adults: A pilot study. *Disability and Rehabilitation, 31*(16), 1353–1361.

Percival, J. (2011). Whole system care and social inclusion of people with sight loss: Implications of key research for policy and service development. *Journal of Integrated Care, 19*(5), 47–57.

Quek, D. T., Koh, V. T., Tan, G. S., Perera, S. A., Wong, T. T., & Aung, T. (2011). Blindness and long-term progression of visual field defects in Chinese patients with primary angle-closure glaucoma. *American Journal of Ophthalmology, 152*(3), 463–469.

Rabello, S., Gasparetto, M. E. R. F., Alves, C. C. D. F., Monteiro, G. B. M., & Carvalho, K. M. D. (2014). The influence of assistive technology devices on the performance of activities by visually impaired. *Revista Brasileira de Oftalmologia, 73*(2), 103–105.

Rees, G., Keeffe, J. E., Hassell, J., Larizza, M., & Lamoureux, E. (2010). A self-management program for low vision: Program overview and pilot evaluation. *Disability and Rehabilitation, 32*(10), 808–815.

Rees, G., Tee, H. W., Marella, M., Fenwick, E., Dirani, M., & Lamoureux, E. L. (2010). Vision-specific distress and depressive symptoms in people with vision impairment. *Investigative Ophthalmology & Visual Science, 51*(6), 2891–2896.

Rees, G., Xie, J., Chiang, P. P., Larizza, M. F., Marella, M., Hassell, J. B., . . . Lamoureux, E. L. (2015). A randomised controlled trial of a self-management programme for low vision implemented in low vision rehabilitation services. *Patient Education and Counseling, 98*(2), 174–181.

Resnikoff, S., Pascolini, D., Etya'ale, D., Kocur, I., Pararajasegaram, R., Pokharel, G. P., & Mariotti, S. P. (2004). Global data on visual impairment in the year 2002. *Bulletin of the World Health Organization, 82*(11), 844–851.

Resnikoff, S., Pascolini, D., Mariotti, S. P., & Pokharel, G. P. (2008). Global magnitude of visual impairment caused by uncorrected refractive errors in 2004. *Bulletin of the World Health Organization, 86*(1), 63–70.

Ricard, P. (2010). *International Agency for the Prevention of Blindness: 2010 report*: London: International Agency for the Prevention of Blindness.

Rollnick, S., & Miller, W. R. (1995). What is motivational interviewing? *Behavioural and Cognitive Psychotherapy, 23*(4), 325–334.

Royal National Institue for the Blind. (2015). *People with sight loss in later life. A systematic review*. London: Author.

Ryan, B. (2014). Models of low vision care: Past, present and future. *Clinical and Experimental Optometry, 97*(3), 209–213.

Saaddine, J. B., Venkat Narayan, K., & Vinicor, F. (2003). Vision loss: A public health problem? *Ophthalmology, 110*(2), 253–254.

Schurink, J., Cox, R., Cillessen, A., van Rens, G., & Boonstra, F. (2011). Low vision aids for visually impaired children: A perception-action perspective. *Research in Developmental Disabilities, 32*(3), 871–882.

Singapore National Eye Center (2013). MyEyeDrops app. Retrieved from http://www.snec.com.sg/Pages/SNEC-Mobile-Apps.aspx

Smith, C., Hancock, H., Blake-Mortimer, J., & Eckert, K. (2007). A randomised comparative trial of yoga and relaxation to reduce stress and anxiety. *Complementary Therapies in Medicine, 15*(2), 77–83.

Stuen, C., & Faye, E. (2003). Vision loss: Normal and not normal changes among older adults. *Generations, 27*(1), 8–14.

Tay, K. C. P., Drury, V. B., & Mackey, S. (2013). The role of intrinsic motivation in a group of low vision patients participating in a self-management programme to enhance self-efficacy and quality of life. *International Journal of Nursing Practice, 20*(1), 17–24.

Torpy, J. M., Lynm, C., & Glass, R. M. (2003). Causes of visual impairment. *JAMA, 290*(15), 2088–2088.

Toseland, R. W., & Rivas, R. F. (2005). *An introduction to group work practice.* (5th ed.) Boston: Allyn & Bacon.

Verstraten, P., Brinkmann, W., Stevens, N., & Schouten, J. (2005). *Loneliness, adaptation to vision impairment, social support and depression among visually impaired elderly.* Paper presented at the International Congress Series.

Vision Australia. (2012). Connecting with others. Retrieved from http://www.visionaustralia.org/living-with-low-vision/connecting-with-others

Wang, J. J., Foran, S., & Mitchell, P. (2000). Age-specific prevalence and causes of bilateral and unilateral visual impairment in older Australians: The Blue Mountains Eye Study. *Clinical & Experimental Ophthalmology, 28*(4), 268–273.

Wittich, W., Canuto, A., & Overbury, O. (2013). Overcoming barriers to low-vision rehabilitation services: Improving the continuum of care. *Canadian Journal of Ophthalmology/Journal Canadien d'Ophtalmologie, 48*(6), 463–467.

World Health Organization. (2012). *Global data on visual impairments 2010.* Fact Sheet 282. Retrieved from http://www.who.int/mediacentre/factsheets/fs282/en/

Zhang, X., Bullard, K. M., Cotch, M. F., Wilson, M. R., Rovner, B. W., McGwin, G., . . . Saaddine, J. B. (2013). Association between depression and functional vision loss in persons 20 years of age or older in the United States, NHANES 2005–2008. *JAMA Ophthalmology, 131*(5), 573–581.

PART III

Innovative Technology and Techniques to Promote Self-Management

20

Telemedicine

KRISTIAN KIDHOLM ■

Telemedicine is often suggested as the answer when the question is raised whether health technologies can be used for improving self-management of individuals with chronic health conditions (Mushcab, Kernohan, Wallace, & Martin, 2015; Vassilev et al., 2015). The objective of this chapter is to describe how different types of telemedicine can be used as a technology to increase self-management of individuals with chronic health conditions. In addition, the potential benefits of telemedicine are described and the challenges in assessment of the value of these technologies are discussed. Hopefully, these descriptions can be useful for managers and healthcare professionals for determining which telemedicine services could be used by their local healthcare systems for improving self-management of individuals with chronic health conditions.

DEFINITIONS OF TELEMEDICINE

In this chapter, "telemedicine" is defined as the delivery of healthcare services through the use of information technologies and communication technologies in a situation where the actors are at different locations (Kidholm et al., 2012). As described by Dinesen et al. (2016), a large number of definitions exist, and generally, a common nomenclature is missing.

In practice, a large number of information and communication technologies can be used as part of a telemedicine service: computers, tablets, smartphones, mobile phones, wireless Internet, telephone lines, video-conferencing systems. The services can be exchanged between the individual with a chronic health condition or relatives and healthcare professionals or between healthcare professionals (e.g., between doctors at a small, local hospital and specialists at a large university hospital).

In this chapter, telemedicine is divided into two different types of services:

- *Synchronous services.* These services require real-time interaction between participants, such as teleconsultation using videoconferencing technology between a provider and an individual with impairment or a provider and subspecialist.
- *Asynchronous services.* These telemedicine services do not involve real-time interaction but rather the storage and forwarding of clinical data between participants. In most cases, home monitoring of individuals with chronic health conditions are asynchronous services.

In practice, these two types of telemedicine services are often combined, for example, when an individual with impairment measures weight, lung function, or blood pressure and stores the information (i.e., asynchronous services) and subsequently discusses the results with a call nurse by video to allow immediate feedback and follow-up questions (i.e., synchronous services).

In addition, telemedicine services can be divided into different types depending on the participant's location:

- Home-based services. These are used in the home of the individual with impairment or in a nursing home.
- Hospital-based services. These are used by a provider who is in contact with an individual with impairment or a medical specialist.
- Mobile health services (m-health). These telemedicine services can be used independently of a specific location (e.g., by use of smartphones or tablets).

TELEMEDICINE AS A TECHNOLOGY TO IMPROVE SELF-MANAGEMENT

As described already, telemedicine consists of several types of services for individuals with many types of chronic health conditions by means of various kinds of technologies. A telemedicine service can be said to be promoting self-management in accordance with the definition of self-management education by Funnel et al. (2007) if telemedicine is used for supporting individuals with chronic health conditions in informed decision-making, self-care behaviors, problem-solving and active collaboration with healthcare professionals or for improving clinical outcomes, health status, and quality of life.

A large number individual studies and reviews of the use of telemedicine to promote self-management for individuals with chronic health conditions can be found in the literature. A few recent examples of systematic reviews for individuals with diabetes, COPD, and chronic heart disease include the following:

- *Diabetes:* Garabedian, Ross-Degnan, and Wharam (2015) have produced a systematic literature review of the effectiveness of m-health interventions for diabetes care and self-management. In the review, 20 studies were analyzed. The studies included self-monitoring of blood glucose with real-time feedback via text messaging or diabetes education, self-management, medication usage programs via smartphone or text-based interventions. Ten studies had HbA1c as primary outcome and, of these, seven demonstrated a statistically significant reduction. On average, the reduction was 0.83% from a baseline average HbA1c level of 8.9%. However, these interventions rarely improved other outcomes, such as self-efficacy or quality of life. Only three studies reported the continuity of the use of m-health during the study period: One study found that 32% discontinued use within two months, another that 66% were not active users after at least six months, and another that 38% did not complete the six planned sessions. The authors concluded that the short-term results from the m-health studies demonstrated promising results, but little evidence was found about the persistent use by individuals with chronic health conditions and about the long-term effectiveness, and therefore more research is needed in that area.

- *COPD:* Lundell, Holmner, Rehn, Nyberg, and Wadell (2015) report a systematic review of the effects of telemedicine on physical activity level, physical capacity, and dyspnea in individuals with COPD. Based on the literature review, nine randomized controlled studies were included. Five of the studies included interventions with the explicit objective of improving self-management. The telemedicine interventions included regular phone calls, mobile phone reminders, text massages, web-based education, or weekly sessions via Skype combined with education and exercise. Dropouts in the telemedicine groups varied from 0% to 52%. By means of meta-analysis, a statistically significant effect was found on physical activity level but not on physical capacity or dyspnea. The authors conclude that although improvement in physical activity level was found, the result should be treated with caution given the heterogeneity in the studies and that further studies are needed.
- *Heart failure:* Radhakrishnan and Jacelon (2012) reviewed studies of the impact of telemedicine interventions on the self-management of individuals with heart failure. Fourteen studies were included, and eight of these were randomized controlled trials. The telemedicine interventions included devices for remote monitoring of vital signs (blood pressure, pulse, weight, electrocardiogram); real-time remote assessment of cardiopulmonary status through videoconferencing, education, and reinforcement of individuals' knowledge regarding heart-failure pathophysiology; chronic health condition management; and information to informal caregiver through a website specific to a chronic health condition. A meta-analysis of the results was not performed, but in 5 of the 14 studies, significant improvement was found in self-care behaviors of the individuals using telemedicine. Five other studies did not find differences between intervention and control groups. The review

concludes that the available evidence supports the use of telemedicine in enabling self-management, but small sample sizes and inadequate measurement methods limit the generalizability of the findings. Flawed design issues were present in several studies.

Based on the aforementioned results, the evidence for the impact of telemedicine on the self-management of individuals with diabetes, COPD, and heart failure seems to be weak and inconsistent. This could reflect the fact that that even though the number of studies is growing, there is still large variation in the content of the telemedicine interventions, and a large proportion of the studies still have flawed design issues. In addition, many interventions still have problems with a large proportion of participants dropping out and being unwilling to continue using the telemedicine services.

The results from studies of telemedicine interventions that had the objective of influencing individuals' degree of self-management are similar to the evidence on telemedicine for individuals with chronic health conditions in general. In a large literature review by Wootton (2012), the value of telemedicine in the management of five chronic health conditions (asthma, COPD, diabetes, heart failure, and hypertension) was described. The review included 141 randomized controlled trials. Of these, 65 studies (46%) reported a statistically significant improvement in the primary outcomes, and 43 studies (30%) reported a statistically significant improvement in one or more secondary outcomes. The studies are generally criticized for only looking at short-term effects and for not taking into account that the effects found can be caused by the increased attention brought on by the experiment (Hawthorne effect) and not by the telemedicine service itself.

Wootton (2012) also analyzed 22 systematic reviews of telemedicine in the five chronic health conditions mentioned already and found that half of them only performed a qualitative, narrative review and that *none* of the reviews concluded negatively that telemedicine was unhelpful. The other half performed a quantitative analysis and provided 23 pooled estimates of the effect of telemedicine. Of these studies, approximately half showed statistically significant outcomes for the users of telemedicine, whereas the other half showed that telemedicine is no better than the treatment in the control group. On this basis, Wootton concludes that research on telemedicine is rather weak and unsatisfactory at the present time.

The fact that the research behind telemedicine interventions, in general, is weak and unsatisfactory has also been considered in a comment in *The New England Journal of Medicine* by Kahn (2015). He pointed out that most telemedicine studies are "methodologically weak before and after studies that rarely examine patient-centered outcomes, instead focusing on feasibility and acceptability to patients" (p. 1684). This is consistent with the finding by Wootton (2012) that only about 1 in 10 published papers on the use of telemedicine are formal randomized controlled trials.

The issue of the cost-effectiveness of telemedicine solutions is also discussed by Wootton (2012), who argues that few studies include the economic consequences of telemedicine and that it is not possible to state whether telemedicine will be cost-effective in the management of one or more chronic health conditions. This view is supported by Mistry (2012), who carried out a systematic review of cost-effectiveness analyses of telemedicine and telecare in general. Eighty economic studies were found. Generally, inadequate study design was used and the reporting of methods and results was not consistent with guidelines for economic evaluation. As an example, most of the studies did not give adequate details about study design or provide sufficient information on how costs were collected, calculated, and reported. Mistry (2012) therefore concluded that "there is no further conclusive evidence that telemedicine and telecare interventions are cost-effective compared to conventional health care" (p. 1). This is supported by a Cochrane review of interactive telemedicine interventions by Flodgren, Rachas, Farmer, Inzitari, and Shepperd (2015). The review included 93 randomized controlled trials, 23 of which were randomized controlled trials targeting self-management; and of these, 9 were able to find lower costs for treating individuals with chronic health conditions using telemedicine. The review also points out that the studies of the costs of telemedicine differ with regard to the types of costs included and therefore are difficult to compare.

TELEMEDICINE AS A STRATEGY FOR THE DEVELOPMENT OF HEALTHCARE SYSTEMS

In spite of the limitations of the scientific evidence for the effectiveness and cost-effectiveness of telemedicine, these innovative technologies have been suggested as a solution to the demographic and economic challenges that healthcare systems worldwide are facing. Many European countries have developed their own national telemedicine or e-health strategy. "E-health" can be defined as the use of information and communication technologies in healthcare prevention, diagnosis, treatment, monitoring, and management. A sample of strategies from European countries can be found at the Momentum homepage (http://www.telemedicine-momentum.eu/europe/). The Momentum homepage describes that, typically, the aims of using e-health and telemedicine in system-level strategies are to enable individuals to become more directly involved in the design and management of their own care, to implement telemedicine at scale, to improve quality of life for individuals with impairments and citizens, and to increase the efficiency and effectiveness of workflows within the healthcare sector.

In the United States, the Health Resources and Services Administration works to increase and improve the use of telehealth to meet the needs of underserved people. Resources are also provided in the United States through the Federal Office of Rural Health Policy and the Office for the Advancement of Telehealth to support regional telehealth technical assistance centers, a national telehealth policy center, and a national telehealth technology assistance center as described by Dinesen et al. (2016). In addition http://www.telehealthresourcecenter.org/ provides assistance, education, and information on telehealth on behalf the US Department of Health and Human Services' Health Resources and Services Administration Office for the Advancement of Telehealth.

A European policy framework and strategy for the twenty-first century called "Health 2020" has been developed by the World Health Organization. The vision of this initiative is to achieve the highest level of health among European countries, improve health for all citizens, reduce health inequalities, empower citizens to take care of their own health, and strengthen people-centered health systems and public health capacity (World Health Organization, 2012). The strategy describes how telemedicine, e-health, and mobile health (m-health) have the potential for reducing costs of care and at the same time increasing participation and empowerment for individuals with chronic health conditions.

The EU Commission (2012) has also launched an e-health action plan for 2012–2020 titled, "Innovative Healthcare for the 21st Century in the EU." This plan describes how telemedicine and eHealth can benefit citizens, individuals with chronic health conditions, healthcare professionals, and health organizations, and that telemedicine can deliver more personalized healthcare, which is more effective and efficient and helps reduce errors and length of hospitalization when applied effectively (European Commission, 2012).

HOW TO ASSESS THE VALUE OF TELEMEDICINE

In a situation where national and international institutions, on the one hand, recommend implementation and use of telemedicine and e-health, and where, on the other hand, the evidence of the effectiveness and cost-effectiveness of these technologies is described as weak and unsatisfactory, primary and secondary healthcare institutions are faced with a challenge. The severity of this challenge is underscored by a lack of national regulation and control over the use of e-health technology in most countries. Whereas pharmaceutical drugs are highly regulated by the national boards of health or similar governmental institutions in most countries, national institutions regulating e-health generally does not exist.

In this situation, hospitals and other healthcare institutions are forced into producing their own assessment of the value of telemedicine. Wade, Gray, and Carati (2016) describe three evaluation frameworks that can be used to assess the effectiveness of a telemedicine service: the National Telemedicine Outcome Indicators Project in Canada (Scott et al., 2007); the three-dimensional model for telemedicine evaluation by Bashshur, Shannon, and Sapci (2005); and the Model for Assessment of Telemedicine (MAST) by Kidholm et al. (2012). Of these models, MAST is the only one that was developed on the basis of healthcare decision-makers' need for information when making decisions on investment in telemedicine. MAST is also the most widely used model in empirical studies. MAST is described further later.

As described in Table 20.1, six European telemedicine studies, including regions in more than 20 European countries, have used MAST as a structure for data collection and reporting. The studies include more than 30,000 individuals with

Table 20.1. EUROPEAN TELEMEDICINE PROJECTS USING THE MODEL FOR ASSESSMENT OF TELEMEDICINE

Project	Design of Studies	Number of Individuals with Chronic Health Conditions
Renewing Health[a]	19 RCT studies	7,000
United4Health[b]	3 observational studies	10,000
SmartCare[c]	1 observational study	9,000
InCASA[d]	5 feasibility studies	150
MasterMind[e]	1 observational study	5,200
Connected4Health[f]	6 feasibility studies	200

[a]http://www.renewinghealth.eu/en/. [b]http://united4health.eu/. [c]http://www.pilotsmartcare.eu/home./. [d]http://www.incasa-project.eu/news.php. [e]http://mastermind-project.eu/. [f]https://ec.europa.eu/digital-single-market/en/news/testing-e-health-services-nordics-connected-health-project-launched

chronic health conditions, and the design of the studies varies from small feasibility studies to large randomized controlled trials and observational studies. A number of scientific publications using MAST can be found, for example, Charrier, Zarca, Durand-Zaleski, Calinaud, and ARS Ile de France Telemedicine Group (2016), Rosenbek Minet et al. (2015), Rasmussen et al. (2015), and Sorknaes et al. (2013).

MODEL FOR ASSESSMENT OF TELEMEDICINE

MAST states that the objective of an assessment of telemedicine applications is both to describe the effectiveness and contribution to quality of care and to produce a basis for decision-making. This requires the relevant assessment to be a multidisciplinary process, which summarizes and evaluates information about the medical, social, economic, and ethical issues related to the use of telemedicine in a systematic, unbiased, robust manner (Kidholm et al., 2012). This definition is based on the definition of Health Technology Assessment in the EUnetHTA Core model (see Lampe et al., 2009).

Two concepts are crucial in this definition. First, the concept of "multidisciplinary" indicates that the assessments should include all important outcomes of the applications for individuals with chronic health conditions, clinicians, healthcare institutions, and society in general. Thus an assessment of a telemedicine intervention should be comprehensive and include information about the effects of the technology, which is relevant from all kinds of perspectives. Second, the concepts of "systematic, unbiased, and robust" imply that assessment of the effectiveness of telemedicine should be based on scientific studies and methods and on scientific criteria for quality of evidence. This means that description of results should follow general guidelines for reporting health research, such as guidelines for reporting of randomized controlled trials and economic evaluation, as described by Simera et al. (2010).

THE THREE STEPS IN ASSESSING TELEMEDICINE

MAST was developed in 2011 based on results from two workshops with key stakeholder groups from the healthcare systems in European countries. At the workshops, the participants were presented with results from a literature review on methods used in the assessment of telemedicine and the content of the EUnetHTA Core Model. However, during the workshops it became clear that the assessment of telemedicine was not just about assessing the effectiveness of the technology according to the participants but also about evaluating the maturity of the telemedicine service and of the transferability of the evidence found. Therefore, using MAST in an assessment of a telemedicine intervention requires not just one step but three steps as illustrated in Figure 20.1.

The idea behind *the first step*, called the preceding assessment, is that the maturity of the telemedicine technology and the organization planning to implement the intervention need to be assessed before an assessment of the effectiveness of the technology is carried out. For instance, if legal issues or problems with reimbursement are present, these need to be handled first. If the development of a telemedicine service is still at an early stage, formative studies including participatory design studies, prototype studies, usability studies, and feasibility studies must be completed. An example of this first step of MAST can be found in Rosenbek

STEP 1: Preceding assessment:
- Are the technology and the organization matured?

STEP 2: Multidisciplinary assessment:
1. Health problem and characteristics of the application
2. Safety
3. Clinical effectiveness
4. Patient perspectives
5. Economic aspects
6. Organizational aspects
7. Sociocultural, ethical, and legal aspects

STEP 3: Transferability assessment:
- Cross-border
- Scalability
- Generalizability

Figure 20.1 The three steps in assessment of telemedicine.

Minet et al. (2015), describing a feasibility study of a telemedicine rehabilitation application for individuals with COPD. If a telemedicine application is still being developed and needs further improvement, a multidisciplinary assessment of the effectiveness of the application should not be started.

After ensuring that the telemedicine application and the organization are mature and ready for implementation, a multidisciplinary assessment of the effectiveness of the technology can be carried out in *the second step*. To assist those who carry out the assessment, the possible multidisciplinary outcomes and aspects of telemedicine have been divided into seven groups or domains. Table 20.2 defines the different domains and describes topics that could be included within each domain as described in Kidholm et al. (2012). Notice that the relation between the domains are strong, for example, the description of the use of resources in the organizational domain and the estimated costs in the economic domain. Therefore, the division of outcomes into domains may be challenging in practice and the description of effects in one domain may supplement the description of outcomes in other domains.

Finally, in *the third step*, an assessment should be made of the transferability of the results found in the second step. If the multidisciplinary assessment is based on a literature review and includes data from studies in other countries or in healthcare institutions of a different type or size, the relevance of the results for the specific institution considering implementation of the service should be considered. Similarly, if a new study of the telemedicine application is carried out at the local institution considering implementation of the service, the generalizability of the results should be described. This can include assessment of generalizability across borders, the scalability of the results (e.g., from a small to a large hospital), and generalizability to other chronic health condition groups.

Figure 20.2 illustrates an example of how MAST can be applied to structure the design and collection of data in a study of the outcomes of telemedicine. In this case, a randomized controlled trial was carried out to assess the effectiveness of a telemedicine solution for individuals with COPD. The study included collection of data on safety, clinical outcomes, individual with chronic health conditions' perception, and economic aspects. In addition, organizational aspects were studied in an interview study with the COPD nurses, and ethical and legal aspects were assessed by a legal expert. The clinical results are reported in Sorknaes et al. (2012).

LEVEL OF EVIDENCE NEEDED

As described in the literature review by Wootton (2012) and the comment by Kahn (2015), most studies of telemedicine are methodologically weak and focus on feasibility and acceptability to individuals with chronic health conditions. This is reflected in many discussions concerning the necessary level of evidence or internal validity in studies of telemedicine.

On the one hand, it is argued that telemedicine and e-health are technologies that are developing and improving too fast and that randomized controlled trials take too long. On the other hand, it is argued that more rapid focus-group studies

Table 20.2. DOMAINS IN THE MODEL FOR ASSESSMENT OF TELEMEDICINE

Domain	Definition	Topics
1. Health problem and description of the application	Description of the health problem of the individuals with chronic health conditions expected to use the telemedicine application and the application being assessed	• Health problem of individuals with chronic health conditions • Description of the application • Technical characteristics
2. Safety	Identification and assessment of harms	• Clinical safety • Technical safety (technical reliability)
3. Clinical effectiveness	Effects on the individuals with chronic health conditions' health	• Effects on mortality, disability, Health-related quality of life • Behavioral outcomes (e.g., exercise) • Utilization of health services
4. Individual with a chronic health condition perspectives	Issues related to the perception of the individual with a chronic health condition or the relatives of the telemedicine application including the individual with chronic health conditions and his or her relatives' acceptance of the technology	• Satisfaction and acceptance • Ability to use the application • Access and accessibility • Empowerment, self-efficacy
5. Economic aspects	A societal *economic evaluation* comparing a telemedicine application with relevant alternatives in terms of costs and consequences and a *business case* describing the expenditures and revenues for the healthcare institutions using the telemedicine application	Economic evaluation: • Amount of resources used • Prices for each resource • Related changes in use of healthcare • Clinical effectiveness Business case: • Expenditures per year • Revenue per year
6. Organizational aspects	Assessment of what kind of resources have to be mobilized and organized when implementing a new technology, and what kind of changes or consequences the use can further produce in the organization.	• Process • Structure • Culture—perception of staff • Management

Table 20.2. CONTINUED

Domain	Definition	Topics
7. Sociocultural, ethical, and legal aspects	The sociocultural aspects include the social-cultural arenas where the individual with a chronic health condition lives and acts during use of the application. The ethical analysis appraises the ethical questions raised by the application itself and by the consequences of implementing it or not. Legal aspects focus on the legal obligations that must be met and any specific legal barriers that may exist to the implementation of the application	• Ethical issues • Legal issues • Social issues

NOTE: Adapted from Kidholm, K., Ekeland, A. G., Jensen, L.K., Rasmussen, J., Pedersen, C.D., Bowes, A., Flottorp, S.A., Bech, M. (2012). A model for assessment of telemedicine applications: MAST. *International Journal of Technology Assessment in Health Care, 28*(1), 44–51.

and expert views have a low degree of internal validity and will not produce trustworthy estimates about the effectiveness of telemedicine.

Liu and Wyatt (2011) have described the arguments for and against the use of randomized controlled trials in studies on clinical information systems, and their discussion is just as relevant for telemedicine. One of their conclusions is that the general principle for selection between the different study designs should be that the design must follow closely from the question. Thus focus-group studies and other qualitative methods are appropriate when the research question is about how individuals feel about a telemedicine application, such as how it can be improved. Similarly, a randomized controlled trial is appropriate when the research question is about the effect of telemedicine on a specific outcome. Thus focus group and other qualitative methods are relevant in the first step of MAST, whereas randomized controlled trials are relevant in the multidisciplinary assessment of outcomes in the second step.

It should be added that randomized controlled trials have specific challenges in studies of the outcomes of telemedicine. First, the blinding of individuals with chronic health conditions during the treatment allocation process is difficult and the fact that the individuals know that they have been selected in a study to be in

Domain	Data collection and outcomes
1. Health problem and description of the application	Description of the individual with chronic health condition, his or her health problems and the telemedicine intervention.
	Based on data from a randomized controlled trial with 266 individual with chronic health conditions:
2. Safety	Outcome: Ability of individual with chronic health conditions to get Internet connection.
3. Clinical effectiveness	Outcomes: Mortality, FEV1, SAT, MRC, BMI, SF-36, chronic health condition exercise.
4. Individuals with chronic health conditions perspectives	Individuals with chronic health conditions acceptability questionnaire and qualitative interviews with individuals with chronic health conditions.
5. Economic aspects	Total costs of telemedicine intervention per individuals with chronic health condition including: Investments, number of consultations, number of readmissions, number of outpatient visits, number of home nurse visits, use of emergency ward. Business case including estimated costs and changes in reimbursement.
6. Organizational aspects	Interview study with nurses. Topics: Task shifts, use of time, satisfaction.
7. Socio-cultural, ethical and legal aspects	Interview with legal expert

Figure 20.2 Example of data collection based on MAST.

"the telemedicine group" may result in a bias. Second, implementation of telemedicine applications sometimes necessitates large organizational changes in order to be able to obtain the full potential of the technology. In that case, it will be difficult to treat both an intervention group and a control group within the same clinical department because this requires for the organization to be changed and maintained at the same time. In this case, randomization at the level of the individuals with chronic health condition is problematic. The solution is randomization at the organizational level, also called cluster randomization, for example, a group of hospitals is randomized to the telemedicine group and another group is randomized to the control group. In this way, effects of organizational changes can be included in the outcome measures.

Another important conclusion from Liu and Wyatt (2011) is that even though a randomized controlled trial is ideally suited to answer questions about effectiveness, it is only necessary if the technology either costs a significant amount of money or may expose individuals with chronic health conditions, healthcare professionals, or health systems to added risk. As an example, a randomized design should be considered if a telemedicine application is being used by individuals with chronic health conditions with a high level of mortality and disability or if a telemedicine service is very costly. On the other hand, if a low-cost telemedicine service is considered for improving the quality of care for individuals with chronic health conditions with limited impact on disability, other types of design can be used because the consequences of a biased result are limited.

CONCLUSION

Telemedicine has the potential to improve the self-management of individuals with chronic health conditions. This has been demonstrated in a number of studies. However, many different types of technologies exist, and the evidence shows large heterogeneity in both the design of studies and the results found. Even though research in telemedicine is improving in identifying the most relevant groups of individuals with chronic health conditions for these technologies and the optimal conditions for a cost-effective implementation, the typical conclusion in most reviews of telemedicine is that "more research is needed."

At the same time hospitals and other healthcare institutions are under strong pressure from local, national, and international e-health strategies to implement more telemedicine services, and telemedicine is generally considered one of the main technological solutions to the demographic and geographic challenges faced by many countries.

Therefore, healthcare institutions need to carry out their own assessments of telemedicine, and the MAST model presented can be used for this purpose. By means of MAST, healthcare decision-makers will get a multidisciplinary assessment of the outcomes of the technologies based on international standards for the quality of scientific studies. Even though these studies take time, hopefully the systematic assessment of new telemedicine services will ensure that only safe, effective, and cost-effective technologies are implemented for the benefit of individuals with chronic health conditions.

REFERENCES

Angel, D., Bjerregaard, J., O'Conner, T., McGuinness, W., Kröger, K., Rasmussen, B. S. R., & Yderstraede, K. B. (2015). The model for assessment of telemedicine (MAST)—evaluation of telemedical solutions. *Journal of Wound Care*, 24(Suppl. 5), S10–S13.

Bashshur, R., Shannon, G., & Sapci, H. (2005). Telemedicine evaluation. *Telemedicine and eHealth*, 11(3), 296–316.

Charrier, N., Zarca, K., Durand-Zaleski, I., Calinaud, C., & ARS Ile de France Telemedicine Group. (2016). Efficacy and cost effectiveness of telemedicine for improving access to care in the Paris region: study protocols for eight trials. *BMC Health Services Research*, 16, 45.

Dinesen, B., Nonnecke, B., Lindeman, D., Toft, E., Kidholm, K., Jethwani, K., ... Nesbitt, T. (2016). Personalized telehealth in the future: A global research agenda. *Journal of Medical Internet Research*, 18(3), 1–18:

European Commission. (2012). *Communication from the Commission to the European Parliament, the Council, the European Economic and Social Committee and the Committee of the Regions: eHealth Action Plan 2012–2020: Innovative healthcare for the 21st century.* Brussels: Author. Retrieved from http://ec.europa.eu/health/ehealth/docs/com_2012_736_en.pdf

Flodgren, G., Rachas, A., Farmer, A. J., Inzitari, M., & Shepperd, S. (2015). Interactive telemedicine: Effects on professional practice and health care outcomes. *Cochrane Database of Systematic Reviews, 9,* CD002098.

Funnell, M. M., Brown, T. L., Childs, B.P., Haas, L. B., Hosey, G. M., Jensen, B., ... Weiss, M. A. (2007). National standards for diabetes self-management education. *Diabetes Care, 30,* 1630–1637.

Garabedian, L. F., Ross-Degnan, D., & Wharam, J. F. (2015). Mobile phone and smartphone technologies for diabetes care and self-management. *Current Diabetes Reports, 15*(109), 1–9.

Kahn, J. M. (2015). Virtual visits—confronting the challenges of telemedicine. *The New England Journal of Medicine, 372,* 1684–1685.

Kidholm, K., Ekeland, A. G., Jensen, L.K., Rasmussen, J., Pedersen, C. D., Bowes, A., ... Bech, M. (2012). A model for assessment of telemedicine applications: MAST. *International Journal of Technology Assessment in Health Care, 28*(1), 44–51.

Lampe, K., Mäkelä, M., Garrido, M.V., Anttila, H., Autti-Rämö, I., Hicks, N. J., ... European Network for Health Technology Assessment. (2009). The HTA core model: A novel method for producing and reporting health technology assessments. *International Journal of Technology Assessment in Health Care, 25,* 9–20.

Liu, J. L. Y., & Wyatt, J. C. (2011). The case for randomized controlled trials to assess the impact of clinical information systems. *Journal of the American Medical Informatics Association, 18,* 173–180.

Lundell, S., Holmner, Å., Rehn, B., Nyberg, A., & Wadell, K. (2015). Telehealthcare in COPD: A systematic review and meta-analysis on physical outcomes and dyspnea. *Respiratory Medicine, 109*(1), 11–26.

Mistry, H. (2012). Systematic review of studies of the cost-effectiveness of telemedicine and telecare. Changes in the economic evidence over twenty years. *Journal of Telemedicine and Telecare, 18*(1) 1–6.

Mushcab, H., Kernohan, G. W., Wallace, J., & Martin, S. (2015). Web-based remote monitoring systems for self-managing type 2 diabetes: A systematic review. *Diabetes Technology & Therapeutics, 17*(7), 498–509.

Radhakrishnan, K., & Jacelon, C. (2012). Impact of telehealth on patient self-management of heart failure: A review of literature. *Journal of Cardiovascular Nursing, 27*(1), 33–43.

Rasmussen, B. S., Jensen, L. K., Froekjaer, J., Kidholm, K., Kensing, F., & Yderstraede, K. B. (2015). A qualitative study of the key factors in implementing telemedical monitoring of diabetic foot ulcer individual with a chronic impairments. *International Journal of Medical Informatics, 84*(10), 799–807.

Rosenbek Minet, L., Hansen, L. W., Pedersen, C. D., Titlestad, I. L., Christensen, J. K., Kidholm, K., ... Møllegård, L. (2015). Early telemedicine training and counselling after hospitalization in patients with severe chronic obstructive pulmonary disease: a feasibility study. *BMC Medical Informatics and Decision Making, 15,* 3.

Scott, R. E., McCarthy, F. G., Jennett, P. A., Perverseff, T., Lorenzetti, D., & Saeed, A. (2007). National Telehealth Outcome Indicators Project. *J Telemed Telecare, 13*(Suppl. 2), 1–38.

Simera, I., Moher, D., Hirst, A., Hoey, J., Schulz, K. F., & Altman, D. G. (2010). Transparent and accurate reporting increases reliability, utility, and impact of your research: Reporting guidelines and the EQUATOR Network. *BMC Medicine, 8,* 24.

Sorknaes, A. D., Bech, M., Madsen, H., Titlestad, I. L., Hounsgaard, L., Hansen-Nord, M., . . . Østergaard, B. (2013). The effect of real-time teleconsultations between hospital-based nurses and patients with severe COPD discharged after an exacerbation. *Journal of Telemedicine and Telecare, 19*(8), 466–474.

Vassilev, I., Rowsell, A., Pope, C., Kennedy, A., O'Cathain A., Salisbury, C., & Rogers, A. (2015). Assessing the implementability of telehealth interventions for self-management support: A realist review. *Implementation Science, 10,* 59.

Wade, V., Gray, L., & Carati, C. (2016). Theoretical frameworks in telemedicine research. *Journal of Telemedicine and Telecare, 23*(1), 181–187.

World Health Organization. (2012). The new European policy for health—Health 2020 policy framework and strategy. Retrieved from http://www.who.int/workforcealliance/knowledge/resources/Health2020_long.pdf

Wootton, R. (2012). Twenty years of telemedicine in chronic disease management—an evidence synthesis. *Journal of Telemedicine and Telecare, 18*(4), 211–220.

Internet Interventions

GERHARD ANDERSSON ■

Modern information technology and, in particular, use of the Internet have had immediate consequences for the practice of medicine and also for the management of chronic health conditions. Clients use the Internet to search for information, communicate with their significant others and with healthcare professionals, and use social media to get support; in addition, increasingly, the Internet is used as a way to deliver psychosocial interventions (Andersson, 2016). The focus of this chapter is on Internet-delivered psychological treatments and in particular, Internet-supported cognitive-behavior therapy (ICBT). This chapter begins by describing how ICBT can be conducted, covering the role of guiding clinicians and different technological solutions and then commenting on the evidence base for ICBT in the management of chronic health conditions. Some hurdles and problems when implementing ICBT into regular practice are then highlighted. The important topic of moderators of outcomes—in other words, "what works for whom?"—is also covered. Finally, some suggestions for future research including the prospect of blending regular face-to-face services and modern information technology are provided.

THE PRACTICE OF INTERNET INTERVENTIONS

As a starting point, Internet interventions, including ICBT, require technological facilities, such as access to the Internet and a platform to reach the Internet (computer, tablet, smartphone, etc.). One distinguishing feature is whether human contact is involved in the intervention. The role of support in ICBT has been a constant topic for discussion since the early studies in the mid-1990s (Andersson, Carlbring, & Lindefors, 2016), with pros and cons of involving support (e.g., more costly with support, reaching fewer than automated treatments but most likely more secure and effective). Computerized psychological interventions predate Internet interventions (Marks, Shaw, & Parkin, 1998), with programs like Eliza

(Epstein & Klinkenberg, 2001) and computerized cognitive-behavior therapy programs like "Beating the Blues" (Proudfoot et al., 2003).

With the emergence of the Internet came the use of email as a way to deliver therapy, which either can be in a real-time "chat" format (Kessler et al., 2009) or through regular, asynchronous email (Murphy & Mitchell, 1998). Surprisingly, there are few randomized controlled studies on email therapy, in spite of being practiced widely across the world for more than 20 years. However, there are hybrids of computerized programs and correspondence between a client and a therapist in an email-like format, and this combination has been surprisingly effective in a large number of controlled trials (Andersson, 2014). Thus, Internet interventions can either be supported or automated, and sometimes the very same program is delivered as either unguided (Christensen, Griffiths, & Jorm, 2004) or guided as an adjunct to face-to-face services (Høifødt et al., 2013).

Most studies to date show that unguided Internet interventions (mostly ICBT) are associated with less completion of the treatment, higher dropout rates, and potentially smaller effects when compared against guided interventions (Baumeister, Reichler, Munzinger, & Lin, 2014). It is important to note that the guidance in ICBT tends to be minimal and often not more time-consuming than 10 minutes per week per client (compared to a face-to-face session, which requires much more time and also administration). Moreover, it may also be that studies on unguided ICBT have used less comprehensive programs, and in studies directly comparing guided versus unguided delivery of the same Internet treatment program, differences in how much of the treatment is completed and in outcomes have been less marked, with sometimes no difference at all found (Berger, Caspar, et al., 2011; Berger, Hämmerli, Gubser, Andersson, & Caspar, 2011; Dear et al., 2015), whereas in other studies, guidance has generated better outcomes (Kleiboer et al., 2015).

The basic idea behind ICBT is to present the same contents as in manualized cognitive-behavioral therapy (CBT) but to do this via text, video (e.g., online lectures), and audio. Interactive features are also possible in the programs, such as quizzes and automated responses. The programs tend to contain information of similar length as a 200-page book and have more or less the same duration as face-to-face therapy (e.g., 10 weeks for a depression program). A vast majority of the Internet interventions have been based on CBT, but there are also programs based on psychodynamic psychotherapy (Johansson, Nyblom, Carlbring, Cuijpers, & Andersson, 2013), mindfulness (Boettcher et al., 2014), interpersonal psychotherapy (Dagöö et al., 2014), and various forms of CBT, such as acceptance-oriented treatments (Lappalainen et al., 2014) and bias modification training (Boettcher, Berger, & Renneberg, 2012).

In this chapter, the focus is on CBT, and these programs commonly start with psychoeducation. Then treatment components are presented along with homework assignments. Depending on the condition(s) treated, these can be of various forms such as behavioral activation scheduling, exposure, relaxation, stress management, and several other components. In order to accommodate the vast co-occurrence between different forms of psychological problems, two different approaches have emerged (Andersson & Titov, 2014). One is transdiagnostic in the sense that one program is used for several problems (Titov et al., 2011). This program is inspired by the unified protocol outlined by Barlow and colleagues (2011) and has been found to generate good outcomes in controlled trials (Johnston, Titov, Andrews, Spence, & Dear, 2011). Another approach to handle co-occurrence of psychological problems has been developed by researchers in Sweden (Carlbring et al., 2010). Instead of having one treatment intended to suit all, the treatment program is tailored according to the symptoms and problems that the client has and also, to some extent, his or her preferences. This treatment format has been tested for anxiety (Carlbring et al., 2010) and depression (Johansson et al., 2012) and partly for other conditions as well, with some elements being tailored (Buhrman et al., 2015). For example, in the treatment of tinnitus (ringing or buzzing in the ears), tailoring was part of the ICBT program early on, as some clients (but not all) experience insomnia, noise sensitivity, and significant hearing problems (Kaldo et al., 2013).

The role of the therapist in guided ICBT has not been studied extensively, but there are studies showing that a therapeutic alliance is formed between the online therapist and the client and that ratings of the alliance are high (Sucala et al., 2012). However, early ratings of the alliance (e.g., by using an adapted version of the Working Alliance Inventory) rarely correlate with treatment outcome (Andersson, 2016). There is also an emerging literature on therapist behaviors, suggesting that the way the support person (not necessarily a therapist) acts makes a difference (Paxling et al., 2013). On the other hand, therapist effects (i.e., differences in outcome between different therapists) tend to be small (Almlöv, Carlbring, Berger, Cuijpers, & Andersson, 2009), and in a series of studies, Titov and colleagues (2010) found that the support could be provided from a practical and technical rather than therapeutic perspective. Thus, even if support has been found to be important in most studies, the way support is provided can be simple. It may be that just having support when needed (on demand) is sufficient to generate good outcomes (Rheker, Andersson, & Weise, 2015) and that some programs with automated reminders can be effective (Dear et al., 2015).

THE ROLE OF TECHNOLOGY IN INTERNET INTERVENTIONS

Originally, most ICBT programs were basically text-based and presented in PDF files. This was motivated by the fact that in 1998, access to broadband Internet connections was rare, and thus, people did not want to spend much time on the Internet. Since then technology has developed and treatment platforms are now capable of much more than delivering PDF files. First, security is high, with encrypted communication and double- authentication procedures at login (Vlaescu, Carlbring, Lunner, & Andersson, 2015). Overall, security is important in Internet interventions and should be considered when implementing ICBT (Bennett, Bennett, & Griffiths, 2010).

Second, treatment platforms need to be flexible as clients move between different platforms (e.g., computers, smartphones, and tablets). In effect, this means that systems need to be responsive and change appearance depending on which device the client is using. This has been available for some time. Another challenge is to have chat (including video chat) embedded in the system (encrypted). It can also be important to have user-friendly data management procedures for researchers. Use of text messages for reminders and quick links to daily registrations (so-called ecological momentary assessment) are other features of some systems, including the one used by the research group in Linköping, Sweden (Vlaescu, Alasjö, Miloff, Carlbring, & Andersson, 2016).

Third, there are thousands of smartphone applications now available. Very few have been tested in research (Donker et al., 2013), but there are exceptions, such as a smartphone application for behavioral activation in the treatment of depression (Ly, Trüschel, et al., 2014). Overall, this is a rapidly changing field with numerous applications for assessment (Areán, Ly, & Andersson, 2016), including mobile sensors and other innovative approaches, such as serious gaming (Mohr, Burns, Schueller, Clarke, & Klinkman, 2013).

Overall, it is hard to predict future use of technology and the role of social media, changing devices, and, in particular, attitudes among both treatment providers and clients. It is not always the case the best technology wins, and sometimes unexpected uses (text messaging is one example) become popular, whereas approaches, such as video telephony, are used to a much lesser extent than expected.

USE OF ICBT IN SELF-MANAGEMENT OF CHRONIC HEALTH CONDITIONS

It is beyond the scope of this chapter to cover all the conditions for which guided ICBT has been developed and tested (Andersson, 2014). In particular, the literature on mild to moderate psychiatric conditions is extensive, basically covering all of the anxiety disorders and several studies on depression. This section gives examples of programs and studies on chronic somatic impairments for which there are programs and controlled studies on guided ICBT. A systematic review on the effects of Internet interventions for somatic health problems was published (Cuijpers, van Straten, & Andersson, 2008) and included only 12 studies; there are now at least twice as many controlled studies on chronic health conditions. A more recent review included more studies (Beatty & Lambert, 2013): 24 were included, covering eight different health problems.

Chronic pain, including headaches, has been the topic for much research. The first headache study was published by my group and was conducted in 1998 (Ström, Pettersson, & Andersson, 2000). When it comes to headache pain, there have been relatively few studies, but in the field of chronic low back pain, there are several controlled trials. We were first with a trial on ICBT for chronic pain (Buhrman, Fältenhag, Ström, & Andersson, 2004) and have since then conducted four additional controlled trials using different programs. The effects of Internet interventions for chronic pain and headaches were summarized in a systematic review (Buhrman, Gordh, & Andersson, 2016), which included 22 trials. Two trials were aimed at children and youth, and five focused on chronic headaches and/or migraines. The rest were on chronic pain. The studies were very heterogeneous, but promising outcomes were observed on measures of interference/disability (Hedge's $g = -0.39$), pain intensity (Hedge's $g = -0.33$), and catastrophizing (Hedge's $g = -0.49$). Even if these effects are smaller than what usually is found in studies on depression and anxiety, they are in line with findings by studies using regular CBT for chronic pain (Williams, Eccleston, & Morley, 2012). One example of an ICBT trial tested a program in which an individualized treatment was delivered for individuals with chronic pain who also had symptoms of anxiety and depression (Buhrman et al., 2015). A total of 52 participants with chronic pain and depression were included and randomized to either ICBT treatment for eight weeks or to a control group that participated in a moderated online discussion forum. Results showed significant decreases regarding depressive symptoms and pain disability in the treatment group. Reductions were also found on a measure of pain catastrophizing. We also included a one-year follow-up, which showed that results were maintained.

Another problem that is disabling for many people is irritable bowel syndrome (IBS). At least two research groups have done studies on ICBT for IBS, and the first controlled trial was conducted in the United States (Hunt, Moshier, & Milonova, 2009). Swedish researchers developed a program for IBS that includes exposure exercises (directed toward avoidance of situations: e.g., going to the cinema). Following a pilot study, a range of controlled trials were published on the 10-week program. Not only has the program been tested against a wait-list group (Ljótsson et al., 2010) but also in an effectiveness study (Ljótsson, Andersson, et al., 2011), against stress management (Ljótsson, Hedman, et al., 2011), and in a study directly comparing ICBT with or without exposure instructions (Ljotsson et al., 2014). An example of a large trial in that series of trials is the one comparing ICBT against stress management. The trial included 195 participants diagnosed with IBS. The two treatments were distinctly different as the ICBT treatment emphasized acceptance of symptoms through exposure to IBS symptoms and mindfulness training. The stress management program, on the other hand, emphasized symptom control through relaxation techniques, dietary adjustments, and problem-solving skills. Results showed a superior results for ICBT on measures of IBS symptoms and also effects on quality of life (Ljótsson, Hedman, et al., 2011).

A third example of a condition for which several ICBT controlled trials have been conducted is insomnia. The first trial was from our Swedish group (Ström, Pettersson, & Andersson, 2004) and has been followed by more trials. These were summarized in a systematic review and meta-analysis (Seyffert et al., 2016), which included 15 trials. The authors found medium effects on sleep efficiency and several other measures. Interestingly, when comparing ICBT against face-to-face therapy, they found no difference between the two formats. One example of a trial comparing face-to-face CBT versus ICBT was conducted in the Netherlands

(Lancee, van Straten, Morina, Kaldo, & Kamphuis, 2016). The trial randomized 90 individuals with insomnia to either guided ICBT, individual face-to-face CBT, or a wait-list control group. Both active treatments were effective, but there was a statistical advantage for the face-to-face treatment on a measure of insomnia severity. A smaller non-inferiority trial from Sweden compared ICBT against group CBT and found that ICBT was non-inferior to group treatment (Blom et al., 2015), but there is a need for more direct comparisons.

Several other chronic health conditions have been the topic of ICBT research, such as diabetes (van Bastelaar, Pouwer, Cuijpers, Riper, & Snoek, 2011), various forms of cancer (David, Schlenker, Prudlo, & Larbig, 2013), hearing problems (Molander et al., 2015), erectile dysfunction (Andersson et al., 2011), multiple sclerosis (Moss-Morris et al., 2012), and fibromyalgia (Vallejo, Ortega, Rivera, Comeche, & Vallejo-Slocker, 2015), among other examples.

HURDLES AND POTENTIAL PROBLEMS WITH INTERNET INTERVENTIONS

In this section, some hurdles and problems are highlighted. First, even if it is now fairly established that clinician-guided ICBT can be effective for a range of problems (Andersson, 2016), and that for some conditions ICBT can be as effective as face-to-face CBT (Andersson, Cuijpers, Carlbring, Riper, & Hedman, 2014), this does not mean that clinicians by default regard ICBT as a suitable complement and alternative to face-to-face interventions. There are a few studies on attitudes toward Internet treatments showing mixed findings from positive (Gun, Titov, & Andrews, 2011), to moderately positive (Mohr et al., 2010), to hesitant (Vigerland et al., 2014). It is likely that clinicians are more positive toward blending services. It is also important to note that diagnostic procedures still need input from clinicians and that most studies to date suggest that some form of guidance (contact with a clinician) leads to better response and fewer dropouts. Stakeholder data (unpublished) collected in eight European countries suggested that blending face-to-face and Internet interventions were perceived as more feasible than ICBT as a stand-alone treatment.

Second, in spite of the evidence base in favor of ICBT, there are few consistent findings regarding moderators and mediators of outcome. In other words, what works for whom and the mechanisms behind treatment outcomes are still uncertain. Several studies have investigated behavioral (self-reported) predictors (Andersson et al., 2015) and mediators (Hesser, Zetterqvist Westin, & Andersson, 2014), cognitive function (Lindner et al., 2016), genetics (Hedman et al., 2012), and even brain imaging (Månsson et al., 2015). Of these, brain-imaging data show some promise, but the research is in its early stages. It is possible that larger data sets with data collected from everyday practice may reveal more about outcome predictors. In this context, it is important to note that the evidence to date suggests that ICBT works under clinically representative conditions (Andersson & Hedman, 2013).

The third hurdle relates to implementation and the need for updates of technology and service-delivery models. Even if there are longstanding implementations of ICBT, for example, for chronic tinnitus (Kaldo et al., 2013) and anxiety/depression (Titov et al., 2015), it is a challenge to find the appropriate service-delivery format. In many countries, healthcare is funded by private insurance, which means that cost-effectiveness is crucial. In countries like the United Kingdom and Sweden, tax-funded healthcare does not necessarily mean that the implementation of new approaches is easier. Some have argued that opportunities are missed here (Bennett & Glasgow, 2009) and that novel approaches are needed (Yardley, Morrison, Bradbury, & Muller, 2015). Moreover, as technology changes, researchers and clinicians need to be updated on the current ways of accessing the Internet, for example, with people using smartphones instead of desktop computers (Ly, Asplund, & Andersson, 2014). Systems also need to be responsive to where the treatment portal is accessed (via tablet, computer, or smartphone; Vlaescu et al., 2015).

FUTURE DEVELOPMENTS

The future of ICBT is hard to predict, but three observations can be made. First, it is increasingly the case that new treatments are developed and tested online instead of transferring old, established CBT interventions to the Internet format. For example, early trials on panic disorder (Carlbring, Westling, Ljungstrand, Ekselius, & Andersson, 2001) were based on previous bibliotherapy, face-to-face studies, and manuals. However, recently novel treatment approaches for conditions like IBS (Ljótsson et al., 2010), infertility distress (Haemmerli, Znoj, & Berger, 2010), procrastination (Rozental, Forsell, Svensson, Andersson, & Carlbring, 2015), and hearing loss (Molander et al., 2015) were tested directly in controlled ICBT trials and not in controlled face-to-face trials. One driving reason could be that ICBT trials are more cost-effective to run (Andersson, 2016) and large data sets can be collected more rapidly. Another possible development will be to focus more on the educational aspects of psychological treatments (e.g., how information is conveyed and if knowledge is gained), as it is known that individuals in treatment may forget the treatment and may not necessarily comprehend the intervention (Harvey et al., 2014). Some developments have already occurred in this area, such as testing knowledge acquisition following completed ICBT for social anxiety disorder (Andersson, Carlbring, Furmark, & SOFIE Research Group, 2012).

A second projection has already been mentioned, namely that blended interventions will be more common. For example, this could be in the form of having a few face-to-face sessions to support the use of a smartphone application (Ly et al., 2015). It will also most likely be the case that paper-and-pencil questionnaires will be replaced with online questionnaires for use in research and clinical evaluations (van Ballegooijen, Riper, Cuijpers, van Oppen, & Smit, 2016), even when the intervention is provided face-to-face.

A third possible future development is that clients will become more involved in treatment development and even support the use of ICBT interventions. Initial evidence suggest that support of ICBT can be provided from a technical perspective (Titov et al., 2010), and there are also suggestions that on-demand support can work (Rheker et al., 2015). In other words, traditional therapist–client roles may change, and this includes the incorporation of significant others in interventions.

CONCLUSION

There are now numerous Internet intervention programs, most of which can be described as ICBT. Several controlled trials show that therapist-guided ICBT can be effective for chronic health conditions and that they can be as effective as face-to-face treatments. The challenge now is dissemination, which includes not only within North America, Australia, and Europe, where most of the research has been made, but also to other countries and continents. The prospect of translating and culturally adapting programs from one setting to another will facilitate the spread of Internet interventions across the world. Novel treatment approaches will be developed more rapidly as they can be tested in randomized controlled trials. Clinical evaluations of treatment outcomes will also be facilitated by means of modern information technology.

REFERENCES

Almlöv, J., Carlbring, P., Berger, T., Cuijpers, P., & Andersson, G. (2009). Therapist factors in Internet-delivered CBT for major depressive disorder. *Cognitive Behaviour Therapy*, 38, 247–254. doi:10.1080/16506070903116935

Andersson, E., Ljótsson, B., Hedman, E., Enander, J., Kaldo, V., Andersson, G., ... Rück, C. (2015). Predictors and moderators of Internet-based cognitive behavior therapy for obsessive–compulsive disorder: Results from a randomized trial. *Journal of Obsessive-Compulsive and Related Disorders*, 4, 1–7. doi:10.1016/j.jocrd.2014.10.003

Andersson, E., Walén, C., Hallberg, J., Paxling, B., Dahlin, M., Almlöv, J., ... Andersson, G. (2011). A randomized controlled trial of guided Internet-delivered cognitive behavioral therapy for erectile dysfunction. *Journal of Sexual Medicine*, 8, 2800–2809. doi:10.1111/j.1743-6109.2011.02391.x

Andersson, G. (2014). *The Internet and CBT: A clinical guide*. Boca Raton, FL: CRC Press.

Andersson, G. (2016). Internet-delivered psychological treatments. *Annual Review of Clinical Psychology*, 12, 157–179. doi:10.1146/annurev-clinpsy-021815-093006

Andersson, G., Carlbring, P., Furmark, T., & SOFIE Research Group. (2012). Therapist experience and knowledge acquisition in Internet-delivered CBT for social anxiety disorder: A randomized controlled trial. *PloS One*, 7(5), e37411. doi:10.1371/journal.pone.0037411

Andersson, G., Carlbring, P., & Lindefors, N. (2016). History and current status of ICBT. In N. Lindefors & G. Andersson (Eds.), *Guided Internet-based treatments in psychiatry* (pp. 1–16). Cham, Switzerland: Springer.

Andersson, G., Cuijpers, P., Carlbring, P., Riper, H., & Hedman, E. (2014). Internet-based vs. face-to-face cognitive behaviour therapy for psychiatric and somatic disorders: A systematic review and meta-analysis. *World Psychiatry, 13,* 288–295. doi:10.1002/wps.20151

Andersson, G., & Hedman, E. (2013). Effectiveness of guided Internet-delivered cognitive behaviour therapy in regular clinical settings. *Verhaltenstherapie, 23,* 140–148. doi:10.1159/000354779

Andersson, G., & Titov, N. (2014). Advantages and limitations of Internet-based interventions for common mental disorders. *World Psychiatry, 13,* 4–11. doi:10.1002/wps.20083

Areán, P. A., Ly, K. H., & Andersson, G. (2016). Mobile technology for mental health assessment. *Dialogues in Clinical Neuroscience, 18,* 163–169.

Barlow, D. H., Ellard, K. K., Fairholme, C. P., Farchione, T. J., Boisseau, C. L., Allen, L. B., & Ehrenreich-May, J. (2011). *Unified protocol for transdiagnostic treatment of emotional disorders: Workbook.* Oxford: Oxford University Press.

Baumeister, H., Reichler, L., Munzinger, M., & Lin, J. (2014). The impact of guidance on Internet-based mental health interventions: A systematic review. *Internet Interventions, 1*(4), 205–215. doi:10.1016/j.invent.2014.08.003

Beatty, L., & Lambert, S. (2013). A systematic review of Internet-based self-help therapeutic interventions to improve distress and disease-control among adults with chronic health conditions. *Clinical Psychology Review, 33,* 609–622. doi:10.1016/j.cpr.2013.03.004

Bennett, G. G., & Glasgow, R. E. (2009). The delivery of public health interventions via the Internet: Actualizing their potential. *Annual Review of Public Health, 30,* 273–292. doi:10.1146/annurev.publhealth.031308.100235

Bennett, K., Bennett, A. J., & Griffiths, K. M. (2010). Security considerations for e-mental health interventions. *Journal of Medical Internet Research, 12*(5), e61. doi:10.2196/jmir.1468

Berger, T., Caspar, F., Richardson, R., Kneubühler, B., Sutter, D., & Andersson, G. (2011). Internet-based treatment of social phobia: A randomized controlled trial comparing unguided with two types of guided self-help. *Behaviour Research and Therapy, 48,* 158–169. doi:10.1016/j.brat.2010.12.007

Berger, T., Hämmerli, K., Gubser, N., Andersson, G., & Caspar, F. (2011). Internet-based treatment of depression: A randomized controlled trial comparing guided with unguided self-help. *Cognitive Behaviour Therapy, 40,* 251–266. doi:10.1080/16506073.2011.616531

Blom, K., Tarkian Tillgren, H., Wiklund, T., Danlycke, E., Forssén, M., Söderström, A., . . . Kaldo, V. (2015). Internet vs. group cognitive behavior therapy for insomnia: a randomized controlled non-inferiority trial. *Behaviour Research and Therapy, 70,* 47–55. doi:10.1016/j.brat.2015.05.002

Boettcher, J., Åström, V., Påhlsson, D., Schenström, O., Andersson, G., & Carlbring, P. (2014). Internet-based mindfulness treatment for anxiety disorders: A randomised controlled trial. *Behavior Therapy, 45,* 241–253. doi:10.1016/j.beth.2013.11.003

Boettcher, J., Berger, T., & Renneberg, B. (2012). Internet-based attention training for social anxiety: A randomized controlled trial. *Cognitive Therapy and Research, 36,* 522–536. doi:10.1007/s10608-011-9374-y

Buhrman, M., Fältenhag, S., Ström, L., & Andersson, G. (2004). Controlled trial of Internet-based treatment with telephone support for chronic back pain. *Pain, 111,* 368–377. doi:10.1016/j.pain.2004.07.021

Buhrman, M., Gordh, T., & Andersson, G. (2016). Internet interventions for chronic pain including headache: A systematic review. *Internet Interventions, 4,* 17–34. doi:10.1016/j.invent.2015.12.001

Buhrman, M., Syk, M., Burvall, O., Hartig, T., Gordh, T., & Andersson, G. (2015). Individualized guided Internet-delivered cognitive behaviour therapy for chronic pain patients with comorbid depression and anxiety: A randomized controlled trial. *Clinical Journal of Pain, 31,* 504–516. doi:10.1097/AJP.0000000000000176

Carlbring, P., Maurin, L., Törngren, C., Linna, E., Eriksson, T., Sparthan, E., . . . Andersson, G. (2010). Individually tailored Internet-based treatment for anxiety disorders: A randomized controlled trial. *Behaviour Research and Therapy, 49,* 18–24. doi:10.1016/j.brat.2010.10.002

Carlbring, P., Westling, B. E., Ljungstrand, P., Ekselius, L., & Andersson, G. (2001). Treatment of panic disorder via the Internet—a randomized trial of a self-help program. *Behavior Therapy, 32,* 751–764. doi:10.1016/S0005-7894(01)80019-8

Christensen, H., Griffiths, K. M., & Jorm, A. (2004). Delivering interventions for depression by using the Internet: Randomised controlled trial. *British Medical Journal, 328,* 265–268. doi:10.1136/bmj.37945.566632.EE

Cuijpers, P., van Straten, A.-M., & Andersson, G. (2008). Internet-administered cognitive behavior therapy for health problems: A systematic review. *Journal of Behavioral Medicine, 31,* 169–177. doi:10.1007/s10865-007-9144-1

Dagöö, J., Persson Asplund, R., Andersson Bsenko, H., Hjerling, S., Holmberg, A., Westh, S., . . . Andersson, G. (2014). Cognitive behavior therapy versus interpersonal psychotherapy for social anxiety disorder delivered via smartphone and computer: A randomized controlled trial. *Journal of Anxiety Disorders, 28,* 410–417. doi:10.1016/j.janxdis.2014.02.003

David, N., Schlenker, P., Prudlo, U., & Larbig, W. (2013). Internet-based program for coping with cancer: A randomized controlled trial with hematologic cancer patients. *Psychooncology, 22,* 1064–1072. doi:10.1002/pon.3104

Dear, B. F., Staples, L. G., Terides, M. D., Karin, E., Zou, J., Johnston, L., . . . Titov, N. (2015). Transdiagnostic versus disorder-specific and clinician-guided versus self-guided Internet-delivered treatment for generalized anxiety disorder and comorbid disorders: A randomized controlled trial. *Journal of Anxiety Disorders, 36,* 63–77. doi:10.1016/j.janxdis.2015.09.003

Donker, T., Petrie, K., Proudfoot, J., Clarke, J., Birch, M. R., & Christensen, H. (2013). Smartphones for smarter delivery of mental health programs: A systematic review. *Journal of Medical Internet Research, 15*(11), e247. doi:10.2196/jmir.2791

Epstein, J., & Klinkenberg, W. D. (2001). From Eliza to Internet: A brief history of computerized assessment. *Computers in Human Behavior, 17,* 295–314.

Gun, S. Y., Titov, N., & Andrews, G. (2011). Acceptability of Internet treatment of anxiety and depression. *Australasian Psychiatry, 19,* 259–264. doi:10.3109/10398562.2011.562295

Haemmerli, K., Znoj, H., & Berger, T. (2010). Internet-based support for infertile patients: A randomized controlled study. *Journal of Behavioral Medicine, 33,* 135–146. doi:10.1007/s10865-009-9243-2

Harvey, A. G., Lee, J., Williams, J., Hollon, S. D., Walker, M. P., Thompson, M. A., & Smith, R. (2014). Improving outcome of psychosocial treatments by enhancing memory and learning. *Perspectives on Psychological Science, 9,* 161–179. doi:10.1177/1745691614521781

Hedman, E., Andersson, E., Ljótsson, B., Andersson, G., Andersson, E. M., Schalling, M., . . . Rück, C. (2012). Clinical and genetic outcome determinants of Internet- and group-based cognitive behavior therapy for social anxiety disorder. *Acta Psychiatrica Scandinavica*, *126*, 126–136. doi:10.1111/j.1600-0447.2012.01834.x

Hesser, H., Zetterqvist Westin, V., & Andersson, G. (2014). Acceptance as mediator in Internet-delivered acceptance and commitment therapy and cognitive behavior therapy for tinnitus. *Journal of Behavioral Medicine*, *37*, 756–767. doi:10.1007/s10865-013-9525-6

Høifødt, R. S., Lillevoll, K. R., Griffiths, K. M., Wilsgaard, T., Eisemann, M., Waterloo, K., & Kolstrup, N. (2013). The clinical effectiveness of web-based cognitive behavioral therapy with face-to-face therapist support for depressed primary care patients: Randomized controlled trial. *Journal of Medical Internet Research*, *15*, e153. doi:10.2196/jmir.2714

Hunt, M. G., Moshier, S., & Milonova, M. (2009). Brief cognitive-behavioral Internet therapy for irritable bowel syndrome. *Behaviour Research and Therapy*, *47*, 797–802.

Johansson, R., Nyblom, A., Carlbring, P., Cuijpers, P., & Andersson, G. (2013). Choosing between Internet-based psychodynamic versus cognitive behavioral therapy for depression: A pilot preference study. *BMC Psychiatry*, *13*, 268. doi:10.1186/10.1186/1471-244X-13-268

Johansson, R., Sjöberg, E., Sjögren, M., Johnsson, E., Carlbring, P., Andersson, T., . . . Andersson, G. (2012). Tailored vs. standardized Internet-based cognitive behavior therapy for depression and comorbid symptoms: A randomized controlled trial. *PLoS ONE*, *7*(5), e36905. doi:10.1371/journal.pone.0036905

Johnston, L., Titov, N., Andrews, G., Spence, J., & Dear, B. F. (2011). A RCT of a transdiagnostic Internet-delivered treatment for three anxiety disorders: Examination of support roles and disorder-specific outcomes. *PLoS One*, *6*, e28079. doi:10.1371/journal.pone.0028079

Kaldo, V., Haak, T., Buhrman, M., Alfonsson, S., Larsen, H.-C., & Andersson, G. (2013). Internet-based cognitive behaviour therapy for tinnitus patients delivered in a regular clinical setting: Outcome and analysis of treatment drop-out. *Cognitive Behaviour Therapy*, *42*, 146–158. doi:10.1080/16506073.2013.769622

Kessler, D., Lewis, G., Kaur, S., Wiles, N., King, M., Weich, S., . . . Peters, T. J. (2009). Therapist-delivered Internet psychotherapy for depression in primary care: A randomised controlled trial. *The Lancet*, *374*, 628–634. doi:10.1016/S0140-6736(09)61257-5

Kleiboer, A., Donker, T., Seekles, W., van Straten, A., Riper, H., & Cuijpers, P. (2015). A randomized controlled trial on the role of support in Internet-based problem solving therapy for depression and anxiety. *Behaviour Research and Therapy*, *72*, 63–71. doi:10.1016/j.brat.2015.06.013

Lancee, J., van Straten, A., Morina, N., Kaldo, V., & Kamphuis, J. H. (2016). Guided online or face-to-face cognitive behavioral treatment for insomnia? A randomized wait-list controlled trial. *Sleep*, *39*, 183–191. doi:10.5665/sleep.5344.

Lappalainen, P., Granlund, A., Siltanen, S., Ahonen, S., Vitikainen, M., Tolvanen, A., & Lappalainen, R. (2014). ACT Internet-based vs face-to-face? A randomized controlled trial of two ways to deliver acceptance and commitment therapy for depressive symptoms: An 18-month follow-up. *Behaviour Research and Therapy*, *61*, 43–54. doi:10.1016/j.brat.2014.07.006

Lindner, P., Carlbring, P., Flodman, E., Hebert, A., Poysti, S., Hagkvist, F., . . . Andersson, G. (2016). Does cognitive flexibility predict treatment gains in Internet-delivered psychological treatment of social anxiety disorder, depression, or tinnitus? *PeerJ*, *4*, e1934. doi:10.7717/peerj.1934

Ljótsson, B., Andersson, G., Andersson, E., Hedman, E., Lindfors, P., Andréewitch, S., . . . Lindefors, N. (2011). Acceptability, effectiveness, and cost-effectiveness of Internet-based exposure treatment for irritable bowel syndrome in a clinical sample: A randomized controlled trial. *BMC Gastroenterology*, *11*, 110.

Ljótsson, B., Falk, L., Wibron Vesterlund, A., Hedman, E., Lindfors, P.-J., Rück, C., . . . Andersson, G. (2010). Internet-delivered exposure and mindfulness based therapy for irritable bowel syndrome—a randomized controlled trial. *Behaviour Research and Therapy*, *48*, 531–539.

Ljótsson, B., Hedman, E., Andersson, E., Hesser, H., Lindfors, P., Hursti, T., . . . Andersson, G. (2011). Internet-delivered exposure based treatment vs. stress management for irritable bowel syndrome: A randomized trial. *American Journal of Gastroenterology*, *106*, 1481–1491. doi:10.1038/ajg.2011.139

Ljotsson, B., Hesser, H., Andersson, E., Lackner, J. M., El Alaoui, S., Falk, L., . . . Hedman, E. (2014). Provoking symptoms to relieve symptoms: A randomized controlled dismantling study of exposure therapy in irritable bowel syndrome. *Behaviour Research and Therapy*, *55*, 27–39. doi:10.1016/j.brat.2014.01.007

Ly, K. H., Asplund, K., & Andersson, G. (2014). Stress management for middle managers via an acceptance and commitment-based smartphone application: A randomized controlled trial. *Internet Interventions*, *1*, 95–101. doi:http://dx.doi.org/10.1016/j.invent.2014.06.003

Ly, K. H., Topooco, N., Cederlund, H., Wallin, A., Bergström, J., Molander, O., Carlbring, P., & Andersson, G. (2015). Smartphone-supported versus full behavioural activation for depression: A randomised controlled trial. *PLoS One*, *10*, e0126559. doi:10.1371/journal.pone.0126559

Ly, K. H., Trüschel, A., Jarl, L., Magnusson, S., Windahl, T., Johansson, R., Carlbring, P., & Andersson, G. (2014). Behavioral activation vs. Mindfulness-based guided self-help treatment administered through a smartphone application: a randomized controlled trial. *BMJ Open*, *4*, e003440. doi:10.1136/bmjopen-2013-003440

Månsson, K. N. T., Frick, A., Boraxbekk, C.-J., Marquand, A. F., Williams, S. C. R., Carlbring, P., . . . Furmark, T. (2015). Predicting long-term outcome of Internet-delivered cognitive behavior therapy for social anxiety disorder using fMRI and support vector machine learning. *Translational Psychiatry*, *5*, e530. doi:10.1038/tp.2015.22

Marks, I. M., Shaw, S., & Parkin, R. (1998). Computer-assisted treatments of mental health problems. *Clinical Psychology: Science and Practice*, *5*, 51–170. doi:10.1111/j.1468-2850.1998.tb00141.x

Mohr, D. C., Burns, M. N., Schueller, S. M., Clarke, G., & Klinkman, M. (2013). Behavioral intervention technologies: evidence review and recommendations for future research in mental health. *General Hospital Psychiatry*, *35*, 332–338. doi:10.1016/j.genhosppsych.2013.03.008

Mohr, D. C., Siddique, J., Ho, J., Duffecy, J., Jin, L., & Fokuo, J. K. (2010). Interest in behavioral and psychological treatments delivered face-to-face, by telephone, and by Internet. *Annals of Behavioral Medicine*, *40*, 89–98. doi:10.1007/s12160-010-9203-7

Molander, P., Hesser, H., Weineland, S., Bergwall, K., Buck, S., Hansson-Malmlöf, J., ... Andersson, G. (2015). Internet-based acceptance and commitment therapy for psychological distress experienced by people with hearing problems: Study protocol for a randomized controlled trial. *American Journal of Audiology, 24,* 307–310. doi:10.1044/2015_AJA-15-0013

Moss-Morris, R., McCrone, P., Yardley, L., van Kessel, K., Wills, G., & Dennison, L. (2012). A pilot randomised controlled trial of an Internet-based cognitive behavioural therapy self-management programme (MS Invigor8) for multiple sclerosis fatigue. *Behaviour Research and Therapy, 50,* 415–421. doi:10.1016/j.brat.2012.03.001

Murphy, L. J., & Mitchell, D. L. (1998). When writing helps to heal: E-mail as therapy. *British Journal of Guidance and Counselling, 26,* 21–32.

Paxling, B., Lundgren, S., Norman, A., Almlöv, J., Carlbring, P., Cuijpers, P., & Andersson, G. (2013). Therapist behaviours in Internet-delivered cognitive behaviour therapy: Analyses of e-mail correspondence in the treatment of generalized anxiety disorder. *Behavioural and Cognitive Psychotherapy, 41,* 280–289. doi:10.1017/S1352465812000240

Proudfoot, J., Swain, S., Widmer, S., Watkins, E., Goldberg, D., Marks, I., ... Gray, J. A. (2003). The development and beta-test of a computer-therapy program for anxiety and depression: Hurdles and lessons. *Computers in Human Behavior, 19,* 277–289.

Rheker, J., Andersson, G., & Weise, C. (2015). The role of "on demand" therapist guidance vs. no support in the treatment of tinnitus via the Internet: A randomized controlled trial. *Internet Interventions, 2,* 189–199. doi:10.1016/j.invent.2015.03.007

Rozental, A., Forsell, E., Svensson, A., Andersson, G., & Carlbring, P. (2015). Internet-based cognitive behavior therapy for procrastination: A randomized controlled trial. *Journal of Consulting and Clinical Psychology, 83,* 808–824. doi:10.1037/ccp0000023

Seyffert, M., Lagisetty, P., Landgraf, J., Chopra, V., Pfeiffer, P. N., Conte, M. L., & Rogers, M. A. (2016). Internet-delivered cognitive behavioral therapy to treat insomnia: A systematic review and meta-analysis. *PloS One, 11*(2), e0149139. doi:10.1371/journal.pone.0149139

Ström, L., Pettersson, R., & Andersson, G. (2000). A controlled trial of self-help treatment of recurrent headache conducted via the Internet. *Journal of Consulting and Clinical Psychology, 68,* 722–727. doi:10.1037/0022-006X.68.4.722

Ström, L., Pettersson, R., & Andersson, G. (2004). Internet-based treatment for insomnia: A controlled evaluation. *Journal of Consulting and Clinical Psychology, 72,* 113–120. doi:10.1037/0022-006X.72.1.113

Sucala, M., Schnur, J. B., Constantino, M. J., Miller, S. J., Brackman, E. H., & Montgomery, G. H. (2012). The therapeutic relationship in e-therapy for mental health: a systematic review. *Journal of Medical Internet Research, 14*(4), e110. doi:10.2196/jmir.2084

Titov, N., Andrews, G., Davies, M., McIntyre, K., Robinson, E., & Solley, K. (2010). Internet treatment for depression: A randomized controlled trial comparing clinician vs. technician assistance. *PloS One, 5,* e10939. doi:10.1371/journal.pone.0010939

Titov, N., Dear, B. F., Schwencke, G., Andrews, G., Johnston, L., Craske, M. G., & McEvoy, P. (2011). Transdiagnostic Internet treatment for anxiety and depression: A randomised controlled trial. *Behaviour Research and Therapy, 49,* 441–452. doi:10.1016/j.brat.2011.03.007

Titov, N., Dear, B. F., Staples, L., Bennett-Levy, J., Klein, B., Rapee, R. M., ... Nielssen, O. (2015). MindSpot Clinic: An accessible, efficient and effective online treatment service for anxiety and depression. *Psychiatric Services, 66,* 1043–1050. doi:10.1176/appi.ps.201400477

Vallejo, M. A., Ortega, J., Rivera, J., Comeche, M. I., & Vallejo-Slocker, L. (2015). Internet versus face-to-face group cognitive-behavioral therapy for fibromyalgia: A randomized control trial. *Journal of Psychiatric Research, 68,* 106–113. doi:10.1016/j.jpsychires.2015.06.006

van Ballegooijen, W., Riper, H., Cuijpers, P., van Oppen, P., & Smit, J. H. (2016). Validation of online psychometric instruments for common mental health disorders: A systematic review. *BMC Psychiatry, 16,* 45. doi:10.1186/s12888-016-0735-7

van Bastelaar, K. M., Pouwer, F., Cuijpers, P., Riper, H., & Snoek, F. J. (2011). Web-based depression treatment for type 1 and type 2 diabetic patients: A randomized, controlled trial. *Diabetes Care, 34,* 320–325. doi:10.2337/dc10-1248

Vigerland, S., Ljótsson, B., Bergdahl, F., Hagert, S., Thulin, U., Andersson, G., & Serlachius, E. (2014). Attitudes towards the use of computerized cognitive behavior therapy (cCBT) with children and adolescents: A survey among Swedish mental health professionals. *Internet Interventions, 1,* 111–117. doi:10.1016/j.invent.2014.06.002

Williams, A. C., Eccleston, C., & Morley, S. (2012). Psychological therapies for the management of chronic pain (excluding headache) in adults. *Cochrane Database of Systematic Reviews, 11,* CD007407. doi:10.1002/14651858.CD007407.pub3

Vlaescu, G., Alasjö, A., Miloff, A., Carlbring, P., & Andersson, G. (2016). Features and functionality of the Iterapi platform for Internet-based psychological treatment. *Internet Interventions, 6,* 107–114. doi:10.1016/j.invent.2016.09.006

Vlaescu, G., Carlbring, P., Lunner, T., & Andersson, G. (2015). An e-platform for rehabilitation of persons with hearing problems. *American Journal of Audiology, 24,* 271–275. doi:10.1044/2015_AJA-14-0083

Yardley, L., Morrison, L., Bradbury, K., & Muller, I. (2015). The person-based approach to intervention development: Application to digital health-related behavior change interventions. *Journal of Medical Internet Research, 17*(1), e30. doi:10.2196/jmir.4055

PART IV

Promoting Self-Management across the Globe

# 22

Systemic Models of Self-Management

ERIN MARTZ ■

Healthcare systems have to evolve by moving toward a model of care that incorporates both acute problems and chronic conditions. Without advances, countries can anticipate increasingly inadequate care and waste of precious resources.
—World Health Organization [WHO], 2002, p. 38

Researchers and healthcare policy analysts (Wagner et al., 2001; Wagner et al., 2005; WHO, 2002) have asserted that systemic change is needed in healthcare systems because those systems are structured around curable health conditions (i.e., an acute-care model). A healthcare system focused on healing curable health conditions is insufficient because it typically does not incorporate long-term planning of care for chronic health conditions. This chapter focuses on systemic approaches that facilitate self-management of chronic health conditions and models that have been created to help integrate healthcare of chronic conditions into healthcare systems that are centered on acute care. Chapter 2 ("Defining Self-Management on the Individual Level") in this volume discusses research about self-management for individuals with chronic health conditions and what that requires of them. In contrast, the present chapter concentrates on discussing the support and healthcare systems that *surround* the individual who is attempting to self-manage.

There is an international movement to create comprehensive, integrated healthcare models that can better assist individuals who have chronic health conditions (Busse, Blümel, Scheller-Kreinsen, & Zentner, 2010). Various terms have been used throughout the world to describe these programs, ranging from "disease management programs" (DMP, especially in Europe) or "chronic disease self-management programs" (CDSM, as originally created in the United States), to "chronic disease management" (CDM), "chronic illness care," or "collaborative management of chronic illness." In view of the philosophical parameters promoted in this volume (see chapter 1), the term "chronic health condition" is preferred over "chronic illness" or "chronic disease," because the former represents a biopsychosocial approach to disability and the latter represents a "medical model" approach to disability by its focus on pathology. This chapter, however, uses some medical-model terminology in order to discuss the programs that have been developed world-wide.

This chapter begins with a discussion of the definition of "self-management support" (SMS) and how it should be distinguished from self-management and then covers the typical components of SMS interventions. Examples of SMS programs are briefly discussed, as well as the studies conducted on the efficacy of such programs. This chapter also covers several systemic models, followed by a brief section on the economic reasons to promote SMS and integrated healthcare.

SELF-MANAGEMENT SUPPORT

"Self-management support" (SMS) is a term that has been defined in numerous ways, and many components of SMS have been proposed; most include a structured form of intervention to facilitate self-management. One group of researchers defined SMS as consisting of the following:

> Self-management support is defined as the systematic provision of education and supportive interventions by healthcare staff to increase [individuals]' skills and confidence in managing their health problems, including regular assessment of progress and problems, goal setting, and problem-solving support (Adams, Greiner, & Corrigan, 2004, p. 57).

The approach adopted in this chapter defines SMS as referring to the varying types of organized support, training, and structured interventions *offered to individuals* to help them cope with and manage their chronic health conditions. SMS should be distinguished from self-management in that self-management is *what individuals do* to regulate and manage their chronic health conditions. That is, SMS consists of the support and training that healthcare providers, healthcare systems, and resources in the community can provide to individuals (Department of Health and Human Services, 2012), whereas self-management involves the range of skills an individual has and behaviors he or she follows (see chapter 2 in this volume) to manage his or her chronic health condition. Adams and Corrigan (2003) noted that SMS posits the individual and his or her family as the source of control, with the healthcare team collaborating with them and providing expertise and tools to facilitate self-management.

SMS programs often involve structured, time-limited, standardized interventions designed to provide condition-specific information and to empower healthcare recipients to take a more active role in managing their chronic conditions. Part II of the present volume contains discussions about interventions for individuals with specific chronic health conditions; these interventions often include condition-specific education, treatment plan development, goal-setting, and problem-solving. Types of SMS programs may include professional-led groups with peers attending; peer-led, in-person groups; peer coaches/mentors; community health workers; support groups (e.g., mutual help groups); telephone-based peer support; and web/email programs (Heisler, 2006).

In a meta-analysis on self-management programs, Chodosh et al. (2005) defined SMS using the following parameters: SMS involves a systematic intervention that is targeted for chronic health conditions and that helps individuals in one or both of the following: (a) self-monitoring of symptoms and physiological processes or (b) decision-making related to managing one's own chronic health condition(s). This view reflects that SMS represents the intersection of the individual with a chronic health condition and the healthcare system. SMS is described as a component contained in most systemic models on managing chronic health conditions (Grover & Joshi, 2015), but systemic models include other elements than SMS, such as decision support and delivery design. These distinctions are described in the "Models Targeting Delivery Systems" section.

Components of Self-Management Support Programs

SMS evolved out of the traditional models of "patient education" (i.e., didactic counseling that emphasized knowledge acquisition). Wagner and colleagues (2001) noted that although individuals' knowledge increased, these patient education programs were insufficient for changing behavior or increasing self-management. SMS interventions provided more than just didactic education about chronic health conditions. The components of SMS typically consisted of teaching condition-specific education, using behavioral-change techniques to promote healthier lifestyle choices, and teaching skill development, such as problem-solving and goal-setting (Rijken, Jones, Heijmans, & Dixon, 2008). Because the definition of self-management (see chapter 2 in this volume) includes problem-solving skills to be used for symptom fluctuation and other issues related to one's chronic health condition (Adams, Greiner, & Corrigan, 2004), then it follows that SMS programs should teach problem-solving. This is one of the main differences from traditional "patient education" that taught condition-specific information: in SMS, problem-solving is emphasized, given that individuals need to micro-manage their own health conditions, while healthcare professionals and the healthcare system provide collaborative support to these individuals in their practice of self-management.

Yet, SMS often involves many more components than just teaching condition-specific knowledge and problem-solving skills. According to Pearson, Mattke, Shaw, Ridgely, and Wiseman (2007), SMS interventions typically include the following two main components: (a) provisions of information about the specific chronic health condition and its symptoms, the benefits of self-management, what areas need self-management (e.g., diet, physical activity, smoking), how to self-manage, using medications and possible side effects, and resources that are available; and (b) provision of support in assessing individuals' motivation, abilities, needs, and goals related to the chronic health condition; help in building motivation and increasing confidence to self-manage; help in collaboratively defining health-related problems and barriers to self-management and setting self-management goals; help in developing problem-solving skills; providing emotional support to individuals; and teaching stress management skills.

Taylor et al. (2014) noted that two of the most common components of SMS interventions, which were mentioned in most of the qualitative meta-reviews for various chronic conditions, were education and psychological support. According to these authors, key SMS activities included (a) provision of knowledge and information about the chronic health condition, (b) psychological strategies to help individuals adjust to living with a chronic health condition, (c) information and support about physical care tailored to the specific chronic health condition, (d) creating action plans for chronic health conditions that may increase in severity and symptoms, and (e) providing appropriate forms of social support.

The US Department of Health and Human Services (2016) delineated the following six competencies for healthcare workers who provide SMS: (a) goal-setting and developing action plans, while revising as needed, (b) assessing information and its applicability for their treatment plans, (c) identifying and accessing community resources related to self-management, (d) helping individuals to learn problem-solving in the context of their chronic conditions, (e) discussing emotional psychological responses to health conditions, and (f) utilizing evidence-based strategies to encourage self-management of chronic health conditions. These competencies of healthcare workers reflect the kinds of content that SMS programs should contain for helping individuals with chronic health conditions.

Theory Underlying SMS

Given that SMS typically attempts to influence people to adopt new behaviors, SMS programs are often based on psychological theories or models of behavior change, such as the Social Cognitive Theory (Bandura, 1986), the Transtheoretical Model (Prochaska & DiClemente, 1982), the Health Belief Model (Maiman & Becker, 1974), and the Locus of Control theory (Lefcourt, 2014), to promote self-management. Rijken, Jones, Heijmans, and Dixon (2008) provide an overview of theories underlying SMS, while suggesting other possible theories to the aforementioned list. Lorig's self-management interventions (see Chronic Disease Self-Management Program section) are described as based on self-efficacy theory (Lorig, Ritter, Moreland, & Laurent, 2015). Part I of the present volume contains two chapters on behavioral change theories to promote self-management: namely cognitive-behavioral theory and motivational interviewing, in addition to two chapters on using hope theory to promote self-management and applying the Illness Intrusiveness theory to self-management of chronic health conditions.

Differing Levels of Support

In a report on SMS, Pearson, Mattke, Shaw, Ridgely, and Wiseman (2007) proposed four models of SMS, reflecting a differing degree of interaction between the healthcare recipient and provider: (a) a primary-care SMS model, in which SMS is provided at local healthcare providers' offices and may involve referrals to additional SMS resources; (b) an external "on-the-ground" model, in which SMS is provided by an entity that is external to the primary-care provider and typically involves face-to-face meetings held outside of the primary-care setting; (c) an external call-center model, in which SMS is provided by an entity (external to the primary-care provider) that provides phone support from a centralized center without face-to-face interaction; (d) a remote model, whereby the Internet or other electronic media are used and a scripted content is offered by using technology (e.g., computer-generated emails or automated phone calls) that does not involve personal interaction.

Rogers and colleagues (2008) described a three-tier system of providing SMS in the United Kingdom: (a) case management, which is provided to individuals with complex health conditions; (b) "disease management," which is provided by primary-care healthcare professionals to individuals at some risk; and (c) self-management support for individuals with low-risk chronic health conditions. This three-tier system is similar to the Kaiser Permanente's care triangle depicting three levels of support (Singh, 2008): (a) supporting self-management for people with a chronic health condition with a low risk of complications, (b) management programs for individuals who need regular follow-up and who are at high risk of complications, and (c) case management for people who have complex needs and who are frequent users of healthcare. Singh asserted that while SMS programs differentially targeting individual needs are important, their effectiveness may increase if integrated into a whole-system approach to managing chronic health conditions.

The Department of Health and Human Services (2012) in Australia also proposed that individuals with chronic health conditions need differing levels of support. Hence, they proposed three models of SMS: (a) a self-directed model of self-management: the individual is "able to make informed decisions to effectively self manage with little input from healthcare and human service professionals" (p. 10); (b) a collaborative model of self -management: support is provided by means of a collaboration between the individual and their healthcare provider for making self-management decisions; and (c) a supported model of self-management: if the individual's abilities to self-manage are diminished, then an array of approaches are used in order to support self-management.

Ecological Model

Fisher and colleagues (Fisher, Brownson, O'Toole, Shetty, Anwuri, & Glasgow, 2005) proposed an ecological approach to self-management that reflects the multiple levels that affect individuals' choices, skills, and what services and support they receive. While this model mentions social, organizational, community, governmental policy, and economic factors affecting care, its components focus on SMS, and thus, this model is mentioned in the section on SMS. These researchers emphasized that individuals with health conditions (their example was diabetes) need resources and supports for self-management that can include individualized assessment, collaborative goal-setting, skills enrichment, follow-up visits, and access to a range of resources. These researchers also mentioned the need for continuity in the quality clinical care.

EXAMPLES OF PROGRAMS TO SUPPORT SELF-MANAGEMENT OF CHRONIC HEALTH CONDITIONS

Chronic Disease Self-Management Program

Lorig's Chronic Disease Self-Management (CDSMP) program, based at Stanford University, has been taught for almost two decades (Lorig et al., 1999). The current form of CDSMP involves a structured 2.5 hour per week, six-week, in-person program and uses trained peer leaders (i.e., lay-people with chronic health conditions) to run small groups. In the CDSMP, the self-management tasks that are promoted include problem-solving, decision-making, utilizing resources, communication and partnership with healthcare providers, making action plans for behavior change, and self-tailoring. Topics such as pain management, exercise, nutrition, and fatigue are also discussed in the small groups.

Lorig, Ritter, Laurent, and Plant (2006, 2008) adapted CDSMP for the Internet. One study (Lorig et al., 2013) involved collaboration with researchers in Australia. They found that there were significant differences on multiple indicators (e.g., decrease of symptoms and healthcare utilization, improvement in health behaviors and self-efficacy) after the Internet-based intervention, and the positive effects of this Internet-based intervention was maintained at one-year postassessment.

Besides in-person small groups and Internet-based interventions, CDSMP programs have been tested by mailing packets to participants (Goeppinger et al., 2009). Lorig, Ritter, Moreland, and Laurent (2015) tested whether a self-study, mailed intervention helped individuals in their self-management and found that the participants of this study exhibited improvements in the "triple aims" of healthcare: improved care (i.e., improved communication with healthcare providers and implementation of treatment recommendations), improved health (e.g., decreased symptoms), and less healthcare utilization at six months follow-up.

Brady and colleagues (2013) conducted a meta-analysis of 23 studies that utilized the CDSMP. Some of the findings of the meta-analysis were that all measures of psychological health improved significantly (with a moderate effect) at a 4- to 6-month follow-up and at a 9- to 12-month follow-up, that energy, fatigue, and self-reported health exhibited small but significant improvements at a 4- to 6-month follow-up (but not at a 9- to 12-month follow-up) and that there was a small but significant decrease in healthcare utilization as measured by the number of hospitalization days or nights at a 4- to 6-month follow-up (but not at a 9- to 12-month follow-up). These researchers suggested that, based on the results, CDSMP can be recommended for implementation in healthcare systems.

Expert Patient Model

The UK Department of Health (2001) published a manuscript titled, *The Expert Patient: A New Approach to Chronic Disease Management for the 21st Century*. The Expert Patients model was based on Lorig's CDSM program. It promoted self-management programs that focused on developing individuals' confidence, motivation, skills, and knowledge to take effective control over their health conditions. The Department of Health noted that the Expert Patients model was "not an anti-professional initiative ... [but was] based on partnership" with healthcare professionals (p. 7). The Expert Patients model stressed that individuals with chronic conditions are experts in their own health, that they have acquired the skills to cope with a chronic condition, and that they can be important collaborators with healthcare providers.

Kennedy and colleagues (2007) examined the effectiveness of the Expert Patients program's lay-led support groups. Results indicated that participants reported greater self-efficacy and energy at six-month follow-up compared to the wait-list control group. No statistically significant reductions were observed in the participants' healthcare service utilization over the six-month period. These researchers reported that it was likely that the intervention was cost-effective over a six-month period of time. In a follow-up article, Rogers and colleagues (2008) discussed the Expert Patients program and suggested that a more systemic approach be used, instead of focusing on one self-management intervention to provide SMS to individuals with chronic health conditions:

> In its current form, the EPP is helpful for some individuals and is valuable as one of a range of options. ... Rather than being concentrated on a single course, central resources for self-management support should also be directed at a variety of systems and interventions (p. S23).

EFFECTIVE SMS PROGRAMS

The successful SMS emphasizes a collaborative process between healthcare recipients and providers "to define problems, set priorities, establish goals, create treatment plans, and solve problems along the way" (Wagner, Davis, Schaefer, Von Korff, & Austin, 2002, p. 70). Wagner and his research team surveyed 72 programs located with healthcare or health maintenance organizations, which were nominated as effective and innovative for helping individuals with chronic health conditions. This research team found that most of these programs had limited effectiveness and relied on traditional education or information-based models rather than SMS. Further, the research team noted that while many of these programs had created linkages to community resources, most exhibited poor linkages to primary healthcare. In this article and other research (Wagner et al., 2001; Wagner et al., 2005), Wagner and colleagues advocated that fundamental changes in most aspects of care delivery were needed in order to better facilitate self-management of chronic health conditions.

In a report for the Institute of Medicine, Adams and Corrigan (2003) listed four qualities of successful SMS programs: (a) healthcare providers reinforce individuals' active and central role in managing their chronic health conditions, (b) healthcare teams utilize standardized assessments, (c) SMS programs utilize evidence-based interventions, and (d) each person develops an individualized care plan by a collaboration with healthcare teams and each person's problem-solving is emphasized.

A "Five As" approach (assess, advise, agree, assist, and arrange) was suggested as a way for SMS to be implemented effectively (Glasgow, Davis, Funnell, & Beck, 2003). This research team also noted that the following perspectives, which are based on the Five As model, can facilitate effective SMS implementation: acknowledging that an individual is an expert in his or her own life, that the individual has responsibility for himself or herself, and that self-management is self-directed and iterative and support should be ongoing; providing evidence-based programs in which individuals can participate and various SMS methods (e.g., in-person group or individual support, support given by electronic or telephonic means); assessing the individual's progress and providing personalized feedback on outcomes; using participatory decision-making with the person; providing learner-directed education that is tailored to both the person and his or her environment; using problem-based learning; listening to the individual; using collaborative goal-setting that is based on the individual's priorities; using action planning targeting specific behavioral changes; using a problem-solving approach; and following up with the individual (e.g., in person, by phone, or by email).

While numerous Cochrane reviews have been published about *educational* interventions for various chronic health conditions (e.g., Effing et al., 2007; Riemsma, Kirwan, Taal, & Rasker, 2003), several Cochrane reviews have been published on self-management (i.e., not just on programs providing condition-specific education). Zwerink and colleagues (2014) examined 29 programs on assisting individuals with chronic obstructive pulmonary disease and found that self-management interventions increased health-related quality of life as measured, decreased both respiratory-related and other-cause hospital admissions, and improved dyspnea symptoms. Peytremann-Bridevaux, Arditi, Gex, Bridevaux, and Burnand (2015) published a Cochrane review on CDM of asthma. While they used the term "CDM," they were essentially investigating SMS programs. Their examination of 20 studies indicated that compared with usual care, CDM resulted in improvements in asthma-specific quality of life, asthma severity scores, and lung function tests.

In a report on SMS, Pearson, Mattke, Shaw, Ridgely, and Wiseman (2007, p. 1) noted that the provision of SMS involves "a complex sequence of effects," in view that SMS attempts to influence individuals' behaviors and improve symptom control. Those improvements should, in turn, lead to better health outcomes and reduced utilization of healthcare services that ultimately should lead to reduced healthcare costs. This description of the chain of events related to SMS elucidates why SMS should be viewed in the context of healthcare systems: just like individuals' self-management is influenced by the type and quality of SMS that they receive, so is SMS provided by healthcare workers influenced by the type and quality of support provided by the healthcare systems in which they are embedded. The following section reviews systemic models that have been proposed that involve chronic health conditions and the healthcare system.

MODELS TARGETING HEALTHCARE DELIVERY SYSTEMS

Due to the interdisciplinary nature of the support provided by SMS programs, systemic models of self-management have been developed over the past few decades in order to help integrate healthcare services for chronic health conditions. Systemic models targeting healthcare delivery systems also were developed because it was observed that the healthcare system was based on an acute-care model, which was reactive to problems when they arise instead of being proactive and structuring care for those with chronic health conditions in an organized manner (Wagner et al., 2001). Wagner and colleagues suggested that one barrier for individuals' self-management was actually a healthcare system that did not meet their needs (e.g., clinical management, psychological support, and condition-specific information), because the healthcare system was focused on resolving acute healthcare issues over providing chronic care support.

Along with an awareness about the growing numbers of chronic health conditions that needed SMS, there came a call to redesign healthcare systems to incorporate the healthcare needs of individuals with chronic health conditions. Wagner and his colleagues helped to clarify that SMS implementation may not work well in acute-care health systems that focus on healing pathology. They emphasized that implementing effective SMS programs would require changes across the *whole* healthcare system, ranging from how services are provided to how healthcare professionals and individuals with chronic health conditions collaborate on self-management.

The incorporation of chronic condition care into the healthcare system also would require attitude changes, which was depicted as:

> [A] fundamental shift from the perception of self-management as an "add-on" to care to its becoming an expected and systematic part of [individual] care. Accomplishing this shift will in turn require transforming physician/provider culture, diffusing these values up to the national level. (Adams, Greiner, & Corrigan, 2004, p. 61)

According to the Department of Health and Human Services (2012) in Australia, five principles are needed in order to integrate SMS into healthcare services and practices: (a) health and well-being are fundamental human rights; (b) individuals and their families are at the center of care; (c) participation of individuals with chronic health conditions is integral to quality improvement, design, and delivery of SMS services; (d) chronic health conditions involve social, physical, and psychological issues; and (e) partnerships and collaboration should occur within healthcare teams and across healthcare sectors.

Public Health Model of Interventions

Before discussing systemic models that are specific to self-management, it is useful to note the public health model of interventions that categorizes three levels of prevention: (a) primary prevention targeting the causes of a range of health conditions (e.g., smoking, obesity); (b) secondary prevention targeting health conditions at the early stage of their occurrence, which includes the acute-care model of healthcare that attempts to cure the health condition; and (c) tertiary prevention targeting health conditions that cannot be cured but that can be treated to reduce the possibility of secondary complications or a progression in severity of or disability related to the health condition (Goldston, 1987). Hence, the healthcare system's treatment of chronic health conditions and SMS would be viewed as tertiary prevention. Self-management also can be viewed as part of tertiary prevention, in view that individuals with chronic health conditions can play active roles in helping to reduce the possibility of secondary complications, such as by implementing treatment plans advised by healthcare providers, and learning how to manage their own symptoms. In the category of tertiary prevention, cure is not the goal, but adapting to one's chronic health condition and managing its symptoms as much as possible are the main goals.

The WHO (2002) stated that individuals with chronic health conditions need coordinated healthcare services across the three types of care (primary, secondary, and tertiary). More specifically, the WHO asserted that a continuum of care was needed for chronic health conditions that included "prevention, long-term maintenance treatment, management of acute symptom exacerbation, rehabilitation, and palliative or hospice care" (p. 77), suggesting that the healthcare system needed to provide a broad spectrum of care.

A report for the Institute of Medicine by Adams and Corrigan (2003) helped to map out priorities for healthcare system transformation. SMS was listed as one of the cross-cutting priority areas. Further, this report provided a four-level model of viewing the functioning of the healthcare system: (a) the experience of individuals; (b) the functioning of small units of healthcare delivery, which can be viewed as micro-systems; (c) the functioning of healthcare organizations that support micro-systems; and (d) the environment of policy, payment, regulation, and accreditation. In a different report, the Institute of Medicine (2012) suggested a "priority pyramid" of interventions, which categorizes intervention strategies based on their target level (i.e., population versus individual) and the intensity to meet the needs of individuals with chronic health conditions. The bottom level of the pyramid refers to social strategies aimed at promoting health and reducing the onset of health conditions, while the top of the pyramid refers to intensive services needed to help individuals in high-priority groups (e.g., minorities, the elderly), as well as those who have multiple chronic conditions.

Disease Management Programs

"Disease management program" (DMP) is a term used in healthcare policy and research, especially in Europe. Also known as "chronic disease management" (CDM) or "population management programs" (Institute of Medicine, 2012), DMP should be distinguished from SMS. DMP is more systemic in nature and focuses on coordinating the delivery of chronic care within healthcare systems, while SMS emphasizes coordinating and providing support (e.g., condition-specific interventions) for individuals to facilitate their self-management efforts. However, these two terms are often used interchangeably in research and policy briefs.

DMP can be defined as providing the organization of care "in multidisciplinary, multi-component programs, with a proactive approach focusing on the whole course of a chronic disease, using evidence-based standards of care" (Velasco-Garrido, Busse, & Hisashige, 2003, p. 4). Further, DMP involves "the coordination of health care, pharmaceutical or social interventions designed to improve outcomes for people and cost-effectiveness. It recognizes that a systematic approach is an optimal and cost-effective way of providing healthcare" (Singh, 2008, p. 4). Thus, while DMP may include SMS programs (i.e., individual-level interventions), DMPs focus on systemic-level organization and delivery issues.

Velasco-Garrido, Busse, and Hisashige (2003) asserted that DMP programs had the following key elements: a knowledge base (for both healthcare provider and recipient), a delivery system containing coordinated care, and a process for continuous improvement. According to these authors, DMP involves the provision of comprehensive care that includes multidisciplinary care for the entire cycle of the health condition, integrated care, a continuum of care, coordination of the different components within the healthcare system, active client–healthcare recipient management tools (e.g., health education, empowerment, self-management), evidence-based guidelines and protocols, information technology, and continuous quality improvement.

Chronic Care Model

The Chronic Care Model (CCM) is a healthcare delivery-system model that was developed because the research team concluded that effective care for chronic health conditions required an organized delivery system that was not just an add-on to the acute-care system, and, as such, comprehensive system changes were needed (Wagner et al., 2001). CCM is a multidisciplinary model for promoting change in healthcare systems in order to integrate care for chronic health conditions (Wagner et al., 2005) into "ambulatory care" (i.e., outpatient) settings. The CCM was described as a synthesis of the best available evidence that can guide quality improvements in healthcare systems, but it was not an "explanatory theory" (Wagner et al., 2001).

Wagner and colleagues (2001, 2002, 2005) described four key components at the level of healthcare practice in the CCM: self-management support (i.e., individual-level support, including group classes, goal-setting, and action-planning), decision support (e.g., using evidence-based treatment guidelines based on scientific evidence, also called evidence-based practices), delivery-system design (ensuring effective and efficient delivery of clinical care), and clinical information systems (organizing data on healthcare recipients and population of specific chronic conditions to inform the delivery of effective healthcare). Two other broader components in the CCM included the healthcare organization (e.g., leadership and commitment, incentives for change) and community resources (e.g., linking community to healthcare system, such as community support groups, Internet resources).

A review by Coleman, Austin, Brach, and Wagner (2009), which included 82 articles on CCM, analyzed evidence and suggested that there was evidence of CCM's effectiveness and that CCM-based programs generally improved the quality of care among individuals with a variety of chronic health conditions. According to Coleman and colleagues, all of the randomized clinical trials using CCM in their analysis provided evidence that the implementation of CCM significantly improved some components (as measured by a range of process and outcome measures) as compared to control groups across a variety of health conditions. These researchers noted that CCM provides a framework for healthcare delivery but that the components may be implemented differently across programs. Coleman and colleagues suggested that there is some evidence accruing that CCM reduces healthcare costs, but that because of the costs involved with transforming healthcare systems and practices, CCM's overall impact on healthcare costs and revenues remains uncertain.

Zwar and colleagues (2006) investigated the implementation of CCM worldwide and conducted a systematic review of studies examining the effectiveness of the six components of the CCM. The authors concluded that the CCM is useful as a conceptual model but that some components, such as the healthcare organization and community resources components, are difficult to assess experimentally. They noted that the evidence does support CCM on the meso-level (i.e., healthcare organizations) and micro-level (i.e., individual level) of care. Evidence ranges from healthcare-service use and physiological measures of health conditions to quality of life and satisfaction measures. Some researchers criticized CCM for not incorporating health promotion and prevention strategies, which led them to propose an expanded CCM (Barr, et al., 2003) that added those two components.

While CCM has been included in this section on health-system delivery models because it targets change on the level of healthcare practice, it does have a community resource component, suggesting that it is a systemic model. The following section discusses even more expansive models related to the care of chronic health conditions.

SYSTEM-LEVEL MODELS

Numerous models have been developed that include broader and wider perspectives on healthcare delivery and thus, include factors that were not contained in the healthcare models mentioned so far in this chapter. These system models include factors such as healthcare policy and leadership, as well as other factors like economic forces.

System-wide Initiatives

Singh (2008) distinguished system-wide management programs from delivery-system models, such as CCM, stating that system-wide programs "build on delivery-system methods but focus more fully on the policy, structures and community resources needed to implement long-term change ... and the aim is to operate across benefit programs, care settings, and providers" (p. 11). Singh noted that system-wide programs often place an emphasis on prevention of health conditions and on health promotion. Singh provided numerous suggestions for implementing chronic care programs on a systemic level, and these ranged from immediate to longer-term steps that can be taken. Some examples include reorganizing the structures of care and its funding, providing financial incentives for collaboration, implementing a proactive approach that promotes health prevention, and involving many sectors and services. Other recommendations by Singh were similar to what was covered by system-delivery models, such as setting up solid information collection and data-sharing procedures, providing different levels of care based on people's needs, and implementing SMS for individuals who have chronic health conditions.

Innovative Care for the Chronic Conditions Framework

The WHO (2002) proposed viewing healthcare systems from three levels and evaluating them using a multidimensional approach: (a) the micro-level, related to individual-level interaction between healthcare recipients and providers; (b) the meso-level, related to healthcare organizations and their services, such as programs for chronic health conditions, and the broader communities; and (c) the macro-level, related to healthcare systems and healthcare policies on a regional, national, or international level. Each level interacts and influences the other two levels in a dynamic way. The WHO noted that when these three levels are integrated, healthcare services improve:

> When micro-, meso- and macro-levels work effectively within themselves, and successfully function in relation to each other, health care is efficient and effective; healthcare recipients experience better health. Dysfunction within and among the levels creates waste and ineffectiveness. Unfortunately,

concerning health care for chronic conditions, dysfunction in the health care system is typical. (2002, p. 31)

The WHO created an Innovative Care for the Chronic Conditions Framework (ICCCF) to represent a systemic, multilevel approach. Six guiding principles of the ICCCF were proposed as fundamental to all three levels of healthcare systems: evidence-based decision-making, population focus (i.e., population management as a long-term, proactive strategy for organizing care), prevention focus (i.e., providing information and skills to reduce health risks), a focus on quality control, integration (i.e., across time, healthcare settings, and health conditions), and adaptability (i.e., flexibility for change). This report recommended eight essential areas for improving care: supporting a paradigm shift, managing the political environment, building integrated healthcare systems, aligning policies of various sectors (e.g., labor practices) to maximize health outcomes, centering healthcare on the person and the family, supporting individuals in their communities, and emphasizing prevention of health conditions. These ideas were summarized in the ICCCF (see Figure 22.1).

The ICCCF also proposed the idea of a healthcare triad that consisted of a partnership among individuals with chronic health conditions and their families, their

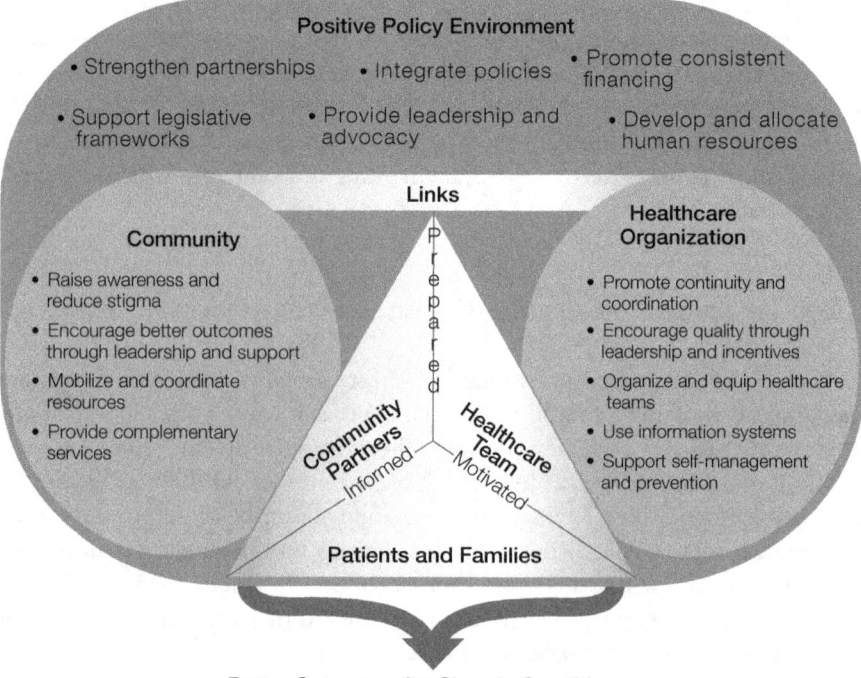

Figure 22.1 Innovative Care for the Chronic Conditions Framework.
Reprinted with permission from World Health Organization (2002). *Innovative care for chronic conditions: building blocks for actions: global report*. Geneva, Switzerland: World Health Organization.

healthcare teams, and community supporters. According to the ICCCF, this triad is affected by healthcare organizations, communities, and the policy environment.

The WHO (2002) noted that many countries have to manage a "dual agenda of healthcare" of providing care for both acute and chronic health problems. The WHO observed that healthcare systems are fragmented in many countries and that both systemic change and a paradigm shift were needed, in view that healthcare systems have evolved with a primary focus on treating acute health conditions. The fundamental perspective offered by the WHO (2002) was that healthcare systems had "to advance beyond the acute care model. Acute care will always be necessary (even chronic conditions have acute episodes), but at the same time health care systems must embrace the concept of caring for long-term health problems" (p. 30).

Chronic Condition Surveillance Model

Ruiz, Brady, Glasgow, Birkel, and Spafford (2014) examined how to set up a national surveillance system on self-management and SMS for chronic conditions in order to track progress in those areas. Their resulting model was a pyramid that contained five levels (see Figure 22.2), which was based on Frieden's

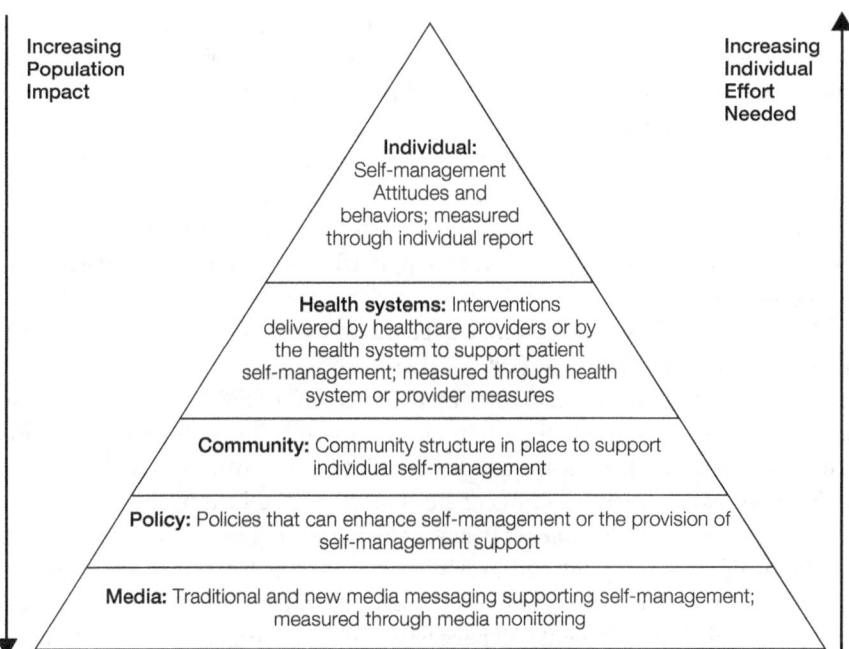

Figure 22.2 Self-management and self-management support pyramid of public health impact.
Reprinted from Ruiz, S., Brady, T. J., Glasgow, R. E., Birkel, R., & Spafford, M. (2014). Chronic condition self-management surveillance: what is and what should be measured? *Preventing Chronic Disease*, 11, E103–E103.

(2010) pyramid of public health impact. They suggested ideas on how to measure the performance at each level: (a) individual level: evaluate individual goal-setting and create health-related action plans; (b) healthcare-systems level: evaluate SMS quality improvement; (c) policy level: measure SMS performance within healthcare systems or plans; (d) community level: assess clinical--community links, e.g., the proportion of individuals being encouraged to attend community programs; and (e) media level: assess SMS media coverage that promotes self-management. While this model was not as extensively documented as the WHO's ICCCF, Ruiz and colleagues provided another multilevel perspective of self-management, SMS, and the environment in which those practices are embedded.

WHY INTEGRATE CHRONIC CONDITION HEALTHCARE?

> Chronic conditions engender increasingly serious economic and social consequences in all regions and threaten health care resources in every country. (WHO, 2001, p. 11)

The costs related to chronic health conditions impact both the individual with the condition and society. On the individual level, there are three types of costs that are created by chronic health conditions. The first is the direct costs (e.g., for treatment); the second involves intangible costs (e.g., the psychological toll related to having a chronic health condition); and the third involves indirect costs (e.g., reduced number of years in the workforce; Nolte & McKee, 2008). Another way of viewing the impact of a chronic health condition is through the lens of microeconomics, which examines how chronic health conditions may impact the economy due to reductions in individuals' consumption of goods, savings, labor productivity, and labor supply (Busse, Blümel, Scheller-Kreinsen, & Zentner, 2010).

One example of a microeconomic explanation is provided by Pearson, Mattke, Shaw, Ridgely, and Wiseman (2007). They described how a SMS program may affect both quality of care and costs by their "chain" of SMS effects (see Pearson et al., 2007, Figure 1, p. 8). The chain of events is as follows: The structure of the SMS influences the healthcare recipient's ability and motivation to improve his or her own care, which affect his or her behavior. The healthcare provider may react to the healthcare recipient's behavior by improving his or her own practices. As the healthcare recipient and provider change their behaviors, the healthcare recipient's chronic condition and its symptoms will likely be better controlled. Thus, the healthcare recipient will have fewer condition-related exacerbations and need less healthcare support (e.g., fewer trips to the emergency room or healthcare provider). Many healthcare recipients will be healthier and thus, more able to decrease their utilization of healthcare services. The healthcare recipient may be more satisfied with his or her life and use fewer healthcare services, which results in cost savings.

A macroeconomic perspective looks at the overall effect of chronic health conditions on the gross domestic product or the rate of gross domestic product growth. Chronic health conditions have been projected as having a major impact due to health conditions and disability-adjusted life years (years lost due to poor health, disability, or early death). But research on the impact is tentative, due to methodological challenges (Busse, Blümel, Scheller-Kreinsen, & Zentner, 2010). Busse et al. also described in depth the payment structures in healthcare systems and suggested that financial incentives were needed to facilitate the implementation of chronic care systems.

With chronic health conditions impacting the economy on both an individual and system level, governments and policymakers have become aware that more investment is needed into systems of managing chronic conditions. For example, in the US Department of Health and Human Services' strategic plan for the fiscal years of 2014–2018, self-management is mentioned in Goals 1 (Strengthen Healthcare) and 2 (Advance Scientific Knowledge and Innovation).

The WHO (2002, p. 85) provided a range of examples of actions that can be taken to finance innovative chronic care, which include (a) passing legislation and policy (e.g., raising taxes on harmful products to decrease unhealthy habits that can lead to chronic conditions); (b) providing healthcare insurance (e.g., adopting a comprehensive benefit package that includes preventive care services, SMS, acute and chronic care services, rehabilitative care, emergency care services, and community-based care); (c) reward efficiency (e.g., using financial incentives and making sure delivery of services occurs in the most appropriate and the most cost-effective setting); (d) promoting systemic quality (e.g., using incentives to encourage quality healthcare and utilize monitoring of quality-of-care factors); (e) engage the private sector (e.g., encouraging fair competition for providing chronic healthcare services); and (f) passing healthcare reforms (e.g., implementing reforms that improve financing for care of chronic conditions).

THE FUTURE OF SELF-MANAGEMENT

Many health systems worldwide have been striving to address the growing population of individuals who have long-term, fluctuating healthcare needs due to chronic health conditions. Policymakers, healthcare analysts, government officials, and researchers continue to dialogue about what changes are needed to merge care for chronic conditions into acute-care models. Many agree that systemic changes are needed in order to integrate chronic care and acute care practices into one system. But one of the major challenges related to changing the healthcare system is how to fund those changes and new practices.

As the creation and use of healthcare technology (e.g., electronic health records, decision tools, SMS provided over the Internet) expands, the costs of providing support to individuals with chronic health conditions may decrease, for example, by reducing the time-intensive models of in-person collaboration between the healthcare provider and recipient. However, despite the rapid advances of technology in healthcare, its usage needs to be examined scientifically in order to determine which system-wide practices are viable and effective in facilitating self-management among individuals with chronic health conditions.

Awareness of self-management and its support (SMS) are entering the radars of healthcare analysts, healthcare organizations, and governments, given the growing prevalence of chronic health conditions throughout the world. As the WHO (2002) noted: "Given the currently available information about the prevention and management of chronic conditions and their complications, the failure to use this knowledge to change healthcare systems is unjustified and reckless with the future of our populations" (p. 87). Let us hope that with more information on the benefits of self-management and self-management support, healthcare systems will do more to integrate chronic-care and acute-care services.

ACKNOWLEDGMENTS

Thank you Dr. Hanoch Livneh and Ms. Joan Martz for providing feedback on this chapter.

REFERENCES

Adams, K., & Corrigan, J. M. (Eds.). (2003). *Priority areas for national action: Transforming health care quality*. Washington, DC: National Academies Press.

Adams, K., Greiner, A. C., & Corrigan, J. M. (Eds.). (2004). *1st Annual Crossing the Quality Chasm Summit: A focus on communities*. Washington, DC: National Academies Press.

Bandura, A. (1986). *Social foundations of thought and action: A social cognitive theory*. Englewood Cliffs, NJ: Prentice Hall.

Barr, V. J., Robinson, S., Marin-Link, B., Underhill, L., Dotts, A., Ravensdale, D., & Salivaras, S. (2003). The expanded chronic care model: An integration of concepts and strategies from population health promotion and the chronic care model. *Hospital Quarterly, 7*(1), 73–82.

Brady, T. J., Murphy, L., O'Colmain, B. J., Beauchesne, D., Daniels, B., Greenberg, M., . . . Chervin, D. (2013). A meta-analysis of health status, health behaviors, and health care utilization outcomes of the chronic disease self-management program. *Preventing Chronic Disease, 10*, 1–14.

Busse, R., Blümel, M., Scheller-Kreinsen, D., & Zentner, A. (2010). *Tackling chronic disease in Europe: Strategies, interventions and challenges*. Observatory Studies Series 20. Geneva: World Health Organization.

Chodosh, J., Morton, S. C., Mojica, W., Maglione, M., Suttorp, M. J., Hilton, L., . . . Shekelle, P. (2005). Meta-analysis: Chronic disease self-management programs for older adults. *Annals of Internal Medicine, 143*(6), 427–438.

Coleman, K., Austin, B. T., Brach, C., & Wagner, E. H. (2009). Evidence on the chronic care model in the new millennium. *Health Affairs, 28*(1), 75–85.

Department of Health. (2001). *The expert patient: A new approach to chronic disease management for the 21st century*. London: Department of Health.

Department of Health and Human Services. (2012). *A framework to support self-management*. Retrieved from https://www.dhhs.tas.gov.au/__data/assets/pdf_file/0019/133480/19122012_FINAL_Self_Management_Framework.pdf

Effing, T., Monninkhof, E. M., Van der Valk, P. D., Van der Palen, J., Van Herwaarden, C. L., Partidge, M. R., . . . Zielhuis, G. A. (2007). Self-management education for patients with chronic obstructive pulmonary disease. *Cochrane Database of Systematic Reviews, 4*, CD002990.

Fisher, E. B., Brownson, C. A., O'Toole, M. L., Shetty, G., Anwuri, V. V., & Glasgow, R. E. (2005). Ecological approaches to self-management: The case of diabetes. *American Journal of Public Health, 95*(9), 1523–1535.

Frieden, T. R. (2010). A framework for public health action: The health impact pyramid. *American Journal of Public Health, 100*(4), 590–595.

Glasgow, R. E., Davis, C. L., Funnell, M. M., & Beck, A. (2003). Implementing practical interventions to support chronic illness self-management. *The Joint Commission Journal on Quality and Patient Safety, 29*(11), 563–574.

Goeppinger, J., Lorig, K. R., Ritter, P. L., Mutatkar, S., Villa, F., & Gizlice, Z. (2009). Mail-delivered arthritis self-management tool kit: A randomized trial and longitudinal followup. *Arthritis Care & Research, 61*(7), 867–875.

Goldston, S. E. (1987). Concepts of primary prevention: A framework for program development. *Sacramento: California Department of Mental Health*.

Grover, A., & Joshi, A. (2015). An overview of chronic disease models: A systematic literature review. *Global Journal of Health Science, 7*(2), 210–227.

Heisler, M. (2006). *Building peer support programs to manage chronic disease: Seven models of success*. Retrieved from http://www.chcf.org/~/media/MEDIA%20LIBRARY%20Files/PDF/PDF%20B/PDF%20BuildingPeerSupportPrograms.pdf

Institute of Medicine. (2012). *Living well with chronic illness: A call for public health action*. Washington, DC: National Academies Press.

Kennedy, A., Reeves, D., Bower, P., Lee, V., Middleton, E., Richardson, G., . . . Rogers, A. (2007). The effectiveness and cost effectiveness of a national lay-led self care support programme for patients with long-term conditions: A pragmatic randomised controlled trial. *Journal of Epidemiology and Community Health, 61*(3), 254–261.

Lefcourt, H. M. (2014). *Locus of control: Current trends in theory & research*. New York: Psychology Press.

Lorig, K. R., Ritter, P. L., Laurent, D. D., & Plant, K. (2006). Internet-based chronic disease self-management: A randomized trial. *Medical Care, 44*(11), 964–971.

Lorig, K. R., Ritter, P. L., Laurent, D. D., & Plant, K. (2008). The Internet-based arthritis self-management program: A one-year randomized trial for patients with arthritis or fibromyalgia. *Arthritis Care & Research, 59*(7), 1009–1017.

Lorig, K., Ritter, P. L., Moreland, C., & Laurent, D. D. (2015). Can a box of mailed materials achieve the triple aims of health care? The Mailed Chronic Disease Self-Management Tool Kit Study. *Health Promotion Practice, 16*(5), 765–774.

Lorig, K., Ritter, P. L., Plant, K., Laurent, D. D., Kelly, P., & Rowe, S. (2013). The South Australia health chronic disease self-management Internet trial. *Health Education & Behavior, 40*(1), 67–77.

Lorig, K. R., Sobel, D. S., Stewart, A. L., Brown Jr, B. W., Bandura, A., Ritter, P., . . . Holman, H. R. (1999). Evidence suggesting that a chronic disease self-management program can improve health status while reducing hospitalization: A randomized trial. *Medical Care, 37*(1), 5–14.

Maiman, L. A., & Becker, M. H. (1974). The health belief model: Origins and correlates in psychological theory. *Health Education & Behavior, 2*(4), 336–353.

Nolte, E., & McKee, M. (Eds.). (2008). *Caring for people with chronic conditions: a health system perspective*. McGraw-Hill Education (UK).

Pearson, M. L., Mattke, S., Shaw, R., Ridgely, M. S., & Wiseman, J. S. H. (2007). *Patient self-management support programs: An evaluation*. Santa Monica, CA: RAND Health.

Peytremann-Bridevaux, I., Arditi, C., Gex, G., Bridevaux, P. O., & Burnand, B. (2015). Chronic disease management programmes for adults with asthma. *Cochrane Database of Systematic Reviews, 5*, CD007988.

Prochaska, J. O., & DiClemente, C. C. (1982). Transtheoretical therapy: Toward a more integrative model of change. *Psychotherapy: Theory, Research & Practice, 19*(3), 276–288.

Riemsma, R. P., Kirwan, J. R., Taal, E., & Rasker, J. J. (2003). Patient education for adults with rheumatoid arthritis. *Cochrane Database of Systematic Reviews, 2*, CD003688.

Rijken, M., Jones, M., Heijmans, M., & Dixon, A. (2008). Supporting self-management. In E. Nolte & M. McKee (Eds.), *Caring for people with chronic conditions: A health system perspective* (pp. 116–142). London: McGraw-Hill Education.

Rogers, A., Kennedy, A., Bower, P., Gardner, C., Gately, C., Lee, V., . . . Richardson, G. (2008). The United Kingdom Expert Patients Programme: Results and implications from a national evaluation. *Medical Journal of Australia, 189*(10), 21–24.

Ruiz, S., Brady, T. J., Glasgow, R. E., Birkel, R., & Spafford, M. (2014). Chronic condition self-management surveillance: What is it and what should it be measured? *Preventing Chronic Disease, 11*, E103–E103.

Singh, D. (2008). *How can chronic disease management programmes operate across care settings and providers?* Copenhagen: Regional Office for Europe of the World Health Organization, European Observatory on Health Systems and Policies. Retrieved from http://www.euro.who.int/__data/assets/pdf_file/0009/75474/E93416.pdf

Taylor, S. J. C., Pinnock, H., Epiphaniou, E., Pearce, G., Parke, H. L., Schwappach, A., . . . Sheikh, A. (2014). A rapid synthesis of the evidence on interventions supporting self-management for people with long-term conditions: PRISMS–Practical systematic Review of Self-Management Support for long-term conditions. Retrieved from https://www.ncbi.nlm.nih.gov/books/NBK263840/pdf/Bookshelf_NBK263840.pdf

US Department of Health and Human Services. (2016). *Self-management support*. Retrieved from http://www.hhs.gov/ash/about-ash/multiple-chronic-conditions/education-and-training/curriculum/module-2-self-management-support/index.html

Velasco-Garrido, M., Busse, R., & Hisashige, A. (2003). *Are disease management programmes (DMPs) effective in improving quality of care for people with chronic conditions?* Copenhagen: WHO Regional Office for Europe. Retrieved from http://www.hcs.tu-berlin.de/fileadmin/a38331600/2003.publications/2003.velasco_HEN.08_DMP.pdf

Wagner, E. H., Austin, B. T., Davis, C., Hindmarsh, M., Schaefer, J., & Bonomi, A. (2001). Improving chronic illness care: Translating evidence into action. *Health Affairs, 20*(6), 64–78.

Wagner, E. H., Bennett, S. M., Austin, B. T., Greene, S. M., Schaefer, J. K., & Vonkorff, M. (2005). Finding common ground: Patient-centeredness and evidence-based chronic illness care. *Journal of Alternative & Complementary Medicine, 11*(Suppl. 1), S7–S15.

Wagner, E. H., Davis, C., Schaefer, J., Von Korff, M., & Austin, B. (2002). A survey of leading chronic disease management programs: Are they consistent with the literature? *Journal of Nursing Care Quality, 16*(2), 67–80.

World Health Organization (2002). *Innovative care for chronic conditions: Building blocks for actions: global report*. Geneva: World Health Organization.

Zwar, N., Harris, M., Griffiths, R., Roland, M., Dennis, S., Powell-Davies, G., & Hasan, I. (2006). *A systematic review of chronic disease management*. Sydney: Australian Primary Health Care Institute.

Zwerink, M., Brusse-Keizer, M., Valk, P. D., Zielhuis, G. A., Monninkhof, E. M., Palen, J., . . . Effing, T. (2014). Self management for patients with chronic obstructive pulmonary disease. *Cochrane Database of Systematic Reviews, 3*, CD002990.

INDEX

Page references for figures are indicated by *f*, tables by *t*, and boxes by *b*.

Acceptance and Commitment Therapy (ACT), tinnitus, 429–430, 431
Acevedo, A., 161
actions, 21
Active Communication Education (ACE), 351
active self-managers, 12
acute-care model, 18–19
acute coronary syndromes, 263
acute stress disorder (ASD), burn injury, 201, 207, 216
Adams, K., 500, 501, 506, 507, 508–509
adaptation, 16
Addiction Severity Index (ASI), 148
addictive behaviors, 147–164
    Alcoholics Anonymous and Narcotics Anonymous, 154–155
    barriers to self-management, 158–161
        affect and substance use, 159–160
        class, status, and power, 161
        co-occurring impairments, 161
        denial, 161
        executive functioning and self-regulation, 160
        mental health conditions, 161
        socioeconomics, race/ethnicity, and family dynamics, 160
        stigma of being "an addict," 158–159
    coping strategies, 162
    diagnosis, 147
    impaired control over substance use, 147
    interventions, evidence-based practices, 148–155
        assessment, 148
        behavioral therapies, 152–153
        community reinforcement approach, 153
        contingency management, 153
        cue exposure and relaxation training, 152–153
        cognitive-behavioral therapies, 150–152
        functional analysis, 151
        intervention mindfulness-based relapse prevention, 150–152
        perspectives, 150
        relapse prevention, 151–152
        group therapy, 154
        pharmacotherapy, 154
        psychodynamic therapies, 153–154
        psychosocial treatments, 148–150
        motivational interviewing, 149
        stages of change model, 149–150
    knowledge, for individual, 155–158
        posttraumatic growth, 155–156
        psychoeducational interventions, 155
        triggers, coping strategies, 157–158
        triggers, understanding, 156–157
    tested techniques, 162–164
        Alcoholics Anonymous and Narcotics Anonymous, 163
        community reinforcement approach, 163

addictive behaviors *(cont.)*
   community reinforcement approach and family training, 163
   couples and family treatments, 164
   harm-reduction approach, 162–163
   value, 162
 tolerance, 147
 withdrawal, 147–148
adherence, 6
adjustment, 16
age, illness intrusiveness, 92, 93*f*, 94, 94*f*
age-related macular degeneration, 444–445
Akeroyd, M., 425
Alcoholics Anonymous, 154–155, 163
Alma, M. A., 449
Andersson, E., 482, 484–488
Andersson, G., 343, 351, 430
Antecedent Target Measure (ATM) approach, 64
antiretroviral therapy (ART), 363, 369
Antonak, R. F., 16, 36, 39, 41, 42, 448–449
Anwuri, V. V., 503–504
anxiety
 arthritis, 176
 burn injury, 204
 cancer, 242*t*, 247*t*
 cardiac-related health issues, 268
 HIV, 369
 multiple sclerosis, 390
 pain, 410
appearance, burn injury, 211–212
Appel, P. R., 414
Arditi, C., 506
Artemiasis, A. K., 393–394
arthritis, 171–186, 225, 226
 barriers to self-management, 177–181
  cognitive vulnerabilities, 178–179
  environmental factors, 180–181
  pain acceptance, 180
  personal factors, 178
  principles, 177–178
  self-efficacy, 179
  self-management, 179
 conditions
  osteoarthritis, 172–173
  rheumatoid arthritis, 173–174
 co-occurring physical conditions, 174–176
  cardiovascular disease, 174–175
  diabetes, 175–176
  respiratory illness, 175
 diagnosis, 171
 education programs, self-management, 181–183, 181–184
  applications, 181
  Arthritis Self-Management Program, 178, 181–185
  Living Well with a Disability, 182–183
  variations, 181
 epidemiology, 171
 pain management, 226–227
 physiological and social factors, 176–177
 research evidence, 183–185
  Arthritis Self-Management Program, 183–185
  Living Well with a Disability, 185
 sequelae, 171
 treatment and course, 171–172
Arthritis Self-Management Program (ASMP), 178, 181–185
A's, Five, 506
assessment
 addictive behaviors, 148
 cognitive-behavioral therapy, 40–41
 tinnitus, 428–429
 vision impairment, 455–456
asynchronous services, 468
atherosclerosis, coronary, 263
audiological education, tinnitus, 422–423
Audulv, Å., 16
aural rehabilitation, 351
Austin, B. T., 505–506, 510
Austin, J. K., 332
Avorn, J., 183
Aw, A. T., 456
awareness, hearing impairment, 346–347

Baguley, D., 421–422, 425
Bair, M. J., 410
Bandura, A., 303, 325
Barefoot, C., 414
Barello, S., 272

INDEX

Barker, F., 343
Barlow, D. H., 33, 59, 484
Barlow, J., 14, 21–22
Bartels, H., 426
Bashshur, R., 472
Beating the Blues, 483
Beatty, L., 432, 433
Beck, A. T., 32, 34, 506
behavior, physical activity
    cancer, 243*t*
    for fatigue, 252
behavioral activation, 35
behavioral component, cognitive-
        behavioral therapy, 33,
        35–36, 45–49
    expressive writing, 49
    fundamentals, 45–46
    monitoring activities, 48
    physical health activities, 46–47
    pleasant activities, 46
    problem-solving, 35–36, 48
    social activities, 47
behavioral management, 5, 12, 21
behavioral therapies, addictive behaviors
    community reinforcement
        approach, 153
    contingency management, 153
    cue exposure and relaxation training,
        152–153
belonging, as core survival need, 210–211
benefits, thinking about, 158
Bennet, P., 268
Berger, S., 450
Bertoli, S., 349–350
Bertoni, A., 272
Bessel, A., 217
Beswick, A. D., 273
Bhargava, P., 388–389
bibliotherapy, 22, 488
    pain, 414
Bilsker, D., 43–45, 48
biomedical philosophy, 18
biopsychosocial model, 21–22
    chronic pain, 176
    disability, 19
Birkel, R., 513–514, 513*f*
Bishop, M., 396

blood glucose self-monitoring, 297–298
Bodenheimer, T., 20
body image, burn injury self-management,
        208–209, 211–212
    factors, 212–214
    outcome impacts, 209–210
    predictors, 209
Bohlmeijer, E. T., 431
Bokhour, B. G., 269
Boldy, D. P., 448
Bombardier, C. J., 397–398
book/manual, self-help, 351–352, 414
Boren, S. A., 300
Bowen, S., 151
Brach, C., 510
Bradley, P. M., 328–329
Brady, T. J., 504–505, 513–514, 513*f*
breathing retraining, 36
Bresnick, M. G., 201–202
Bridevaux, P. O., 506
Brief, D. J., 433
brief motivational interviewing, 128, 129*b*
broaden and build theory, 62
Browne, J. L., 288–289
Brownson, C. A., 503–504
Bucholz, E., 272
Buelow, J. M., 22, 324–325, 332
Burnand, B., 506
burn injury, 197–219
    barriers to self-management, 207–214
        appearance, social stigmatization, and
            social exclusion, 211–212
        body image and social adjustment,
            208–210, 212–214
        post-traumatic stress disorder,
            207–208
        resilience and social support, 208
        social belonging, 210–211
        stigmatization, 208–209
        visibility hypothesis, 214
    coping
        practices and interventions, 205–206
        self-efficacy, 201–203
    emotional impact, 201–205
    epidemiology, 197
    evidence-based practices, improving
        health outcomes, 198–199

burn injury (*cont.*)
  functional limitations, 197–198
  hypertrophic scars, 198
  interventions and peer support, 214–218
    professional assistance to survivor and family, 216–218
    survivor assistance to other survivors, 214–216
  knowledge, 200–201
  pain, 197, 198, 199, 203
  severity and functional limitations, 197–198
  techniques promotion self-management, 206–207
Busse, R., 509
Butler, M., 19–20

Cain, K. C., 414
Calhoun, L. G., 155–156
Campos-Melady, M., 163
cancer, 225–254
  barriers to self-management, 253
  chronic conditions *vs.*, 226–227
  chronic disease self-management, 227
  collaboration, 226
  considerations and future directions, 253–254
  empowerment, 235–236
  illness trajectory, 229
  impairments, 227
  implementation and integration into cancer care, 254
  interventions, 239–248, 240*t*–247*t*
    anxiety and depression, 242*t*, 245*t*, 247*t*
    cognitive pain-related barriers, 241*t*
    distress, physical, 245*t*
    distress, psychological, 240*t*, 243*t*, 246*t*
    distress, symptom, 247*t*
    empowerment, 246*t*
    fatigue, 232, 233, 234–235, 247*t*
    mental adjustment, 242*t*
    mood states, 244*t*
    pain, 231, 245*t*
    pain intensity and analgesic use, 244*t*
    pain interference, 244*t*
    physical activity behavior, 243*t*
    psychological adjustment, 246*t*
    quality of life, 241*t*–245*t*, 247*t*
    self-efficacy, 242*t*, 245*t*, 247*t*
    social support, 245*t*
    symptom limitations, 241*t*
    symptom severity, 246*t*
    weight loss and 2-year survival, 240*t*
    well-being, psychological, 247*t*
  lifestyle changes, 226
  literature, 231
    nonsubstantiated findings, 252–253
  patient activation, 235–238
  physical activity for fatigue, 252
  prehabilitation, 238–239
  programs, 227–228
  progression, 225
  psychoeducation, 235
  quality of life, 249*t*–251*t*
  self-efficacy, 249*t*, 250*t*
  self-management *vs.* self-regulation, 253
  sexual health, 249*t*
  signs and symptoms, 225–226
  survivors, HOPE Programme, 64–67
  targets, 231–239
    primary, 231, 232
    quaternary, 232, 238–239
    secondary, 232, 233–235
    tertiary, 232, 235–238
  tasks and skills, 228–231
  treatment goals, 225
  works in progress, 248–253, 249*t*–252*t*
    distress, psychological, 251*t*
    empowerment, 251*t*
    fatigue, 248, 249*t*
    health behaviors, 250*t*
    lifestyle behaviors, 250*t*
    pain intensity, 250*t*
    quality of life, 249*t*–251*t*
    self-efficacy, 249*t*, 250*t*
    sexual health, 249*t*
Capoccia, K., 295–296
Carati, C., 472
cardiac arrest, 263
cardiac prevention and rehabilitation programs (CPRP), 267–268, 271, 273

cardiac-related health issues, 262–274
    barriers to self-management, 266–269
        gender-related, 267–268
        psychological, 268–269
        systemic and sociocultural, 266–267
    chronic conditions, 263
    conclusions and limitations, 273
    lifestyle areas for intervention, 264–266
        eating habits, 265
        exercise, 264–265
        medication-taking, 265–266
        smoking cessation, 264
    nature and prevalence, 262–263
    partner support, 272–273
    practices and interventions, 269–272
        formal, 270–272
            cardiac prevention and
                rehabilitation programs, 271
            web-based, 271–272
        knowledge, 269–270
    prevalence, 263
    recommendations, 273
    types, 262–263
cardiovascular disease, 262–263
    with arthritis, 174–175
Carlbring, P., 484
Carr, S., 60
cataracts, 444
catastrophic thinking, 44
    arthritis, 178
    pain, 412–413
cell phone apps, 305
    diabetes, 305
    HIV support, 372–373
    pain, 415
    vision impairment, 458
Changing Faces, 214
Chawla, N., 151
Chiang, P. P., 447, 449, 453, 453t, 456
Chiaravalloti, N. D., 385
Chisolm, T., 341–342
Chodosh, J., 501
Chronic Care Model (CCM), 509–510
chronic condition surveillance model,
    513–514, 513f
chronic disease management
    (CDM), 509

chronic disease self-management, 227,
    504–505
chronic health conditions
    behavioral management, 2, 5, 12
    definition, 5–6
    emotional management, 5, 12, 21
    increased, global, 2–3
    medical management, 5, 12, 21
    multiple chronic conditions, 2
    untreated, danger, 3
chronic obstructive pulmonary disease
    (COPD), telemedicine, 469
chronic pain. *See also specific disorders*
    internet-supported cognitive-behavior
        therapy, 485–486
Clark, D. P. A, 343
Clark, K. A., 324
Clark, M., 450
Clark, N. M., 12, 17, 21, 59
cognitive appraisal, burn injury, 202
cognitive-behavioral therapy (CBT), 31–53
    addictive behaviors, 150–152
        functional analysis, 151
        intervention mindfulness-based
            relapse prevention, 150–152
        perspectives, 150
        range of treatments, 150–151
        relapse prevention, 151–152
    behavioral component, 33, 35–36
    burn injury, 205, 217
    cancer, 235
    central notion, 33
    chronic conditions, rationale, 32–33
    cognitive component, 33, 34–35
    conditions treated, 32
    definition, 150
    delivery formats, 50–52
    effectiveness, 32
    functional analysis, 151
    fundamentals, 31
    HIV, 363
    homework practice, 36–37
    interactive model, 33–34
    intervention mindfulness-based relapse
        prevention, 150–152
    physical activity, 46–47
    physiological, 33, 36

cognitive-behavioral therapy (CBT) (cont.)
  psychoeducation, 33
  relapse prevention, 151–152
  self-management, 31
  self-management promotion, 39–50
    assessment, 40–41
    behavioral, 45–49 (see also behavioral component, cognitive-behavioral therapy)
    cognitive, 42–45
    overview, 39–40
    pain, 39–40
    physiological, 49–50
    psychoeducation and goal-setting, 41–42
    setting and delivery, 40
  short-term, 33
  termination of therapy, 37
  tinnitus, 429, 430–431
  vicious cycle, 37–39, 38f
cognitive component
  cognitive-behavioral therapy, 33, 34–35, 42–45
  pain, 412–413
cognitive pain-related barriers, cancer, 241t
cognitive vulnerabilities, arthritis, 178–179
Colberg, S. R., 291–292
Coleman, K., 510
collaborative care, 19–21
  definition and components, 20
  Expert Patients Program, 20–21
  individual–health care provider, 11, 19–20
  motivational interviewing, 127
  synonyms, 19–20
communication environment and needs, hearing impairment, 348–349
community reinforcement approach (CRA), addictive behaviors, 153, 163
community reinforcement approach and family training (CRAFT), 163
compliance, 6
computer-based interventions, diabetes, 305
concerned significant others, 163

confidence, self-care abilities, 58
consequences, thinking about, 158
contextual factors, illness intrusiveness, 82–83, 82f, 84
contingency management, addictive behaviors, 153
convulsions, 320. See also epilepsy
co-occurring conditions
  addictive behaviors, 161
  arthritis, 174–176
  hearing impairment, 349–350, 350f
Coping Effectiveness Training (CET), 425, 429
coping skills and strategies, 16, 21, 31
  addictive behaviors, 157–158, 162
  burn injury, 201–203, 205–206
  definition, 16
  diabetes, 301–302
  epilepsy, 326–327, 329–330, 351–352
  hearing impairment, 351–352
  HIV, 371–372
  multiple sclerosis, 393–395
  pain, 411–413
  tinnitus, 427–430
  vision impairment, 452–455
Corbin, J. M., 12, 21
core beliefs, 31, 34, 40, 43–45
coronary artery bypass grafting (CABG), 269
coronary atherosclerosis, 263
Corrigan, J. M., 500, 501, 506, 507, 508–509
Coster, S., 407
cost-of-caring phenomenon, 99
costs, chronic health conditions, 3–4
counseling, tinnitus, 424
couples treatment, addictive behaviors, 164
Cowie, R. I. D., 344
Cox, H., 156
Crawford, J. D., 394
Creer, T. L., 14
Cronin, L., 270
Crowley, M., 448
cue exposure, addictive behaviors, 152–153
Cukor, J., 216

cultural syndromes, illness intrusiveness, 97–99, 98f, 102f–103f
Curry, S. J., 20
Cushman, M., 264

Davidson, B., 342
Davies, E. J., 264
Davis, A., 345
Davis, C. L., 506
Davis, D., 505–506
delirium, burn injury, 206–207
Dellasega, C., 136
DeLuca, J., 385–386
de Lusignan S., 343
denial, 16, 39
  addictive behaviors, 161, 163
  diabetes, 287
  vision impairment, 448–449, 456
depression
  arthritis, 176–177
  cancer, 242t, 245t, 247t
  cardiac-related health issues, 268
  HIV, 369
  illness intrusiveness, 88–90, 94, 94f
  Lewinsohn's theory, 88–89
  multiple sclerosis, 390
  pain, 410
  vision impairment, 449
Devellis, B. M., 302, 303
Devellis, R. F., 302, 303
DeWall, C. N., 210–211
Dhaliwal, S. S., 448
diabetes, 284–306
  with arthritis, 175–176
  biological aspects, 285–286
  epidemiology, 284
  psychological aspects, 286–287
  self-management, 289
  self-management behaviors, 289–302
    blood glucose self-monitoring, 297–298
    coping and psychosocial adaptation, 301–302
    diet, 293–294
    exercise, 289–293
    medication, 294–296
    problem-solving, 298–299

  risk reduction, 299–301
  social aspects, 287–289
  strategies, 303–306
    education programs, 303–304
    technology-based interventions, 304–306
  telemedicine, 468–469
  types and pathogenesis, 284
Diabetes Numeracy Test, 299
Diabetes Self-Management Program (DSMP), 303–304
diabetic retinopathy, 445
diaphragmatic breathing, 36
DiClemente, C. C., 149–150
didactic approach, 126
Didsbury, L. P., 51, 52
diet, diabetes, 293–294
Difede, J., 216
DiIorio, C., 324, 325, 326, 331
Dimidjian, S., 46
Dinesen, B., 467, 471
disability, 19. *See also specific types*
  adaptation to, 16
  biopsychosocial model, 6, 19
  illness intrusiveness, 86
Disability Centrality Model, 101
disclosure, HIV, 366, 367–368
disease management program (DMP), 509
disease-modifying therapies (DMTs), multiple sclerosis, 386
distraction, 157–158
distress, physical, cancer, 245t
distress, psychological
  cancer, 240t, 243t, 246t, 251t
  HIV, 361–362, 367, 369
  multiple sclerosis, 390
distress, symptom, cancer, 247t
Dixon, A., 502
Dobie, R., 426
Donato, S., 272
Donovan, D. M., 151
Doorenbos, A., 236
Drury, V., 447–449, 455–458
Du, S., 407, 414
Dunn, D. W., 332
Dunn, M., 388–389
Dwyer, E., 321

eating habits, cardiac-related health issues, 265
ecological model, 503–504
economics, chronic health conditions, 3–4
Edmondson-Jones, M., 425
education. *See* knowledge; psychoeducation
Edwards, L. M., 63
Edwards, R. R., 206
Edwards, S. A., 330
e-health. *See also* telehealth; telemedicine
   definition, 471
   tinnitus, 432–434
   U.S., 471–472
   WHO and European Union, 472
Eldridge, S. E., 183
Eliza, 482–483
Elliott, L., 343
Ellis, R. B., 22
email therapy, 483. *See also* Internet-based interventions
Emmons, K. M., 126, 128
emotional approach coping, 202
emotional avoidant coping, 202
emotional impact
   burn injury, 201–205
   hearing impairment, 344–345
   HIV, 368–370
   illness intrusiveness, 99
   multiple sclerosis, 389–390
   pain, 410–411
   tinnitus, 426–427
   vision impairment, 448–450
emotional management, 5, 12, 15–17, 21
   adaptation, 16
   adjusting, 16
   coping, 16
   multiple sclerosis, 389
   psychological support, 15
   self-management, 17
   stress-management strategies, 15
emotional regulation, 202
emotions. *See also* anxiety; depression; mood states
   addiction and substance use on, 159–160
   functionalist perspective, 202–203

employment, epilepsy, 322
empowerment, cancer, 235–236, 246*t*, 251*t*
Enders, C., 414
endurance, 158
Engdahl, B., 426
Engel, G. L., 19
environmental factors, arthritis, 180–181
epilepsy, 319–334
   accidents, 323
   barriers to self-management, 325–327
      coping, 326–327
      life management, 327
      seizure medications, 325–326
      seizure triggers, 326
   case study, 327–328
   coping strategies, 329–330, 351–352
   definition and description, 319–320
   diagnosis, 320
   impact, 320–323
      employment and social isolation, 322
      physical, 320–321
      psychological and social, 321
      risk management, 322–323
      stigma, 321–322
   interventions
      evidence-based practices, 328–329
      reported, 330–332
   knowledge, 323–325
   mortality, 323
   tested techniques, 332–334, 352–353
      Managing Epilepsy Well network, 333–334
      Modular Service Package Epilepsy, 332
      Self-Management Education for Adults with Poorly Controlled Epilepsy, 332–333
   trauma, 323
Erlandsson, S., 426
Ersek, M., 414
escape, 157
executive functioning, addiction and substance use, 160
exercise. *See* physical activity
expert patient program, 20–21, 505
expressive writing, 49

FaceIT, 214
family support
  multiple sclerosis, 390
  partner, cardiac-related health issues, 272–273
  vision impairment, 450, 454
family treatment, addictive behaviors, 164
Farmer, A. J., 471
fatigue
  cancer, 232, 233, 234–235, 247t, 248, 249t, 252
  multiple sclerosis, 394–395
Fatigue: Take Control, 394
Fauerbach, J. A., 201–202
fear avoidance, arthritis, 178, 186
Featherstone, D., 433
Ferguson, M. A., 342, 343, 345
Finlayson, M., 391–392, 393, 398
Fisher, E. B., 302, 303, 503–504
Fitzpatrick, S. L., 299
5 Year Forward View, 58–59
Five As, 506
Fix, G. M., 269
Flinders model, 382–383
Flodgren, G., 471
Flor, H., 407
Folkman, S., 16, 427–428
Foroushani, P. S., 215–216
Foster, G., 20, 183
Franklin, B. A., 264
Fraser, R., 387
Frederick, M. T., 347
Fredrickson, B. L., 62
Frenzel's Tinnitus Coping Questionnaire (TCQ), 428
Frieden, T. R., 513–514
functional analysis, addictive behaviors, 151
Funnell, M. M., 297–298, 468, 506
Fydrich T., 407

Gagné, J., 347
Gahm, G. A., 433
Garabedian, L. F., 468–469
Garnefski, N., 345, 352
Gatchel, R. J., 407
Gemmell, L., 298–299, 303

gender
  cardiac-related health issues, barriers, 267–268
  illness intrusiveness, 92–95
gender dystony, 86
gender syntony, 86
Geocze, L., 427
Germann, G., 217
Gex, G., 506
Ghahari, S., 394
Gianopoulos, I., 345
Giordano, A., 396–397
Girdler, S., 448
Glasgow, R. E., 503–504, 506, 513–514, 513f
Glass, P., 49
glaucoma, 445–446
goal-setting, cognitive-behavioral therapy, 41–42
Golm, D., 431
Gomez, R. G., 351
Goobermann-Hill, R., 348
Graffigna, G., 272
Graham, J. E., 49
Gray, L., 472
Gray-Donald, K., 414
Greenwell, K., 433
Greeson, J. M., 162
Gregory, P. C., 267
Greiner, A. C., 500, 501, 507
Grenness, C., 342
Griffin, K. W., 162
Griffiths, C. J., 183
Gross, J. J., 202
group therapy
  addictive behaviors, 154
  pain, 414
Gruman, J., 20

Hadjistavropoulos, T., 411
Hägnebo, C., 351
Hainsworth, J., 14
Halban, P. A., 285
Hall, D., 425, 430–431
Hallberg, L. R., 426
Han, K. D., 427
handicap, 19

HARKing, 253
harm-reduction approach, 162–163
Harrop-Griffiths, J., 426
Hartmann, B., 217
Haselkorn, J. K, 391, 392–393
Hassell, J., 448
headache pain, internet-supported cognitive-behavior therapy, 485–486
health
  definition, 1
  as self-management, 1
health behaviors, cancer, 250t
healthcare provider, changing role, 20
Heapy, A. A., 407–408, 414
hearing-aid use, successful, 353
hearing impairment, 340–353
  associations, 340–341
  barriers to self-management, 346–350
    awareness, 346–347
    communication environment and needs, 348–349
    co-occurring conditions, 349–350, 350f
    self-efficacy, 347–348
    skill, 349
    social support, 348
  consequences, 341
  coping strategies, 351–352
  definition and diagnosis, 340
  emotional impact, 344–345
  interventions, evidence-based practices, 341–343
  knowledge, 345–346
  prevalence, 340
  sensorineural, 340
  tested techniques
    aural rehabilitation, 351
    hearing-aid use, successful, 353
    online peer discussion forum, 352–353
    self-help book/manual, 351–352
    telephone support, 353
heart failure, telemedicine, 469–470
Heesen, C., 396–397
Heijmans, M., 502

Heine, M., 394
Help to Overcome Problems Effectively (HOPE), 58–74. *See also* HOPE Programme
Hennessy, M., 324
Henry, J. A., 422, 424, 425
Henry, J. L., 428–429
Henshaw, H., 342, 343
Hesser, H., 430, 433
Hickson, L., 341, 342, 347
hidden scar hypothesis, 214
Hill-Briggs, F., 298–299, 303
Hisashige, A., 509
HIV, 360–374
  barriers to self-management, 370–371
  coping strategies, 371–372
  emotional impact, 368–370
  evidence-based practices, 362–365
    beyond medication, 364–365
    medication-taking, 363–364
  functional limitations, 361–362
  global overview, 360–361
  knowledge needs and self-management tasks, 365–368
    disclosure, 366, 367–368
    knowledge, 365–367
    medication management, 367
    stigma, 367, 369
    transmission, 366–367
  medication-taking, 363–364
  multidimensional approach, 362
  risk factors, 362
  tested techniques, 372–373
Hixson, J. D., 331
Ho, P. M., 270
Hoare, D. J., 425, 430–431, 433
Hobson, J., 423
Hofmann, S. F., 34
Hogden, A., 136–138
Holman, H., 228–229, 382, 391
Holmner, Å, 469
Holroyd, K. A., 14
home-based services, 468
homework practice, cognitive-behavioral therapy, 36–37
hope
  definitions, 61–62

INDEX

measurement, 61–62
recovery, 60–61
resilience, 61
therapy outcome, 61
HOPE Programme, 58–74
  cancer survivors, 64–67
  concept and definition, 60–62
  delivery, 67
  discussion, 71–72
  implications, self-management research and practice, 73
  limitations, 72–73
  origins, 60
  outcome improvements, across interventions, 67–71, 68t, 70t
  positive psychology, 62–63
  program development, 63–64
  self-management fundamentals, 58–60
hope theory, vs. self-efficacy theory, 62
hospital-based services, 468
Huber, M., 1
Huffman, J. C., 268
Human immunodeficiency virus. See HIV
Hunziker, J., 391, 392–393
Hutchinson, S., 16
Hwang, S. H., 427
hyperopia, 443–444
hypertrophic scars, 198

illness intrusiveness, 80–114
  age, 92, 93f, 94, 94f
  cultural syndromes, 97–99, 98f, 102f–103f
  definition, 80
  depression, 88–90, 94, 94f
  disability, 86
  disabling and life-threatening conditions, 81–83, 82f
  disease factors, 81, 82f, 84
  emotional reactions, family and friends, 99
  empirical evidence, 83–102
    associations, statistically significant, 83–84
    contextual factors, 86–88
    disease and treatment factors, 84–86, 87–88
    findings not predicted by framework, 101
    personal control, 91–92
    psychological, social, and contextual variables, medical condition and treatment effects, 92–93, 93f
    psychological, social, and contextual variables, subjective well-being, 93–101, 94f–96f, 98f, 100f, 102f
    subjective well-being, 88–91
    theoretical refinements, 101–103
    treatment factors, 86
  etiology, 81
  future directions, 105–106
  gender, 92–93, 94–95
  gender dystony, 86
  gender syntony, 86
  Illness Intrusiveness Ratings Scale, 81–82, 106–114 (see also Illness Intrusiveness Ratings Scale (IIRS))
  intervening variable, 82, 82f, 84
  interventions, 80
  maximizing healthcare outcomes, 80–81
  MaxLife, 104–105
  personal control, 81, 82, 82f, 84
  positive psychological states, 89–90
  psychological, social and contextual factors, 82–83, 82f, 84
  race, 92
  self-concept, as "chronic patient," 96–97, 96f
  self-management of medical conditions, 103–105
  social support, perceived, 92–93
  stigma, 95–96, 95f
  symptom interference, 103–104
  targets, 81
  theoretical framework, 82, 82f
  treatment factors, 81, 82f, 84
Illness Intrusiveness Ratings Scale (IIRS), 81–82, 106–113, 114t
  chronic disease group statistics, 107, 108t–111t
  factor structure and factorial invariance, 112–113
  fundamentals, 106–107

Illness Intrusiveness Ratings
Scale (IIRS) (cont.)
psychometric properties
concurrent validity, 111–112
discriminant validity, 112
reliability, 107, 111
test–retest reliability, 111
subscales
instrumental life domains, 107, 108t–111t, 112
intimacy, 107, 108t–111t, 112
relationships and personal development, 107, 108t–111t, 112
translations and alternative instruments, 113
impairment, 19
Improved Access to Psychological Therapies (IAPT), 71–72
individual–health care provider alliance, 19–20. *See also* collaborative care
individual-level self-management, 10–25. *See also specific theories and interventions*
active *vs.* passive, 12
acute-care model, 18–19
balancing act, 10–11
collaborative care, 11, 19–21
components, 14–15
education, 14
emotional management, 15–17 (*see also* emotional management)
good self-managers, 12–13
holistic care, 19
macro-decisions, 11
micro-decisions and micro-management, 11
problem-solving, 14
processes, 13
psychological support, 14–15
self-management *vs.* self-care, 17–18
self-managers, 12–13
shift, philosophy, 18–19
social support, practical, 15
targets, four levels, 15
treatment implementation support, 15
tripartite model, 12

tripartite model, expanded, 21–24, 24f (*see also* tripartite model, expanded)
Ingram, B. O., 365
Innovative Care for the Chronic Conditions Framework (ICCCF), 511–513, 512f
insomnia, internet-supported cognitive-behavior therapy, 486–487
instrumental life domains, 107, 108t–111t, 112
insulin-replacement therapy, diabetes, 294–296
interactive model, cognitive-behavioral therapy, 33–34
interference, symptom, 103–104
International Classification of Functioning, Disability, and Health (ICF), 19
Internet-based interventions
cardiac, 271–272
diabetes, 305
face-to-face, 483
pain, 414
tinnitus, 432–434
unguided, 483
Internet-supported cognitive-behavior therapy (ICBT), 51–52, 482–489
approaches, 483–484
basic idea, 483
chronic pain and headache pain, 485–486
future developments, 488–489
hurdles and potential problems, 487–488
insomnia, 486–487
irritable bowel syndrome, 486
practice, 482–484
technology role, 484–485
therapeutic alliance, 484
therapist role, 484
intervening variable, 82, 82f
illness intrusiveness, 82, 82f, 84
intervention mapping, 64
intimacy, 107, 108t–111t, 112
Inzitari, M., 471
irritable bowel syndrome, internet-supported cognitive-behavior therapy, 486
ischemic heart disease, 262–263

Jacelon, C., 469–470
Jastreboff, G. P., 422–423, 424
Jeans, M. E., 414
Jennings, M., 347
Jennings, M. B., 346
Jerant, A. F., 12, 206
Johnson, C. S., 332
Johnson, J., 325
Jones, M., 502
Jones, S., 343
Joo, Y. H., 427
Joseph, S., 63

Kahn, J. M., 470, 475
Kalb, R., 388–389
Kang, J. M., 427
Kang, S., 343, 430–431
Kannel, W. B., 264
Karoly, P., 414
Karwoski, L., 63, 65
Katon, W., 426
Kavookjian, J., 292
Keeffe, J. E., 448
Keidser, G., 344
Keller, R. J., 330
Kelly, T. B., 348, 349
Kelly-Campbell, R. J., 347
Kemp, C. A., 414
Kendall, E., 73
Kennedy, A., 505
Kephart, G., 16
Kerr, P. C., 344, 345
Khan, A., 347
Khan, F., 396–397, 398
Khanna, S., 162
Khantzian, E. J., 153–154
Kidholm, K., 472, 473, 475
knowledge, 14, 21
　addictive behaviors, 155–158 (*see also* *under* addictive behaviors)
　application, 23
　arthritis, 181–183
　burn injury, 200–201
　cancer, 235
　cardiac-related health issues, 269–270
　condition-specific, acquiring, 22–23
　diabetes, 303–304
　epilepsy, 323–325
　hearing impairment, 345–346
　HIV, 365–368
　multiple sclerosis, 386–389
　tinnitus, 424–426
　vision impairment, 450–451
Kocur, P., 395
Köpke, S., 396–397
Kowalkowski, V., 430–431
Kraaij, V., 345, 352
Kremastinos, D., 264
Kristjánsdóttir, Ó. B., 37
Krog, N., 426
Kröner-Herwig, B., 428, 431
Kroon, F. B. P., 183–184
Kwakkel, G., 394

Lalloo, C., 415
Lambert, M. J., 61
Lambert, S., 432, 433
Lamoureux, E., 448
Lampert, M., 347
Langguth, B., 421–422, 424, 426
language, person-first, 6–7
Laplante-Lévesque, A., 341, 342, 346
Larizza, M. F., 448
Lasiter, S., 22
Laurent, D. D., 504
LaValley, M. P., 183
LaVeist, T. A., 267
Lawn, S., 136
Lawrence, J. W., 214
Lazarus, R., 16, 427–428
Leahy, N., 216
LeFort, S. M., 414
leisure activities, vision impairment, 450
Leroux, T., 347
Leszcz, M., 65
Lewinsohn, P. M., 88
life management, epilepsy, 327
lifestyle
　cancer, 226, 250*t*
　cardiac-related health issues, 264–266
Lim, P. S. H., 447, 449, 453, 453*t*
Lind, C., 347
Lindberg, P., 343
Lindsay, B., 328–329

Linley, P. A., 63
Lippe, B., 407
Liu, J. L. Y., 477–479
Living Well with a Disability (LWWD), 182–183, 185
Livneh, H., 7, 16, 36, 39, 41, 42, 448–449
Ljótsson, B., 486
Lobel, M., 49
Lockey, K., 346
locus of care, shift, 25
Lokshina, I., 49
Lomas, P., 59–60
loneliness, vision impairment, 449
Lopez, S. J., 63
Lorig, K. R., 60, 62, 73, 228–229, 303–304, 382, 391, 504
Lorig's Chronic Disease Self-Management (CDSMP) program, 504
Lovelock, K., 347
Lundell, S., 469
Lyttkens, L., 430

Mackenzie, E., 343
Mackey, S., 447–449, 455–458
macro-decisions, 11
macro-level, 511
Madey, S. F., 351
Maes, I., 422
Magyar-Mor, J. L., 63
Management Information Decision Support Epilepsy Tool (MINDSET), 333–334
Managing Epilepsy Well (MEW) network, 333–334
Managing Fatigue, 394
Mann, E. G., 180
Manteuffel, B., 324
Marlatt, G. A., 151
Martin, F., 64
Martinez Devesa, P., 430
Martz, E., 16, 427, 429, 449
Mason, S. T., 209
Mathiowetz, V., 394–395
Mattila, E., 42
Mattke, S., 501–503, 507, 514
MaxLife, 104–105
May, T. W., 332

McAlpine, L., 51, 52
McAndrew, L., 297–298
McCarty, E., 331
McCormack, A., 427
McFerran, D., 424
McGeary, C. A., 407
McGeary, D. D., 407
McIvor, G. P., 394
McKibben, J. B., 204–205, 207
McMillan, A., 347
Meade, M. A., 270
meaningful activity, 80
medical management, 5, 12, 21
medical model, 18
medical nutrition therapy (MNT), diabetes, 293–294
medication-taking
  cardiac-related health issues, 265–266
  diabetes, 294–296
  epilepsy, 325–326
  HIV, 363–364, 367
Melin, L., 343
mental adjustment, cancer, 242*t*
meso-level, 511
Meyer, C., 342, 347
Meyers, R. J., 163
m-health, 468. *See also* telemedicine
  tinnitus, 433–434
micro-decisions, 11
micro-level, 511
micro-management, 11
Miller, D., 391, 392–393
Miller, K. M., 294
Miller, W. R., 22, 125–128, 130*b*, 132–133, 132*b*, 133*b*, 136, 447
Minden, S. L., 395
mindfulness-based approaches
  addictive behaviors, 150–152
  burn injury, 206
Mistry, H., 471
mobile health services, 468
  tinnitus, 433–434
mobile phones. *See* cell phone apps
Model for Assessment of Telemedicine (MAST), 472–478, 473*t*
  data collection, 475, 478*f*
  development, 474

domains, 475, 476t–477t
evidence needed, level of, 475–479
three steps, 474–475, 474t
Modular Service Package Epilepsy (MOSES), 332
Momentum, 471
monitoring activities, cognitive-behavioral therapy, 48
mood states. *See also* anxiety; depression
cancer, 244t
Moore, M., 12
Moreland, C., 504
Moskowitz, J. R., 16
Moss-Morris, R., 51, 52
motivational interviewing (MI), 126–140
addictive behaviors, 149
brief, 128, 129b
burn injury, 206
collaboration, 127
definition, 126
vs. didactic approach, 126
effectiveness, 128, 131t
focus, clarifying, 128, 130b
guiding principles, 127–128
history, 127
HIV, 363
Motivational Interviewing Treatment Integrity (MITI) scale, 133b
strategies, practice, 128
using, key considerations, 138–139, 139t
using, practice, 130–138
clinician perspectives, 135
fidelity, assessing, 133, 133b
healthcare, 134
implementation barriers, 137–138
individuals' perspectives, 136
promoting chronic impairment self-management, 134–135
strengths, 136–137
training, 132–134, 132b
vision impairment, 447, 456–457
Motivational Interviewing Treatment Integrity (MITI) scale, 133b
Moyers, T. B., 132–133, 132b, 133b
Mozaffarian, D., 264
Mulcahy, K., 299, 300
multidimensional perspective, 22

multidisciplinary, 473
multiple chronic conditions, prevalence, 2–3
multiple sclerosis, 382–398
barriers to self-management, 395–396
clinical courses, 384–385
coping strategies, 393–395
fatigue, 394–395
stress management interventions, 393–394
disease overview, 383–384
emotional impact, 389–390
epidemiology and etiology, 384
evidence-based research, 391–393
knowledge, 386–389
managing MS, 388–389
people with, perspectives, 387
research, 387–388
person-centered multiple sclerosis care, 383
symptoms and functional limitations, 385–386
techniques, 396–398
information, 396–397
telehealth and telerehabilitation, 397–398
treatment, 386
Multiple Sclerosis Self-Management Scale, 388
Munday, D., 61
Myers, P. M., 425
myopia, 443–444

Nachtegaal, J., 344
Narcotics Anonymous, 154–155, 163
negative emotionality, cardiac-related health issues, 268
Nelson, W. J., 330
Nocentini, U., 385–386
Norman, I., 407
Nothwehr, F., 324
nutrition, HIV, 364
Nyberg, A., 469
Nyenhuis, N., 431

Odegard, P. S., 295–296
Oliviera, V. C., 407

online peer discussion forum, hearing impairments, 352–353
osteoarthritis, 172–173. *See also* arthritis
O'Toole, M. L., 503–504
Otto, M. W., 156–157

pacing, activity, pain, 412
Packer, T. L., 16, 448
pain, 406–415
  acceptance, arthritis, 180
  acute *vs.* chronic, 406
  barriers to self-management, 409–410
  cancer, 231, 245t
    analgesic use, 244t
    cognitive pain-related barriers, 241t
    intensity, 244t, 250t
    interference, 244t
  coping strategies, 411–413
    cognitive, 412–413
    complementary approaches, 413
    pacing, activity, 412
    pain diaries, 411
    problem-solving, 412
    relaxation strategies, 411
    social and pleasant activities, 413
    support, 413
    treatment participation, 411
  definition, 406, 408
  diaries, 411
  emotional impact, 410–411
  evidence-based approaches, 407–408
  functional limitations, 406
  HIV, 361
  knowledge, 408–409
  prevalence, 406
  tested approaches, 413–415
Panagiotakos, D. B., 264
Panoulas, V. F., 175
Papesh, M., 347
Parise, M., 272
partner support, cardiac-related health issues, 272–273
passive self-managers, 12
Paterson, R., 48, 49
pathway thoughts, 62
patient, 6
patient activation, cancer, 235–238

Pearson, M. L., 501–503, 507, 514
Pedrotti, J. T., 63
peer support
  burn survivor, 215
  HIV, 364–465
  vision impairment, 454–455
Pennebaker, J. W., 49
Perkins, S. M., 332
personal control, illness intrusiveness, 81, 82, 82f, 84, 91–92
personal factors, arthritis, 178
person-first language, 6–7
Pettersson, R., 485, 486
Peytremann-Bridevaux, I., 506
Pfafflin, M., 332
pharmacotherapy
  addictive behaviors, 154
  definition, 154
Phillips, J., 424
Phoenix Society for Burn Survivors, 214–215
physical activity
  cancer, 243t, 252
  cardiac-related health issues, 264–265
  cognitive-behavioral therapy, 46–47
  diabetes, 289–293
  HIV, 364
  multiple sclerosis, 389
  scheduling, 46–47
physiological component, cognitive-behavioral therapy, 33, 36, 49–50
Pichora-Fuller, M., 423, 431
Pinto, P., 427
Pitsavos, C., 264
Plant, K., 504
pleasant activities
  cognitive-behavioral therapy, 46
  pain, 413
Plow, M., 391–392, 393, 398
Positive and Negative Affect Scale (PANAS), 62
positive psychological states, illness intrusiveness, 89–90
positive psychology, 62–63
posttraumatic growth, addictive behaviors, 155–156

post-traumatic stress disorder (PTSD), burn injury, 201–205, 207–208, 216
Pots, W. T. M., 431
POWER problem-solving process, 453, 453t
Practical Systematic Review of Self-Management Support for Long- Term Conditions (PRISMS), 14–15
prehabilitation, cancer, 238–239
primary targets, 81
 cancer, 231, 232
problem-solving, 14
 cognitive-behavioral therapy, 35–36, 48
 diabetes, 298–299
 epilepsy, 331
 pain, 412
 vision impairment, 453, 453t
processes, 13
Prochaska, J. O., 149–150
Program to Encourage Active, Rewarding Lives for Seniors (PEARLS), 334
progressive muscle relaxation (PMR), 36
 multiple sclerosis, 394
 pain, 411
 vision impairment, 454
Progressive Tinnitus Management, 422
PRO-SELF Pain Control Program;, 235
Pryce, H., 348
psychodynamic therapies, addictive behaviors, 153–154
psychoeducation. *See also* knowledge
 addictive behaviors, 155
 cancer, 235
 cardiac-related health issues, 269–270
 cognitive-behavioral therapy, 33, 41–42
 tinnitus, 422–423
psychological factors
 arthritis, 176–177
 cancer, 246t
 cardiac-related health issues, 268–269
 epilepsy, 321
 illness intrusiveness, 82–83, 82f, 84
  medical condition and treatment effects, 92–93, 93f
  subjective well-being, 93–101, 94f–96f, 98f, 100f, 102f
 pain, 408–409

psychological interventions and support, 14–15
 HIV, 465
 tinnitus, 430–431
psychological thriving, 177
psychosocial integration, 23–24
 diabetes, 301–302
psychosocial treatments, addictive behaviors, 148–150
 motivational interviewing, 149
 stages of change model, 149–150
psychotherapy. *See also specific types*
 success, factors, 61
 tinnitus, 424
public health model of interventions, 508–509

quality of life
 cancer, 241t–245t, 247t
 vision impairment, 449
quaternary targets, cancer, 232, 238–239

race, illness intrusiveness, 92
Rachas, A., 471
Radhakrishnan, K., 270, 469–470
Radnitz, C. L., 47
Rae-Grant, A. D., 391, 392–393
Rallidis, L. S., 264
Ramsay, J., 183
Ravesloot, C., 185
Realising the Value Programme, 59
recovery, hope in, 60–61
Rees, G., 448
Reger, M. A., 433
Reges, O., 266–267
Rehn, B., 469
reinforcement, 151
Reisinger, E. L., 331
relapse prevention, addictive behaviors, 151–152
relapse prevention (RP) therapy, 151–152
relationships and personal development, 107, 108t–111t, 112
relaxation techniques and training
 addictive behaviors, 153
 pain, 411
 vision impairment, 454

Renneberg, B., 217
resilience
  burn injury, 208
  hope, 61
respiratory illness, arthritis, 175
Reynard, A. K., 393
Rezac, M., 391–392, 393, 398
rheumatoid arthritis, 173–174. *See also* arthritis
Richard, A. A., 17
Ridgely, M. S., 501–503, 507, 514
Ridgway, J., 347
Rietberg, M. B., 394
Rijken, M., 502
Ripper, S., 217
risk management, epilepsy, 322–323
Ritter, P. L., 504
Roberts, A. W., 330
Roberts, J. I., 321
Roger, K. S., 16
Rogers, A., 503, 505
Rollnick, S., 126, 127–128, 129b, 130b, 447
Rosenbek Minet, L., 474–475
Ross-Degnan, D., 468–469
Rotheram-Borus, J. J., 365
Rowat, K. M., 414
Rozansky, A., 270
Ruehlman, L. S., 414
Ruiz, F., 431
Ruiz, S., 513–514, 513f
Russo, J., 426
Ryder, J. A., 63

Saaddine, J. B., 431t–432t, 440
Sacks, J., 61
Safety, Meaning, Activation, and Reappraisal Therapy (SMART) study, 216–217
Safren, S., 33, 39, 46, 48, 49–50
Saito, H., 344
Sakai, C., 426
Sapci, H., 472
Satisfaction with Appearance Scale (SWAP), burn injury, 209
Saunders, G. H., 347
Schaefer, J., 20, 505–506
Schechter, M. A., 425

Schiller, J. S., 2–3
Schoo, A., 136
Schulman-Green, D., 13
Schumann, K. P., 299
Scott, B., 343
secondary targets, 81
  cancer, 232, 233–235
Seehausen, A., 217
seizures, 320. *See also* epilepsy
  triggers, 326
self-care
  abilities, confidence, 58
  definition, 17
  vs. self-management, 17–18
self-concept, as "chronic patient," 96–97, 96f
self-determination, in recovery, 60–61
self-efficacy, 228, 269
  arthritis, 179, 186
  cancer, 228, 242t, 245t, 247t
  hearing impairment, 347–348
  vs. hope theory, 62
self-help book/manual
  hearing impairments, 351–352
  pain, 414
self-management, 1–8. *See also specific disorders*
  categories of activities (behaviors), 12
  complex intervention, 11
  components, 225
  coping skills, 31
  definitions, 2, 5, 13, 17, 21–22, 59, 181, 382
  efficacious, 31
  focus, research and practice, 60
  fundamentals, 58–59, 58–60
  health as, 1
  intervention models, 59
  life-time task, 10
  multidimensional perspective, 22
  outcomes, maximizing healthcare, 80–81
  promoting, rationale, 2–4
  recovery, 60–61
  scope, 10, 31
  vs. self-care, 17–18
  vs. self-regulation, cancer, 253
  skills, 15

Self-Management Education for Adults
with Poorly Controlled Epilepsy
(SMILE), 332–333
self-management support (SMS), 500–504
  components, 501–502
  definitions and elements, 500
  ecological model, 503–504
  effective programs, 505–507
  levels of support, 503
  models targeting healthcare delivery
    systems, 507–510
  theory, 502
self-managers, 12–13
self-monitoring of blood glucose, 297–298
self-regulation
  addiction and substance use, 160
  cancer, *vs.* self-management, 253
self-talk, 158, 453
  addictive behaviors, 158
  cognitive-behavioral therapy, 34
  vision impairment, 453–455
Seligman, M. E. P., 62
sensorineural hearing impairment, 340.
    See also hearing impairment
Seo, J. H., 427
Sereda, M., 425
service design, HIV, 373
sex. *See* gender
Seyffert, M., 486
shame, HIV, 370
Shannon, G., 472
Shaw, L., 346
Shaw, R., 501–503, 507, 514
Shea, K., 17
Sheasby, J., 14
Shepperd, S., 471
Sher, T., 272
Shetty, G., 503–504
short-term therapy, cognitive-behavioral
    therapy, 33
Silverman, S., 347
Simera, I., 474
Simpson, C., 267
Singh, D., 511
skills. *See specific types*
Sloan, A., 391, 392–393
Smail, D., 65

Smith, J. E., 153
Smith, M. T., 201–202, 206
Smith, P., 345
Smith, S. L., 346
smoking cessation, cardiac-related health
    issues, 264
Snyder, C. R., 60, 61, 62, 69
Snyder's Adult State Hope Scale (ASHS),
    67–69, 70*t*
social activities
  cognitive-behavioral therapy, 47
  pain, 413
social adjustment, burn injury, 208–209
  factors, 212–214
  outcome impacts, 209–210
  predictors, 209
social belonging, 210–211
social costs and exclusion
  burn injury, 211–212
  chronic health conditions, 3–4
  epilepsy, 321, 322
social factors
  arthritis, 176–177
  illness intrusiveness, 82–83, 82*f*, 84
social support
  burn injury, 208
  cancer, 245*t*
  cardiac-related health issues, 272–273
  hearing impairment, 348
  illness intrusiveness, perceived, 92–93
  practical, 15
  vision impairment, 450, 454
sociocultural barriers, cardiac-related
    health issues, 266–267
Solari, A., 396–397
Solomon, D. H., 183
Sommers, M. S., 341
Song, Y., 270
sound therapy, tinnitus, 423
Southall, K., 347, 348
Spafford, M., 513–514, 513*f*
Spence, M. K., 51, 52
Spijkerman, M. P. J., 431
stages of change model. *See also* self-
    management support (SMS)
  addictive behaviors, 149–150
Stefanadis, C., 264

Stephens, D., 345
stepped-care, tinnitus, 422
stigma
   being "an addict," as treatment barrier, 158–159
   burn injury, 208–209, 211–212
   definition, 321
   epilepsy, 321–322
   HIV, 367, 369
   illness intrusiveness, 95–96, 95f
Strauss, A., 12, 21
stress management interventions, 15. *See also* distress; *specific types*
   multiple sclerosis, 393–394
   tinnitus, 425–426, 429–430
Ström, L., 485, 486
subjective well-being, illness intrusiveness, 88–91
substance use. *See also* addictive behaviors
   impaired control over, 147
sudden unexpected death in epilepsy (SUDEP), 323
suicide, tinnitus, 427
Sullivan, A. B., 393
Sullivan, M., 426
support. *See also specific types*
   epilepsy, 331
   pain, 413
support groups
   HIV, 372
   vision impairment, 454–455
Survivor Outreach to Assist in Recovery of the Phoenix Society for Burn Survivors, 214
Swendenman, D., 365
symptom
   cancer
      decreased limitations, 241t
      severity, 246t
   interference, 103–104
synchronous services, 468
systematic, unbiased, and robust, 473–474
systemic barriers, cardiac-related health issues, 266–267
systemic model, 499–516
   examples

      chronic disease self-management program, 504–505
      expert patient model, 505
   fundamentals, 499–500
   future of self-management, 515–516
   integrating chronic condition healthcare, rationale, 514–515
   international movement, 499–500
   models targeting healthcare delivery systems, 507–510
      attitude changes, 507–508
      Chronic Care Model, 509–510
      disease management program, 509
      public health model of interventions, 508–509
   self-management support, 500–504
      components, 501–502
      definitions and elements, 500
      ecological model, 503–504
      effective programs, 505–507
      levels of support, 503
      theory, 502
   system-level models, 511–514
      chronic condition surveillance mode, 513–514, 513f
      Innovative Care for the Chronic Conditions Framework, 511–513, 512f
      system-wide initiatives, 511

Tambs, K., 344, 426
Tasiemski T., 395
Tay, P., 447–449, 455–458
Taylor, D. C., 321
Taylor, J. D., 61
Taylor, S. J., 14–15, 183
Taylor, S. J. C., 502
Tedeschi, R. G., 155–156
telehealth
   multiple sclerosis, 397–398
   vision impairment, 458
telemedicine, 467–479. *See also* Model for Assessment of Telemedicine (MAST)
   asynchronous services, 468
   data collection, 475, 478f
   definitions, 467–468

evidence needed, level of, 475–479
Model for Assessment of Telemedicine, 472–478, 473*t*
self-management improvement, 468–471
    chronic obstructive pulmonary disease, 469
    cost-effectiveness, 470–471
    diabetes, 468–469
    heart failure, 469–470
    strategy for healthcare system development, 471–472
synchronous services, 468
value assessment, 472–473, 473*t*
telephone education and support
    epilepsy, 331
    hearing impairment, 353
telerehabilitation, multiple sclerosis, 397–398
termination of therapy, cognitive-behavioral therapy, 37
tertiary targets, 81
    cancer, 232, 235–238
text messaging, HIV support, 373
Teyber, E., 149
therapeutic alliance
    collaborative care, 19–20 (*see also* collaborative care)
    internet-supported cognitive-behavior therapy, 484
therapy outcome, hope in, 61
thinking about benefits and consequences, 158
Thombs, B. D., 200
Thompson, P. J., 321
Thompson, R. A., 202
Thorén, E. S., 352–353
Thorpe, C. T., 302, 303
three-component model. *See also specific components*
    cognitive-behavioral therapy, 33–34
thriving, psychological, 177
time limitations, healthcare professionals, 4
tinnitus, 420–434
    barriers to self-management, 432
    coping skills and strategies, 427–430
    assessment instruments, 428–429
    stress-management, 429–430
definition and symptoms, 420
emotional impact, 426–427
etiology, 420
evidence-based approaches, 421–424
    audiological education, 422–423
    counseling, 424
    multidisciplinary, 421–422
    sound therapy, 423
    stepped-care, 422
functional limitations, 421
knowledge, 424–426
    auditory, 425
    psychological, 425–426
prevalence, 421
psychological interventions, 430–431
tested approaches, 432–434
traumatic brain injury, 421
Tinnitus Coping Questionnaire (TCQ), 428
Tinnitus Coping Strategy Questionnaire (TCSQ), 428–429
Tinnitus Coping Training (TCT), 425, 428
tinnitus masking (TM), 424
Tinnitus Retraining Therapy (TRT), 422–423, 424
Titov, N., 484
tolerance, 147
Tolley, J. S., 215–216
total burn surface area (TBSA), 197–198
treatment factors, illness intrusiveness, 81, 82*f*, 84, 86
treatment implementation support, 15
triggers
    addictive behaviors
        coping strategies, 157–158
        understanding, 156–157
    seizures, 326
tripartite model, 12
tripartite model, expanded, 21–24, 24*f*
    Barlow's biopsychosocial definition, 21–22
    knowledge, acquiring condition-specific, 22–23
    knowledge, application, 23
    multidimensional perspective, 22
    psychosocial integration, 23–24

Tunkel, D. E., 420, 421–422, 424–425
Turk, D. C., 407
Turner, A., 14
Turner, A. P., 391, 392–393
Turner, de S., 156
Turner, J. A., 414

uncorrected refracted errors, 443–444
Unger, W. R., 325
Using Practice and Learning to Increase Favorable Thoughts (UPLIFT), 333

van de Port, I., 394
van Eijken, M., 345
van Wegen, E. E. H., 394
Velasco-Garrido, M., 509
vicious cycle, chronic conditions, 37–39, 38f
visible hypothesis, 214
vision, normal, 443
vision impairment, 440–459
　age-related macular degeneration, 444–445
　barriers to self-management, 452
　cataracts, 444
　classifications, 440–443
　coping skills and strategies, 452–455
　　peer-support programs, 454–455
　　POWER problem-solving process, 453, 453t
　　relaxation techniques, 454
　　self-talk, 453–454
　　social support, 454
　demographics, 440
　diabetic retinopathy, 445
　emotional impact, 448–450
　　leisure activities, 450
　　mental wellness, 448–449
　　quality of life, 449
　evidence-based practices, 446–448
　　common elements, 447–448
　　history, 446–447
　　motivational interviewing, 447, 456–457
　eye conditions, 443
　functional limitations, 441t–442t, 446

　glaucoma, 445–446
　global burden, 443
　healthcare professional role, 451–452, 451f
　knowledge, 450–451
　neglect, 440
　prevalence, 440
　strategies, 455–458
　　assessment, 455–456
　　interventions, individuals in state of readiness, 457–458
　　interventions, individuals not in state of readiness, 456–457
　　phone apps, 458
　　readiness and motivation for change, assessing, 456
　　telehealth, 458
　uncorrected refracted errors, 443–444
vision rehabilitation, 446–447
vital exhaustion, burn injury, 206–207
Vital Exhaustion (VE) construct, 206
von Friederichs-Fitzwater, M. M., 12
Von Korff, M., 20, 505–506

Wade, V., 472
Wadell, K., 469
Wagner, E. H., 18, 20, 59, 501, 505–506, 507, 510
Wallhagen, M., 345
Wang, P. S., 183
Ward, B. W., 2–3
Warsi, A., 183
web-based interventions
　cardiac-related health issues, 271–272
　epilepsy, 331–332
Web Epilepsy, Awareness, Support, and Education (WEBEASE), 333
Weise, C., 430
well-being, psychological, cancer, 247t
West, R. L., 346
Westin, V. Z., 430
Wharam, J. F., 468–469
Wicks, P., 331–332
Wilski, M., 395
Wilson, P. H., 428–429
Wilson, P. W., 264
Wind, G., 217

Wiseman, J. S. H., 501–503, 507, 514
withdrawal, 147–148
Wittich, W., 452
Wootton, R., 470–471, 475
Worrall, L., 341
Wright, C., 14
writing, expressive, 49
Wyatt, J. C., 477–479
Wyka, K., 216

Yalom, I., 65
Yeager, K. A., 331
Yu, C.-H., 394–395
Yurt, R., 216

Zachriat, C., 428
Zaugg, T. L., 425
Zwar, N., 510
Zwerink, M., 506